Janet Wilkie

KT-557-343

James Wolke

Medicine for Anaesthetists

Medicine for Anaesthetists

EDITED BY

M. D. VICKERS

*Professor of Anaesthetics
Welsh National School of
Medicine, Cardiff*

FOREWORD BY

WILLIAM W. MUSHIN CBE

*Emeritus Professor of Anaesthetics,
Welsh National School of
Medicine, Cardiff*

SECOND EDITION

BLACKWELL SCIENTIFIC PUBLICATIONS

OXFORD LONDON EDINBURGH
BOSTON MELBOURNE

© 1977, 1982 by
Blackwell Scientific Publications
Editorial offices:
Osney Mead, Oxford, OX2 0EL
8 John Street, London, WC1N 2ES
9 Forrest Road, Edinburgh, EH1 2QH
52 Beacon Street, Boston
    Massachusetts 02108, USA
99 Barry Street, Carlton
    Victoria 3053, Australia

All rights reserved. No part of this
publication may be reproduced, stored
in a retrieval system, or transmitted,
in any form or by any means,
electronic, mechanical, photocopying,
recording or otherwise
without the prior permission of
the copyright owner

First published 1977
Reprinted 1978, 1979
Second edition 1982

Printed in Great Britain by
Billing & Sons Ltd
Guildford and London
and bound at
Kemp Hall Bindery, Oxford

DISTRIBUTORS

USA
    Blackwell Mosby Book Distributors
    11830 Westline Industrial Drive
    St Louis, Missouri 63141

Canada
    Blackwell Mosby Book Distributors
    120 Melford Drive, Scarborough
    Ontario, M1B 2X4

Australia
    Blackwell Scientific Book Distributors
    214 Berkeley Street, Carlton
    Victoria 3053

British Library
Cataloguing in Publication Data

Vickers, M. D.
    Medicine for anaesthetists. – 2nd ed.
    1. Pathology
    I. Title
    616'.0024617   RB111

    ISBN 0–632–00737–0

Contents

Contributors

A. P. ADAMS PhD, MB, BS, FFARCS, *Professor of Anaesthetics, Guy's Hospital, London.*

D. R. BEVAN, MA, MB, MRCP, FFARCS, *Associate Professor, McGill University, Royal Victoria Hospital, Montreal, Quebec, Canada.*

G. W. BLACK MD, PhD, FRCPI, FFARCS, *Consultant Anaesthetist, Royal Belfast Hospital for Sick Children and Royal Victoria Hospital, Belfast.*

M. A. BRANTHWAITE MD, MRCP, FFARCS, *Consultant Physician and Anaesthetist, Brompton Hospital (National Heart and Chest Hospitals); Honorary Senior Lecturer in Thoracic Medicine, Cardiothoracic Institute.*

J. S. CRAWFORD MB, ChB, FFARCS, *Consultant Anaesthetist, Birmingham Maternity Hospital; Honorary Lecturer in Obstetric Anaesthesia and Analgesia, University of Birmingham.*

F. R. ELLIS PhD, MB, ChB, FFARCS, DObst RCOG, *Reader in Anaesthesia in the Department of Anaesthetics, University of Leeds; Honorary Consultant Anaesthetist, Leeds A.H.A.*

CHRISTINE EVANS MB, BS, DPM, *Psychiatrist, Cardiff.*

D. E. N. EVANS MB, BS, FFARCS, *Consultant Anaesthetist, University Hospital of Wales, Cardiff.*

S. A. FELDMAN BSc, MB, BS, FFARCS, *Consultant Anaesthetist, Magill Department of Anaesthetics, Westminster Hospital, London.*

R. F. FLETCHER PhD, FRCP, *Consultant Physician, Dudley Road Hospital; Senior Clinical Lecturer, University of Birmingham.*

T. M. HAYES FRCP, *Consultant Physician, University Hospital of Wales, Senior Lecturer, Welsh National School of Medicine, Cardiff.*

T. H. HOWELLS MB, ChB, FFARCS, *Director and Honorary Senior Lecturer, Department of Anaesthesia, The Royal Free Hospital, London.*

J. N. LUNN MD, FFARCS, *Senior Lecturer in the Department of Anaesthetics, Welsh National School of Medicine, Cardiff.*

K. MASHITER BSc, PhD, *Lecturer in Medicine and Chemical Pathology in the Department of Medicine, Royal Postgraduate Medical School, London.*

MERLIN MARSHALL BA, MB, BChir, FFARCS, *Consultant Anaesthetist, Regional Neurological Centre, Newcastle General Hospital, Newcastle upon Tyne.*

B. McCONKEY DM, BM, BCh, FRCP, *Consultant Physician, Dudley Road Hospital, Birmingham, Senior Lecturer in the Department of Medicine, University of Birmingham.*

D. A. D. MONTGOMERY CBE, MD, DSc, FRCP, FRCPI, FRCOG, *Chairman, Northern Ireland Council for Postgraduate Medical Education. Honorary Consultant Physician, Royal Victoria Hospital, Belfast. Formerly Professor of Endocrinology, Queen's University, Belfast.*

J. R. MUIR DM, FRCP, *Senior Consultant Cardiologist, Military Hospital, Riyadh, Saudi Arabia.*

K. W. PETTINGALE MD, MB, BS, MRCP, *Senior Lecturer in the Department of Medicine, King's College Hospital Medical School, London; Honorary Consultant Physician, King's College Hospital.*

J. E. PETTIT MD, FRCPA, MRCPath, *Associate Professor of Haematology, University of Otago Medical School, Dunedin, New Zealand.*

R. J. POWELL MB, MRCP, *Consultant Immunologist, Queen's Medical Centre, Nottingham.*

C. PRYS-ROBERTS PhD, MA, DM, MB, BS, FFARCS, *Professor of Anaesthetics in the University of Bristol; Honorary Consultant Anaesthetist, Avon A.H.A. (T).*

L. STRUNIN MD, MB, BS, FFARCS, *Director, Department of Anaesthesia, Foothills Hospital, Calgary, Canada.*

M. D. VICKERS MB, BS, FFARCS, *Professor of Anaesthetics, Welsh National School of Medicine, Cardiff.*

J. G. WHITWAM PhD, MB, ChB, MRCP, FFARCS, *Reader in Clinical Anaesthesia in the Department of Anaesthetics, Royal Postgraduate Medical School, London.*

Foreword

Of the many factors which affect the safety of anaesthesia, the careful and accurate assessment of the health of the patient by the anaesthetist must rank high in importance. By this means not only can the best type of anaesthetic be selected but any hazards to which the patient will be exposed by virtue of his pre-existing general medical disease can be avoided or minimized. Prophylactic measures can be taken preoperatively, extra vigilance for warning signs can be maintained during and after operation, and any special drugs or instruments kept ready in case of need. There is therefore a high priority for every anaesthetist to be sufficiently well versed in general medicine to play his proper part in bringing the patient safely through the anaesthetic and surgical operation. This need was recognized by the Faculty of Anaesthetists at its inception of the FFARCS diploma, by the inclusion in it of a test in clinical medicine in relation to anaesthesia, by clinical, oral, and written examination.

However, instruction in this field, to say nothing of source material in the literature, is not easy to come by. Practising internists have, by and large, little opportunity for acquiring knowledge or experience of the problems posed by their patients when subjected to anaesthesia, or of the risks they face. As a result, in the past, such advice as they gave was often absurd, perhaps ludicrous, and sometimes downright dangerous. Textbooks on internal medicine are no better. They either omit all mention of anaesthesia, or refer to it so sparsely that they give little help to the clinical anaesthetist.

Nearly all the authors of this book are anaesthetists and they have undertaken their task with courage, knowledge, and enthusiasm. They show courage in entering with confidence a field of medicine to which others might claim territorial rights, but which in reality belongs to all physicians, not least to anaesthetists. Their knowledge has been acquired in the most fruitful of places in medicine—the bedside. The present day anaesthetist has long ago extended his activities beyond the operating theatre and the description of him as the clinical physiologist of the surgical team is apt. The authors are enthusiastic fortunately, for a new venture such as this book (it is the first of its kind in this country) needs that quality of vigour which only enthusiasts, sure of their objectives, can give it.

This book instructs both learner and teacher. It will be an invaluable source of reference for research and practise alike. It will raise the standard of knowledge of clinical medicine among anaesthetists. As a result, the standard of anaesthesia will still further improve, leading to safer anaesthesia, more successful surgery, and improved health in the community.

William W. Mushin, CBE, MA, MBBS, FRCS, FFARCS
Emeritus Professor of Anaesthetics,
Welsh National School of Medicine, Cardiff

1*

ix

Preface to Second Edition

The success of the first edition of this book has been gratifying and not a little surprising, and reflects credit on the contributors rather than on any efforts of mine. With the steady increase in knowledge in many fields of medicine, it seems worthwhile therefore to bring out a new edition.

The same basic format has been retained and most of the original contributors: however, I have exercised an editor's prerogative to bring in some new authors, three of whom have written completely new chapters which replace previous ones on broadly the same topics. In addition, two chapters have been added on topics not previously covered: that on immunological-related diseases includes an explanation of the current understanding of the immune mechanisms and the laboratory investigations which are now employed together with a wide range of conditions in which these mechanisms are deranged; that on psychological aspects of anaesthesia should help to refocus the attention of the trainee anaesthetist on the crucial importance of understanding the whole patient and not just his pathology and the immense influence that the anaesthetist can have on the patient's experience of surgery.

The contributors have retained the emphasis on the common and routine rather than the rare and unexpected and kept matters of anaesthetic technique restricted to interactions between the medical condition and the choice of method. I have tried to achieve a more uniform approach to the use of references (which have been converted to Vancouver style) and improve the clarity of the illustrations.

I should like to thank all the reviewers of the first edition for the many valuable comments which they made. All have been carefully considered and, whenever appropriate, modifications have been made.

I remain convinced that the speciality needs, first and foremost, good physicians; whether they then administer the anaesthetic themselves or supervise others is of lesser importance. I hope this book will assist this trend.

1982   *M. D. Vickers*

Preface to First Edition

Unless the anaesthetist is also a physician, his expertise is ultimately technical. The last 20 years have indeed seen great technical advances in anaesthesia and this has been founded on the application of physiological and pharmacological knowledge. It would now be fair to claim that an individual in normal health is exposed to no measurable risk from modern anaesthesia.

The extension of this degree of safety to the unfit is unlikely to be achieved by any mere technical advances. This will require an understanding of the pathophysiology of all those conditions which render a patient less than optimally fit; in short, a knowledge of medicine in its widest sense.

To be able to cope safely with all such patients the truly professional practitioner of the art and science of anaesthesia has to have the breadth of approach of a general physician. Medicine, however, has seen the growth of specialisms and has led to the evolution of the cardiologist, neurologist, gastroenterologist, rheumatologist, nephrologist and many other '-ologists'. The anaesthetist cannot hope to match such specialists in their own field, nor should he try to do so. He must, however, keep sufficiently up to date with all of them to know the importance of their knowledge to the practice of anaesthesia.

This is the justification for a textbook of medicine for anaesthetists. But what form should it take? A standard test, even if simplified or of restricted scope is not what anaesthetists need. They rarely need, for example, to make initial diagnoses and their approach is much more problem-orientated than that of the traditional physician. They are less concerned with what the problem *is*, as with what it *means* in terms of function. Can the patient be improved in the time available? How does one decide when the situation is optimal? What else *might* go wrong with the patient? These are the sort of questions to which anaesthetists need to know the answers.

The structure of the book has resulted from an attempt to obtain this perspective. Some subjects have been covered by individuals who are acknowledged authorities in both the anaesthetic and medical aspects of their subject. Most have been tackled by a team of two in which an anaesthetist has chosen a physician or other expert colleague to assist him. I have invited three physician colleagues to contribute chapters on their respective fields and in these chapters the anaesthetic viewpoint is my own.

Multiple authorship inevitably brings the problem of sub-dividing integrated subject matter into more or less logical parts and introduces problems of deciding where to cover topics which can be put into more than one place: cross-referencing may save space but it does so at the expense of readability; on occasions it has seemed better to allow some duplication in order to allow a more complete presentation of a subject. This has added a little additional length to what I fear is already a rather overlong work. I hope the reader will find that it improves his understanding, assessment and management of the medical status of all those patients who are presented to him with chronic or acute illnesses. It is these patients to whom we need to give our most expert attention and who offer the greatest margin for improvement in current anaesthetic practice.

M. D. Vickers

Chapter 1
Heart Disease

J. N. LUNN AND J. R. MUIR

Studies of the results of surgery in patients with cardiac disease have revealed that the overall hospital mortality is significantly greater in patients with heart disease than in other patients. The mortality increases with increasing severity of functional impairment. However, the surgical and anaesthetic techniques are usually completely exonerated since these deaths do not customarily occur within the first 24 hours after surgery. The mortality is, furthermore, not clearly related to the duration of the surgery; indeed, there is some evidence of a negative correlation between the incidence of postoperative death and duration of surgery for specific operations [21]. The majority of patients who die do so as a result of recognizable complications of heart disease such as pulmonary embolus, intractable cardiac failure or myocardial ischaemia. In one series [9] nine clinical features were identified which indicated a significant statistical risk of complication or death of cardiac origin. The important aspect of this study was that the authors did not concentrate merely upon single disorders (e.g. myocardial infarction) which have an adverse influence upon outcome but demonstrated that sufficient interaction exists between several disorders so that good risk patients can be separated from bad risk ones.

It is this increased hospital mortality following surgery in patients with coincidental heart disease which makes the study of cardiology so important for anaesthetists. Recognition that heart disease is present in an individual patient is an important step in the identification of risk and in the anticipation of the probable effects of anaesthesia upon cardiac function.

THE ASSESSMENT OF THE PATIENT

The assessment of patients who may have heart disease involves the careful integration of information derived from the history, the physical examination, the electrocardiogram, the chest X-ray and other special investigations. All these parts of the assessment are of value, but the history and the physical examination are the most important, since they determine the type and scope of special investigations. In the particular context of the work of the anaesthetist the history and physical examination are essential. Detailed diagnostic features are not however relevant and for this purpose standard textbooks are recommended at the end of this chapter.

THE HISTORY

The importance of a clear history will be readily understood if it is appreciated that the diagnosis of severe coronary arterial disease may be dependent solely on a history of angina pectoris, when the physical examination and electrocardiogram may be entirely normal.

Cardiac ischaemic pain results from an inadequate supply of oxygen to the myo-cardium, and it may take the form of angina pectoris, acute coronary insufficiency or acute myocardial infarction.

Angina pectoris, characteristically described as a crushing 'band-like' pain or discomfort across the chest, this may radiate to one or both arms, into the neck or the jaw. The pain is usually closely associated with effort, precipitated by exertion but relieved by rest within a few minutes. In patients with severe coronary arterial disease, it may occur at rest, be precipitated by excitement or emotional disturbance or in bed at night when it is due to the increase in cardiac output required in the supine position. Voluntary restriction of exertion by the patient may result in the absence of a history of angina of exertion and yet nocturnal angina may occur.

Acute coronary insufficiency is more severe and lasts longer but does not cause myo-cardial necrosis which is the end result of *acute myocardial infarction*. Myocardial ischaemic pain is usually the result of arteriosclerotic narrowing or obstruction but may also result from the increased afterload caused by aortic stenosis or systemic hypertension. Hyperkinetic states (thyrotoxicosis or severe anaemia) can cause angina when the coronary artery disease is mild.

The importance of a clear diagnosis of the origin of chest pain cannot be over-stressed. The damage to a patient that may follow an incorrect label of cardiac ischaemic pain is incalculable, for, once the spectre of coronary arterial disease has been raised it is extremely difficult to restore the patient's confidence in his heart.

Dyspnoea is an important and usually progressive symptom and is graded according to the New York Heart Association Scale (Table 1.1). In heart disease dyspnoea is usually related to a rise in the pulmonary venous pressure, but it may also occur in patients with primary pulmonary hypertension or severe pulmonary stenosis when the pulmonary venous pressure is normal.

Table 1.1. New York Heart Association functional classification.

Grade 1	No limitation of activity.
Grade 2	Some limitation on heavy exertion, but patient can climb 1 flight of stairs or walk three blocks without shortness of breath.
Grade 3	Some limitation on ordinary activity with difficulty walking 3 blocks or climbing 1 flight of stairs.
Grade 4	Shortness of breath at rest.

When a subject lies flat there is a temporary increase in the stroke volume of the right ventricle as compared to that of the left and the left atrial pressure increases. *Orthopnoea* is dyspnoea in the supine position usually found in a patient who already has Grade 3 or 4 dyspnoea as a result of mitral valve disease or left ventricular disease. In *paroxysmal nocturnal dyspnoea* the patient is awoken from sleep with life-threatening dyspnoea and florid pulmonary oedema may develop.

Haemoptysis is an important symptom and may be due to pulmonary infarction, rupture of a small intrapulmonary bronchial vein, or be associated with paroxysmal nocturnal dyspnoea or pulmonary oedema. Recurrent winter bronchitis is a common presenting feature of mitral stenosis, and blood streaking of the sputum may occur.

Syncope is associated in particular with complete heart block (Stokes–Adams attacks) and is also an important symptom of aortic stenosis, atrial myxoma and pulmonary embolus.

Palpitations do not necessarily indicate cardiac pathology. They may be due to paroxysmal tachycardia (including paroxysmal atrial fibrillation) or recurrent extrasystoles. Attacks of *paroxysmal tachycardia* usually start and end suddenly, lasting from a few seconds to many hours. The patient may be conscious of a rapid regular palpitation and may feel faint if the heart rate is very high. When paroxysmal tachycardia is associated with dyspnoea or ischaemic pain the possibility of occult heart disease exists. *Paroxysmal atrial fibrillation* usually indicates significant underlying disease (commonly rheumatic heart disease, ischaemic heart disease or thyrotoxicosis) and the patient is aware of the irregularity. *Recurrent extrasystoles* occur both in normal subjects and in those with heart disease. The sufferer is conscious of a sudden heavy beat, which is the accentuated post-extrasystolic beat since the filling and emptying of the ventricle following the premature extrasystole is of greater volume than normal. When extrasystoles occur in runs the patient may complain of episodes of completely irregular palpitation, which are then historically indistinguishable from atrial fibrillation.

Oedema is a relatively late symptom of cardiac failure and does not usually appear until right heart failure with elevation of the jugular venous pressure has developed, but this is not the principal cause of oedema. There is an abnormal retention of sodium by the kidneys which results in a secondary retention of water with a consequent increase in the extracellular and plasma volumes. In heart failure there is a particularly marked reduction in renal blood flow due to renal arteriolar constriction and it may fall to 25 per cent of control levels. The diminished glomerular filtration and consequent increased tubular reabsorption of sodium is not as marked as the reduction in cardiac output, and therefore it appears unlikely that it is an important factor in sodium retention.

Hyperaldosteronism occurs in some patients with severe failure and in these cases the increased retention of sodium and excretion of potassium and hydrogen, due to the action of aldosterone on the distal tubule, certainly increases the severity of the oedema. In the majority of patients with cardiac failure, however, there is no evidence of hyperaldosteronism and the mechanism underlying the increased retention of sodium is unknown.

The retention of water is almost always secondary to sodium retention: Active retention of water, however, occasionally results in a reduction in the serum sodium concentration. This may be due to an inappropriate secretion of antidiuretic hormone (ADH).

Other causes of peripheral oedema which need to be distinguished are venous incompetence, deep venous thrombosis, inferior vena-caval obstruction, lymphatic obstruction, low serum albumin, pre-eclamptic toxaemia and acute glomerulo-nephritis.

Ascites may occur in advanced failure; the fluid is a transudate with a low protein content ($<$ 30 g/litre). Ascites is particularly common when the venous pressure is very high (tricuspid incompetence and constrictive pericarditis). The very high jugular venous pressures can result in the development of cardiac cirrhosis and hypertension, and this may play a part in the development of ascites which is disproportionate to the degree of peripheral oedema.

PHYSICAL EXAMINATION

Inspection

The general appearance and build of patients with heart disease is usually unremarkable. However, a tall thin individual whose arm span exceeds his height, with a high-arched palate, and dislocation of the lens, probably has Marfan's syndrome, which is associated with cystic medial necrosis of the aorta. Similarly, certain types of congenital heart disease are often associated with other congenital abnormalities. One such association is the frequent occurrence of abnormalities of the endocardial cushion with Down's syndrome.

Cardiac disability may be secondary to another disease process. For example, anaemia secondary to bleeding from a carcinoma may cause angina or cardiac failure; rapid atrial fibrillation in a patient with a thyroid mass should suggest thyrotoxicosis, rather than primary heart disease.

Clubbing of the fingers occurs in cyanotic congenital heart disease, chronic suppuration in the chest, carcinoma of the bronchus, subacute bacterial endocarditis and occasionally in hepatic cirrhosis. It may also rarely be congenital.

Peripheral cyanosis is due to an increased extraction of oxygen in the tissues as a result of reduced flow of blood through the capillary beds in the skin. This occurs when the cardiac output is substantially reduced or, in normal people, as a result of peripheral vasoconstriction due to cold. In *central cyanosis* the skin is warm and the discoloration is readily apparent in the tongue: desaturated blood mixes with oxygenated blood in the heart, great vessels or lungs. Ventilation-perfusion abnormalities in the lungs cause central cyanosis which can be distinguished from that due to cardiac abnormalities because high inspired concentrations of oxygen reduce the cyanosis.

Abnormal haemoglobins, such as methaemoglobin or sulphaemoglobin, can cause a blue colour in the skin and are usually due to drugs, but on very rare occasions, methaemoglobinaemia may be congenital.

Arterial pulse

The carotid is superior to the radial for the detection of abnormalities of character

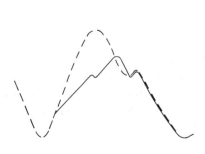

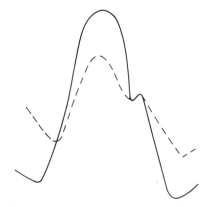

Fig. 1.1. Diagram of aortic pressure trace of a plateau pulse. (A normal trace is shown in broken lines for comparison.) The normal dicrotic notch is seen on both traces.

Fig. 1.2. Diagram of a collapsing pulse.

and volume of the pulse because alterations occur as the pulse wave is propagated peripherally. Low cardiac output states or severe mitral stenosis cause a small-volume pulse with a normal upstroke. Aortic stenosis causes a slow upstroke and a sustained plateau (Fig. 1.1).

A large volume <u>collapsing pulse</u> (Fig. 1.2) occurs in any condition in which the <u>total resistance in the systemic arterial system is low</u>. This may be due to exercise, fever, pregnancy: it is characteristic of aortic regurgitation, patent ductus arteriosus, aortopulmonary window, large arteriovenous fistulae, severe anaemia and thyrotoxicosis.

Jugular venous pulse

The level of the jugular venous pressure and the character of its waveform (Fig. 1.3) reflects changes in the right side of the heart and is also altered by rhythm disturbances. In the normal subject it can be just seen in the supraclavicular fossa with the subject reclining at 45°.

The *a* wave is caused by atrial contraction; it is absent in atrial fibrillation. Cannon waves are caused by the atrium contracting against a closed tricuspid valve,

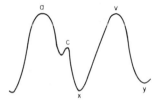

Fig. 1.3. Diagram of a normal jugular venous pulse.

when atrial and ventricular contraction are completely dissociated and are seen in complete heart block. A prominent *a* wave is characteristic of right ventricular hypertrophy with sinus rhythm. This may be caused by any condition which causes a rise in pulmonary arterial pressure. If the tricuspid valve is incompetent the *x* descent is replaced by a high *c-v* wave due to the transmission of the ventricular pressure pulse to the right atrium across the incompetent valve.

The cardiac impulse (*apex beat*)

This is normally situated in the fifth intercostal space within the mid-clavicular line. Reliable assessment of its character demands considerable experience but the cause of any displacement is more important than its precise location which is merely the best bedside guide to the size of the heart. Displacement can be caused by extracardial factors. Hypertension or aortic stenosis causes a sustained heave of the left ventricle due to pressure-overload. Volume-overload occurs in aortic or mitral regurgitation and causes the left ventricular pulse to be hyperdynamic.

The heart sounds

The most important step in auscultation of the heart is the correct identification of the first and second heart sounds. The carotid pulse should be felt routinely during auscultation. Precise differentiation between diseases of different valves by auscultation is properly the province of cardiologists. Anaesthetists seldom need to make diagnoses in this field but they do need to be able to recognize that the heart is abnormal. There are up to four normal heart sounds: the first two are caused by turbulent blood flow at the closure of valves, but the third and fourth (atrial), which are not easily heard, are believed to be caused by the flow of blood into the ventricle and their presence in patients aged over thirty years indicates heart disease.

Splitting of both first and second heart sounds into components, which arise from each valve, occurs. A split first sound is seldom pathological; a split second sound may be normal, if the degree of splitting varies with respiration but if it does not, or if there is a long interval between the components, it is pathological. The *opening snap,* which is diagnostic of mitral stenosis, occurs early in diastole at the time when the mitral valve opens, and it is thought that it is caused by vibrations set up in the mobile, but stenosed, valve. The opening snap is best heard either at the apex or just medial to it. *Systolic clicks* can be divided into two groups, early or 'ejection' clicks, and mid- and late-systolic clicks. Early clicks occur immediately after the first heart sound and are always heard in significant aortic or pulmonary valvular stenosis when the valves are mobile. They may also occur in systemic or pulmonary hypertension. Mid- or late-systolic clicks are often of no significance, and a certain number of them may be exocardial in origin.

Murmurs

Murmurs also result from turbulence in blood flow: increased resistance to flow, increased velocity and changed viscosity of the blood all increase turbulence.

Systolic murmurs may be pan-systolic, late-systolic or mid-systolic in timing. *Pan-systolic* murmurs are of constant volume, occupy the whole of systole and are always pathological. Mitral regurgitation typically produces an apical pan-systolic murmur but on occasions the murmur may be *late-systolic* and incidates mildre flux. *Mid-systolic* ejection murmurs are usually best heard at the base of the heart and are frequently not pathological. The loudness of a mid-systolic ejection murmur is of some help in distinguishing between a benign flow murmur due to turbulence and a murmur indicating pathology, but *important murmurs may be relatively quiet.* Turbulence is increased by increased blood flow so that flow murmurs may be heard in exercise, anxiety, pregnancy or thyrotoxicosis. Benign flow murmurs are frequently heard in young children, in whom they are due to a combination of thin build and relatively high cardiac output. The essential clinical differentiation between pathological and benign murmurs depends on the presence or absence of other physical signs.

Other ejection systolic murmurs indicate severe cardiac disease.

Diastolic murmurs may be early, mid or late (presystolic) in timing. Diastolic murmurs, unlike systolic murmurs, are *always* indicative of cardiac pathology. *Early diastolic murmurs* start immediately after the aortic or the pulmonary component of the second heart sound, and are due to incompetence of either the aortic or the pulmonary valve. The murmur diminishes in volume as the pressure declines between the ascending aorta or the pulmonary artery and the left or right ventricle declines throughout diastole. Aortic and pulmonary regurgitation give rise to soft, high frequency murmurs best heard with the diaphragm of the stethoscope. Pulmonary regurgitation is uncommon and is usually secondary to severe pulmonary hypertension. The murmur is then called the Graham Steel murmur. *Mid-diastolic murmurs* do not start immediately after the second heart sound. The low-pitched rumbling diastolic murmurs of mitral stenosis is best heard at the apex with the bell of the stethoscope. Mid-diastolic murmurs arising from the mitral valve may also be heard in pure mitral incompetence or in the presence of ventricular septal defects or patent ducts with large left to right shunts, which cause increased flow through the left side of the heart. A left to right shunt at atrial level causes an increased flow across the tricuspid valve, which gives rise to a murmur similar to that of tricuspid stenosis.

Presystolic murmurs occur in patients with either mitral or tricuspid stenosis who are in sinus rhythm and disappear when atrial fibrillation develops. They are caused by the atria contracting and expelling blood into the ventricle just before the onset of ventricular systole. The murmurs increase in intensity up to the first heart sound.

Continuous murmurs continue from systole to diastole. It is important to distinguish them from venous hums which are normal in young children. These noises arise in the large veins in the upper thorax or neck and they can be abolished by postural changes or by rotation of the head.

A pericardial rub produces a superficial scratching noise and does not have a fixed relationship to systole or diastole. Its intensity and character may be altered by posture, or by varying the pressure with which the diaphragm of the stethoscope is applied to the chest wall. It is usually audible for only a few hours or days.

THE ELECTROCARDIOGRAM (ECG)

The ECG is a graphical recording of the electrical potential changes in the heart muscle obtained through electrodes placed on the surface of the body. These voltages have both direction and magnitude which are reflected in the recording. The conventional scalar ECG consists of twelve leads, which are divided into three groups: the standard limb leads, the augmented limb leads and the chest leads. In standard lead I the left arm is positive relative to the right; in lead II the left leg is positive relative to the right arm; and in lead III the left leg is positive relative to the left arm.

The three augumented (unipolar) limb leads are referred to as aVR, aVL and aVF. In these leads, the exploring (positive electrode) is placed on the right arm (aVR), the left arm (aVL) or the left leg (aVF) and connected to an indifferent electrode which is itself formed by connecting all the three limb electrodes together through a $5k\Omega$ resistance to form a central electrode of zero potential.

For the recording of the chest (unipolar) leads the electrode is placed on the chest wall over the precordium and connected to the same indifferent electrode used for recording the augmented limb leads. Six sites are usually chosen. These are:

V_1 the fourth intercostal space just to the right of the sternal edge;
V_2 the fourth intercostal space just to the left of the sternal edge;
V_3 midway between V_2 and V_4;
V_4 the fifth intercostal space in the mid-clavicular line;
V_5 the left anterior axillary line on the same level as V_4;
V_6 the left mid-axillary line on the same level as V_4 and V_5.

On occasions other chest leads may be recorded, and in particular in children V_3R and V_4R which correspond on the right side of the chest to V_3 and V_4 may be of particular value. The ECG is normally recorded at a paper speed of 25 mm/sec, and

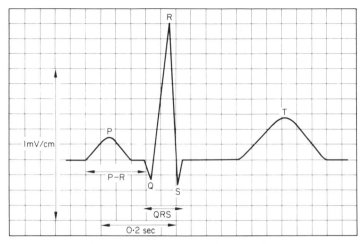

Fig. 1.4. An idealized normal electrocardiogram.

at a calibration of 1 mV/cm. The normal ECG (Fig. 1.4) can be divided into three separate waves, the P wave, the QRS complex and the T wave. The P wave is caused by atrial depolarization, and while it is usually positive (upright), in some leads it is negative (aVR) or occasionally biphasic (V_1). It is followed by a short iso-electric line, the P–R interval, which separates it from the QRS complex. The P–R interval corresponds to the passage of the depolarizing wave through the atrio-ventricular node and down the bundle of His and the bundle branch and Purkinje systems to the ventricular muscle. The QRS complex is caused by ventricular depolarization. The shape of the normal QRS varies widely from lead to lead, but it is usually made up of three parts, the Q, the R and the S wave. The initial negative deflection, the Q wave, should not exceed 25 per cent of the succeeding positive R wave in magnitude, or 0·04 s in duration. The positive R wave may be followed by a second negative wave, the S wave. The total duration of the QRS complex should be not more than 0·10 s. Following the inscription of the QRS complex the ECG record returns to the iso-electric line for a short period. This part of the record is called the S–T segment and is followed by the T wave, which represents ventricular repolarization. The T wave is less in magnitude and longer in duration than the preceding QRS complex, but in the normal ECG the direction of the QRS and T waves is the same.

The actual configuration of the ECG waveform in each lead depends on both the magnitude and direction of the intracardiac potential changes relative to the lead in question. Minor variations may therefore occur as a result of either differing body proportions or shifts in the position of the heart in the thorax.

It is very important that the value and limitations of ECG should be clearly understood. It is of particular value in the diagnosis of dysrhythmias and in the recognition of certain conduction abnormalities such as the Wolff–Parkinson–White syndrome and bifasicular block, which may predispose to the development of a dysrhythmia.

The ECG is also of help in identifying chamber hypertrophy, whether atrial or ventricular. The resting ECG may be abnormal in patients with ischaemic heart disease although the presence of an entirely normal ECG does not rule out this diagnosis. *Indeed it is now well recognized that patients with severe stenosis of all the major coronary arteries may have an entirely normal ECG.* This has led to the increasing use of exercise or stress ECG. An exercise ECG is recorded during or immediately after a period of exercise performed on a bicycle ergometer, a treadmill or on a standard step (Master's test). When exercise testing is done to confirm the diagnosis of ischaemic heart disease by the production of an obviously ischaemic record, the end point of the exercise is the development of chest pain or the inability of the patient to exercise further. One of the pitfalls of the exercise ECG is that the recordings taken with conventional leads are often uninterpretable due to poor recording. It is now a widespread practice therefore to record the ECG immediately after the exercise. The sensitivity of the technique is thus greatly reduced and interpretation of a negative result should be guarded. The changes of myocardial ischaemia which may occur are a 2 mm ST–T depression (which lasts about 0·8 s) and T wave inversion. These changes are seen in the chest leads particularly V_4 and V_5. If these changes are easily produced the disease is probably extensive. If hypotension occurs simultaneously multi-vessel disease is likely. Unfortunately, the correlation with coronary angiography is not 100 per cent: the exercise ECG may, uncommonly, be positive whilst angiography is negative and *vice versa*. Nevertheless in about three-quarters of cases there is agreement between both investigations. Drugs, particularly digitalis, can cause false positives.

THE CHEST RADIOGRAPH

The study of the chest X-ray is an integral part of the cardiological examination. The features which should be particularly noted include the size and shape of the heart and great vessels, the pattern of the vascular shadows in the lung fields, the presence or absence of calcification within the heart, great vessels or lung fields, and other changes such as linear shadows or avascular areas within the lung fields. The borders of the normal heart shadow are made up from above downwards by the aortic knuckle, the pulmonary artery and the ventricle on the left, and by the superior vena cava and the right atrium on the right. (Fig. 1.5)

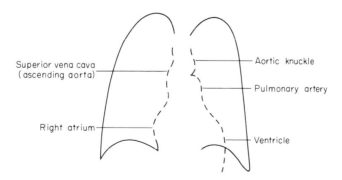

Fig. 1.5. The normal cardiac silhouette.

In a good quality postero-anterior (P–A) chest film taken in deep inspiration, the heart size should not exceed 50 per cent of the maximum internal diameter of the normal thoracic cage.

Enlargement of the left atrium, which occurs in mitral valve disease, is best seen in a penetrated P–A film (Fig. 1.6), when the left atrium appears as a dense shadow in the middle of the heart. The enlarged left atrium pushes posteriorly between the bronchi,

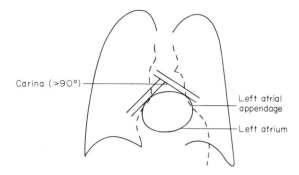

Fig. 1.6. Diagram of a penetrated P–A film showing enlargement of the left atrium.

pushing up the left bronchus so that the angle of the carina becomes greater than 90°. The left atrial appendage also enlarges to cause a bulge on the left border of the heart between the pulmonary artery and the ventricle. When the right atrium enlarges, the lower half of the right border of the heart extends to the right.

Enlargement of the ventricles may lead to an increase in the size of the cardiac shadow. The cardiac silhouette may suggest that the enlargement is due to one or other of the ventricles, but it is impossible to be absolutely certain on a P–A chest X-ray which ventricle is enlarged.

Increase in size of the pulmonary artery is shown in Fig. 1.7.

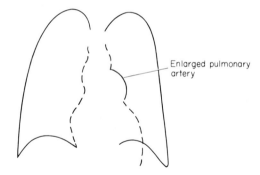

Fig. 1.7. Cardiac silhouette showing enlargement of the main pulmonary artery.

In normal subjects under the age of 40, the ascending aorta is not usually visible on the P–A chest film. However, in the older age group, or in some diseases, the dilated ascending aorta becomes visible to the right in the upper part of the cardiac shadow, displacing the superior vena cava (Fig. 1.8).

Calcification may occur in the mitral or aortic valves (Fig. 1.9). It is usually best seen in penetrated films. While mitral valve calcification is easy to see on both P–A and lateral films, aortic valve calcification is often obscured by the spine in the P–A projection.

Mild degrees of valve calcification may be better appreciated on cardiac screening because the characteristic movement of the valves can be seen.

The appearance of the lung fields on the chest X-ray gives valuable information about the pulmonary circulation. When pulmonary venous hypertension is present,

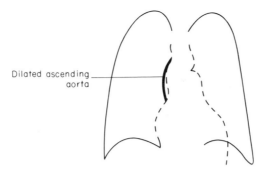

Fig. 1.8. Cardiac silhouette showing enlarged ascending aorta.

there is increased <u>dilatation of the pulmonary veins,</u> particularly in the <u>upper zones</u> of the lung fields. The fluid, which exudes from the capilliaries as a result of the rise in the pulmonary venous pressure, is at first confined to the pulmonary interstitial tissue. This interstitial oedema causes haziness around the vascular shadows and bronchi (<u>peribronchial oedema</u>). Short, thin, horizontal lines (<u>Kerley *b* lines</u>) due to <u>septal oedema</u> may also appear just above the costophrenic angles. When the pulmonary oedema becomes worse, the exudation of fluid into the alveoli produces a <u>fluffy</u> appearance which is more marked in the areas of the lung adjacent to the <u>hila.</u> This distribution of the opacities may give rise to a 'butterfly' or '<u>bat's wing</u>' appearance. In severe pulmonary hypertension the vascular markings in the peripheral lung fields may be sparse. This, coupled with the prominence of the proximal pulmonary arteries

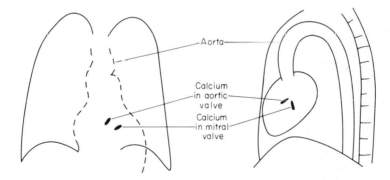

Fig. 1.9. Diagrams of P–A and lateral chest films showing calcification in aortic and mitral valves.

that occurs in this condition, produces an appearance of 'pruning' in the pulmonary vascular pattern. When the pulmonary blood flow is greatly increased in patients with large left to right shunts the main and the peripheral pulmonary arteries are dilated giving an appearance of pulmonary plethora.

   <u>Wedge-shaped shadows</u> and <u>linear scars</u> in the lung fields may be caused by <u>small pulmonary emboli</u>, whereas large pulmonary emboli which lodge in the proximal pulmonary arteries may produce either avascular (translucent) areas, or no radiological change at all. Calcification in the lung fields, due to secondary ossification in focal accumulations of haemosiderin, may occur in mitral valve disease with severe pulmonary hypertension.

SPECIAL INVESTIGATIONS

The special investigations used in cardiac assessment can be grouped into non-invasive and invasive.

Non-invasive investigations

Phonocardiography is the recording of the heart sounds and murmurs. It is extremely useful for teaching auscultation and of value in timing certain of the cardiac sounds. However, it does not detect murmurs and sounds of importance that are inaudible to the skilled clinician, and is not a substitute for careful auscultation.

Echocardiography is now one of the most important investigative techniques in clinical cardiology whose potential is not yet fully realized. The underlying principle is not new. High frequency (2 MHz) sound waves (ultrasound) are reflected from an interface between two tissues of different density. This is the same principle which was utilized in the Asdic detection of submarines in World War II. Intermittent bursts of sound waves are emitted from a piezo-electric crystal. After a burst has been emitted the crystal becomes the receiver and detects the echo. The receiver transduces this echo into an electric signal which can be recorded. The time between emission and return indicates the thickness of the tissue.

There are several techniques employed. Intensity can be displayed on the X or Y axis of an oscilloscope or as the varying brightness of the light spot (Z axis). Conventionally motion echocardiography (M scan) displays intensity on the Z axis, distance of the various tissue planes from the transducer (emitter/receiver) on the Y axis, and time on the X axis. The most recent development is the B scanner which moves in two directions (at 90 degrees) so that a two-dimensional picture is obtained.

The velocity of sound waves through body tissues varies but is about 10^{-5} times that of X-rays. The wavelength is longer. Both these factors contributed to the poor definition of images.

The technique is simple and non-invasive and can be used dynamically. It is of particular value in the diagnosis of a <u>pericardial effusion,</u> in which condition an echo-free gap can be identified between the posterior pericardium and the back of the heart. The speed of closure of the mitral valve can be easily followed by recording echoes reflected from the anterior cusp of the valve. This speed is progressively reduced as the severity of mitral stenosis increases. Echocardiography is also of value in other acquired valve disease, in congenital heart disease, in cardiomyopathy, and in the assessment of left ventricular function.

Vectorcardiography. The conventional ECG records the magnitude of the electrical forces moving through the myocardium in one direction only, either towards or away from the exploring electrode. It is possible to record these changes as a vectorcardiogram in two directions, that is, in one of the planes of the body, either horizontal, frontal or sagittal. Loops are obtained in place of the simple wave forms of the standard ECG. Vectorcardiography is of considerable theoretical interest, but it is not of much practical importance in routine clinical cardiology outside the study of certain conduction defects and complex paediatric cardiology.

Nuclear medicine. During the last few years the techniques of nuclear medicine have been applied on a qualitative basis to cardiology. The use of isotopes as a non-invasive method for the diagnosis and measurement of the size of intracardiac shunts is established. Intravenous injection of an isotope-labelled substance is followed by direct scanning of the heart aided by computer analysis of the output. New developments in this growing area include the measurement of the <u>ejection fraction of the left ventricle</u> and of coronary flow, and the 'imaging' of myocardial infarcts with isotopes that are selectively taken up either by active or by dead tissue. The use of radio-isotopes in cardiology is an exciting and promising field but the definition that is possible with the imaging techniques now available is not sufficiently good to permit the use of radio-isotopes in place of radio-opaque contrast medium.

Systolic time intervals are derived values from records of the ECG, the phono-cardiogram and the carotid pulse waveform. Fig. 1.10 shows diagrammatically how these values are calculated.

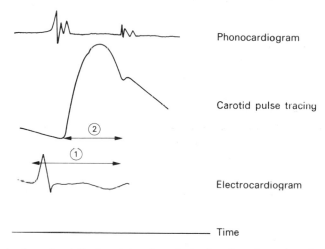

Phonocardiogram

Carotid pulse tracing

Electrocardiogram

Time

Fig. 1.10. Determination of systolic time intervals: 1 is the duration of systole, 2 is the left ventricular ejection time (see text).

The left ventricular ejection time (LVET) represents, as its name suggests, the duration of ejection of blood from the left ventricle. It starts with the beginning of the carotid pulse and ends with the closure of the aortic valve. The duration of systole is taken to be from the Q wave on the ECG to the same end point (closure of the aortic valve). The pre-injection period (PEP) is the difference between these two times. Left ventricular function is sometimes represented by PEP/LVET and is normally about 0·3 s; it increases in cardiac failure. However, systolic time intervals have not proved to be a reliable index of left ventricular function.

Invasive investigations

There are a number of measurements of cardiac and vascular variables which are important clinically to anaesthetists in their work in the operating room and in intensive therapy. Some of these are also used in the quantitative assessment of patients with cardiac disease together with more elaborate tests which have little application outside the catheter laboratory. The range of the latter group is quite wide and selection of a particular series of investigations is a personal one of the cardio-logist.

There are two *peripheral*, as opposed to intracardiac, invasive measurements which are well known to anaesthetists and their details will not be elaborated here. (References 26, 28 and 31 should be consulted.)

Central venous pressure is used in intensive therapy to differentiate between the arterial hypotension of cardiac failure, of hypovolaemia, and of gross vasodilatation. Trends of changes in central venous pressure are more readily and reliably interpreted than isolated values and simultaneous observation of the arterial pressure is required as well as a full clinical assessment.

Peripheral arterial pressure is occasionally required as an invasive investigation in clinical cardiology, for instance in order to record a patient's response to the Valsalva manoeuvre in the presence of autonomic neuropathy.

Intracardiac invasive measurements

The pressure in central veins represents the filling pressure of the *right* side of the heart. When right heart function is adequate for its venous return this pressure is not raised. When left heart function is impaired for any reason the imbalance between the two sides is reflected in a rise at first in pulmonary venous pressure and later in pulmonary arterial pressure. If the rise in pressure exceeds the oncotic pressure in the capillaries pulmonary oedema results.

Pulmonary arterial pressure. Pulmonary arterial catheterization with a flow-directed catheter is used to determine this pressure (and also, when a thermistor is incorporated in the catheter, for cardiac output measurements). If the catheter is advanced until it will pass no further into the pulmonary circulation and the balloon at the end of the catheter inflated, the 'wedge-pressure' (PAWP) is obtained. This wedge-pressure is used as an indicator of left atrial pressure (LAP), that is the filling pressure of the left ventricle. Unfortunately this is not always reliable, particularly when left ventricular filling is abnormal (e.g. mitral stenosis), or when parenchymal lung disease is sufficient to cause pulmonary vascular changes.

The presence of an intracardiac catheter may cause dysrhythmias, but removal usually restores normal rhythm.

Cardiac catheterization and angiography. In spite of the development of valuable non-invasive techniques such as echocardiography, cardiac catheterization and angio-cardiography still remain the most important special investigations in cardiology. Cardiac catheterization and angiocardiography establish the degree of haemodynamic abnormality in the circulation and identify the anatomical abnormalities responsible for the haemodynamic disturbance. This is achieved by recording pressures within the heart and the great vessels; by establishing the presence of intracardiac shunts; and by the use of angiocardiography to classify the anatomy and to study the dynamics of chamber function. Pressure gradients across valves cannot be fully interpreted without a knowledge of the cardiac output, and thus this measurement is an important part of cardiac catheterization. Specific angiocardiographic findings in various cardiac conditions are beyond the scope of this book. Those patients who have congenital defects, obstructive lesions or abnormal communications should have the investigation at least as confirmation of the clinical diagnosis. Table 1.2 gives some reference values.

Table 1.2. The pressures and oxygen saturation levels in the chambers of the heart and great vessels.

	Pressures		% Oxygen saturation
	mmHg	kPa	
Right atrium	0–8	0–1	60–70
Right ventricle	15–30/0–8	2–4/0–1	60–70
Pulmonary artery	15–30/5–15	2–4/0·6–2	60–70
Pulmonary wedge (indirect left atrial)	5–13	0·6–1·7	100
Left atrium	4–12	5–1·6	100
Left ventricle	90–140/4–12	12–19/0·5–1·6	97
Aorta	90–140/60–90	12–19/8–12	97

'Myocardial contractility'

Various indices derived from haemodynamic studies have been described but none is widely accepted and none represents a significant advance in our understanding. For example although under physiological conditions aortic peak velocity and maximum acceleration correlate well with stroke volume they do not discriminate between groups of patients with varying impairment of left ventricular function. Furthermore, if the behaviour of papillary muscle is representative of all cardiac muscle, it appears that the contractility is not an intrinsic function but depends also upon fibre length.

Finally, the absence of an independent measure of contractility with which comparisons may be made has led most clinicians almost to abandon or to ignore the use of these indices in clinical assessment. [13, 17, 18]

CARDIAC FAILURE

AETIOLOGY

There is unfortunately no comprehensive definition of cardiac failure. From the clinical standpoint, however, the most useful definition is probably that of the late Dr Paul Wood who has observed that '(Cardiac failure) is a state in which the heart fails to maintain an adequate circulation for the needs of the body despite a satisfactory venous filling pressure.' This definition excludes conditions in which the cardiac output is reduced secondary to salt, plasma or blood loss from the intravascular compartment.

Cardiac failure is usually divided clinically into three types, left, right and congestive (combined left and right) cardiac failure. In left heart failure the symptoms are the result of pulmonary venous hypertension and capillary engorgement and include dyspnoea, orthopnoea and paroxysmal nocturnal dyspnoea. The manifestations of right heart failure are largely the result of systemic venous engorgement and include raised jugular venous pressure, peripheral oedema, hepatic engorgement and ascites. Right heart failure is frequently secondary to left heart failure, but it may be due to primary disease of the lungs as well as of the right side of the heart. Cardiogenic shock is simply an extreme example of acute cardiac failure.

When the heart is subjected to an intolerable pressure or volume load or when the function of cardiac muscle is impaired, failure of the heart as a pump may occur.

Pressure overload on the left heart is caused by severe aortic stenosis or systemic hypertension; pulmonary stenosis and pulmonary hypertension have the same effect on the right side. This increased afterload causes the ventricular muscle to hypertrophy, to provide compensation, for many years. Eventually the load is intolerable and decompensation with ventricular dilatation and reduced output occurs. Decompensation of the ventricle may occur very suddenly, and the mechanism underlying this sudden failure is not well understood. It may be that the increased size of the contractile fibres, which underlies the hypertrophy, is itself harmful as it results in an increase in the distance between the capillary and the centre of the contractile cell. This may lead to relative hypoxia in the centre of the cell. Recent experimental work has suggested that myocardial hypertrophy is accompanied by a reduction in the enzyme activity of the contractile protein, myosin. This enzyme catalyses the splitting of adenosine triphosphate (ATP) and therefore controls the final stage in the conversion of chemical energy to mechanical work. At the stage of final failure there is not only overload but also myocardial muscle impairment.

Volume overload (*pre-load*) is usually gradual and the ventricle responds with an increase in stroke volume and later by hypertrophy. Compensation lasts for many years, but the ventricle eventually fails as the function of the cardiac muscle deteriorates. In accordance with Laplace's law, as the ventricular cavity increases in size, the wall tension required to generate a given pressure increases. The oxygen requirement of the ventricular muscle inevitably rises because wall tension is one of the important determinants of myocardial oxygen consumption. The increased wall tension may act as a trigger for hypertrophy.

Relative volume overload occurs when the demands for cardiac ouput are greater than can be met, for example in anaemia, thyrotoxicosis, pregnancy, Paget's disease or in arteriovenous fistulae. The fact that the cardiac output may at this time be normal or at least not reduced has led to the use of the paradoxical term 'high output failure' to describe this situation.

Intrinsic disease of the myocardial muscle causes impairment of function which may also be the primary cause of cardiac failure in cardiomyopathy, myocarditis, or when patchy destruction of the muscle occurs as a result of ischaemic heart disease.

In the early stages of failure, the resting cardiac output is normal, but fails to rise sufficiently in response to exercise. This failure to respond progresses and eventually output is below normal at rest. There is a compensatory increase in sympathetic nervous activity which causes tachycardia and venous and arterial constriction and there is an associated redistribution of blood flow. Blood flow is maintained to muscle, cerebral and coronary vessels but there is a substantial reduction in renal and skin blood flow.

Failure in patients with otherwise compensated disease may be precipitated by a number of factors which may not only have this effect outside the usual spheres of work of the anaesthetist but also in the operating room and intensive therapy unit. The factors likely to be important in the latter situations are respiratory infections, dysrhythmias, saline infusions, fluid overload, corticosteroid therapy, or the use of β-adrenergic blocking drugs. Pulmonary embolism or myocardial infarction are two of the common causes in other locations.

TREATMENT

The management of cardiac failure aims to reduce the work of the heart by rest, to improve the function of the cardiac muscle with cardiac glycosides and to correct salt and water retention with diuretics. Precipitating factors are treated by appropriate specific therapy.

Rest

Cardiac work is reduced by rest, and in many patients this alone results in a considerable improvement. Prolonged bed rest in patients with cardiac failure is, however, associated with an increased incidence of deep venous thrombosis and pulmonary embolism. Strict bed rest is only indicated for patients with severe failure, and these patients are usually more comfortable if they are nursed in the sitting position. In patients with mild cardiac failure bed rest should not be enforced, but activity should be restricted. When cardiac failure is controlled, exercise that does not produce symptoms should be encouraged.

Cardiac glycosides

These drugs increase myocardial contractility both in the normal and the failing myocardium. The glycosides inhibit the sodium–potassium ATP-ase enzyme, which is located in the external membrane of the muscle cell and it is thought that this inhibition results in a secondary increase in the intracellular calcium ion concentration which in turn increases contractility. Increase in contractility is normally accompanied by a rise in the oxygen consumption of the heart, but in the failing heart the decrease in end-diastolic volume, which follows the improvement in contractility, leads to a reduction in oxygen demand. The cardiac glycosides also slow the ventricular rate by a combination of vagal stimulation and prolongation of the refractory period of the atrioventricular node; this is useful in uncontrolled atrial fibrillation. Cardiac glycosides also reduce the refractory period of both atrial and ventricular muscle.

Digoxin, either orally or intravenously, is adequate for almost all cases, but in special circumstances, when a very rapid and short action is required, ouabain may be indicated.

The action of digoxin starts within a half hour following oral administration and reaches its peak after 6 hr. It is excreted unchanged by the kidneys, but even in the presence of normal renal function its half life in the body is 50 hr. When renal function is impaired, this is greatly prolonged. Particular care must therefore be taken in patients with poor renal function or in the elderly. The oral dosage regimen for digoxin depends not only on these factors, but also on the rapidity with which full digitalization is required.

Intravenous administration should only be used in emergencies when it is certain that the patient has not received any digitalis preparation within the preceding 14 days. The adult intravenous dose of digoxin is 0·5–1·0 mg, and of ouabain is 0·25–0·5 mg. The onset of action is approximately 15 min after administration of digoxin, and 5 min for ouabain. The peak action occurs after 2 hr and 1 hr respectively.

The symptoms of *digitalis toxicity* include anorexia, nausea, vomiting, diarrhoea and rarely xanthopsia, but the more serious effects are disturbances of cardiac rhythm and intracardiac conduction. The different effects of the glycosides on the refractory period of atrial and ventricular muscle, and on the atrioventricular node, predispose to the development of dysrhythmias. Almost every abnormality of rhythm or conduction has been recorded in patients suffering from digitalis toxicity, but the most frequent is the appearance of frequent ventricular ectopic beats, which are often coupled with normal sinus beats to produce ventricular bigeminy. Other frequent abnormalities are paroxysmal atrial tachycardia with varying atrioventricular block, ventricular tachycardia, junctional rhythm, first degree heart block and second degree heart block of the Wenckebach type. Complete heart block and ventricular fibrillation may occasionally occur.

Reduction in total body potassium facilitates the appearance of digitalis-induced dysrhythmias. The frequency with which these complications are encountered has increased dramatically since the introduction of the powerful diuretics, all of which cause some degree of potassium loss. The serum potassium level does not necessarily reflect loss in intracellular potassium, and potassium depletion should always be considered as a precipitating factor in patients with digitalis toxicity. Digitalis should be stopped and potassium supplements given either orally or intravenously. Tachy-dysrhythmias should be treated with a β-blocking drug, such as propanolol. DC counter-shock should only be used to correct ventricular fibrillation if it occurs, since its use in the presence of cardiac glycosides may be followed by the appearance of severe dysrhythmias. A smaller dose of cardiac glycoside may be given after the patient has been free of symptoms or signs of toxicity for at least 48 hr.

The achievement of satisfactory digitalization is easily recognized in the presence of atrial fibrillation by the slowing of the heart, but its recognition may be more difficult when the patient is in sinus rhythm. In these circumstances the improvement in the symptoms and signs of heart failure usually provides a satisfactory guide.

Diuretics

Diuretics increase sodium excretion by the kidney and this is accompanied by an increased excretion of water. The thiazide diuretics exert their major effect by the inhibition of sodium reabsorption in the distal tubule and most patients can be well controlled with them. Side effects are uncommon; they include hyperglycaemia, hyperuricaemia and rarely agranulocytosis, thrombocytopenia and skin rashes.

The 'loop' diuretics, such as frusemide and ethacrynic acid, inhibit sodium retention in the distal tubule, in the proximal tubule and in the ascending limb of the loop of Henle.

The effect of an oral dose of frusemide starts within 1 hr, and is complete within 8 hr. The diuresis starts within minutes when the drug is given intravenously. When patients are not responsive to frusemide, ethacrynic acid may be used.

All these diuretics increase the excretion of potassium and sodium. The loss of potassium relative to that of sodium is more marked with thiazide drugs, but with both types of diuretics the total loss is considerable and supplements should therefore be given.

The aldosterone antagonist, spironolactone, is particularly useful when there are high circulating levels of aldosterone, for example in severe right heart failure with ascites. It promotes sodium loss and potassium retention. It is relatively ineffective as a sole diuretic but in combination with either a thiazide or a 'loop' diuretic it may be very effective and less potassium supplementation is then required. It takes between three and four days to exert its full effect.

Other diuretics such as the mercurials, triamterene and acetazolamide are less commonly used.

ACUTE LEFT VENTRICULAR FAILURE

Patients in acute left ventricular failure are severely breathless and should be nursed in the sitting position. The accumulation of fluid in the pulmonary interstitial tissue and the alveoli decreases diffusion of oxygen so that arterial hypoxaemia occurs and hypoxic hyperventilation may follow. In the absence of concurrent lung disease hypocapnia results. There is, therefore, no contraindication to the administration of oxygen in high concentration to patients with left ventricular failure. Morphine or diamorphine, aminophylline, and frusemide or chlorthiazide should be given intravenously. The classical treatment in the undigitalised patient used to include intravenous digoxin. There is now clinical evidence that better results can be achieved by the continuous intravenous infusion of nitrites in order to reduce the afterload on the left ventricle. If there is no response within a short time, intermittent positive pressure ventilation (IPPV) (with positive end-expiratory pressure) should be used. The old-fashioned technique of venesection (500 ml) may still occasionally have a place when IPPV is not available. As soon as the emergency is controlled attempts should be made to establish and correct the causes underlying the pulmonary oedema. Conditions which typically give rise to acute left ventricular failure include hypertension, rapid atrial fibrillation in tight mitral stenosis, severe aortic valve disease and acute myocardial infarction.

CARDIOGENIC SHOCK

Cardiogenic shock is a clinical condition in which cardiac output is very low in spite of an adequate filling pressure for the left ventricle. The clinical manifestations are systemic hypotension (systolic < 80 mmHg), tachycardia, peripheral cyanosis, vasoconstriction, oliguria (< 20 ml/hr), and mental confusion. The usual cause of cardiogenic shock is acute myocardial infarction, and the mortality is very high (95–100 per cent) regardless of the type of treatment even when this includes IPPV and counterpulsation with an aortic balloon pump.

THE DYSRHYTHMIAS

The dysrhythmias can be considered conveniently in two groups: disorders of rhythm and rate and disorders of conduction.

DISORDERS OF RHYTHM AND RATE

The normal pacemaker of the heart is the sino-atrial node, which undergoes spontaneous, rhythmic depolarization. There are other potential pacemakers, but the rate of their automaticity is usually slower than that of the sino-atrial node. They may take over control of the heart rate if the sino-atrial rate is depressed below their intrinsic rate or if their excitability is increased.

Re-entry is another important mechanism for the generation of tachycardias. This mechanism requires that adjacent areas of myocardium have different refractory periods, such as may occur in myocardial ischaemia. An impulse may thus be able to stimulate one of the adjacent areas, but not the other which is still refractory from the previous impulse. When this second area ceases to be refractory, it may allow the impulse to pass in a retrograde direction and to depolarize the first area again if that is now receptive. Thus a re-entry movement may be set up. The majority of the tachycardias which follow acute myocardial infarction are due to re-entry mechanisms.

ABNORMAL SINUS RHYTHMS

Sinus tachycardia is present when the sinus rate exceeds the upper range of normal. In adults this is 100/minute but in neonates and infants, rates of up to 160/minute would be regarded as normal. Sinus tachycardia is a normal response to exercise and anxiety. When it occurs in association with anaemia, thyrotoxicosis or heart failure, it is the underlying disease that requires treatment.

Sinus bradycardia is said to be present when the sinus rate falls below 60/minute and is a normal finding in some people. It is commonly seen after acute myocardial infarction when it is usually due to parasympathetic overactivity. Under these circumstances bradycardia may permit the escape of another pacemaker, which may take control of the heart rate; furthermore the damaged ventricle may be unable to compensate for the decrease in rate by an increase in stroke volume, and the cardiac output may thus decrease. Sinus bradycardia after an infarction usually responds to atropine. It is also associated with hypothyroidism, hypothermia, raised intracranial pressure and certain drugs, in particular digitalis and β-blocking agents.

Sinus bradycardia may also occur when there is disease of the sinus node, the sick sinus syndrome. This condition is being increasingly recognized in the elderly in whom it may present as bradycardia in an otherwise symptom-free patient, or as bradycardia associated with syncopal attacks, or finally as bradycardia complicated by recurrent tachycardias. In the presence of symptoms the treatment is the implantation of a permanent cardiac pacemaker coupled, on occasions, with the use of β-blocking drugs to control the tachycardias.

Sinus arrhythmia is a variation in the rate of the sinus node discharge; the rate increases during inspiration and decreases during expiration. It is a normal finding, being particularly marked in children and teenagers.

ABNORMAL ATRIAL RHYTHMS

Atrial ectopic beats arise from a focus in the atria, other than the sino-atrial node. The beat is premature and therefore causes an occasional irregularity of the pulse. The impulses spread through the atria in an abnormal direction, giving rise to an abnormally shaped P wave but the QRS is usually normal since conduction through the ventricles takes place in the normal manner (Fig. 1.11). Atrial ectopic beats frequently occur in normal individuals and do not require treatment.

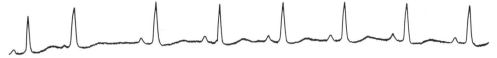

Fig. 1.11. Atrial ectopic. The second beat is an atrial ectopic. The beat is premature, the P wave is abnormal in shape but the QRS and T waves are the same as in the sinus beats.

Atrial tachycardia results from the rapid discharge of an abnormal focus in the atria at a rate of between 140 and 220/minute. Conduction at the atrioventricular node is usually normal and therefore each atrial contraction is followed by a ventricular contraction. The P wave is different in shape from normal but it may on occasions be difficult to identify the P wave in the standard ECG (Fig. 1.12) as it becomes buried

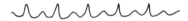

Fig. 1.12. Atrial tachycardia. The ventricular rate is 180/minute.

in the preceding T wave. The QRS is usually normal in configuration, but aberrant conduction may result in a widening of the complex. Atrial tachycardia may be precipitated in normal people by undue consumption of tea, coffee, alcohol, cigarettes or by emotion. Other causes are the Wolff–Parkinson–White syndrome (see below), thyrotoxicosis, rheumatic and ischaemic heart disease.

The attacks usually last for only a few seconds, but they may continue for hours or even days. They usually start and end suddenly. The patient may be unaware of the attack, although he usually complains of rapid regular palpitation and occasionally of dizziness or even syncope. The attacks may precipitate angina pectoris or dyspnoea in patients with established heart disease, or if prolonged, cardiac failure may develop. Attacks may be sometimes terminated by carotid sinus pressure or by the Valsalva manoeuvre; sedation by itself may be effective. If the condition of the patient deteriorates, a β-blocker or digoxin may be given intravenously or synchronized DC shock used.

Atrial flutter is usually associated with heart disease. The atria contract at rates between 250 and 350/minute and there are varying degrees of atrioventricular block; the ventricles respond in a 2:1, 3:1 or 4:1 ratio. Occasionally there is a 1:1 atrioventricular response and this usually leads to a rapid deterioration in haemodynamic function.

Atrial flutter usually presents as a regular tachycardia and 'flutter' waves may be visible in the jugular venous pulse.

The ECG (Fig. 1.13) is characteristic; the rapid regular atrial complexes

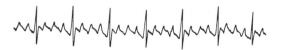

Fig. 1.13. Atrial flutter.

(250–350/minute) give the record a saw-toothed appearance which is best seen in leads II, III and V_1. Carotid sinus pressure may cause a sudden increase in the degree of atrioventricular block, but the ventricular rate almost always returns to its former level when the pressure is released.

Individual attacks are best treated with digoxin; this slows the ventricular response by increasing the degree of atrioventricular block and may in fact restore sinus rhythm, but if the haemodynamic condition of the patient is deteriorating the attack can almost always be rapidly terminated by synchronized DC shock. The long-term management of patients with chronic or recurrent paroxysmal atrial flutter is difficult, since this dysrhythmia is notoriously unstable. The drug of choice is still digoxin but β-blockers are also useful.

Atrial fibrillation. Here the atrial muscle is contracting rapidly (> 300/min), irregularly, and without coordination. The common causes of atrial fibrillation are rheumatic heart disease, ischaemic heart disease and thyrotoxicosis, but it may also occur in association with acute lung infections, the involvement of the mediastinum and pericardium by malignant disease, lung surgery, myocarditis and the cardiomyopathies. It occasionally occurs in the absence of other evidence of heart disease.

Atrial fibrillation may be paroxysmal but it usually becomes established and persists for the rest of the patient's life. The onset of atrial fibrillation has three adverse effects. Firstly, since there is usually no delay in atrioventricular conduction, the ventricular rate is very rapid. Secondly, the contribution of atrial contraction to ventricular filling disappears. This is not usually of great importance but in some patients with severe left ventricular disease and low ventricular compliance, it makes an important contribution to ventricular filling in diastole. In these patients the cardiac output remains reduced even following the control of the ventricular rate with digoxin. The third hazard is the development of mural thrombi in the atria, since the cessation of co-ordinated atrial contraction causes some stasis of blood in the atria, which is particularly marked when there is associated mitral valve obstruction. The mural thrombi may become dislodged causing systemic emboli.

Patients with atrial fibrillation may only complain of irregular palpitations, but it is more usual for the symptoms of pulmonary venous congestion to develop either

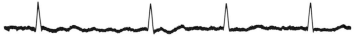

Fig. 1.14. Atrial fibrillation.

gradually or rapidly. On examination the arterial pulse is irregular both in rhythm and volume and remains so on exercise. (Multiple ectopic beats, a dysrhythmia which may be confused with fibrillation, disappear on exercise.)

The ECG of atrial fibrillation is characteristic (Fig. 1.14). There are no P waves, but the disordered atrial activity produces an irregular wavy base line, and the QRS complexes are completely irregular in timing.

The drug of choice in the management of atrial fibrillation is digoxin supplemented if necessary by a β-adrenergic blocking drug. Restoration of sinus rhythm can be achieved, at least temporarily, in most patients with synchronized DC shock. The probability of sinus rhythm being restored for any length of time is remote if the patient has been in atrial fibrillation for more than 2 years, even if drugs, such as quinidine, are used after cardioversion.

ATRIOVENTRICULAR NODAL (JUNCTIONAL) RHYTHM

These rhythms originate in the tissue of the atrioventricular node. Nodal ectopic beats and nodal bradycardia and tachycardia are not uncommon. They may occur in normal people or in association with underlying heart disease particularly immediately following an acute myocardial infarction. Excessive vagal tone is a common precipitating factor. They should be treated in the same manner as other atrial dysrhythmias from which they can be distinguished by the ECG (Fig. 1.15). The site of origin of the impulse is low down in the atria, so the P wave is opposite in direction from the normal P wave. The P wave may precede, be buried in or follow the QRS complex.

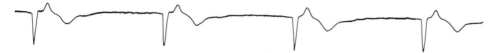

Fig. 1.15. Nodal rhythm.

ABNORMAL VENTRICULAR RHYTHMS

Ventricular ectopic beats may arise from a focus in any part of either ventricle. They may occur in healthy subjects but are more commonly seen in patients with heart disease, and particularly following acute myocardial infarction.

The QRS complex of the ventricular ectopic beat is wide and abnormal in appearance (Fig. 1.16). The succeeding T wave is inverted. The ectopic beat is followed by a compensatory pause.

No specific treatment is usually required unless the patient is very distressed by the sensation of palpitation. Treatment is required following an acute myocardial infarction since otherwise ventricular tachycardia or ventricular fibrillation may develop. Ventricular ectopics require treatment when they occur soon after the preceding beat and coincide with the sensitive part of the T wave; when they are multifocal in origin; when the ratio of their frequency to that of the normal beats exceeds 1 in 6; and when they are increasing in frequency. The most useful drug for the suppression of ventricular ectopic beats is intravenous lignocaine, initially as a bolus dose of 1 mg/kg and subsequently as a continuous intravenous infusion of 1–2 g/24 hr. Procainamide or sustained release quinidine may be used to suppress chronic ventricular ectopics.

Ventricular tachycardia. Here the rate is between 140 and 230/minute. The paroxysms may last from a few seconds to hours or days. The symptoms are the same as those of atrial tachycardia, but the frequency with which ventricular tachycardia precipitates severe symptoms, such as ischaemic pain, dyspnoea or shock is greater, because this dysrhythmia is almost always associated with severe heart disease.

Carotid sinus pressure has no effect on ventricular tachycardias: the diagnosis is confirmed by the ECG which shows a tachycardia with widened QRS complexes of either left or right bundle branch block pattern, depending on the site of the ventricular focus (Fig. 1.17). Ventricular tachycardia is usually slightly irregular as compared with the strict regularity of atrial tachycardia.

The development of ventricular tachycardia is, almost without exception, an emergency situation which requires immediate treatment since this dysrhythmia frequently precedes the development of ventricular fibrillation. The drug therapy is the same as that for multiple ventricular ectopics both for the attack and for prophylaxis.

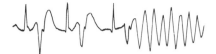

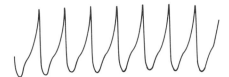

Fig. 1.16. The second, fourth and sixth beats are ventricular ectopics. The last of these falls on the sensitive area of the T wave of the preceding beat and precipitates ventricular fibrillation.

Fig. 1.17. Ventricular tachycardia.

Intravenous practolol may also be of value if lignocaine or procainamide fails to stop the dysrhythmia. If the patient's condition is rapidly deteriorating synchronized DC cardioversion should be used immediately. DC cardioversion has no effect on the cause of the dysrhythmia and therefore successful cardioversion must be followed by the immediate use of an antidysrhythmic drug, such as lignocaine. Other possible precipitating factors such as hypoxia, hypercarbia or acidosis should be corrected.

Ventricular fibrillation is characterized by a totally disorganized electrical activity of the ventricles at a rate between 300 and 500/minute (Fig. 1.16). The ventricular muscle does not contract in a coordinated fashion and the heart ceases to pump; management will be described in the section on cardiac arrest.

DISORDERS OF CONDUCTION

Disorders of impulse conduction can occur at any point in the conducting system of the heart—from the sino-atrial node to the fascicles of the right and left bundles beyond the bundle of His.

DELAYED CONDUCTION

Sino-atrial block. The impulse, generated in the sino-atrial (S–A) node, fails to escape from the node to activate the atria. This causes a dropped beat. Both the P wave and the QRS complex are absent on the ECG (Fig. 1.18). However, since the S–A node

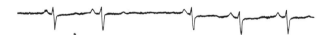

Fig. 1.18. Sino-atrial block.

has discharged, the distance between the P wave preceding the blocked beat and that following it is an exact multiple of the normal P–P interval. S–A block may occur in digitalis toxicity or it may be part of the 'sick sinus' syndrome. Patients are usually free of symptoms but, if the period of block is prolonged, they may feel dizzy or faint. If the patient has symptoms and the block is not due to drug therapy, the correct treatment is the implantation of a permanent pacemaker.

Sinus arrest. Here the sinus node fails to discharge. If the arrest is intermittent, sinus rhythm is restored but the interval between the preceding P wave and that following the period of arrest is not an exact multiple of the normal P–P interval (Fig. 1.19). If

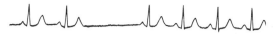

Fig. 1.19. Sinus arrest.

the arrest is prolonged either a nodal or ventricular escape rhythm may develop. If there is a long delay before the escape rhythm appears, the patient may be dizzy or may faint. The treatment is the implantation of a permanent pacemaker.

Atrioventricular block. The usual site of an atrioventricular (A–V) block is either in the A–V node or in the fascicles of the right and left bundle branch system. The block may, on rare occasions, occur in the bundle of His itself. There are four types of A–V block; first degree block; second degree block; third degree (or complete) block, and bundle branch block.

First degree A–V block is an electrocardiographic diagnosis. In this condition the

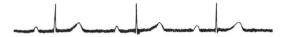

Fig. 1.20. First degree atrioventricular block.

P–R interval is prolonged (> 0.2 s) (Fig. 1.20). It may be a sign of digitalis toxicity or may precede higher degrees of block following acute myocardial infarction.

Second degree A–V block. There are two varieties—Wenckebach (Mobitz I) and Mobitz II. In the Wenckebach type the P–R interval becomes gradually prolonged over a series of beats until a P wave is not followed by a QRS complex (Fig. 1.21).

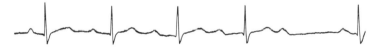

Fig. 1.21. Second degree atrioventricular block; Wenckebach (Mobitz I).

The next P–R interval is of normal length and the cycle is then repeated. In the Mobitz II variety there is no change in the P–R interval before a QRS complex is suddenly dropped (Fig. 1.22). The causes of second degree heart block include digitalis toxicity, myocarditis, ischaemic heart disease, particularly acute myocardial infarction, and idiopathic fibrosis of the conducting system. Patients with second degree A–V block may develop complete A–V block and periods of asystole. This is

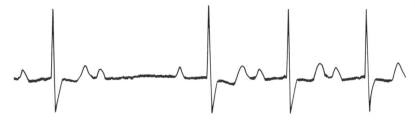

Fig. 1.22. Second degree atrioventricular block (Mobitz II). First degree heart block with intermittent Mobitz II block.

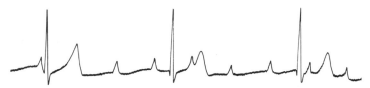

Fig. 1.23. Complete (third degree) atrioventricular block.

more common with the Mobitz II variety. Second degree block may be abolished by atropine particularly if it has developed after an acute myocardial infarction.

In third degree or complete block the conduction of impulses from the atria to the ventricles is completely blocked (Fig. 1.23). and the ventricular rate is controlled by a pacemaker situated in the A–V node, the bundle of His or more distally in the fascicles or the Purkinje system. The rate of the ventricular pacemaker is slow, usually less than 30 per minute in acquired complete block, or up to 50 per minute in the rare cases of congenital complete block.

Acute complete A–V block is commonly caused by acute myocardial infarction but other causes are acute myocarditis, cardiac surgery and digitalis toxicity. The development of complete block is serious because the heart may be unable to maintain an adequate cardiac output since the diseased ventricle may be unable to increase its stroke volume. There is, in addition, a considerable risk of ventricular standstill.

The heart rate may be temporarily increased by an infusion of isoprenaline. Isoprenaline increases the oxygen demand of the heart; a temporary pacemaker is a more appropriate treatment.

Chronic complete A–V block is occasionally congenital in origin but most cases occur in the elderly. It is usually due to idiopathic fibrosis of the conducting system. It may be completely asymptomatic, in which case it requires no specific treatment. The patients, however, may have syncopal attacks (Stokes–Adams attacks) or, less commonly, develop cardiac failure due to the slow heart rate.

The prognosis following the development of symptoms is poor in the absence of treatment: 50 per cent of patients die within one year. A few patients may do well with long-acting isoprenaline derivatives but these drugs often produce troublesome palpitations and they do not appear to alter the prognosis. The prognosis following the implantation of a permanent pacemaker is good.

Bundle branch block

Delay in conduction may occur in either the left or the right bundle branches beyond the bundle of His.

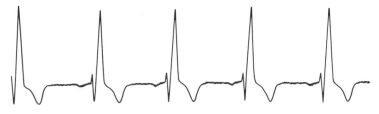

Fig. 1.24. Right bundle branch block (V$_1$).

Right bundle branch block. There is a delay in conduction in the right bundle and therefore delayed activation of the right ventricle. If the QRS complex is not widened ($<$ 0·12 s) the condition is partial but if it is widened it is called complete right branch block. The P–R interval is normal. The ECG pattern of right bundle branch block is characteristic (Fig. 1.24) there being an rs R pattern in V_1 and q Rs in V_6. It is not uncommon in normal people and it also occurs in certain types of congenital heart disease (e.g. atrial septal defects), in the cardiomyopathies and ischaemic heart disease.

Left bundle branch block may also be either partial or complete and also produces characteristic ECG changes (QrS in V_1 and rs R in V_6) (Fig. 1.25). It can be regarded as an indicator of heart disease since it rarely occurs in a normal heart.

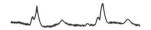

Fig. 1.25. Left bundle branch block (V_6).

The left bundle branch is more diffuse than the single discrete right branch and consists of two principal subdivisions, an anterior (or superior) branch and a posterior (or inferior) branch. Discrete blocks can occur in either of these two divisions and their presence will produce characteristic changes in the ECG. Block in the anterior division produces a marked swing of the QRS vector to the left ($> -45°$), while block in the posterior division swings the vector to the right ($> +125°$).

These fascicular blocks are most commonly seen after acute myocardial infarction but they are sometimes chronic. Their recognition is important, particularly when complete right bundle branch block is also present, as this pattern of *bifascicular* block may be the precursor of complete heart block. The management of asymptomatic patients with bifascicular block is controversial, but if Stokes–Adams attacks develop, a permanent pacemaker should be implanted.

Prolonged QT interval syndrome is a rare condition in which congenital deafness is associated with the ECG finding and syncopal attacks which culminate in sudden death due to ventricular fibrillation. A prolonged QT interval can be acquired following myocarditis, myocardial infarct, sinus tachycardia, hypokalaemia, hypocalcaemia and overdosage of drugs. The cause of the congenital variety is unknown but there are a number of hypotheses. The condition is diagnosed when the QT interval is greater than 0·4 s [24].

ATRIOVENTRICULAR DISSOCIATION

There is no delay in conduction in this dysrhythmia but it is considered here since it is frequently confused with A–V block. The atria are controlled by a pacemaker in the atria and the ventricles by one in the ventricles. Both pacemaker rates are similar and nearly synchronous and the territory of each pacemaker is refractory to the impulses of the other. This dysrhythmia is quite frequently found after acute infarction, and it carries a good prognosis. It can usually be abolished by the use of atropine which speeds up the atrial rate sufficiently to capture the ventricles.

ACCELERATED CONDUCTION

The speed of conduction of the impulse from the atria to the ventricles may occasionally be faster than normal ($<$ 0·12 s). This condition is referred to as pre-excitation

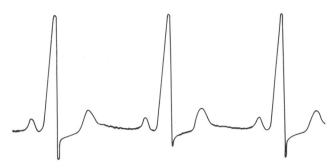

Fig. 1.26. Wolff–Parkinson–White syndrome.

(Wolff–Parkinson–White syndrome). It is thought that most cases are due to the presence of an aberrant conducting pathway, which bypasses the atrioventricular node. The ECG is characteristic (Fig. 1.26), the P–R interval is less than 0·12 s and the initial deflection of the QRS is slurred. This slurring is called the *delta* wave and is due to early excitation (pre-excitation) of part of the ventricular muscle. The ECG may mimic that of acute anteroseptal infarction or severe right ventricular hypertrophy. Some patients with this condition are prone to develop supraventricular tachycardia due to re-entry. This may be difficult to treat, the most useful drugs being the *β*-blocking agents.

STOKES–ADAMS ATTACKS

Syncopal attacks of the Stokes–Adams variety are associated with several disturbances of rhythm. They may, on occasions, be preceded by a brief period of dizziness, although frequently they occur without warning. The sufferer loses consciousness and falls to the ground, and the attack may be associated with convulsions. The attack usually lasts for less than 30 sec and the patient recovers quickly following the restoration of the heart beat. In old patients the attack may be followed by a period of mental confusion of varying duration. The patient is pale at first but peripheral cyanosis develops rapidly if the period of circulatory arrest persists, and reactive hyperaemia occurs after the circulation is restored. The frequency of Stokes–Adams attacks varies widely from patient to patient, but the prognosis of such patients is poor, 50 per cent die within one year of the onset of the attacks, in the absence of specific treatment.

Stokes–Adams attacks are usually the result of ventricular asystole, although they may occasionally be due to a short run of very rapid ventricular tachycardia or even ventricular fibrillation. The attacks most commonly occur in patients with second or third degree heart block, but they may also be associated with bundle branch block, particularly of the bifascicular variety, or disorders of the sinus node, such as the 'sick sinus' syndrome. They may rarely occur in patients with normal sinus ryhthm. During an attack normal rhythm may be restored by a single blow over the precordium but, if this fails, the management is the same as for cardiac arrest.

CARDIAC ARREST

Cardiac arrest may be due to either ventricular fibrillation or ventricular asystole. It frequently occurs without warning but it may be preceded by the appearance of less severe disturbances of cardiac rhythm, such as ventricular ectopics, ventricular tachycardia or conduction disturbances; it most frequently occurs after acute myocardial infarction.

Management of cardiac arrest must be skilful and prompt since irreversible brain damage will occur if the <u>cerebral circulation is not restored within 4 min.</u> A single firm blow over the precordium may on occasions restore normal rhythm, but external cardiac massage is usually needed. If this is to be effective, it must be done correctly. It is essential that the patient should be lying on a firm surface, either on a special intensive care bed with a rigid base and firm mattress or with a board behind the chest or else moved on to the floor. Two hands are placed one on the other over the lower sternum and the pressure applied through the heel of the underneath hand. The heart is thus compressed between the posterior surface of the sternum and the vertebral column. The amount of blood that can be ejected from the heart during each compression is limited even during correctly performed cardiac massage (approximately 30 ml) and so the cardiac output is principally dependent upon the rate of massage, which should be not less than 80 per minute. In old patients, or in a patient with a barrel-shaped chest due to emphysema, effective cardiac massage will frequently result in the fracture of ribs. Undue damage which might result in lacerations of underlying organs, such as the liver and spleen, should be avoided but the achievement of an adequate cardiac output takes precedence.

Respiratory resuscitation should be commenced at the same time as cardiac massage since it is the delivery of oxygenated blood to the tissues which is required. Expired air resuscitation should be used as a first aid measure; manual ventilation with oxygen-enriched air administered with a self-filling bag and face mask should be the next stage and finally, when the necessary apparatus and skill are available the airway should be protected by an endotracheal tube. A brief pause by the person performing cardiac massage allows proper ventilation of the lungs. Satisfactory rates will be achieved if this is done every 5–7 compressions and the lungs inflated 12–16/minute.

Metabolic acidosis develops within minutes after the cessation of the circulation, and sodium bicarbonate (100 mmol for an adult) should be given intravenously to counteract this, and an arterial blood sample should then be taken to ensure that the blood gases and the acid–base balance of the blood are maintained within the reference ranges. Inadequate correction of acidosis, hypoxia and hypercarbia are important factors in the failure of electrical defibrillation and in the recurrence of an unstable cardiac rhythm following initially successful defibrillation.

The ECG should be recorded as soon as external cardiac massage and ventilation have been successfully started. If the cardiac arrest is due to ventricular fibrillation immediate DC shock should be used. It may sometimes be impossible to convert low voltage ventricular fibrillation with electric shock and in these cases intravenous or even intracardiac adrenaline may be of use since conversion is more successful when the fibrillation waves become coarse.

Isoprenaline, adrenaline, calcium and cardiac pacing may be needed in the management of ventricular asystole. In spite of these measures, the results of resuscitation of asystolic cardiac arrest are much worse than those of cardiac arrest due to fibrillation.

Considerable care must be exercised in the management of patients after successful resuscitation, since the correction of the immediate emergency may not have influenced the underlying cause of the cardiac arrest. Factors which may have played a part in the genesis of the arrest include hypoxia, acidosis, and the development of ventricular ectopics, either unifocal or multifocal, occurring in runs or on the sensitive area of the T wave. Management should be directed to their correction.

2*

The duration for which artificial ventilation should be continued after cardiac arrest must be judged in each individual case. If there is any doubt it is better to ventilate the patient. Adequate oxygenation can usually be achieved and the work of breathing is abolished. IPPV with a positive end-expiratory pressure or spontaneous ventilation with a continuous positive airway pressure may also be helpful in the management of pulmonary oedema which is the inevitable accompaniment of cardiac arrest and external cardiac massage.

CONGENITAL HEART DISEASE

Congenital anomalies of the heart and the great vessels occur in approximately 0·6 per cent of all live births. Half of these children die within the first few months of life, and many within the first few weeks. Those who survive to the second year usually remain well until early adult life, when symptoms begin to appear; few patients with severe disease survive beyond the fifth decade.

The 5th–8th weeks of gestation are very important in the development of the heart, and errors in development at this stage may cause major cardiac abnormalities. No clear aetiology can be established in most cases but the occurrence of maternal viral infections, particularly rubella, during the first trimester is followed by a high incidence of congenital cardiac abnormalities. Cardiovascular abnormalities are frequently multiple. Musculoskeletal abnormalities (kyphoscoliosis, syndactyly, polydactyly, arachnodactyly ect.) are commonly associated with congenital heart lesions.

ABNORMAL COMMUNICATIONS

ATRIAL SEPTAL DEFECTS

In 25 per cent of normal subjects it is possible to pass a cardiac catheter from the right atrium to the left atrium through the foramen ovale. The pressure in the left atrium normally exceeds that in the right and the valvular action of the foramen ovale prevents blood from flowing from one atrium to the other. Functional communications (atrial septal defects) between the two atria are nonetheless common congenital cardiac defects. There are two types: secundum defects and primum defects. The former are the more common variety and can, in turn, be further subdivided into fossa ovalis defects, sinus venosus defects, and low atrial septal defects. This subdivision is important surgically since a sinus venosus defect is frequently associated with one or more pulmonary veins draining into the right atrium (anomalous pulmonary venous drainage), and a low secundum atrial septal defect may on occasion have no inferior border, the defect sitting over the entrance of the inferior vena cava into the right atrium.

Primum atrial septal defects are due to a developmental abnormality of the septum primum, which is part of the endocardial cushion. The mitral and tricuspid valves and the interventricular septum also develop from the endocardial cushion and therefore valvular incompetence, ventricular septal defect, or a common atrioventricular canal can be associated with an ostium primum defect.

At birth the right and the left ventricular walls are approximately the same thickness, and the ventricles have the same compliance. There is therefore no reason why blood should pass from the left to the right atrium, and thence to the right ventricle during diastole even if there is a communication between the two atria. However, as the infant grows the left ventricular wall becomes thicker than the right and there is therefore a change in the relative compliance of the two ventricles. A left to right shunt at atrial level develops during diastole. In consequence, uncomplicated atrial septal defects are rarely detected during the first year of life.

After the first year of life the left to right shunt is usually large, and pulmonary blood flow is at least two to three times greater than the systemic blood flow. This does not lead immediately to a large rise in pulmonary arterial pressure since the pulmonary arterioles are relatively distensible, but over many years structural changes occur in the pulmonary vascular bed which result in an increase in the pulmonary vascular resistance and severe pulmonary hypertension. This is occasionally so severe that the right atrial pressure exceeds the left and the shunt is reversed. The patient is then cyanosed. In uncomplicated atrial septal defects the development of severe pulmonary hypertension is uncommon before the fourth or fifth decade.

The symptoms of an uncomplicated atrial septal defect are usually minimal in childhood and early adult life, but they may include recurrent palpitations and winter bronchitis. Severe symptoms usually develop in the fourth and fifth decades, and consist of increasing breathlessness and fatigue. The development of atrial dysrhythmias, particularly atrial fibrillation, is a very frequent occurrence at this stage of the disease and it usually precipitates the development of severe congestive cardiac failure. Symptoms occur earlier and are more severe in patients with ostium primum defects with associated mitral or tricuspid valve abnormalities.

The arterial pulse is usually of small volume and the venous pressure is normal. The right ventricular impulse is hyperdynamic, and on auscultation there is a soft ejection systolic murmur best heard at the left sternal edge. The second heart sound is widely split and the two components do not move with respiration. A soft mid-diastolic murmur, accentuated by inspiration, can frequently be heard at the lower left sternal edge. This murmur is due to a large flow of blood across the tricuspid valve. In ostium primum defects the murmurs of mitral or tricuspid incompetence may also be heard.

The ECG helps to distinguish between secundum and primum defects. In secundum defects the ECG shows right axis deviation and partial right bundle branch block. In primum defects the partial right bundle branch block is almost always accompanied by left axis deviation. The chest X-ray shows a slightly enlarged heart with considerable enlargement of the pulmonary artery. The right atrium may also be prominent. The aorta is small, and there is marked pulmonary plethora (Fig. 1.27).

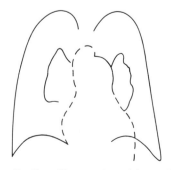

Fig. 1.27. Cardiac silhouette in atrial septal defect.

The degree of the shunt should be established by cardiac catheterization. Mean pressures in the left and right atria are the same. The higher the oxygen saturation in the pulmonary arterial blood the greater the pulmonary blood flow. The defect is significant when pulmonary blood flow is twice that of the systemic flow. There is often a small pressure difference across the pulmonary valve due to the high blood flow which disappears when the defect is closed. However, pulmonary vascular resistance tends to rise with age in patients with large defects and the risk of surgery also then increases. Angiography is not necessary in patients with secundum defects but it is essential in patients with primum defects since it enables the degree of mitral regurgitation to be established and demonstrates the endocardial cushion defect.

In spite of the relative lack of symptoms in the first three decades, the prognosis of patients with atrial septal defects is not good; few patients survive beyond the end of the fifth decade. Operation should be recommended in all patients with this condition who have a shunt of more than two to one since the mortality of closure of secundum defects is small. The operative mortality in primum defects is higher because of the associated abnormalities, but if the shunt is substantial, surgery should be recommended. In the absence of raised pulmonary vascular resistance the overall mortality of surgery should be less than 1 per cent but if the resistance is raised the mortality may be around 10 per cent.

VENTRICULAR SEPTAL DEFECT

The interventricular septum is derived from three components: the muscular septum, the membranous septum, which is part of the endocardial cushion, and the bulbus cordis which divides the outflow tract into the right and left ventricle. The majority of defects are situated in the membranous septum and many close early in childhood.

The size of ventricular septal defects varies widely. The degree of haemodynamic abnormality depends on the size of the defect and on the pulmonary vascular resistance. If the defect is small, the flow of blood in systole from the high pressure left ventricle to the low pressure right ventricle is small, and therefore the pulmonary blood flow is only slightly greater than the systemic blood flow. These patients have no symptoms but their physical signs are remarkable. There is a loud pansystolic murmur, usually with a thrill, best heard at the left sternal edge in the third to fifth intercostal spaces. The second heart sound is normal.

If the defect is large and the pulmonary vascular resistance is low a large left to right shunt develops immediately after birth and left ventricular failure may occur within the first few months of life. If the shunt is large, but not large enough to produce failure in infancy, there are usually few symptoms until adult life when breathlessness, fatigue and eventually cardiac failure develop. Examination in these patients reveals hyperdynamic left and right ventricles and a pansystolic murmur at the lower left sternal edge. There is usually a mid-diastolic murmur at the apex, which is due to the large diastolic flow across the mitral valve.

In some patients with large defects there is a high pulmonary vascular resistance. The pulmonary arterial and right ventricular pressures are therefore high and the left to right shunt is often small. The pulmonary vascular resistance may be high in some infants from birth but in others it becomes high during infancy and childhood, the high pulmonary flow through a low resistance changing to a low flow through a high resistance. Recognition that this change may occur is vitally important since the risks of surgery increase rapidly once the pulmonary vascular resistance rises, and if it exceeds the systemic vascular resistance surgery is contraindicated. The symptoms then include breathlessness, fatigue and cyanosis (Eisenmenger syndrome—see below).

The ECG is normal in small ventricular septal defects but when the left to right shunt is large there is usually evidence of biventricular hypertrophy. When pulmonary hypertension becomes severe the pattern of right ventricular hypertrophy develops on the ECG. When the shunt is large the pulmonary artery and left atrium are enlarged on chest X-ray and pulmonary plethora can be seen.

The prognosis of small ventricular septal defects is excellent, apart from the risk of infective endocarditis. Large ventricular septal defects often cause trouble in infancy. Surgery should be recommended in patients who have such a large left to right shunt at ventricular level that pulmonary blood flow is twice the systemic flow. The question of surgery in patients in whom the pulmonary vascular resistance is elevated requires special consideration.

PATENT DUCTUS ARTERIOSUS

The ductus arteriosus normally closes within a few hours of birth but in a few instances it remains open and allows a large left to right shunt between the aorta and the pulmonary artery. This may precipitate left ventricular failure within the first few weeks of life and ligation of the duct may be required as an emergency procedure.

If the shunt is insufficient to produce trouble during the first weeks of life it is usually not detected until a routine examination in early childhood. The persistent duct provides a site for infective endocarditis. Patients with large shunts may develop left ventricular failure or pulmonary hypertension in adolescence or early adult life.

The pulse is collapsing in nature if the shunt is large. There is left ventricular enlargement and the impulse is hyperdynamic. If pulmonary hypertension has developed there is also right ventricular hypertrophy. On auscultation in the area between the second left intercostal space at the left sternal edge and left clavicle a murmur can be heard, sometimes referred to as a 'machinery murmur' or a Gibson murmur. It starts soon after the first heart sound, reaches a crescendo at the second heart sound and spills over into diastole. It usually ends before the end of diastole.

The ECG is unremarkable if the shunt is small but may show evidence of left ventricular hypertrophy if the shunt is large. The chest X-ray shows a prominent aortic knuckle, a very large proximal pulmonary artery and pulmonary plethora (Fig. 1.28). Catheterization (right) is not essential for the diagnosis of the uncomplicated condition but where multiple abnormalities are suspected it is essential. The severity of the

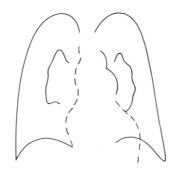

Fig. 1.28. Cardiac silhouette in patent ductus arteriosus.

haemodynamic condition is revealed: a 2:1 increase in pulmonary blood flow suggests a significant shunt. Left heart catheterization can be used to differentiate aorto-pulmonary window defects (which are associated with other severe lesions) from simple ductus arteriosus. The operative risks of direct ligation and division are extremely small in infants but are greater in adults.

OBSTRUCTIVE LESIONS

COARCTATION OF THE AORTA

Coarctation of the aorta is a narrowing of the aortic lumen and there are two types; the infantile or preductal, and the adult type. The preductal type of coarctation of the aorta is usually part of the hypoplastic left heart syndrome, in which there is poor development or even atresia of the left ventricle and ascending aorta. However, on occasions the preductal coarctation is an isolated lesion and may produce severe left ventricular failure in the first few weeks of life. Surgical correction may be an emergency procedure.

The more usual form of coarctation of the aorta is the adult variety, which is often associated with a bicuspid aortic valve. In this variety of coarctation the obstruction is situated at or just below the site at which the ductus arteriosus entered the aorta. The obstruction may be severe, there being little or no flow of blood from the ascending to descending aorta. In these cases blood reaches the lower part of the body through an extensive collateral system developed through the internal mammary arteries and the intercostal arteries. The systolic blood pressure in the vessels above the obstruction is elevated. If the condition remains unrelieved the hypertension causes left ventricular hypertrophy and eventually left ventricular failure. These patients are also at risk from endocarditis involving either the site of the coarctation or, more commonly, the associated bicuspid aortic valve. There is frequently associated cystic medial necrosis of the aorta above the coarctation and there is a definite risk of rupture of the aorta in unrelieved cases. Rupture of intracranial aneurysms is also a frequent complication.

On examination, the blood pressure in the upper limbs is higher than in the lower limbs and the femoral pulses are reduced in volume and delayed relative to the radial pulses. The collaterals can frequently be felt pulsating at the back of the chest. The left ventricle is usually enlarged and a murmur can be heard posteriorly in the fourth and fifth intercostal spaces to the left of the spine over the site of the coarctation.

The ECG may either be normal or show evidence of left ventricular hypertrophy. The chest X-ray is usually normal in children but in adults shows a prominent aortic knuckle and notching of the underside of the ribs due to the large intercostal arteries. In severe cases the left ventricle may also be enlarged. The diagnosis can usually be made clinically but aortography may be necessary to outline the anatomy accurately. The correct treatment is surgical relief.

AORTIC STENOSIS—see page 43

PULMONARY STENOSIS

Pulmonary stenosis may occur either at the valve or immediately below the valve in the region of the right ventricular infundibulum. In the latter case the obstruction is due to hypertrophy of the infundibular muscle. Pulmonary valve stenosis is the more common lesion although infundibular stenosis is frequently associated with other congenital heart defects such as a ventricular septal defect. Obstruction to the right ventricular outflow causes a systolic gradient between the right ventricle and the pulmonary artery. If the gradient is severe, right ventricular hypertrophy occurs and right ventricular failure may follow.

Although severe pulmonary stenosis may cause cardiac failure in infancy or early childhood, it is more usual for the patient to be asymptomatic until early adult life, when in severe cases breathlessness and syncope may develop. When the condition is mild the patients have no symptoms and have a normal life expectancy.

On physical examination the jugular venous pressure is normal in mild cases but shows a dominant *a* wave in severe cases. On palpation there is right ventricular hypertrophy and on auscultation in the pulmonary area there is an ejection systolic murmur. If the obstruction is at valve level this murmur is preceded by an ejection click. The pulmonary component of the second heart sound is soft and delayed if the obstruction is severe.

The ECG is normal in mild cases but in severe cases evidence of right ventricular hypertrophy is found. Chest X-ray may be normal but in moderate or severe cases when the obstruction is at the pulmonary valve level there is post-stenotic dilatation of the proximal pulmonary artery. A pulmonary artery catheter is passed and the pressures recorded during withdrawal to determine the severity of the lesion. If the systolic gradient between the right ventricle and the pulmonary artery exceeds 50 mmHg at rest (normally 10–15 mmHg) surgical relief of the stenosis should be advised, because right ventricular hypertrophy and eventual right ventricular failure will almost certainly follow.

TRICUSPID ATRESIA

This is a rare condition in which there is no direct communication between the right atrium and the right ventricle. It is frequently associated with varying degrees of hypoplasia of the right ventricle. For the infant to survive beyond birth there must be associated lesions including atrial septal defect and usually a ventricular septal defect. The infant is cyanosed at birth and the ECG shows left axis deviation and left ventricular hypertrophy. Some improvement can be produced surgically by increasing flow to the pulmonary artery but these operations can only be regarded as palliative.

DISPLACEMENT OF CHAMBERS, VESSELS OR VALVES

TRANSPOSITION OF THE GREAT ARTERIES

In this condition the aorta rises from the right ventricle and the pulmonary artery from the left ventricle. There is therefore a 'split' circulation, and the condition is incompatible with life after delivery unless there are associated lesions, such as an atrial septal defect, ventricular septal defect or patent ductus arteriosus which permit the pulmonary and systemic circulations to mix.

Transposition of the great arteries is the commonest cardiac cause of cyanosis at birth. Increasing cyanosis, dyspnoea and cardiac failure develop rapidly; death usually occurs within the first weeks or months of life. On auscultation there is a systolic murmur heard over most of the precordium. On X-ray the heart may be of normal size at birth although it may enlarge over the succeeding days or weeks. The lung fields may show either pulmonary plethora or avascularity. The ECG is usually unhelpful.

As the outcome of transposition of the great vessels is so poor without definitive treatment, it is mandatory to catheterize these infants within a few hours of the diagnosis being suspected. If the infant is densely cyanosed due to poor mixing between the pulmonary and systemic circulations, temporary improvement can be obtained by rupture of the atrial septum with a balloon catheter (Rashkind catheter). Definitive surgery can be performed at approximately one year of age.

EBSTEIN'S ANOMALY

This is an uncommon condition in which the septal cusp of the tricuspid valve is displaced into the right ventricle. There is often an associated atrial septal defect. Patients with Ebstein's anomaly may be entirely asymptomatic but if the tricuspid valve is very incompetent they may be cyanosed due to a right to left shunt through the associated atrial septal defect. They are also prone to dysrhythmias from which they may die. In severe cases with gross tricuspid reflux cardiac failure may develop. Surgery may be indicated in severe cases.

DEXTROCARDIA

In dextrocardia the heart is displaced into the right side of the chest and it is a mirror image of the normal situation. There is usually transposition of all the viscera and in these cases the heart is almost always normal apart from its malposition. If, however, the heart alone is displaced (Situs Solitus) there are usually complex cardiac abnormalities.

LAEVOCARDIA

Laevocardia is said to be present when the heart is in its normal position in the left side of the thorax but all the other viscera are transposed. Once again complex cardiac abnormalities are usual.

COMBINED CONGENITAL HEART DISEASE

Congenital abnormalities of the heart are often multiple: one of the most common combinations is pulmonary stenosis with a ventricular septal defect. The size of the defect and the severity of the obstruction may vary widely, but when the pulmonary stenosis is severe and the right ventricular pressure equals left ventricular pressure, blood is shunted from right to the left ventricle, and the patient is cyanosed. The combination of these two abnormalities with severe right ventricular hypertrophy and an aorta over-riding the ventricular septal defect, constitutes Fallot's Tetralogy.

FALLOT'S TETRALOGY

Fallot's Tetralogy is the most common form of cyanotic congenital heart disease in children after the first year of life. The obstruction to the right ventricular outflow tract is usually both at the level of the valve and of the infundibulum but rarely is it solely at valve level.

When the obstruction to the right ventricle is extreme, symptoms appear very soon after birth. More usually, the degree of obstruction is less marked and central cyanosis, dyspnoea and fatigue become apparent during the second year of life. In severe cases dense cyanotic attacks occur, unconsciousness and convulsions may follow due to spasm of the infundibular outflow tract. Dyspnoea is frequently relieved by squatting; the mechanism by which this occurs is not known but it is thought that compression of the abdominal aorta and femoral arteries increases the peripheral systemic resistance and therefore decreases the degree of right to left shunt at the level of the ventricular septum. Venous return is increased by squatting; pulmonary blood flow therefore increases, cyanosis decreases and systemic arterial pressure increases.

There is usually dense cyanosis and marked clubbing of the fingers. The jugular venous pressure is usually normal. There is palpable right ventricular hypertrophy, and there is an easily audible systolic ejection murmur at the left sternal edge in the second intercostal space. The second heart sound is single, since the pulmonary component is unaudible. In very severe cases when the flow through the pulmonary valve is very low the murmur is quiet, and during severe cyanotic attacks the murmur may disappear.

The ECG shows right axis deviation and moderate to severe right ventricular hypertrophy. The chest X-ray usually shows a characteristic boot-shaped appearance of the heart due to absence of the normal pulmonary artery shadows, and the lung fields are relatively oligaemic (Fig. 1.29).

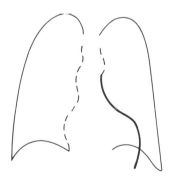

Fig. 1.29. Cardiac silhouette in Fallot's tetralogy.

Right heart catherization is essential prior to surgery and demonstrates that the right intraventricular pressure is the same as the aortic pressure. The catheter frequently passes through the ventricular defect into the pulmonary artery where flow is much less than normal.

The prognosis of Fallot's tetralogy is poor: the patients rarely live beyond the third decade. In severe cases infants or children may die during a cyanotic attack, usually as a result of cerebrovascular accident following cerebral thrombosis. Other causes of death include infective endocarditis and cerebral abscess. Cardiac failure rarely develops in Fallot's tetralogy in the absence of subacute bacterial endocarditis or anaemia.

Severe cyanotic attacks with fainting are best treated by intravenous β-blockers although cyclopropane also relieves the muscle spasm. Almost all patients with Fallot's tetralogy require corrective surgery. In most children surgery can be deferred until the age of five, at which age complete correction can be carried out. If, however, severe cyanotic attacks occur earlier, it may be necessary for a palliative 'shunt' operation to be performed, although recently total correction has been successful in infants.

THE EISENMENGER SYNDROME

This condition is relatively rare but it merits special mention since it illustrates certain important physiological and pathophysiological principles. The syndrome, as originally described, consisted of a ventricular septal defect in which the flow of blood was from right to left following the development of severe pulmonary hypertension due to high pulmonary vascular resistance. However, this term is now used to describe any reversed shunt (right to left) at atrial, ventricular or duct level, when the reversal of the shunt is due to an increase in pulmonary vascular resistance. The reason why this high resistance develops is not clear, but a number of factors are known to be important. These include the maintenance of the fetal type of pulmonary vasculature into adult life, and the prolonged exposure of the pulmonary vascular bed to high pulmonary flows.

Patients with the Eisenmenger syndrome remain relatively free of symptoms until late in the natural history of the condition when, three to five years before death, symptoms develop. Survival is rare beyond the third decade. The symptoms include fatigue, increasing dyspnoea on exertion, angina on effort and syncope. Signs of right heart failure develop. The patients are cyanosed and there are signs of right ventricular hypertrophy. On auscultation the murmurs may be unremarkable because blood flow through the abnormal channel has lessened, and the characteristic murmurs of a patent ductus arteriosus, ventricular septal defect, or atrial septal defect disappear. The closure of the pulmonary valve is accentuated and there may be a soft ejection systolic murmur best heard in the pulmonary area. There is frequently a pulmonary ejection click and on occasions the murmur of pulmonary incompetence. The ECG shows evidence of right ventricular and right atrial hypertrophy. Chest X-ray shows enlarged proximal pulmonary arteries with peripheral pruning of the pulmonary arterial tree. Right ventricular and right atrial enlargement may also be obvious.

The prognosis is poor; common causes of death being pulmonary infarction, pulmonary thrombosis and intractable right heart failure. It is one of the few cardiac conditions in which pregnancy is contraindicated, since patients rarely come successfully to term. Maternal mortality is high and even if the mother survives pregnancy, the clinical course is usually rapidly downhill following delivery. Patients should therefore be strongly advised against pregnancy and if pregnancy occurs, early termination should be recommended. The contraceptive pill is absolutely contraindicated in these patients, as in all other women with severe pulmonary hypertension.

Surgery has nothing to offer since closure of the defect is followed rapidly by the development of intractable right heart failure. Conventional treatment for cardiac failure may be of some temporary help in these patients and if deep venous thrombosis or pulmonary infarction should occur anticoagulants should be advised.

ACUTE RHEUMATIC FEVER

Acute rheumatic fever is a rare complication of infections probably due to hypersensitivity to Group A *β*-haemolytic streptococci or to one of its products. The disease is still important in developing countries where these organisms may be responsible for a third of all upper respiratory tract infections and, although the general standard of living is an important causative factor, there may also be a genetic element (suggested by the fact that the disease is frequently seen in several members of one family).

The rheumatic process affects particularly the endothelium lining the blood vessels, the endocardium, the pericardium and the synovial membranes. There is oedema and lymphocytic infiltration around the collagen fibres. Later, Aschoff bodies (granulomatous collections of round cells, fibroblasts and giant cells) occur throughout the myocardium. The cusps of the cardiac valves become oedematous and infiltrated with capillaries during the acute phase and vegetations occur along the lines of closure particularly of the mitral and aortic valves. A fibrinous pericardial effusion may occur.

The condition is, in its acute phase, relatively without significance for anaesthetists, since it is extremely unlikely that assessment prior to surgery would be required at this stage but it is a very important medical condition (see Further Reading list). Nevertheless, the disease may become chronic and severe damage to cardiac valves may occur particularly when rheumatic carditis develops (50 per cent of patients during their first attack). Some children develop Sydenham's chorea (St Vitus' Dance) (see Chapter 8) but this is less commonly followed by chronic rheumatic heart disease.

RHEUMATIC AND CHRONIC VALVE DISEASE

Rheumatic pericarditis heals without residual damage to the heart, but the sequelae of rheumatic valvulitis are often severe. Regurgitation may occur both during acute rheumatic carditis and during the healing process when the valve cusps become distorted and shrink. Obstruction only occurs during healing which causes the cusps to become thickened and adherent. There is fusion of the valve commissures, shortening of the chordae tendineae and eventually valve calcification may occur. Although the acute rheumatic process is not confined to the endothelium and indeed, in severe cases, acute myocarditis is a major feature, myocardial damage rarely plays a part in chronic cases.

The mitral valve is the valve most frequently involved in chronic rheumatic heart disease. The valve orifice may be stenosed with little or no mitral regurgitation, but a mixture of mitral stenosis and mitral regurgitation is not uncommon. After the mitral the aortic is the most commonly affected valve; then the tricuspid and rarely the pulmonary valves.

MITRAL STENOSIS

Mitral stenosis is almost always due to the fusion of the mitral valve leaflets at the commissures during the healing process of acute rheumatic carditis, and may be associated with shortening and thickening of the chordae tendineae. It may rarely be congenital.

Normally, after the mitral valve opens, the pressure in the left atrium rapidly falls to that in the left ventricle. However, when the mitral valve orifice is narrowed, the pressure in the left atrium remains higher than that in the left ventricle throughout diastole. In relatively mild cases both the left atrial pressure and the cardiac output are normal at rest, but on exercise the cardiac output fails to rise even though the left atrial pressure increases. When the obstruction at the mitral valve is more severe, the cardiac output at rest is depressed and the pressure in the pulmonary veins and pulmonary capillaries rises. When the pressure in the pulmonary capillaries exceeds the osmotic pressure of the plasma proteins (approximately 25 mmHg), fluid exudes from the capillaries into the pulmonary interstitial space and eventually into the alveoli as pulmonary oedema.

If, however, the rise in pressure in the pulmonary capillaries is gradual, there is an increase in the lymphatic drainage from the lungs. In addition, the chronic exudation of fluid into the pulmonary interstitial tissue is followed by thickening of the capillary basement membranes and an increase in the collagen within the interstitial tissue. This results in the development of an actual barrier between the pulmonary capillaries and the alveolar air space. The combination of these two mechanisms permits some patients to tolerate raised pulmonary venous pressure without the development of frank pulmonary oedema.

The elevation of the pulmonary venous pressure and the pulmonary capillary pressure naturally results in a moderate elevation of the pulmonary arterial pressure. However, in approximately 25 per cent of patients with mitral stenosis there is a much greater increase in the pulmonary arterial pressure due to a rise in the pulmonary vascular resistance, caused by an increase in the tone of the pulmonary arterioles and constriction of the small pulmonary arteries. In these cases the pulmonary vascular resistance decreases following successful mitral valvotomy but rarely returns to normal levels. The changes in the pulmonary vasculature result in a decrease in lung compliance and an increase in the work of breathing.

Patients with mitral stenosis usually remain symptom-free for 15–20 years after the first attack of acute rheumatic fever. This is followed by the onset of mild dyspnoea on exertion. Thereafter, the symptoms gradually progress, the patient taking about 3–4 years to pass through each grade of the New York Heart Association scale of dyspnoea. The untreated patient can therefore be expected to be breathless at rest (Grade 3 NYHA) approximately 12–16 years after the onset of symptoms. Orthopnoea and paroxysmal nocturnal dyspnoea are frequent symptoms associated with Grade 3 and Grade 4 dyspnoea on exertion. Signs of right heart failure only occur late in the natural history of the disease, by which time the patient is severely limited by breath-lessness. In Asia and in developing countries 'accelerated' mitral stenosis is not uncommon; signs and symptoms of severe stenosis appear within months after the attack of acute rheumatic carditis.

Acute pulmonary oedema may be precipitated in previously symptom-free patients who have had mitral stenosis for many years because atrial fibrillation occurs. The reason for this change in rhythm is unknown. Diastolic filling of the ventricle is reduced because the heart rate rises and atrial contraction ceases. Thus left atrial pressure may rise rapidly. Palpitations may be experienced by the patient and these are due to the recurrent atrial ectopics of atrial fibrillation.

The dyspnoea is not only due to pulmonary venous congestion but also to con-comitant deterioration in lung function. Airways resistance is increased, (reduced forced expiratory volume in 1 second) pulmonary compliance reduced, and evidence of restrictive lung disease (reduced vital capacity) are found. The work of breathing is thus increased. Perfusion of the lungs is abnormal: the gravity-dependent perfusion of the lower zones of the lungs is lost and blood flow to the apices of the lungs is increased. These changes show themselves as recurrent attacks of winter bronchitis. Hypoxic hyperventilation develops later so that arterial tensions of both oxygen and carbon dioxide may then be reduced. Haemoptysis is another important symptom; the patient may cough up pink frothy sputum during an attack of acute pulmonary oedema; bright red blood from rupture of a pulmonary bronchial vein, or haemoptysis may be due to pulmonary infarction.

Stasis of blood in the distended left atrium predisposes to the formation of thrombus, particularly within the appendage, and systemic embolus may follow. Pulmonary emboli and infarction are common complications of severe mitral stenosis; venous thrombosis is encouraged by the low cardiac output and decreased mobility of the patient.

The classical malar flush, due to a combination of the low cardiac output and vasoconstriction, is seldom seen nowadays. The arterial pulse is usually normal, but it is reduced in volume in severe cases. The jugular venous pressure is normal unless right-sided heart failure develops or there is severe pulmonary hypertension. The cardiac apex is characteristically tapping in nature and, if severe pulmonary hypertension is present, there is also a right ventricular lift to the left of the sternum. The first heart sound is loud and if the patient is in sinus rhythm it is preceded by a pre-systolic murmur. The second heart sound is followed by an opening snap unless the valve is heavily calcified and immobile. The opening snap is followed by a rumbling diastolic murmur that extends for a variable length into diastole. The closeness of the opening snap to the second heart sound reflects the severity of the mitral valve obstruction. If the patient has severe pulmonary hypertension, the pulmonary component of the second heart sound is accentuated and in rare cases the murmur of pulmonary incompetence (Graham Steell murmur) may be heard.

The ECG is usually unhelpful unless the patient is in sinus rhythm when the P wave is bifid and prolonged in duration due to left atrial hypertrophy (P mitrale). Signs of right ventricular and possibly atrial hypertrophy may also be present. The X-ray appearances of mitral stenosis have already been discussed (see page 9).

The haemodynamic significance of mitral stenosis may be assessed by cardiac catheterization. Cardiac output, duration of diastole and the pressure gradient across the valve need to be determined. PAWP at rest is significantly raised in symptomatic mitral stenosis.

Left ventricular angiography is necessary to assess the degree of any co-existing mitral regurgitation.

The development of atrial fibrillation, pulmonary oedema, pulmonary infarction or congestive cardiac failure should be treated in the conventional manner. Prophylaxis against systemic emboli with anticoagulants, unless there are strong contraindications, is essential when atrial fibrillation occurs.

The risks of closed mitral valvotomy are now extremely small (less than 0·1 per cent) and symptomatic isolated mitral stenosis should be treated in this way. If there is significant mitral regurgitation, or if the valve is heavily calcified, valve replacement is necessary.

Patients who have very mild mitral stenosis insufficient to cause any dyspnoea on exertion, may occasionally have repeated systemic emboli in spite of adequate anticoagulants. Valvotomy and removal of the left atrial appendage usually prevents recurrences.

MITRAL REGURGITATION

Mitral regurgitation is usually rheumatic in origin and associated with some degree of mitral stenosis, but it may occasionally be due to other causes (e.g. weakness or rupture of the papillary muscles following myocardial infarction, spontaneous rupture of the chordae tendineae, dilatation of the mitral valve ring due to left ventricular dilatation or congenital). Congenital mitral regurgitation is usually associated with abnormalities of the endocardial cushion.

The reflux of blood into the left atrium due to mitral regurgitation produces a high *v* wave in the left atrium, but if there is no mitral stenosis the left atrial pressure falls rapidly after ventricular systole to equal that in the left ventricle. Therefore, even though the *v* wave may be very high, the mean pressure in the left atrium is often normal or only slightly elevated. If the mitral regurgitation is severe, left ventricular failure eventually develops and the left ventricular end-diastolic pressure becomes elevated. At this stage the mean left atrial pressure and the pulmonary capillary pressure rise.

The symptoms of mitral regurgitation include dyspnoea on exertion, orthopnoea and paroxysmal nocturnal dyspnoea. Palpitations are also a common complaint and atrial fibrillation frequently develops. Symptoms of mitral regurgitation of rheumatic origin are usually insidious in onset, but when the regurgitation has developed acutely due to rupture of a chorda tendineae or a papillary muscle, severe symptoms usually develop rapidly, sometimes within a few minutes or hours.

The pulse is usually of normal volume and may be regular or irregular due to either multiple extrasystoles or to atrial fibrillation. The venous pressure is normal until congestive cardiac failure develops. The apex beat is left ventricular in character and hyperdynamic which indicates that the left ventricle is having to cope with an increased volume. The first heart sound is unremarkable or soft, unless there is associated mitral stenosis. There is an apical systolic murmur which is typically pansystolic, but in mild cases the murmur may start in mid or late systole and increase in volume up to the second heart sound. The murmur usually radiates to the axilla but if the reflux is due to papillary muscle dysfunction, it may radiate towards the left sternal edge. There is usually an easily audible left ventricular third heart sound and if mitral reflux is severe there may also be a soft mid-diastolic murmur even in the absence of organic mitral stenosis. This mitral diastolic murmur is due to the increased volume of blood that has to cross the mitral valve in diastole.

The ECG may show the presence of left atrial enlargement if the patient is in sinus rhythm and left ventricular hypertrophy if regurgitation is severe. The chest X-ray shows an increase in the cardiac shadow due to left ventricular enlargement. On a penetrated PA film left atrial enlargement can be clearly seen. The lung fields may show the changes of pulmonary venous hypertension and, in some cases, of pulmonary arterial hypertension. In cases of mitral regurgitation of recent onset the chest X-ray may show no changes apart from those of pulmonary oedema.

The diagnosis can be confirmed by echocardiography which is capable of revealing minor degrees of mitral valve dysfunction. Right and left heart catheter studies may also be necessary particularly following sudden rupture of a chorda or papillary muscle.

Patients with chronic mitral regurgitation may remain asymptomatic for many years. However, when left ventricular failure does develop, the prognosis is poor. The risk of systemic emboli is less in patients with mitral regurgitation than in those with mitral stenosis but it is still real, especially if there is any degree of mitral valve obstruction. Subacute bacterial endocarditis is a particular risk and chemoprophylaxis for dental treatment or other 'dirty' surgery is mandatory in these patients. Fifty per cent of patients with incompetence due to papillary muscle rupture following myocardial infarction die in acute pulmonary oedema within 24 hr. Those who survive usually remain in refractory left ventricular failure.

The medical management of mitral reflux is the same as that of mitral stenosis. The indications for surgery in chronic rheumatic mitral incompetence, or in mixed mitral valve disease where incompetence is more than minimal, depend on the severity of symptoms. The mortality of mitral valve replacement is between 5 and 10 per cent, and since there is still a morbidity with valve prostheses, valve replacement should not be recommended in patients unless their symptoms are Grade 3 on the NYHA Scale in spite of adequate medical treatment. The results of valve replacement become worse as the left ventricular function declines. The selection of patients for mitral valve replacement following papillary muscle rupture after myocardial infarction has to be decided on an individual basis but in view of the high mortality of conservative treatment it is becoming a more widely-accepted operation. Valvuloplasty is an alternative which has the advantage that long-term anticoagulation is not then required. The surgery of congenital mitral incompetence is usually determined by the associated lesions.

AORTIC STENOSIS

Obstruction to the left ventricular outflow tract is usually at the level of the aortic valve, but it may (1 per cent of cases) be subvalvar (due to a web or to hypertrophic obstruction cardiomyopathy) or supravalvar (often associated with hypercalcaemia and mental subnormality).

Aortic valve stenosis may be rheumatic, congenital or sclerotic in origin. Rheumatic disease is almost always associated with some degree of aortic regurgitation and frequently with mitral valve disease. Many of the cases of isolated calcific aortic stenosis presenting in middle age are not rheumatic in origin but are the result of gradual thickening and calcification of aortic valves which were originally either bicuspid or only mildly stenotic.

There is considerable hypertrophy of the left ventricular muscle due to the obstruction to the left ventricular outflow, but there is little dilatation of the left ventricular cavity in isolated aortic stenosis until the final stages of the disease, when the ventricle fails and dilates.

The symptoms of aortic stenosis are angina pectoris, dyspnoea on exertion and syncope. Effort dyspnoea is eventually followed by orthopnoea and paroxysmal nocturnal dyspnoea and finally congestive cardiac failure appears. Syncope is important and characteristically it also occurs on effort. The precise cause of syncope is often difficult to determine, but it may be due either to a dysrhythmia or to an inadequate systemic pressure in the presence of the vasodilatation of exercise.

The pulse is usually regular but atrial fibrillation suggests co-existent mitral valve disease. The carotid pulse is characteristically small and sustained in volume with a slow upstroke. The jugular venous pressure is not elevated until congestive cardiac failure develops. The cardiac impulse is left ventricular in character but is not usually displaced unless regurgitation or cardiac decompensation is present. On auscultation there is an ejection systolic murmur which is best heard in the 2nd–3rd left intercostal spaces. The murmur is preceded by an early systolic ejection click, unless the valve is calcified or the obstruction is above or below the valve. The aortic component of the second heart sound is quiet or inaudible, and therefore the second heart sound may be single on auscultation.

The ECG shows evidence of left atrial and left ventricular hypertrophy. The chest X-ray may be normal, but the ascending aorta is usually prominent due to post-stenotic dilatation, which does not occur if the obstruction is subvalvar. Enlargement of the left ventricle and calcification may be visible. Radiological changes of left ventricular failure may be apparent.

The diagnosis of aortic stenosis is not always easy particularly when cardiac failure causes the murmur apparently to be insignificant. Left heart catheter studies are important in order that haemodynamically insignificant stenosis may be eliminated. The orifice of the valve is reduced to as little as 25 per cent of its normal area before this significance appears. Echocardiography demonstrates immobility of the valve but an invasive study is the means whereby quantitation is possible. Measurements of left ventricular and aortic pressures at the same time as cardiac output determination are useful. If left ventricular failure has developed there is also a raised pulmonary vascular resistance shown by an increased PAWP.

The prognosis of mild stenosis is relatively good, but once symptoms have developed the prognosis is poor, many patients dying within three years. There is also a significant incidence of sudden death in asymptomatic patients with severe aortic stenosis.

Medical treatment has almost nothing to offer in the management of aortic stenosis. If the obstruction is severe, whether the patient has symptoms or not, aortic valve replacement should be recommended since the mortality for this operation in the absence of cardiac failure is now less than 5 per cent.

AORTIC REGURGITATION

Aortic regurgitation is usually rheumatic in origin. It may occasionally be congenital (associated with congenital aortic or subaortic stenosis or ventricular septal defect), or it may follow infective endocarditis, Marfan's syndrome, syphilitic aortitis, ankylosing spondylitis, Reiter's syndrome, or dissection of the aorta. Severe systemic hypertension may also cause mild degrees of aortic regurgitation. The valve is incompetent either as a result of damage to the aortic cusps themselves as in rheumatic heart disease or because of dilatation or damage to the aortic valve ring (syphilitic aortitis or dissection of the aorta).

Symptoms of aortic regurgitation may not develop for many years after the reflux has started. The more common symptoms are dyspnoea on exertion, palpitation and fatigue. When regurgitation is severe, angina pectoris, orthopnoea and paroxysmal nocturnal dyspnoea also occur. In the late stages the signs and symptoms of right heart failure also develop.

On examination, the carotid pulse has a large volume and may be collapsing in nature. It is usually regular. The presence of atrial fibrillation should alert the clinician to the possibility of associated mitral valve disease. The apex beat is left ventricular in character, hyperdynamic and is displaced towards the axilla.

On auscultation the second heart sound is usually single and is followed by an immediate diastolic murmur, which is best heard at the left sternal edge in the second to fourth intercostal spaces. The murmur is high-pitched in character and diminishes in volume throughout diastole. It starts immediately following the second heart sound. In severe aortic regurgitation a mid-diastolic murmur (Austin Flint murmur) can often be heard at the apex which is caused by the jet of regurgitant blood pushing the anterior cusp of the mitral valve backwards in diastole. Relative obstruction through the mitral valve is thus produced but there is neither the opening snap nor the loud first heart sound of mitral stenosis.

The ECG confirms the presence of left ventricular hypertrophy and left atrial enlargement if the regurgitation is severe, and in these cases the chest X-ray shows considerable cardiac enlargement, due to left atrial dilatation.

The pressure changes revealed by cardiac catheterization studies depend not only on the severity of the lesion but also upon its chronicity. The acute onset of regurgitation causes much more dramatic increases in pulmonary vascular resistance than are found in chronic cases. Both pulmonary wedge pressures and left ventricular end-diastolic pressures are raised to the extent (more than 30 mmHg) that pulmonary oedema is to be expected. As the condition becomes chronic the ventricle dilates and these pressures tend to decline. Chronic cases may show much lower diastolic pressures. Dye studies complete the essential investigation in this condition. It is important to eliminate lesions causing similar signs to those of aortic incompetence (ruptured sinus of Valsalva) prior to cardiac surgery.

The decision to recommend surgery is a fine one. Valve replacement is technically difficult in these patients and the diagnosis of asymptomatic aortic incompetence is not yet an indication for prosthetic surgery. Long term digitalis for cardiac failure is also contraindicated since when decompensation has started the patient needs a new valve. Severe symptoms (Grade 3 or 4 NYHA scale) indicate that this is the case. At the moment there is no satisfactory index of left ventricular function which can determine that the moment for surgery has arrived.

The prognosis of mild aortic regurgitation is excellent, but there is a considerable risk of subacute bacterial endocarditis. In moderate or severe cases the patients may be symptom-free for many years, but when symptoms do eventually develop, usually during the fourth or fifth decade, the deterioration may be rapid. In contrast to severe aortic stenosis the incidence of sudden death in asymptomatic patients is uncommon.

TRICUSPID STENOSIS

Tricuspid stenosis in adults is almost always rheumatic in origin and occurs in approximately 10 per cent of patients with rheumatic heart disease. Significant stenosis is however rare, and when it does occur it is almost always associated with involvement of other valves, particularly the mitral valve. The physiological effects of tricuspid stenosis are an increase in right atrial pressure and a decline in cardiac output. Hepatic distension, ascites and peripheral oedema develop. The symptoms of any associated valve lesion may also occur.

The physical findings are characteristic. When the patient is in sinus rhythm there is a high *a* wave in the jugular venous pressure, which is followed by a slow *x* descent. In severe tricuspid stenosis the whole of the jugular venous pressure is elevated. Presystolic pulsations may be palpable over the enlarged liver. On auscultation at the lower left sternal edge murmurs almost identical to those of mitral stenosis with sinus rhythm can be heard, and in addition the first heart sound may be loud and an opening snap may be present. However, in contrast to the auscultatory findings of mitral stenosis, they are increased by inspiration.

The ECG shows signs of right atrial enlargement (tall P wave) if the patient is in sinus rhythm, but is otherwise unhelpful. Enlargement of the right atrium and the superior vena cava may be seen on the chest X-ray, but the radiological changes of the associated valve lesions usually dominate.

The outlook in mild tricuspid valve stenosis is good but if the obstruction is severe, right-sided cardiac failure gradually worsens and death follows. The management of patients with tricuspid stenosis is usually dominated by the presence or absence of other associated valve disease, particularly mitral valve disease. Valve replacement is the preferred surgical treatment for severe obstruction since valvotomy usually results in severe regurgitation.

TRICUSPID REGURGITATION

Most cases of tricuspid regurgitation are functional and due to dilatation of the tricuspid valve ring following the development of pulmonary hypertension and right ventricular failure. However tricuspid regurgitation may occasionally be rheumatic in origin, or congenital defects of the valve may be associated with defects of the endocardial cushion or with Ebstein's anomaly (see page 36). The distinction between organic rheumatic tricuspid regurgitation and tricuspid regurgitation secondary to dilatation of the tricuspid ring may be difficult, but the persistence of marked regurgitation following effective medical treatment in the absence of severe pulmonary hypertension, should suggest organic valve disease.

The symptoms of severe tricuspid incompetence are those of right-sided heart failure. On examination the jugular venous pressure is elevated with a high flicking *v* wave. There is a parasternal, right ventricular lift, and on auscultation at the lower left sternal edge there is a pansystolic murmur which increases on inspiration. The physical signs of pulmonary hypertension may or may not be present.

The ECG is usually unhelpful although the absence of right ventricular hypertrophy suggests that the regurgitation is organic. Although the right atrium may be considerably enlarged on the chest X-ray, the dominant radiological features are usually those of other associated valve lesions.

Tricuspid reflux is usually well tolerated for many years, although in severe cases gross oedema and ascites develop. The timing of cardiac surgery should be determined by the severity of the associated valve lesions.

The **pulmonary valve** is very rarely involved by rheumatic heart disease. The symptoms, signs and management of congenital pulmonary stenosis have been dealt with above.

DISEASE OF THE PERICARDIUM

PERICARDITIS

Disease of the pericardium may be a primary disorder, secondary to local disease, or a manifestation of a generalized disease process. Pericarditis may be acute or chronic.

ACUTE PERICARDITIS

The commonest type of acute pericarditis is acute 'benign' pericarditis. Most of the cases are probably viri in origin, usually the Coxsackie B, but several other viruses have also been incriminated including mumps, chicken pox, measles and influenza. The prognosis of this variety of acute pericarditis is usually good, although the term 'benign' is unfortunate since there is some involvement of the myocardium in most cases. The pericardium may also be involved in bacterial infections which usually spread to the pericardium from adjacent structures such as tuberculous mediastinal lymph glands, or a pyogenic infection of the lung. Other causes of acute pericarditis include myocardial infarction, rheumatic fever, neoplastic invasion of the pericardium, accidental or surgical trauma, the post-pericardotomy and post-infarction syndromes, uraemia and the collagenoses (e.g. SLE, polyarteritis and rheumatoid arthritis).

The principal symptom is pain, which is usually severe and of very sudden onset. Its site is lower retrosternal although it may sometimes radiate to the shoulder if the diaphragmatic pericardium is involved. It differs from ischaemic pain in that it is often eased by sitting up and made worse by lying down or by a deep breath if the adjacent pleura is involved.

The diagnostic physical finding is a pericardial friction rub which is usually widespread but occasionally very localized. There may be a pericardial effusion or cardiac tamponade (see below).

The ECG shows a characteristic concave elevation of the ST segment. After 48–72 hr the ST segment returns to the isoelectric line and the T wave becomes inverted.

Treatment consists of the relief of pain and the management of the underlying disease. Viral pericarditis, which is usually a short illness, requires no specific treatment unless either the symptoms are prolonged, when a course of steroids may help, or when an associated myocarditis leads to congestive cardiac failure or the development of dysrhythmias.

PERICARDIAL EFFUSION

The fluid of a pericardial effusion may be a transudate, as in cardiac failure, an exudate, as in acute pericarditis, purulent, as in pyogenic pericarditis, or haemorrhagic following surgical or accidental trauma, and malignant disease.

Small effusions cannot be detected clinically. Large effusions increase the area of cardiac dullness even beyond the apex beat. The heart sounds are often quiet and there may be a pericardial friction rub.

A sudden increase in cardiac size on the chest X-ray is very suggestive of a pericardial effusion particularly if the increase is not associated with the other radiological signs of cardiac failure. The heart shadow is characteristically pear-shaped, and there is little movement on screening.

The treatment is that of the underlying disease unless cardiac tamponade develops.

Acute cardiac tamponade is caused by the accumulation of fluid within the pericardial cavity at a pressure sufficient to restrict the filling of the cardiac chambers. It may occur as a result of a penetrating or a blunt injury to the chest, cardiac surgery or rarely cardiac catheterization; it carries a high mortality. The rise in intrapericardial pressure restricts the ability of the atria and the ventricles to fill in diastole. There is therefore a reduction in cardiac output and an elevation of both the jugular and pulmonary venous pressures. A reflex sinus tachycardia develops in an attempt to maintain an adequate cardiac output. Both the arterial pulse and jugular venous pressures move paradoxically with respiration, and in severe cases the peripheral arterial pulse may be impalpable during inspiration (pulsus paradoxus). If the fluid accumulates rapidly the patient may faint or die within minutes. The most important differential diagnosis of acute cardiac tamponade is a pulmonary embolus, the presentation and physical signs of which may be very similar. The absence of a right-sided atrial gallop and the presence of marked arterial paradox should suggest tamponade.

The chest X-ray may be unhelpful as the cardiac shadow may not be much increased in the presence of critical tamponade. However, a pulmonary embolus sufficient to produce such severe haemodynamic disturbance is almost certain to be associated with characteristic changes in the ECG. The most useful investigation in the diagnosis of acute tamponade is echocardiography.

The outcome of untreated acute tamponade is almost invariably fatal, and if the diagnosis is seriously entertained but cannot be confirmed due to the lack of facilities, the patient must be treated as a case of acute tamponade. The treatment is the removal of the pericardial fluid either by aspiration or more usually by formal operation, when the source of the fluid can be located and treated.

CHRONIC CONSTRICTIVE PERICARDITIS

Chronic constrictive pericarditis is now a comparatively uncommon condition in Western Europe. In the past it was almost invariably the end result of tuberculous pericarditis, but, while this is still the case in the countries of the Third World, it is no longer true in the developed countries. In many cases the aetiology may remain uncertain; it may follow viral pericarditis or haemorrhagic pericardial effusion.

The haemodynamic effects are similar to those of acute tamponade but start more slowly. They result from thickening and stiffening of the pericardium which prevent adequate filling of the atria and ventricles during diastole. The pericardium may become calcified (Fig. 1.30).

The constriction usually involves both the right and the left side of the heart but the dominant symptoms are most commonly those of right-sided failure. Dyspnoea and the other symptoms of pulmonary venous hypertension may dominate the clinical picture occasionally.

On examination there is usually marked ascites, and the liver is enlarged and frequently tender. The arterial pulse is small in volume, of normal character, and may show paradox. The jugular venous pressure is grossly elevated, and increases on

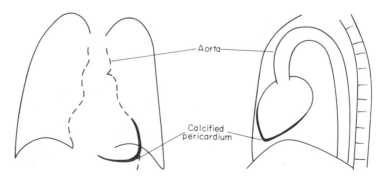

Fig. 1.30. Cardiac silhouettes of calcification in the pericardium.

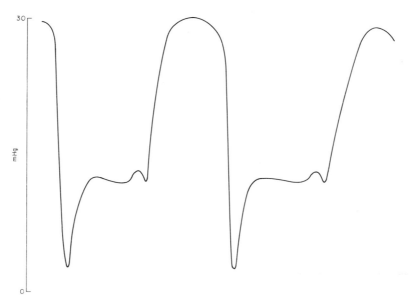

Fig. 1.31. Right ventricular pressure tracing in constrictive pericarditis.

inspiration. On auscultation the heart sounds are usually quiet, apart from a loud third heart sound which is almost invariably present.

The ECG shows low voltage QRS complexes and sometimes left atrial hypertrophy. The chest X-ray may show calcification of the pericardium which is seen best in the lateral projection. The heart is not usually enlarged.

The haemodynamic findings on cardiac catheterization are the same in all conditions which restrict filling of the cardiac chambers during diastole with a characteristic early 'dip' in the ventricular diastole pressure followed by an elevated plateau throughout the remainder of a diastole (Fig. 1.31).

The most important conditions which may be confused with constrictive pericarditis are cirrhosis of the liver and restrictive cardiomyopathy. In the latter condition the heart is usually enlarged but the correct diagnosis may be made only at thoracotomy.

The management is pericardectomy. The underlying cause of the pericardial disease, for example tuberculosis, must also be treated.

DISEASES OF THE MYOCARDIUM

MYOCARDITIS

Myocarditis may be caused by infection or toxins. Many viruses have been incriminated, but the most commonly involved is probably Coxsackie B. Other important causes of myocarditis include acute rheumatic fever, diphtheria and Chagas' disease.

In mild cases the only findings are a non-specific inappropriate tachycardia and non-specific ECG changes. Severe cases may present with heart failure or cardiogenic shock. Dysrhythmias of all types may occur.

The treatment of acute myocarditis is the treatment of its complications, which include dysrhythmias and cardiac failure; some authorities recommend the use also of <u>steroids.</u>

CARDIOMYOPATHIES

The cardiomyopathies are chronic conditions which involve the myocardium and which are not secondary to coronary arterial disease, hypertension, valve disease, intracardiac shunts or thyrotoxicosis. In most cases, the heart is the only organ involved, although cardiomyopathy may also be a part of a wide range of generalized diseases which include haemochromatosis, sarcoidosis, the collagenoses, amyloidosis and certain neuromuscular diseases.

The aetiology of most types of cardiomyopathy is unknown. Classification is based on the clinical and haemodynamic findings into four types: <u>congestive,</u> <u>hyper-trophic</u>, <u>constrictive</u> and <u>obliterative.</u> The latter two are rare in this country.

Congestive cardiomyopathy presents with the symptoms and signs of <u>cardiac failure</u>. Dilatation of the ventricles may be severe and may cause stretching of the atrio-ventricular valve rings. The murmurs of mitral and tricuspid reflux may therefore be present. The chest X-ray confirms the presence of generalized cardiomegaly and usually shows evidence of pulmonary venous congestion. There may be changes in the ST segments and the T waves of the ECG. The <u>diagnosis is made by the exclusion</u> of other causes of congestive cardiac failure. There is no specific treatment.

Hypertrophic cardiomyopathy is sometimes <u>familial</u>. Gross hypertrophy occurs in both ventricles but in the left usually more than the right and the <u>intraventricular septum</u> is often seriously affected. When the papillary muscles are involved the anterior cusp of the mitral valve moves not backwards but forwards during ventricular systole. Abnormal movement of the anterior cusp of the mitral valve and the asymmetric hypertrophy of the septum may together obstruct the outflow tract of the left ventricle during systole (<u>hypertrophic *obstructive* cardiomyopathy</u>). Inflow tract obstruction occurs less often. Ventricular compliance is reduced so the ventricle is difficult to fill.

Hypertrophic cardiomyopathy may present with exertional dyspnoea, angina pectoris, syncope, palpitations, congestive cardiac failure, systemic emboli and sudden death. Dyspnoea and chest pain occur together rather than separately as in classical angina. When there is obstruction of the left ventricular outflow tract, the carotid pulse is characteristically jerky due to a rapid ejection of blood early in systole being followed by sudden obstruction of the outflow late in systole. The *a* wave of the jugular venous wave may be increased, and evidence of left ventricular hypertrophy can usually be detected on palpation. Right ventricular hypertrophy is present less frequently. A palpable atrial sound is a common finding, and this may result in a 'double apex beat'. The obstruction to the left ventricular outflow tract causes a mid-systolic ejection murmur, which is well conducted to the carotid arteries. Murmurs of mitral reflux and mitral valve obstruction (due to left ventricular inflow obstruction) may also occur, but are less frequent.

The ECG usually shows evidence of marked left ventricular hypertrophy. In those cases with <u>severe septal hypertrophy Q waves</u> may be present in the anterior chest leads, thus producing the appearance of an anteroseptal myocardial infarction. The heart is usually of normal size on the chest X-ray until a late stage of the disease. Outflow tract obstruction can be confirmed by cardiac catheterization, angiography and echocardiography. The <u>degree of obstruction is increased by inotropic agents</u>, such as isoprenaline, and by the potentiated post-ectopic beat. It is reduced by <u>β-adrenergic blocking drugs.</u> The left ventricular end-diastolic pressure may be normal or elevated and it is characteristically increased by isoprenaline.

The prognosis is not good, many patients dying in the fourth or fifth decade. Death may be sudden due to a dysrhythmia. The onset of atrial fibrillation usually presages a rapid deterioration in the patient's condition with the development of congestive cardiac failure.

Treatment is difficult. Although β-blockers may lead to an improvement in symptoms, there is little evidence that they improve the prognosis of the condition. Complications should be treated in the conventional manner. Surgical resection of the subvalvar obstruction has been recommended by some groups; this may be appropriate for the few cases with very severe discrete obstruction but its place in the management of the majority of patients is controversial.

Constrictive cardiomyopathy is rare. It resembles constrictive pericarditis since the stiff myocardium impedes the filling of the ventricle. <u>Leukaemic infiltration</u> of the myocardium, <u>haemochromatosis</u> and <u>amyloidosis</u> are causes of this condition. The heart is usually enlarged in constrictive cardiomyopathy and it may be impossible to differentiate this condition from constrictive pericarditis. This differentiation is very important from the therapeutic point of view and it may be necessary to resort to thoracotomy to establish the diagnosis. The treatment is symptomatic and the prognosis is poor.

Obliterative cardiomyopathy is almost always the result of <u>endomyocardial fibrosis,</u> which is a disease involving both the endocardium and the myocardium. It is a relatively common cause of heart disease in certain parts of <u>Africa and South India.</u> The endocardium and the inner part of the myocardium are replaced by dense fibrous tissue, which may reduce the cavity of the ventricle to a narrow rigid tube. The prognosis is poor, the patient dies either of intractable congestive cardiac failure or of embolization.

DISEASES OF THE ENDOCARDIUM

These are usually inflammatory except endocardial fibroelastosis which is a disease almost entirely confined to neonates. The endocardial layers of the left ventricle and left atrium are replaced by thick plaques of elastic tissue and collagen which often involve the mitral valve. The cause is unknown but it is frequently associated with other congenital cardiac defects and the prognosis is very poor.

INFECTIVE ENDOCARDITIS

The endocardium may be involved in bacterial, fungal or *Rickettsial* infection. There is almost always some underlying abnormality of the heart. The condition is usually subacute and involves pre-existing mixed mitral disease, aortic valve disease, ventricular septal defect and patent ductus arteriosus. Pure mitral stenosis and secundum atrial septal defects are rarely complicated by the development of infective endocarditis but even the smallest defect may be affected.

Streptococcus viridans, originating from the <u>mouth,</u> is still the most common organism responsible for infective endocarditis. *Streptococcus faecalis* is becoming an increasingly important cause of the disease particularly in the elderly. The *Staphylococcus* usually causes a very virulent form of the disease, particularly in patients with prosthetic heart valves or in those with a reduced resistance, such as heroin addicts. Fungal and *Rickettsial* infections are rare.

The infection leads to the formation of friable vegetations, which consist of platelets, fibrin, white cells, red cells and the infecting organisms. The valve cusps may become ulcerated and perforated and aortic or mitral reflux result. Vegetations may break off and cause emboli; large emboli may cause cerebral, renal or splenic infarcts, while microemboli may be widespread and may occur in showers. If the infection is long-standing, glomerulonephritis may develop due to an immunological response.

SUBACUTE BACTERIAL ENDOCARDITIS

The clinical presentation with malaise and a low grade fever is often insidious. The patient becomes increasingly anaemic and develops clubbing, widespread petechiae, splenomegaly, microscopic haematuria and varying cardiac murmurs. Splinter haemorrhages in nail beds and infected microemboli in the pulps of the fingers, which cause tender red swollen spots (Osler's nodes), are characteristic. Cardiac failure may appear either gradually or rapidly following the rupture of an aortic or mitral valve cusp. The occurrence of a coronary artery embolism will be followed by cardiac ischaemic pain and the ECG appearances of an acute myocardial infarction. Large cerebral emboli cause hemiplegia or other gross neurological defects whereas multiple small cerebral emboli may produce confusion, dementia or other psychiatric disturbance. Nowadays the florid clinical picture of subacute bacterial endocarditis is frequently masked by the administration of short inadequate courses of antibiotics. A five- or ten-day course of antibiotics in patients with a pyrexia of unknown origin in the presence of established valvar or congenital heart disease makes the diagnosis of endocarditis difficult and may lead to the emergence of strains of infecting organisms which are resistant to many antibiotics.

Laboratory investigations shows a normocytic normochromic anaemia, a moderate polymorpholeucocytosis, and a raised sedimentation rate. Red cells can be found in *fresh* urine specimens in 90–95 per cent of cases. The diagnosis can be confirmed by blood culture.

Ideally, treatment should not be commenced until the identity of the infecting organism has been established. Appropriate bactericidal antibiotics should then be given parenterally for not less than six weeks. Blood assays must be employed to ensure that bactericidal levels of antibiotic are maintained. If the organism cannot be identified a combination of penicillin (8 M-units/24 hours i.v.) and streptomycin (0·5 g b.d.) may be used. Intractable cardiac failure is almost always due to gross valvar regurgitation and may require emergency valve replacement. Infective emboli may lead to the development of mycotic aneurysms which may rupture. Anticoagulants should therefore be avoided.

The importance of eliminating the original source of infection cannot be overemphasized otherwise recurrence may occur.

The mortality of subacute bacterial endocarditis remains approximately 30 per cent in spite of antibiotic therapy and prevention of infection in susceptible patients is of great importance.

ISCHAEMIC HEART DISEASE

Arterial blood reaches the myocardium through the coronary arteries. The left coronary artery arises from the left coronary sinus of Valsalva and immediately divides into the circumflex branch, which supplies the lateral and posterior aspects of the left ventricle, and the anterior descending branch, which supplies the interventricular septum and the anterior wall of the left ventricle. The inferior wall of the left ventricle, the right ventricle, the sinus node, the atrioventricular node and the bundle of His are usually supplied by the right coronary artery which arises from the right coronary sinus of Valsalva. The major arteries run on the surface of the heart and give off branches which penetrate into the heart muscle.

The heart differs from other organs in the body in that almost all the oxygen in the arterial blood is extracted so that the oxygen saturation of the blood draining from the myocardium is about 20 per cent. Increased oxygen demands by the heart must therefore be met by an increase in coronary blood flow. The pattern of blood flow in the myocardium is also different from that in other organs since the arteries within the myocardium are compressed during systole and therefore the bulk of coronary flow takes place during diastole. Coronary flow is determined by two factors at any one moment; the diastolic pressure in the aorta and, more importantly, the diameter of the coronary vessels.

Ischaemic heart disease is said to be present when the supply of oxygen to the myocardium is insufficient to meet its needs and when this restriction is due to atherosclerosis involving the coronary arterial tree. The coronary arteries may be involved in other disease (e.g. congenital abnormalities, coronary embolism, syphilitic stenosis of the coronary ostia, and polyarteritis nodosa), but these are not considered to be part of the syndrome of ischaemic heart disease.

Ischaemic heart disease is now the commonest form of heart disease in the Western World and is the most frequent cause of death in men over the age of 40, causing approximately 40 per cent of all deaths in men over this age. There also appears to have been an increase in the incidence of the disease over the last two decades. This is a genuine increase despite simultaneous increases in both the frequency of diagnosis and the average age of the population.

The pathological changes which occur in the coronary arteries due to atherosclerosis are the same as those that occur in the other arteries of the body. Cholesterol is deposited in patches in the intima of the arteries, frequently at bends or points of division. The deposition of lipid within the intima results in a fibrous reaction and atrophy of the underlying media. The atheromatous plaque thus formed leads to a narrowing of the lumen of the vessel and ulceration may follow. Platelets and fibrin become deposited on the plaque. This may eventually lead to the development of a thrombus which occludes the coronary artery. If this does occur the thrombus may eventually become organized and the vessel recanalized. Arteriographic studies have shown that significant disease may involve only one of the three principal arteries even in patients with severe symptoms.

If the supply of arterial blood to an area of the myocardium remains critically insufficient for a considerable period of time, muscle necrosis occurs. An acute myocardial infarction is then said to have occured. Most episodes probably follow the complete occlusion of a coronary artery but sometimes it may occur simply from severe coronary arterial spasm. Minimal pathological changes occur if death follows rapidly. However, if the patient survives, the infarcted area becomes pale and surrounded by a hyperaemic area. The healing process including scar formation is complete after about 6–8 weeks. The infarcted area may occasionally rupture during the first 10 days–2 weeks after the acute attack. If the infarct extends through the full thickness of the ventricular wall, thrombus may form on the endocardial surface and a pericardial reaction may develop on the epicardial surface. The scar tissue formed in the infarcted area of muscle is usually firm but on occasions it may be weak and a left ventricular aneurysm may eventually develop.

ANGINA PECTORIS

The characteristics of this pain are well known: a crushing 'bandlike' pain or discomfort is felt across the chest which may radiate into one or both arms, into the neck or the jaw. It is caused by an inadequate supply of oxygen to the myocardium, which is usually due to atherosclerosis of the coronary arteries, but it may occur in other conditions (e.g. aortic stenosis or regurgitation, pulmonary hypertensive mitral stenosis, syphilitic aortitis with coronary ostial stenosis and rarely in cyanotic congenital heart disease). Systemic hypertension, severe anaemia and thyrotoxicosis, may precipitate angina in patients with relatively mild coronary atherosclerosis, which itself would not be severe enough to produce symptoms.

The diagnosis of angina pectoris is made on the history. It is usually clearcut, but may take some considerable time to elucidate. Particular attention should be paid to the site of the pain, its character, its relationship to exercise or emotion, and its duration. Physical examination of the patient is usually normal. The ECG may be abnormal in patients with angina, but it cannot be overemphasized that the record may be entirely normal in patients with severe angina due to extensive coronary atherosclerosis. The abnormalities that may occur include non-specific T wave flattening or inversion, and possibly the signs of an old myocardial infarction. If the ECG is recorded during an acute attack of angina, the ST segment is usually horizontally depressed, although it may rarely be elevated (Prinzmetal variant). The value of exercise ECGs has already been discussed (page 8). In the rare cases in which diagnosis of angina cannot be clearly established from the history and the ECG, it is sometimes justifiable to use coronary arteriography as a diagnostic procedure. The risks are now extremely small in skilled hands (mortality 1 in 1,000) and arteriography is regarded as an essential preoperatively in patients for coronary arterial surgery, but otherwise the procedure should not be used lightly.

It is vital to distinguish angina pectoris from inframammary pain due to anxiety. This lasts for a considerable length of time and does not occur on effort although it may *follow* physical exertion. Musculoskeletal chest pain may be precipitated by lifting or by movement of the thorax. Tender spots can often be found in palpation over the ribs. Intermittent chest pain may also arise from oesophagitis or oesophageal spasm, peptic ulceration or gall bladder disease.

The prognosis of angina pectoris is very variable; some patients may live for many years with little increase in the severity of their symptoms, but others may die within a few days from myocardial infarction. However, most patients with angina pectoris have a good prognosis, the annual mortality of those patients with a normal ECG is probably under 2 per cent. If the ECG at rest is abnormal, the annual mortality is about 10 per cent. In those patients in whom only one coronary artery is significantly affected the five-year mortality is between 10 and 13 per cent; when two vessels are significantly involved the mortality is between 35 and 40 per cent, and when all three vessels are significantly diseased or when the left main coronary artery is involved the five-year mortality is between 50 and 60 per cent. Nonetheless, the prognosis in any one patient presenting with angina pectoris is usually good. Most patients survive five years after the onset of their symptoms and almost 40 per cent live for 10 years.

The overall management of the patient with angina pectoris is extremely important since the anxieties which this diagnosis creates may be very considerable. Since the expectation of life is relatively good, patients should be reassured that they should be able to continue in full-time employment and to live a normal life. Exercise that does not produce chest pain is not harmful and may in fact be beneficial. Strenuous exercise, particularly in cold weather, and after a heavy meal should be avoided. Sexual intercourse is not harmful as long as it does not precipitate angina pectoris.

There is no evidence that low fat diets are of any value in patients with established coronary arterial disease. The patient should, however, avoid obesity. There is clear evidence that heavy cigarette smoking may provoke angina pectoris and may precipitate an acute myocardial infarction.

Sublingual glyceryl trinitrate is effective in that it not only stops an attack within a few minutes, but also may prevent attacks. The drug causes peripheral vasodilatation and this reduces the load on the left ventricle which leads to a reduction in the myocardial demand for oxygen. Nitrates cause dilatation of the normal coronary arteries but there is little evidence that they increase oxygen delivery to the ischaemic myocardium in patients with coronary arterial disease.

Beta-adrenergic blocking drugs are important in the management of angina pectoris although they have not displaced glyceryl trinitrate. These drugs reduce the oxygen demand of the heart by slowing it, by causing hypotension and by decreasing the contractility of the myocardium. There is some variation between the different drugs but all may occasionally precipitate bronchospasm in patients with obstructive airways disease and cardiac failure in patients whose cardiac reserve is already reduced.

Coronary arterial bypass grafts may be advised for patients with severe angina pectoris who do not respond to medical treatment and in whom the arterial obstructions are discrete. The operative mortality is less than 1 per cent. However, the operations should not be recommended in patients whose ventricular function is poor since the mortality is high in this group. Angina is completely relieved in approximately 80 per cent of cases but the effect of the operation on prognosis is not clear.

Unstable (crescendo) angina

The term unstable angina is used to describe a number of conditions in which the pattern of angina pectoris changes rapidly. These include an increase in frequency, duration or severity of the attacks. This pattern may develop in patients who have had pre-existing stable angina pectoris or it may appear *de novo*. The pain may occur at rest and may last for a prolonged period of time. The ECG may show ST segment depression, or T wave changes, which may also persist, but the serum enzymes are not elevated.

The prognosis of unstable angina is not good, approximately 15–20 per cent of patients suffer a major myocardial infarction within a year of the first symptom in spite of medical treatment, and 4 per cent of patients die within this period.

The treatment of unstable angina is the subject of considerable controversy. Traditional management of the condition is similar to that of a minor myocardial infarction. It has, however, recently been suggested that emergency coronary arterial surgery should be considered.

ACUTE MYOCARDIAL INFARCTION

The pain of acute myocardial infarction is usually maximal in the retrosternal region, but it may radiate to both sides of the chest, to one or both arms, up into the neck, into the jaw, and less frequently to the epigastrium or the back. The pain is described as 'band-like', 'gripping', 'vice-like', 'a pressure', 'like indigestion' or simply as a discomfort. It is rarely stabbing in character and one should be suspicious of pain that is described as being 'knife-like'. The pain usually lasts for at least half an hour but rarely for more than 12 hours. It is not relieved by rest or by glyceryl trinitrate.

In patients under the age of 65, pain is the usual dominant feature and also in 30 per cent of elderly patients. However, acute pulmonary oedema, congestive cardiac failure, syncope, confusion, cerebrovascular accidents or symptoms of systemic emboli are common presenting features in the elderly.

The patient looks ill, frightened and distressed. He is pale and vasoconstricted, and there may be either a bradycardia or a tachycardia. The reduction in stroke volume which follows a myocardial infarction induces a compensatory sinus tachycardia in order to maintain the cardiac output. This tachycardia rarely exceeds 110–115 per minute and does not indicate the development of cardiac failure.

The blood pressure may be normal or in severe cases it may fall rapidly. There is usually a small fall in blood pressure over the first week, but it gradually returns to the pre-infarction level over the next few months.

The jugular venous pressure is usually normal immediately after myocardial infarction, but rises if cardiac failure develops. The apex beat may be normal but in patients with extensive infarction the cardiac impulse may feel diffuse and 'flabby' due to the paradoxical pulsation of the infarcted area. The heart sounds may be normal, but in severe cases they are soft and the splitting of the second heart sound may be reversed. In almost all patients an atrial (fourth) sound is audible at some time during the first 36–48 hr after infarction. A third heart sound or a gallop rhythm is associated with the development of left ventricular failure or cardiogenic shock. Transmural infarction may be accompanied by a pericardial friction rub within 24 hr. The appearance of a pansystolic murmur indicates the development of mitral reflux due to rupture or dysfunction of the papillary muscle, or rupture of the interventricular septum. Basal crepitations not cleared by coughing, which persist for more than a few hours, indicate the development of pulmonary oedema secondary to left ventricular failure.

Most patients develop a low grade fever (up to 39°C) which persists for 48–72 hr. There is a moderate polymorpholeucocytosis and elevation of the ESR. These are the response to myocardial necrosis.

ENZYME CHANGES

Certain enzymes, which are normally present in large quantities in the myocardium are released into the blood following myocardial necrosis. Different enzymes are used for diagnosis by different laboratories and the reference values vary from laboratory to laboratory. However, a rise to twice the reference level for that particular laboratory and its subsequent fall to within the reference range can be considered important.

Serum creatinine phosphokinase (CPK). Creatine phosphokinase occurs in myocardial and skeletal muscle and in brain tissue, and is released into the blood following damage. It begins to appear in the serum within six hours of a myocardial infarction, reaches a peak within 24 hours and then falls to within the reference range over the succeeding 3–4 days. This enzyme is particularly useful in diagnosis, but muscle trauma, intramuscular injections, exercise or epileptic fits, are all sufficient to cause an increase and is occasionally raised after pulmonary embolus. More recent isolation of an isoenzyme of CPK (CPK–MB) which is specific to the myocardium has proved of considerable value. The total amount of CPK released into the blood following acute myocardial infarction can be measured. This is being used in attempts to measure the amount of myocardial necrosis and, therefore, the size and prognosis of the myocardial infarction.

Serum glutamic-oxalo-acetic transaminase (SGOT). (Aspartate aminotransferase.) This enzyme occurs in heart and skeletal muscle, brain, liver and kidney. The rise in the level in the serum after an acute myocardial infarction occurs between 12 and 24 hr after infarction, and reaches its peak after 36–48 hr. It falls to the reference level within 5 days.

Serum lactic dehydrogenase (LDH). Lactic dehydrogenase is present in the myocardium and in red cells. The level in the serum rises late after myocardial infarction, reaches its peak between 48 and 72 hr and may remain raised for 10–14 days. It is therefore of value in the diagnosis of myocardial infarction some days after the acute incident.

ECG CHANGES

Acute myocardial infarction is almost always associated with changes in the standard 12 lead ECG. The changes may be permanent or relatively transient and therefore it is extremely important that serial ECGs be taken. There are three types of change.

ST segment changes are the first to appear. Convex elevation upwards of the ST segments occurs within a few hours in those ECG leads which overlie the damaged myocardium. They return to the isoelectric line over the next 2–4 days. Persistent elevation of the ST segment beyond this time should arouse suspicion of the development of a left ventricular aneurysm.

Q or QS waves only appear if the myocardial infarction has involved the full thickness of the ventricular wall. Pathological Q waves develop in the leads which are over the myocardial infarction and are more than 0·4 s in duration and greater than 25 per cent of the amplitude of the succeeding R wave. Q waves do not develop immediately the pain occurs but only when muscle necrosis has developed and therefore their appearance is usually delayed for some hours. The Q waves diminish in size during healing but they usually persist.

T wave. This becomes symmetrically and often deeply inverted as the ST segment begins to return to the isoelectric line. The degree of inversion becomes less over the next 2–3 months and the T waves may eventually become upright or they may remain inverted permanently.

In inferior infarctions the ECG changes are best seen in leads II, III and AVL, and in anterior infarctions in leads I, AVL and the chest leads. If the anterior infarction is anteroseptal, leads V_1 to V_3 show the maximal changes, whereas if it is anterolateral,

V_4 to V_6 are maximally affected. On some occasions extensive infarcts affect all the anterior chest leads.

The differential diagnosis of acute myocardial infarction is wide. It can be distinguished from angina pectoris and unstable angina by the persistence of the pain associated with an elevation of the temperature, the sedimentation rate and the serum enzymes, and the presence of persistent changes in the ECG.

Other conditions which must be distinguished from acute myocardial infarction include pulmonary embolism, acute pericarditis, dissecting aneurysm of the aorta, pneumothorax, Bornholm disease, 'shingles' (Herpes Zoster), perforated duodenal ulcer, oesophageal pain and acute cholecystitis.

EARLY COMPLICATIONS OF MYOCARDIAL INFARCTION

The early complications occur within the first 4 weeks of an infarct and include disturbances of rate, rhythm and conduction, cardiogenic shock, left ventricular failure and pulmonary oedema, congestive cardiac failure, pulmonary embolism and infarction, systemic embolism, dysfunction or rupture of a papillary muscle, and rupture of the interventricular septum or the free wall of the ventricle.

Almost all disorders of rate, rhythm and conduction may occur within the first few days following an acute myocardial infarction. The majority of patients develop a dysrhythmia but only approximately half require specific treatment.

Sinus tachycardia is a physiological response whose rate reflects the severity, and therefore the prognosis, of the infarction.

Sinus bradycardia frequently occurs, particularly after inferior infarction, and is usually caused by vagal overtone. It may be aggravated by the overuse of opiates, particularly morphine. It is usually harmless but it contributes to the decrease in cardiac output and hypotension and encourages the development of ectopic rhythms.

Atrial (supraventricular) tachycardia is relatively common in the first few days after an acute infarction and may precipitate cardiac failure or cardiogenic shock in patients with major infarctions. Atrial fibrillation is surprisingly uncommon.

Ventricular ectopics are common and may be of little importance. However, they are dangerous if they are multifocal; if they occur at a frequency of more than 6 per minute or in runs of more than 3, if they occur early after a preceding beat, particularly if they fall on the sensitive part of the T wave of that preceding beat, when they may precipitate ventricular fibrillation. The occurrence of ventricular tachycardia is serious and may precipitate cardiogenic shock or ventricular fibrillation.

Ventricular fibrillation occurs in about 10 per cent of patients who are admitted to hospital with acute myocardial infarction. It is often preceded by the appearance of ventricular ectopics or ventricular tachycardia and is more frequent in patients with cardiogenic shock and severe left ventricular failure. However, it may also occur without warning (primary ventricular fibrillation).

Some degree of heart block occurs in about 7 per cent of patients. It is particularly common in those with inferior or posterior infarcts in whom it is relatively benign. In almost all such patients, conduction is restored to normal if the patient survives the acute infarction. The appearance of heart block of any degree in patients with anterior myocardial infarction carries a poor prognosis (despite the use of a temporary pacemaker) because heart block only appears in extensive anterior infarctions which involve the conducting system below the bundle of His.

Cardiogenic shock. This clinical state (see page 19) is caused by a low cardiac output in the presence of a high peripheral vascular resistance. The depressed cardiac output is usually the result of extensive myocardial damage and occurs in spite of an adequate or even high left ventricular filling pressure (primary cardiogenic shock). However, in a few cases it may be due to an inadequate left ventricular filling pressure (relative hypovolaemia) which may follow previous diuretic therapy, or it may be secondary to the development of a dysrhythmia.

Left ventricular failure and pulmonary oedema. A mild degree of left ventricular failure is present in the majority of patients following acute myocardial infarction but in most of these cases, the prognosis is reasonable. If, however, frank pulmonary oedema develops, the mortality is approximately 40 per cent.

If the infarction involves one or other of the papillary muscles some degree of mitral regurgitation may develop. If the papillary muscle actually ruptures, torrential mitral regurgitation develops immediately and 50 per cent of patients die within 24 hr. The survivors usally remain in chronic severe left ventricular failure. The interventricular septum may also rupture, particular after an anteroseptal myocardial infarction with a similar prognosis. The free wall of the left ventricle may also occasionally rupture and this is invariably fatal.

Pulmonary infarction and pulmonary embolism are common complications of acute myocardial infarction. Less commonly systemic arterial emboli originating from a mural thrombus in the left ventricle may occur.

LATE COMPLICATIONS OF MYOCARDIAL INFARCTION

A left *ventricular aneurysm* develops when the fibrous tissue which replaces the infarcted myocardium is weak. This causes a gradual expansion of the weak fibrotic area which results in extra work for the remaining myocardium. Many left ventricular aneurysms do not produce symptoms but, if they are large, they may cause left ventricular failure. Mural thrombi may form within the aneurysm and give rise to systemic emboli. The presence of an aneurysm may predispose to the development of ventricular dysrhythmias. The physical signs are the persistence of an abnormal systolic pulsation for more than 3 weeks after the acute myocardial infarction, and the presence of a loud apical third heart sound. The ECG shows persistent ST segment elevation. The bulge may be seen on chest X-ray, and on screening, paradoxical movement of the cardiac shadow may be obvious.

Post-infarction (Dressler's) syndrome develops between 3 and 5 weeks after acute infarction. It is thought to be due to hypersensitivity to cardiac muscle and it is characterized by fever, pericardial pain and a pericardial rub, pleuritic pain and a pleural rub, leucocytosis, and a considerably elevated ESR. Although the condition may be painful and troublesome, it is benign and usually resolves spontaneously.

Frozen shoulder develops in a few patients after infarction but it may persist in these cases for many months. The cause of this condition is unknown. The left shoulder is usually involved and there is considerable limitation in movement of the joint with pain and tenderness over it.

PROGNOSIS OF MYOCARDIAL INFARCTION

The overall mortality of acute myocardial infarction is approximately 30 per cent, but it is lower in the younger age group and rises rapidly above the age of 60. Two-thirds of those patients who are going to die from an acute myocardial infarction do so within 2 hr after the onset of symptoms and 75 per cent die within the first 12 hr. These early deaths are mostly due to serious dysrhythmias and a certain number occur in patients in whom the myocardial infarction is itself small.

The prognosis of myocardial infarction is usually good if the patient survives 48 hr and does not develop cardiogenic shock or severe left ventricular failure. The long-term prognosis of patients who survive an acute infarction is also quite good. About 50 per cent live for 10 years and over 25 per cent live for 20 years. The vast majority of survivors should be able to return to their previous work within 3 months.

MANAGEMENT OF ACUTE MYOCARDIAL INFARCTION

Over the last few years the value of admitting patients with acute myocardial infarction to specialized coronary care units has been questioned and recent studies have suggested that the overall benefit of such units is marginal. There is, however, no doubt that life-threatening dysrhythmias can be corrected more effectively in individual patients within a Coronary Care Unit (CCU). The majority of these dysrhythmias occur within 12 hr of the onset of symptoms and it is therefore reasonable to admit patients less than 65 years old, who are seen within this period, to a CCU provided that the journey to hospital is not too long. Patients over this age, or younger patients who are seen more than 12 hr after the acute episode, may be nursed at home if there is no evidence of cardiac failure, cardiogenic shock or persistent dysrhythmias.

In view of the risk of early deaths which are largely due to dysrhythmias there has been an increasing interest in the possible value of *mobile* CCUs. These might reduce the delay before specialist treatment is started.

The management of a patient within a CCU is not difficult. Undue excitement and alarm should be avoided since dysrhythmias may be precipitated. The most important immediate treatment of myocardial infarction is the relief of pain. This usually requires either morphine or diamorphine. Both drugs should ideally be given intravenously, since peripheral constriction and low cardiac output may delay the absorption of intramuscular drugs. Opiate overdose must be avoided since this may lead to severe bradycardia and hypotension. It is traditional to give patients oxygen but the value of its routine administration in the absence of left ventricular failure or cardiogenic shock is doubtful.

Serious ectopic beats should be treated in the manner discussed in the preceding section on dysrhythmias (page 23).

Heart block of any degree after an inferior infarction will usually respond to atropine but a few cases are resistant and may require treatment with a temporary pacing wire. Heart block following anterior infarction does not usually respond to atropine. The routine use of temporary pacemakers in such patients probably does not alter the prognosis but it may be justifiable.

The treatment of cardiogenic shock depends on the aetiology. If cardiogenic shock is secondary to a rapid dysrhythmia, this should be treated and the outcome may be good. Cardiogenic shock due to relative hypovolaemia can only be identified by measurement of the left ventricular filling pressure either indirectly, through a pulmonary arterial catheter, or directly by retrograde left ventricular catheterization. These patients sometimes do well following the infusion of a volume expander, such as low molecular weight dextran or salt-free albumin. It is important to identify these two groups of patients in view of the poor prognosis of primary cardiogenic shock.

All patients with cardiogenic shock should receive IPPV since, by this means, the oxygen cost of breathing can be reduced and the arterial oxygenation controlled. It is usual to give muscle relaxants or narcotics to ensure full control of the ventilation. Alpha-adrenergic blocking drugs reduce the work of the heart and improve the peripheral perfusion, including that of the kidney. Other drugs which have been used include digoxin, isoprenaline, dopamine and other inotropic agents. The place of mechanical support to the circulation by, for example, counterpulsation, is controversial but may eventually find a place. In spite of all these measures, either individually or collectively, the prognosis of primary cardiogenic shock is extremely bad.

Complications are treated conventionally. Surgical replacement of the mitral valve or repair of the interventricular septum may have to be considered. A left ventricular aneurysm which causes persistent left ventricular failure or recurrent dysrhythmias may need to be resected. Post myocardial infarction syndrome (Dressler's syndrome) is treated symptomatically but occasionally a short course of steroids may be given.

The rehabilitation of patients following infarction is extremely important. There is no evidence that prolonged bed rest is beneficial and, in fact, it is probably dangerous since the development of deep vein thrombosis and pulmonary embolism is encouraged. Patients without evidence of left ventricular failure or persistent ischaemic pain should be mobilized within 5 days of the acute episode and be ready for discharge from hospital after 10 days. Their activities should be gradually increased over the succeeding 6 weeks, after which they should return to normal activity within 10 weeks and, in most cases, to their previous employment. They should be told that sexual relations are permissible as long as angina is not provoked. The risk factors in the genesis of coronary arterial disease should be explained. There is no evidence that longterm anticoagulant therapy influences the prognosis of either acute or chronic ischaemic heart disease unless there is clear evidence of deep vein thrombosis or pulmonary infarction.

THE PREVENTION OF ISCHAEMIC HEART DISEASE

The exact aetiology of ischaemic heart disease is still not fully understood, but a certain number of risk factors have been clearly identified. These include cigarette smoking, systemic hypertension, and hyperlipidaemia. Less important factors include a sedentary mode of life, a strong family history of coronary artery disease, obesity, diabetes mellitus and, possibly, mental stress. While some of these factors are not correctable, others are capable of modification either by alterations in the patient's way of life or by therapeutic measures. Their detailed management is outside the scope of this book.

PULMONARY HEART DISEASE

Pulmonary heart disease (cor pulmonale) includes all types of heart disease which are secondary to primary disorders of the lungs. A number of factors in lung disease cause a rise in pulmonary vascular resistance and therefore in the pulmonary arterial pressure. These are a reduction in the alveolar oxygen tension which causes pulmonary arterial constriction; a permanent reduction in the size of the pulmonary vascular bed due to rupture of alveoli which causes destruction of capillaries; and air trapping with resultant raised alveolar pressures with compression of the pulmonary capillaries.

3*

Increased pulmonary vascular resistance causes pulmonary hypertension, right ventricular hypertrophy and eventually, in severe cases, right heart failure. Alveolar hypoxia and arterial hypoxaemia are essential prerequisites for the development of cor pulmonale; the arterial carbon dioxide tension is also raised when there is alveolar hypoventilation. Secondary effects include polycythaemia and cerebral vasodilatation, due to hypercapnia.

The most common type of lung disease which results in cor pulmonale is chronic obstructive airways disease with or without emphysema. In this condition there is mismatching between ventilation and perfusion with resultant hypoxaemia. In patients with chronic obstructive airways disease the pulmonary arterial pressure may be only mildly elevated or even normal for much of the time, but hypertension may become severe during episodes of bronchial infection when small airway obstruction becomes more marked and further hypoxaemia develops. Pulmonary fibrosis, secondary to pulmonary tuberculosis or irradiation, may cause cor pulmonale particularly if there is associated emphysema.

A number of conditions (including pulmonary granulomata, sarcoidosis, malignant infiltration of the lungs and the pulmonary manifestations of the collagenoses) cause thickening of the alveolar membrane and a so-called 'diffusion defect'. However, random reductions in lung compliance which cause further ventilation-perfusion abnormalities and frank loss of alveoli for gaseous exchange are more probable causes for the hypoxaemia than different rates of diffusion for oxygen and carbon dioxide. Hypocapnia is not uncommon and is due to hypoxaemic hyperventilation. Hypoxaemia causes pulmonary arterial constriction; pulmonary hypertension follows and eventually the right heart fails.

Any disease which causes pulmonary hypoventilation may lead to hypoxaemia and hypercarbia with the subsequent development of cor pulmonale. These disorders include severe kyphoscoliosis, pleural fibrosis, obesity with alveolar hypoventilation (Pickwickian syndrome), and chronic weakness of the respiratory muscles (poliomyelitis).

Pulmonary heart disease, including thromboembolic pulmonary disease, is discussed in Chapter 3.

DISEASES OF THE AORTA

DISSECTION OF THE AORTA

When blood enters the media of the aorta through a tear in the intima, it may track either distally or proximally and strip the intima and part of the media away from the remaining media and the adventitia. The dissection may spread a considerable distance and obstruct the origins of the arteries, including the coronaries, which arise from the aorta. The attachment of the aortic valve may be damaged causing aortic regurgitation. The dissection usually ruptures into the mediastinum, pleura, pericardium or the retroperitoneal space, but it may re-enter the true lumen of the aorta through a further tear in the intima. Dissection of the aorta usually occurs in late middle-aged and elderly people with moderate to severe systemic hypertension, but in younger patients it may be a complication of Marfan's syndrome.

The principal symptom of dissection of the aorta is sudden, severe 'tearing' pain. It is usually maximal between the shoulder blades but it tends to move as the dissection spreads. Occasionally the patient may present with syncope or severe dyspnoea. On examination the patient is pale and sweaty; the blood pressure may be elevated or normal but in severe cases the patient is hypotensive. Examination of the cardiac impulse and the retinal vessels may show changes associated with long-standing systemic hypertension. One or other of the peripheral pulses may be absent. The other physical findings depend on which of the arteries arising from the aorta has been damaged and include hemiplegia, haematuria, signs of pleural effusion and of peritonitis. If the dissection has spread proximally to involve the aortic root, the murmur of aortic regurgitation may be audible. There may be a pericardial friction rub if blood has leaked into the pericardium. The ECG is of little help but the chest X-ray frequently shows a wide mediastinum and an irregular aortic arch. The most important differential diagnosis is an acute myocardial infarction.

Death may occur immediately or within a few hours; some patients survive for two weeks but most die within three. A few patients in whom re-entry has occurred may survive to leave hospital.

Management of this serious condition has caused controversy. Immediate surgical repair of the dissection has been proposed but recent evidence suggests that the results are no better than those of medical management. The latter includes the urgent reduction of the systolic blood pressure to below 100 mmHg, with trimetaphan or sodium nitroprusside given by an intravenous infusion for 48–72 hr, and then replaced by oral hypotensive agents. Surgery should be considered if a limb is jeopardized or if there has been severe damage to the aortic valve.

ANEURYSMS

Aneurysms of the aorta are mostly arteriosclerotic but, in the younger age group, Marfan's syndrome may be the cause. Syphilis should not be forgotten as a cause of aneurysms of the ascending aorta.

If the aneurysms are asymptomatic, the prognosis is good and specific treatment is not required. Pressure on surrounding organs may, however, cause symptoms which include pain, cough, wheeze or hoarseness of the voice if the aneurysm presses on bone, the trachea, bronchus or larynx. The outlook for symptomatic aortic aneurysms is poor but because they usually appear in the older age group in whom there is associated severe vascular disease, surgery should only be considered for those patients who have severe symptoms or in whom the aneurysm is rapidly enlarging.

Aneurysm of the sinuses of Valsalva may also occur. These may rupture into the left ventricle, when they produce the signs and symptoms of severe aortic regurgitation, or they may rupture into the right side of the heart when the signs of a left to right shunt are associated with those of aortic reflux. Rupture of a sinus of Valsalva aneurysm should be repaired surgically.

HEART DISEASE IN PREGNANCY

Seventy years ago the maternal mortality in cardiac patients was 50 per cent; it is now less than 0·1 per cent. This change has not been due to any single alteration in management but to a steady improvement in both antenatal care and in the management of labour. These improvements have been based on an increased understanding of the physiology of pregnancy.

Blood volume and cardiac output normally increase steadily throughout pregnancy and these changes present special problems to the cardiac patient.

The most frequent cardiac disease encountered during pregnancy is <u>mitral stenosis</u>. In severe cases the obstruction at the valve limits the degree to which the stroke volume can increase. The increase in cardiac output which occurs in pregnancy is therefore associated with a <u>disproportionate increase in heart rate</u>. The consequent reduction of left ventricular diastolic filling time leads to a marked rise in left atrial pressure which may precipitate pulmonary congestion.

Few patients with mitral stenosis who have grade 3, or more, dyspnoea on exertion conceive but, if they do, they almost always develop frank cardiac failure in the first trimester and miscarry.

Most of those women with mitral stenosis who pass through the first trimester without developing cardiac failure will come to term and deliver spontaneously, provided that they rest if necessary, and continue under close medical supervision. Ten years ago a considerable number of patients had <u>mitral valvotomy</u> during the <u>middle trimester</u> but there appear to be fewer patients now whose symptoms are severe enough to warrant this. This is probably because potent diuretics are now employed. Nevertheless, occasional patients continue to have severe symptoms of pulmonary congestion in spite of full medical treatment and may, therefore, require valvotomy. If this is necessary it should be performed in the middle trimester since valvotomy in the first trimester almost always precipitates a miscarriage and, in the last trimester, premature labour. Mitral valvotomy should only be performed in patients with pure mitral stenosis. Valve replacement using cardiopulmonary bypass has occasionally been performed successfully during pregnancy, but it should be avoided if possible.

Patients with mitral stenosis should be seen at monthly intervals in the cardiac clinic for the first five months of pregnancy and at two-weekly intervals thereafter. Particular note should be taken of <u>dyspnoea</u> which is disproportionate to the stage of pregnancy, and of a <u>persistently raised pulse rate</u> (more than 90/min) at rest. These indicate <u>decompensation</u> and the need for <u>digitalis</u> and <u>diuretics</u>. The management should include <u>bed rest if</u> the symptoms continue in spite of these drugs. The occurrence of palpitations, however mild, often precedes atrial fibrillation and again indicates the need for digitalization. The onset of atrial fibrillation may be followed by the occurrence of systemic emboli and anticoagulants should therefore be considered. However, these drugs should be avoided if possible in the first trimester since they may make a threatened miscarriage complete. After the end of this period of pregnancy, oral anticoagulants may be used, if indicated, since the risks to the mother of systemic emboli outweigh those to the fetus from the placental transfer of these drugs. Deep venous thrombosis or pulmonary emboli should also be treated with anticoagulants with the same caution.

The expectant mother should be admitted electively between one and two weeks before the expected date of delivery. Intravenous heparin should be substituted for oral anticoagulants. Labour should be allowed to proceed normally either following spontaneous or artificial rupture of the membranes. Most patients with mitral valve disease deliver rapidly. If, however, the labour is prolonged, consideration may have to be given to delivery by Caesarean section. Parenteral antibiotics should be started using a bactericidal agent which is effective against Gram-negative organisms when the membranes rupture.

During labour the mother should be nursed <u>sitting up</u> for as long as possible, and should be given oxygen in high concentrations. Reassurance and adequate analgesia form an important part of the therapy since tachycardia may precipitate pulmonary congestion. A pulse rate above 100/min, even during a contraction, suggests trouble and that delivery should be expedited. Intravenous saline infusion should be avoided.

Pulmonary congestion and oedema most commonly develop during the third stage of labour following the delivery of the placenta. This is due to the relative increase in the circulating blood volume. Ergometrine should be avoided because this drug may cause widespread venoconstriction with resultant pulmonary congestion. Oxytocin has a briefer action than ergometrine and causes less venoconstriction; it is therefore the preferred drug.

Women with other cardiac diseases may present during pregnancy and their management is simple *if* the underlying cardiac physiology is understood. Expert help should be sought. Aspects of the obstetric management and the control of pain in labour are described in Chapter 6.

ANAESTHESIA FOR PATIENTS WITH CARDIAC DISEASE

Much of the knowledge about the effects of anaesthesia on patients with cardiac disease has been acquired in the field of cardiac surgery but the derived lessons can probably be applied to the vastly more numerous patients who are suffering from intercurrent cardiac disease whilst undergoing other types of surgery.

Preoperative assessment

The functional end result of pathology in the heart is cardiac failure and anaesthetists therefore wish to assess how close any patient is to failure. The functional reserve of the heart can be gauged from the degree to which dyspnoea or angina occur at various levels of activity. In the case of dyspnoea, the more severe it is the greater the risk that some relatively trivial mishap, such as a modest circulatory overload, may be followed by deterioration during, or after, operation. Thus the presence of cardiac dyspnoea is alone sufficient to warn that decompensation is not far off and it is therefore appropriate to consider prophylaxis with digitalis.

The need to prevent emotional stress by proper psychological and pharmacological preparation of a patient with angina is obvious; sedatives should be given for several days preoperatively; in some patients, β-blockers may be indicated; glyceryl trinitrate may also be used.

Prophylactic digitalization

There is considerable controversy about the use of digitalis in the preparation of elderly patients, who have diminished cardiac reserve, for non-cardiac surgery. Those who oppose the routine use of digitalis point out that the factors which predispose to dysrhythmias and cardiac failure associated with surgery increase sensitivity to digitalis and thus the clinical picture may be unnecessarily complicated in the period immediately after surgery, if digitalis therapy has recently been started. Rather than expose the patients to these risks, many anaesthetists advocate careful monitoring of the central venous pressure and arterial blood pressure during surgery and in the event of cardiac failure, the use of rapidly-acting cardiac glycosides or, more properly, diuretics. However, change in central venous pressure does not provide warning of left ventricular failure and the pulmonary artery pressure would need to be measured for this aim to be met. Furthermore, although preoperative preparation with digitalis was associated with a decrease in mortality from cardiac failure in patients having non-cardiac *thoracic* surgery, it increased the mortality from dysrhythmias [11]. Many anaesthetists and physicians recommend withdrawal of these drugs 36 hours prior to cardiopulmonary bypass operations [27].

However, digitalis does have an effect on both the failing and non-failing heart [20] and does decrease mortality from cardiac failure. In the authors' opinion, prophylaxis with digitalis can do no harm, may be beneficial, and unless there is overwhelming urgency, two or three days should be spent in achieving full digitalization. There are several clinical series which support this view [3, 4, 15].

Physiological and pharmacological aspects of anaesthesia for non-cardiac operations

It is virtually impossible to collect a large personal experience of particular cardiac conditions which are intercurrent with non-cardiac surgical conditions. Thus, although patients with cardiac disease might be anticipated to suffer from any adverse effects more than patients without such disease, in fact little is known about the effects of anaesthesia and surgery in patients with cardiac disease. General and regional anaesthesia have identifiable effects on the heart and circulation and it is desirable to choose an anaesthetic method which is as harmless for the function of the heart as possible. The choice of premedicant, induction, muscle relaxant and analgesic drugs, whilst partly dependent upon personal familiarity, is affected by pharmacological desirability. No particular combination of drugs is totally safe and the various operative factors must be judged individually for each patient and different decisions may be reached in different circumstances although the medical condition is the same.

All the inhaled anaesthetic agents depress myocardial activity but the effects on cardiac output, after-load and heart rate vary from agent to agent [10, 29]. The effects on isolated cardiac muscle, on conducting tissue, on intact animals, or on patients *without* simultaneous surgical stimulation can be misleading and one must beware of the ready acceptance of data in this field particularly when the interpretation goes beyond the limits of the experimental protocol. Even nitrous oxide may not be as free from harm as is sometimes assumed although studies so far have been with the simultaneous use of other drugs. Intravenous morphine in large doses, or neuroleptanaesthetic techniques, including the use of butyrophenone drugs to modify peripheral vasoconstriction and thus to lessen cardiac work, are currently used in many cardiac centres. Pancuronium and gallamine should be avoided in patients with ischaemic heart disease unless β- blocking drugs have been used in the preparation of the patient for surgery. When an intravenous analgesic forms the basis of the anaesthetic technique, hypertension is more likely and the minor ganglion blocking action of tubocurarine is useful.

Dysrhythmias

Sinus rhythm is not an essential prerequisite for all surgical patients preoperatively. Disturbances of cardiac rhythm should, nevertheless, be identified and a preoperative ECG is valuable for comparison with the ECG during anaesthesia if there is any suspicion that cardiac disease may be present. The importance of any dysrhythmia to the anaesthetist is the effect of that dysrhythmia on cardiac output and the possible interactions of the antidysrhythmic agent with subsequent anaesthesia.

Hypoxia and hypercarbia must be avoided or the dysrhythmia will be aggravated. Continuous monitoring of the ECG, preferably the CM5 disposition of electrodes [12], should start before induction and continue at least until the patient leaves the recovery room. Preoxygenation (four maximal deep breaths of 100 per cent oxygen is as effective as five minutes ordinary breathing [8]) and postoperative oxygen therapy are essential for all patients with dysrhythmias. Dysrhythmias are common under anaesthesia but are without serious import unless they are associated with a haemodynamic effect. Frequent and irregular ventricular ectopics herald more serious complications and in a patient with recognized cardiac disease should not be ignored. Antidysrhythmic drugs (lignocaine, disopyramide, β-adrenergic blocking agents) should be available.

Bradycardia with hypotension should be treated with atropine. Sinus tachycardia may be associated with inadequate anaesthesia and this can be managed appropriately: tachycardia with hypertension in patients with ischaemic heart disease is particularly undesirable since permanent damage to subendocardial muscle may follow [30]. The rate-pressure product (systolic, arterial *or* aortic pressure, $\times$ cardiac frequency) correlates well both with coronary perfusion and myocardial oxygen consumption and with the onset of angina [16]. If the rate-pressure product exceeds 15–20,000, ischaemic changes on the ECG are more likely [25] and indicate the need for active treatment. β- adrenergic blocking drugs, either preoperatively or at induction, may be used to prevent the increased demand for oxygen by the myocardium which a tachydysrhythmia causes. Afterload can be reduced by halothane [5].

One important element of technique is intermittent positive pressure ventilation of the lungs (IPPV). Its cardiovascular effects have been reviewed by Foëx [6] but the effect of raised intrathoracic pressures may be less in patients with cardiac failure than in those without. This is because atrial pressures are already higher than normal and any effect of raised intrapulmonary pressure on venous return is less than normal. An increase in intrathoracic pressure also impedes pulmonary blood flow and this will aggravate a right-to-left shunt with a subsequent increase in arterial hypoxaemia. A positive end expiratory pressure (PEEP) is sometimes employed in patients with cardiac failure in order to improve arterial oxygenation: with some ventilators this can reduce the overall tidal ventilation unless the machine is suitably adjusted. Adverse effects of PEEP on cardiac output mean that the delivery of oxygen to the tissues may be impaired by this manoeuvre: the level of PEEP which achieves the best compromise is called 'best PEEP' [22].

Regional anaesthesia with large volumes of local analgesic solutions should be avoided since systemic absorption of local analgesic drugs causes depression of myocardial conductivity and dysrhythmias.

Electrolyte shifts and hydrogen ion changes

Changes in the concentration ratio of potassium across the cell membrane cause changes in the excitability or the conduction velocity in nervous or cardiac muscle: hence the dysrhythmias associated with hypokalaemia and digitalis. Acidosis causes hyperkalaemia (and therefore reduces intracellular potassium) in the conscious subject and is a myocardial depressant: it also reduces the effectiveness of adrenergic stimulation. Patients with cardiac disease are thus especially at risk from sudden changes in electrolyte or hydrogen ion concentrations caused by accidental hypovolaemic hypotension during anaesthesia. Diuretics, which cause potassium loss, should not be used indiscriminately. Sodium-containing solutions should be administered very cautiously to patients whose salt excretory mechanisms are already inefficient: on most occasions 5 per cent dextrose solution is adequate.

The desirability of monitoring the filling pressure of the left ventricle has already been mentioned (see page 14). Recent myocardial infarction, severe ischaemic heart disease, congestive cardiac failure and pulmonary hypertension are cardiac conditions in which it has been suggested that this invasive technique should be considered [14]. Where the facilities exist, the value of this technique has been appreciated. On the other hand, one must remember that premature ventricular contractions, atrial dysrhythmias, atrioventricular block, pulmonary infarction and pulmonary haemorrhage have all occurred in association with the presence of pulmonary artery catheters. Thus the risk/benefit ratio must be carefully considered in each case: nevertheless, the prevalence of early postoperative death in patients with these conditions suggests that a positive approach to these problems might have beneficial effects.

Cardiac failure

Many patients in established, but controlled, cardiac failure are subjected to the risks of elective surgery and anaesthesia and survive without incident. Each case must be judged individually bearing in mind the nature of the surgery and the cardiac reserve. Whilst cardiac failure should ideally be controlled preoperatively, essential life-saving surgery is never contraindicated, and attempts should be made to improve the patient's condition within whatever time is available.

There is an established clinical impression that general anaesthesia lessens the signs of congestive cardiac failure. Improved ventilation-perfusion ratios, improved tissue perfusion due to vasodilatation, reduction of sympathetic tone, improved myocardial function because of reduced myocardial afterload, improved oxygenation as a result of increased inspired oxygen concentrations and the raised intrathoracic pressure of automatic ventilation which improves incipient pulmonary oedema are all possible mechanisms which may be important during anaesthesia. Patients in cardiac failure have a high mortality postoperatively; venous engorgement predisposes to thromboembolic phenomena and pulmonary infections are common.

Cardiac glycosides should be used cautiously in the period immediately before or after surgery since the sensitivity of patients to these drugs is increased postoperatively. This is partly due to the perioperative decrease in renal function which results in higher plasma levels and is particularly important in elderly patients. A negative potassium balance makes the development of digitalis toxicity more likely.

Ischaemic heart disease

All of the reports concerning the influence of a previous recent infarction upon the outcome of surgery emphasize the increased risk of a second infarct which exists. This risk decreases with time and appears to be similar to that in the normal surgical population after 1–3 years. In general, it is wise to defer 'cold' surgery for at least six months after an ischaemic incident.

Between 35 and 70 per cent of patients who have a subsequent infarct in association with surgery die. If it is necessary to operate on a patient within days of a coronary occlusion then a delay of even a day improves the prognosis since both the risk of dysrhythmias declines and the reparative processes begin. A very high mortality indeed can be anticipated if the interval is less than two weeks.

If the choice of agent and technique are rationally based it is unlikely that a significant difference in results between various methods would be detectable. Nevertheless, the anaesthetic method is probably important since a comparative study [1] has failed to show a significant re-infarction rate amongst a group of patients who had surgery (ophthalmic) under local analgesia. This group were at substantial risk when compared with a similar and earlier group reported from the same institution [23]. A similar conclusion can be drawn from another study [19].

The picture is complicated by the effect of surgery. In one study, 50 patients with evidence of earlier infarction, who underwent major surgery, had a hospital mortality of 38 per cent; in 10 similar patients who received anaesthesia for minor and endoscopic surgery or diagnostic radiology, the mortality was zero [7]. As to timing, in one large series of more than 30,000 surgical patients, the third postoperative day showed the highest incidence of postoperative infarct [23].

Infarction *during* anaesthesia is fortunately rare. The onset of otherwise inexplicable non-specific changes in the clinical state (hypotension, rise in central venous pressure or sweating), the appearance of ST changes in the ECG or of dysrhythmias, are signs which might be observed. In the unlikely event of a myocardial infarction occurring during anaesthesia and being diagnosed, it would be advisable to continue, or institute, mechanical ventilation post operatively in order to remove the work of breathing: this would certainly be indicated in the event of haemodynamic embarrassment.

Conduction disorders

Heart block. The risks of ventricular fibrillation or cardiac arrest are such that it is doubtful if any patient with complete AV block should be anaesthetized for any condition, other than a life-threatening one, without facilities for cardiac pacemaking. Long-acting β-adrenergic stimulators have been advocated in the past, but in general, these drugs are no longer in use since the advent of pacemakers. Second degree AV block readily progresses to complete block and transvenous pacemakers should ideally be inserted as a precaution into surgical patients with partial AV block, of whatever type, prior to operation. Many of these pacemakers may never need to be used, but in the event of block occurring during surgery or recovery, the flick of a switch can control what could be a life-threatening disaster. Right bundle branch block as an isolated finding is not very serious and can safely be ignored. Left bundle branch block, however, is potentially serious and expert cardiological advice should be sought in individual cases, particularly with regard to the decision about the use of a temporary transvenous pacemaker.

Surgical diathermy and pacemakers. Total avoidance of surgical diathermy is the safest course of action when a patient is dependent on a pacemaker. When the surgery demands the use of diathermy, it is important for each member of the theatre team to be aware of the risk. Isoprenaline, a transvenous pacemaker and a defibrillator must be available. Monitoring the haemodynamic condition of the patient should employ methods which are not affected by diathermy, such as intra-arterial pressure measurement or a peripheral pulse meter. Factors known to increase the myocardial threshold for stimulation by the pacemaker, and which therefore reduce the effect of this stimulation, should be avoided; these include suxamethonium, hyperkalaemia and metabolic acidosis. Fresh blood should always be used and it is important that blood volume be maintained. Regional techniques should be employed when possible. Displacement of the tip of a permanent transvenous pacing electrode is theoretically possible but very unlikely after the first month since its insertion.

Some types of on-demand pacemakers are sensitive to radiofrequency interference: specialist advice, including that of the manufacturer, should be sought before patients with these units are anaesthetized.

Wolff–Parkinson–White phenomenon. These patients may suddenly develop paroxysmal tachycardia. Atropine can precipitate these changes in susceptible patients and should be avoided in favour of hyoscine or glycopyrrolate.

First degree heart block either indicates organic disease or it may be the effect of parasympathetic overtone. If the latter, it can be abolished by atropine and is of no great significance to anaesthetists.

Defibrillation

Electric shock plays an important part in the management of tachydysrhythmias and is an essential tool in the correction of ventricular fibrillation. The brief application of a high energy shock across the myocardium usually results in complete and simultaneous depolarization of the myocardium. This is usually followed by the restoration of sinus rhythm. However, if the shock occurs on the upstroke of the T wave during natural repolarization, ventricular depolarization may be incomplete and this may permit 're-entry'. Ventricular tachycardia or fibrillation may therefore be precipitated. The impulse should be accurately controlled and usually the shock is timed to occur 20 ms after the peak of the R wave.

Although AC shock can be used for cardioversion, it causes more myocardial damage and is more likely to precipitate ventricular fibrillation than DC shock. Therefore AC cardioverters should only be used in a grave emergency when a DC unit is not available. All patients should receive anticoagulants for at least four weeks before an elective DC cardioversion. It is customary to withdraw digitalis 24–48 hours beforehand.

Electrical cardioversion is painful and light general anaesthesia should always be used unless the patient is already unconscious.

Intracardiac shunts, valve disease, and previous cardiac surgery

The immediate effect of an intravenous drug in a patient with a shunt is modified by dilution with shunted blood. This also occurs when either the mitral or aortic valves are grossly incompetent. Overdosage with intravenous induction agents should be avoided by giving repeated small doses and each increment should be delayed until sufficient time has elapsed to observe the effect of the previous dose. The action of suxamethonium may be both delayed, diminished, and unaccompanied by fasciculation. This is not only due to the dilutional effect but also due to prolongation of the time for which the drug is exposed to the action of plasma cholinesterase.

Both left-to-right shunts and a low cardiac output reduce the rate of uptake of inhaled anaesthetics.

Shunt reversal may occur in patients with atrial septal defects if the afterload on the ventricles is altered. If pulmonary blood flow is markedly reduced by IPPV a pathological left-to-right shunt may be reduced (cf. shunt reversal in patients with small atrial septal defects in response to a Valsalva manoeuvre). Conversely, if systemic vasoconstriction occurs a left-to-right shunt may be increased. Both are undesirable.

Patients with chronic mitral stenosis or aortic stenosis have an increased central blood volume and increased pulmonary extravascular water: transfusion is thus hazardous. Pulmonary compliance is reduced and therefore PEEP should be used during IPPV.

Coronary perfusion may be jeopardised in patients with aortic stenosis if there is a sudden reduction in afterload as a result of widespread vasodilatation. Management should be similar to that for any patient with a fixed cardiac output.

The prevention of endocarditis following surgery in susceptible patients (see page 51) is very important. There are two groups of patients to be considered: those having surgery which itself leads to bacteraemia (dental, colonic, rectal or gynaecological procedures) and those who have poor dental hygiene but having surgery which of itself would not be expected to cause bacteraemia.

All patients susceptible to subacute bacterial endocarditis should have antibiotic cover for all dental treatment. Ideally a dental swab should be taken a week prior to the dental appointment; this should be cultured and the sensitivity of the organisms to antibiotics determined. The appropriate antibiotic should be given parenterally not more than one hour preoperatively and again in the evening. Alternatively, crystalline penicillin, 0·5 M units one hour before dental treatment and once again afterwards should be given as a routine. Unfortunately a substantial number of strains of *Streptococcus viridans* are insensitive to this drug. Rectal, colonic, genito-urinary or gynaecological surgery should be preceded by the administration of a bactericidal antibiotic active against Gram-negative organisms (ampicillin 0·5 g, one hour before surgery, and four times a day for five days). Non-absorbable antibiotics should, in addition, be given before colonic surgery in an attempt to sterilize the bowel.

The place of prevention of subacute bacterial endocarditis in the second group of patients is less well defined. Nonetheless, pressure on the teeth which may inevitably occur during the administration of anaesthesia can lead to bacteraemia; chemoprophylaxis is therefore practiced widely and seems advisable.

Anticoagulants should be continued until just before the operation in all patients who have prosthetic valves. Since heparin anticoagulant therapy is so readily controlled, long-term coumarin derivatives should be withdrawn and heparin substituted. Treatment with intravenous heparin should be managed by determination of the clotting time; if haemorrhage is likely to be serious, protamine sulphate can be given until the clotting time is more than 25 per cent of normal. Regional, and particularly epidural, anaesthesia should be avoided in such patients.

Cardiomyopathy

The occasional association of 'idiopathic' cardiomyopathy with Friedriech's ataxia or myotonic dystrophy should be noted since these conditions are themselves associated with problems. β-adrenergic blockade may be used in therapy for the angina of cardiomyopathy but otherwise cardiac failure is managed conventionally. β-adrenergic stimulating drugs are contraindicated. Specific experience of anaesthesia for patients with cardiomyopathy of any type is necessarily limited but the advice to avoid bradycardia seems sensible [2].

REFERENCES

1 BACKER CL, TINKER JH, ROBERTSON DM. Myocardial reinfarction following local anesthesia. *Anesthesiology* 1979; **51**: 61S.

2 BOWERS JR. Anesthesia and cardiomyopathies: report of two cases. *Anesth Analg (Cleve)* 1971; **50**: 1013–16.

3 CHRISTIANSEN J, BROCKNER J. Prophylactic preoperative digitalization in old surgical patients. *Dan Med Bull* 1967; **14**: 38–40.

4 DEUTSCH S, DALEN JE. Indications for prophylactic digitalization. *Anesthesiology* 1969; **30**: 648.

5 FLETCHER R. Coronary disease and anaesthesia. *Anaesthesia* 1980; **35**: 27–34.

6 FOËX P. The mechanical effects of raised airway pressure. In: Prys Roberts C, ed. *The Circulation in Anaesthesia*. Oxford: Blackwell Scientific Publications, 1980.

7 FRASER JG, RAMACHANDRAN PR, DAVIS HC. Anesthesia and recent myocardial infarction. *JAMA* 1967; **199**: 318–20.

8 GOLD MI, MURAVCHICK S. A four-breath preoxygenation technique. *Anesthesiology* 1979; **51**: 358S.

9 GOLDMAN L, CALDERA DL, NUSSBAUM SR, *et al*. Multifactorial index of cardiac risk in non-cardiac surgical procedures. *N Engl J Med* 1977; **297**: 845–50.

10 JEWELL BR. A reexamination of the influence of muscle length on myocardial performance. *Circ Res* 1977, **40**: 221–30.

11 JULER GL, STEMMER EA, CONNOLLY JE. Complications of prophylactic digitalization in thoracic surgical patients. *J Thorac Cardiovasc Surg* 1969; **58**: 352–60.

12 KAPLAN JA, KING SB. The precordial electrocardiographic lead (V5) in patients who have coronary artery disease. *Anesthesiology* 1976; **45**: 570–74.

13 KOLETTIS M, JENKINS BS, WEBB-PEPLOE MM. Assessment of left ventricular function by indices derived from aortic flow velocity. *Br Heart J* 1976; **38**: 18–31.

14 LAPPAS DG, POWELL WWJ, DAGGETT WM. Cardiac dysfunction in the perioperative period. *Anesthesiology* 1977; **47**: 117–37.

15 McCORD BL. The digitalization of elderly patients with cardiovascular disease requiring colectomy. *J Kans Med Soc* 1967; **68**: 295–99.

16 NELSON RR, GOBEL FL, JORGENSEN GW, WANG K, WANG Y, TAYLOR HL. Hemodynamic predictors of myocardial oxygen consumption during static and dynamic exercise. *Circulation* 1974; **50**: 1179–89.

17 NOBLE MI. The Frank-Starling curve. *Clin Sci Mol Med* 1978; **54**(1): 1–7.

18 POOLE-WILSON PA. Interpretation of haemodynamic measurement. *Br J Hosp Med* 1978; **20**: 371–2, 376–7, 380–2.

19 SAPALA JA, PONKA JL, DUVERNOY WFC. Operative and non-operative risks in the cardiac patient. *J Am Geriatr Soc* 1975; **23**: 529–34.

20 SELZER A, KELLY JJ Jr, GERBODE F, KERTH WJ, OSBORN JJ, PAPPER RW. Case against the routine use of digitalis in patients undergoing cardiac surgery. *JAMA* 1966; **195**: 549–53.

21 SKINNER JF, PEARCE ML. Surgical risk in the cardiac patient. *J Chronic Dis* 1964; **17**: 57–72.

22 SUTER PM, FAIRLEY HB, ISENBERG MD. Optimum end-expiratory airway pressure in patients with acute pulmonary failure. *N Engl J Med* 1975; **292**: 284–9.

23 TARHAN S, MOFFITT EA, TAYLOR WF, GIULIANI ER. Myocardial infarction after general anesthesia. *JAMA* 1972; **220**: 1451–4.

24 WIG J, BALI IM, SINGH RG, KATARIA RN, KATTRI HN. Prolonged Q-T interval syndrome. Sudden cardiac arrest during anaesthesia. *Anaesthesia* 1979; **34**: 37–40.

25 WILKINSON CJ. Halothane anaesthesia is preferable to morphine. In: Eckenhoff JE, ed. *Controversy in Anaesthesia*. Saunders, 1979.

FURTHER READING

26 BRADLEY RD. *Studies in acute heart failure*. London: Arnold, 1977.

27 BRANTHWAITE M. *Anaesthesia for cardiac surgery*. Oxford: Blackwell Scientific Publications, 1980.

28 BRAUNWALD E. *Heart disease*. London: Saunders, 1980.

29 PHILBIN DM. *Anesthetic management of patients with cardio-vascular disease.* International Anesthesiology Clinics, 1979.

30 PRYS ROBERTS C. *The circulation in anaesthesia.* Oxford: Blackwell Scientific Publications, 1980.

31 SOKOLOW M, McILROY MB. *Clinical cardiology.* Los Altos USA: Lange, 1977.

Chapter 2
Hypertension and Systemic Arterial Diseases

C. PRYS-ROBERTS

Hypertension and atheromatous vascular disease are the leading causes of death in most advanced nations. Involvement of the coronary, cerebral and peripheral arteries in the atherosclerotic process accounts for about half of all deaths in Europe and North America, with coronary arterial disease accounting for two thirds of this mortality. High arterial pressure is not necessarily a feature of atherosclerotic disease, but a number of epidemiological studies have shown that high arterial pressure accelerates and aggravates the process of atherosclerosis, and significantly influences the mortality from coronary and cerebral arterial disease. Conversely, coronary artery disease and its consequences are the main complication associated with high arterial pressure, pathological evidence of substantial coronary arterial lesions being found in more than 60 per cent of hypertensive patients at autopsy. Coronary artery disease is the cause of death in more than one half of all patients with high blood pressure, and is becoming more predominant as a cause of morbidity and mortality as other causes have declined as a result of successful antihypertensive therapy [22, 26]. Vascular disease in cerebral arteries is also common in patients with high arterial pressure and there is a relationship between the incidence of such disease in cerebral and coronary arteries [35]. The mortality from unclassified cerebral vascular accidents or strokes accounts for between 30 and 40 per cent of all deaths in untreated hypertensive patients, though the incidence of cerebral vascular accident has decreased by more than 50 per cent as a result of antihypertensive therapy.

It is generally agreed that ischaemic heart disease, either alone or in association with high arterial pressure, is associated with a significant risk of morbidity and mortality during and after anaesthesia and surgery. Consequently, the pre-existence of atheroclerosis causing cerebral or coronary arterial disease, and of hypertension, are of considerable importance to the practising anaesthetist.

The management of anaesthesia in patients with hypertension or systemic arterial disease demands a full understanding of the pathophysiology of these conditions, and that of associated coronary arterial disease and its manifestations. Also important is a full appreciation of the drug therapy of these disease states and the possible interactions of these drugs with those used during anaesthesia.

PATHOPHYSIOLOGY

Pathological changes in the aorta, major arteries and arterioles can be classified according to three main processes.

Aging, arteriosclerosis and calcification

The main process of aging in the arterial system is a gradual loss of elastic tissue (elastin and collagen) and its replacement by fibrin, with the associated hyaline degeneration which leads to fibrinoid necrosis. This general process is often over-shadowed by the concurrent development of the atheromatous process so that the effects of organ ischaemia tend to preponderate. However, the anaesthetist who deals with an elderly clientele must recognize the patient with <u>rigid arterial disease</u> who presents few of the specific stigmata of true hypertension or of coronary artery disease. These patients typically have arterial pressures of about 160/80 mmHg in a relaxed state, but often present in the anaesthetic room, or during the preoperative visit with <u>high systolic arterial pressures (180–220 mmHg) but with normal or low diastolic pressures (75–90 mmHg)</u>. The high pulse pressure under conditions of stress indicates the ejection of <u>increased stroke volume</u> into a <u>rigid arterial system</u> having a <u>high resistance.</u> These patients often show patchy calcification in their major arteries, and must be clearly distinguished from patients who have true diastolic hypertension, and also from those who have Mönckeberg's medial sclerosis.

Atheromatous vascular disease

The development of the characteristic lesion, the atheromatous plaque, in the major vessels (Chapter 1) produces changes in the perfusion of organs as the plaque and its attendant thrombus encroaches on and occupies a progressively larger proportion of the arterial lumen. Common sites at which these plaques obliterate major arteries to cause distal organ ischaemia, either at rest or under working conditions, follow.

> Coronary arteries (Chapter 1)
> Carotid arteries—at the bifurcation of the common carotid artery
> Abdominal aorta and its bifurcation
> Iliac, femoral and popliteal arteries
> Mesenteric arteries
> Renal arteries

Although atheromatous disease can involve the arteries of the upper limb, the incidence of consequential upper limb ischaemia is very low, especially when compared with that of lower limb ischaemia from aorto-iliac or aorto-femoral disease.

As the general pathology of the atheromatous lesion has been dealt with in Chapter 1, only those aspects of atheromatous disease affecting the peripheral arteries and the interaction with hypertension will be dealt with in this chapter.

Hypertension

The characteristic acquired lesions of small arteries and arterioles in patients with high arterial pressure, especially those with the accelerated or 'malignant' phase of the conditions, have been variously described as the miliary aneurysms of Charcot and Bouchard and the nodular arteriosclerosis of Councilman. These features had been described long before arterial pressure could be measured in man, and the pathological features which we now associate with hypertension, vascular thickening and fibrinoid degeneration, were linked to high arterial pressure by Volhard and Fahr [60]. It is now recognized that these changes are the end-stages of damage to arteries caused by sustained high arterial pressure [16, 17]. The major pathological change which occurs early in response to sustained high arterial pressure, whatever its cause, is hypertrophy of the inner layer of smooth muscle in the arterial media. Folkow [12, 13] has de-scribed this hypertrophy as an adaptive phenomenon to protect the systemic capillaries from the damaging effects of high arterial pressure. Associated with this hypertrophy there is increased deposition of acid mucopolysaccharides, fibrin and elastin in the arterial wall [16]. Further is an increase in the arterial wall content of salt and water. The end result is a progressive <u>thickening of the arterial wall relative to the internal radius of the arterial lumen.</u>

Where high arterial pressure is associated with atheromatous disease the development of the latter is accelerated and aggravated [23] so that in the white populations of the world, coronary artery and cerebrovascular disease contribute to more than 90 per cent of the death rate in hypertensive patients. Negro and many other coloured populations are particularly prone to hypertension, but not to atheromatous disease. In these races the causes of death in patients with hypertension are more related to long-term heart failure and renal failure.

HYPERTENSION

Pickering [36] emphasized that high arterial pressure is a quantitative phenomenon and not a disease entity in itself. He has stressed the difficulties in defining criteria which differentiate between 'normotensive' and 'hypertensive' patients, as arterial pressure is a continuously distributed quantity. Nevertheless, high arterial pressure has grave consequences to the cardiovascular system, and the higher the arterial pressure the worse the prognosis. Life insurance companies have long recognized that mortality ratios increase as a function of departure from average blood pressures and that the higher mortality rates among patients with high arterial pressures are largely due to associated cardiovascular and renal disease. Of those patients who present with signs and symptoms related to high arterial pressure, about 15 per cent are found to have specific disease states as an aetiological factor of their hypertension (Table 2.1) whereas the remaining <u>85 per cent </u>do not appear to have any recognizable pathological entity

Table 2.1. Classification of hypertension by cause.

I Secondary hypertension

---

1 Diseases of the <u>kidneys and urinary tract</u>
  (*a*) acute nephritis
  (*b*) chronic pyelonephritis
  (*c*) renal arterial disease
  (*d*) polycystic kidney
  (*e*) renal stone or other causes of urinary tract obstruction
  (*f*) interstitial nephritis
  (*g*) diabetes mellitus
  (*h*) connective tissue diseases involving the kidney:
    polyarteritis nodosa
    disseminated lupus erythematosus
  (*i*) certain renal tumours
2 Coarctation of the aorta
3 Phaeochromocytoma
4 Cushing's Syndrome
5 Primary hyperaldosteronism (Conn's Syndrome)
6 Toxaemia of pregnancy
7 Miscellaneous conditions affecting the autonomic nervous system:
  tetanus
  polyneuropathy (Guillain–Barré Syndrome)

II Essential hypertension

---

and a diagnosis of 'essential' hypertension is retained. Most authorities acknowledge the futility of a statistical differentiation between normal and high arterial pressures, most have accepted a pragmatic indication for an arbitary definition of the limits of normal arterial pressure, this need being well summarized by Grimley-Evans and Rose, '. . . in an operational sense, hypertension should be defined in terms of blood pressure levels above which investigations and treatment do more good than harm'. Based on such arbitrary criteria, it is clear that hypertension is a common phenomenon affecting between 15 and 20 per cent of the adult population in most communities [26, 36, 47].

The prognosis of arterial hypertension

Based on a careful epidemiological survey (The Framingham Study), Kannel, Schwartz and McNamara [25] concluded that '. . . few conditions so easily detected and readily controlled are more potent than arterial hypertension as a menace to health'. Life expectancy in both men and women is decreased in the presence of raised arterial pressure. The incidence of morbid events related to this high arterial pressure is almost three times as high in untreated hypertensive patients with modestly raised arterial diastolic pressures as in the treated patients with nearly normal arterial pressure [58, 59]. Reduction of elevated arterial pressure prevents the development of the cardiovascular lesions and their manifestations such as stroke, congestive heart failure, renal insufficiency and coronary artery disease. Even when therapy is instituted at a late stage, subsequent morbidity and mortality are significantly reduced. While evidence of the value of antihypertensive therapy in malignant hypertension has been amply demonstrated since the late 1950s, the effectiveness of antihypertensive therapy in reducing the morbidity and mortality associated with lesser degrees of hypertension has been disputed. However, the recent results of the studies carried out by the Veterans Administration Co-operative Study Group on antihypertensive agents [57, 58] have indicated that antihypertensive therapy exerted a significant beneficial effect not only in severe hypertension (diastolic pressures between 115 and 129 mmHg) but also in moderate hypertension (diastolic pressures between 90 and 114 mmHg). Treatment of hypertension has been shown to be more effective in reducing the incidence of congestive heart failure and of stroke than in preventing the complications related to coronary artery disease, confirming the conclusions of Hodge and Smirk [22]. Despite the findings of these and other surveys, the impact of antihypertensive therapy on the course of medical management has been by no means universal. Kaplan [26] concluded that between 20 and 60 per cent of the patients with hypertension did not know of their condition; of those who knew, about one in three were receiving therapy, and fewer than one in five were under good blood pressure control.

The haemodynamic basis of high arterial pressure

The overall systemic resistance cannot be measured directly and is no more than a convenient way of describing the ratio of mean arterial pressure to the mean blood flow or cardiac output. Nevertheless, this ratio represents the main criterion by which patients with most forms of high arterial pressure can be differentiated from those with normal pressures. It has been widely established that patients with essential hypertension have cardiac outputs at rest which do not differ significantly from those of patients with normal arterial pressures. Based on their re-examination of the haemodynamics of hypertension, Frohlich, Tarazi and Dustan [14] suggested that previous investigators had not differentiated sufficiently between patients with essential and other forms of hypertension, and had not differentiated between patients with or without cardiac hypertrophy. They found that in patients with untreated essential hypertension, cardiac hypertrophy was associated with a lower than normal cardiac output. Patients with hypertension of renovascular origin had higher cardiac output than normal, whereas patients with hypertension associated with renal parenchymal disease had normal cardiac output. Patients with primary hyperaldosteronism (Conn's syndrome) have significantly higher cardiac output than matched patients with essential hypertension of a comparable degree, and a similar hyperdynamic state to that of Conn's syndrome, though undoubtedly one of different origin, has been described in patients with labile hypertension. While systemic vascular resistance at rest may be normal in patients with labile hypertension, their values during exercise are significantly higher than those of normotensive subjects, indicating that they have some abnormality of peripheral vasculature which does not allow the normal degree of arterial dilatation during exercise. The nature of the peripheral lesion which causes an increased flow resistance in hypertension has recently received considerable attention since the role of the impedance to left ventricular injection has been clarified as an important determinant of left ventricular performance. In patients with hypertension, the systemic vascular resistance is raised because of increased flow resistance in peripheral arterioles, whereas the major changes in the pulse wave in hypertension are due to changes in aortic impedance reflecting the decreased vascular distensibility secondary to degeneration of the vessel walls. The relationship between flow resistance in peripheral arteriolar segments, and the 'tone' or smooth muscle shortening of these vessels is important in the understanding of the basic abnormality of the blood vessels in hypertensive

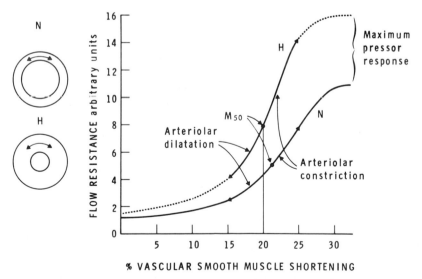

Fig. 2.1. Vascular reactivity explained in terms of flow resistance through arterioles as a function of their calibre and muscle 'tone' or degree of smooth muscle shortening. The cross-sectional representations on the left, of arterioles from normotensive (N) and hypertensive (H) subjects, indicate that for a given external diameter of vessel, the internal diameter of hypertensive vessels is less than that of vessels from normotensive subjects, thus at any given degree of smooth muscle shortening the flow resistance in hypertensive vessels is greater. Stimuli causing vasoconstriction or dilatation will induce greater changes of resistance to blood flow in blood vessels of hypertensive patients than in those of normotensive patients, and will cause correspondingly greater changes of blood pressure in either direction. (After Folkow 1971; with permission of *Clinical Science*.)

patients, and of the effects of drugs and anaesthetics on such vessels. For years it has been believed that the blood vessels of hypertensive patients are hyper-reactive, because these patients develop greater changes in arterial pressure in response to drug and reflex stimulation than do patients with normal blood pressures. However, it is now appreciated from the work of Folkow and his colleagues [13] that such hyper-reactivity is not due to increased sensitivity of the vascular smooth muscle to neurotransmitter. Folkow has developed the concept that the high vascular resistance in hypertensive patients is due to thickening or adaptive hypertrophy of the arterial media to such an extent that the luminar diameter of arterioles is reduced without alteration of the resting length of vascular smooth muscle. Thus the high flow resistance is the result of decreased vessel calibre, not due to abnormal vasoconstriction, but due to medial thickening. This implies that when arterioles of hypertensive patients are maximally vasodilated the resistance they offer to blood flow is greater than that of their normotensive counterpart, yet retaining a complete range of vasodilatation/vasoconstriction within the confines of a different flow resistance/smooth muscle shortening relationship as shown in Fig. 2.1. The importance of this relationship lies in the more marked response to any stimulus which causes dilatation or constriction of such vessels in patients with high blood pressure, which has been termed 'hyper-reactivity' in the past. The enhanced effects of sympathetic nerve stimulation, or of catecholamine infusions, changes in transmural pressure, changes in carbon dioxide or oxygen levels in the perfusing blood, and the effects of many drugs, can therefore be attributed to the higher slope of the resistance/shortening relationship in the patients with high blood pressure.

Effects of high arterial pressure on the heart

The end result of sustained high arterial pressure on the heart is left ventricular failure. This well-documented complication may arise by one of two main mechanisms (Fig. 2.2). In order to maintain cardiac output in the face of a persistently raised systemic vascular resistance, the left ventricular muscle must develop very high wall tensions during systole. Thus myocardial work and oxygen uptake are both increased, to a greater extent than if the cardiac output were increased in the face of a normal or low systemic vascular resistance. Persistently raised myocardial wall tension leads to hypertrophy of the muscle and demands increased coronary blood flow to support the increased myocardial oxygen uptake. The development of coronary atherosclerosis [23] seriously impairs the availability of blood flow to certain areas of myocardium, especially to the subendocardial layer where the increase in wall tension and myocardial oxygen uptake is greatest [24]. Myocardial ischaemia may lead indirectly to left ventricular failure, either due to loss of functioning muscle secondary to infarction, or due to dysrhythmia, which may be due to hypoxic muscle or to impaired blood flow to the normal pacemaking cells.

The left ventricle adapts to the increased load presented by the high systemic vascular resistance by hypertrophy of the muscle. As the ventricular wall becomes thickened, its diastolic distensibility decreases and thus a given end-diastolic length of the ventricular myofibrils can be attained only at a higher filling pressure. The function (Frank-Starling) curve of the left ventricle is displaced to the right of that of a normotensive individual. Thus under normal conditions, the hypertensive patient can maintain a normal stroke volume and cardiac output in the face of a chronically increased systemic vascular resistance only by maintaining a high left ventricular end-diastolic pressure (8–15 mmHg) by comparison with his normotensive counterpart (4–8 mmHg).

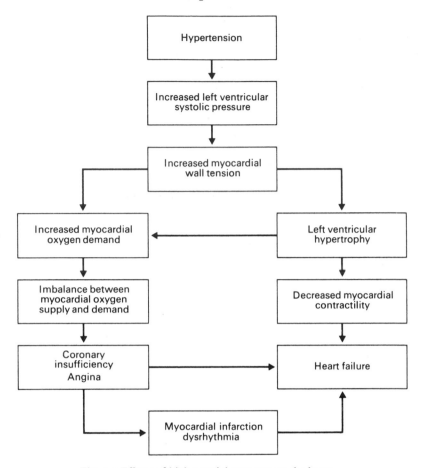

Fig. 2.2 Effects of high arterial pressure on the heart.

Acute increases of systemic vascular resistance, induced either by increased sympathetic nervous activity or by vasoconstrictor drugs, impose a much greater load on the hypertrophied muscle. If these are sustained, a state of chronic left ventricular failure ensues, with decreased cardiac output despite elevated left ventricular end-diastolic pressures. Where coronary artery disease is associated with the development of left ventricular failure, subendocardial ischaemia caused by the high diastolic intracavitary pressure (see later section) contributes to the impairment of left ventricular performance.

The renin-angiotensin-aldosterone system (RAS)

This is an important part of the renal mechanism for regulation of arterial pressure, sodium balance and the volume of the extra-cellular space. Together with the antidiuretic hormone system, the RAS constitutes the single feedback mechanism having a long enough time-constant to be effective as a regulator of major perturbations of arterial pressure [52]. The RAS is the major feedback system which prevents the development of structural adaptation to high arterial pressure by regulating those factors tending to cause the persistent high arterial pressure. Thus disordered function of the RAS may play a major part in the development of primary hypertension.

The activity of the enzyme renin in producing Angiotension I and the conversion of the latter to Angiotension II in the lung, and the pressor activity of Angiotensin II, are all modified by the state of sodium balance of the patient. The pressor effect of Angiotensin II is enhanced by sodium loading, and impaired by sodium depletion [52]. Plasma renin activity (measured in terms of the amount of Angiotensin II produced) is usually increased in patients with hypertension of renovascular or renal parenchymal origin, and the increased activity of Angiotensin II can be observed as a decrease of arterial pressure in response to a specific Angiotensin II inhibitor: Sar^1-ala^8-angiotensin II (Saralasin).

A high proportion of patients with accelerated or malignant hypertension show increased PRA, but only a small percentage of patients with primary hypertension (10–15 per cent) can be shown to have elevated PRA values [52].

We may therefore summarize that the main features of hypertensive heart disease which may directly influence the administration of anaesthesia to these patients, are:

1 their altered vascular reactivity to drugs, which is due to the altered flow resistance/smooth muscle shortening relationship in the arterioles of hypertensive patients. This is of much greater significance than drug interactions in the causation of hypertensive and hypotensive responses during anaesthesia and surgery;

2 the pre-existence of atheromatous arterial disease, especially involving the coronary and cerebral vessels, pre-disposing the hypertensive patient to myocardial ischaemia and cerebral ischaemia as potential problems during induction, maintenance and recovery from anaesthesia;

3 left ventricular hypertrophy with the attendant consequence of acute or chronic left ventricular failure;

4 renal dysfunction associated with impaired renal perfusion, sometimes associated with dysfunction of the renin–angiotensin–aldosterone system.

DRUG MANAGEMENT OF HYPERTENSION

The therapeutic use of drugs which exert a hypotensive effect is empirically based and does not usually aim to treat the cause of the hypertension. Nevertheless the overall success of therapy has been considerable, and has contributed to the reduction in mortality in patients with high arterial pressure. Drugs used in the management of hypertension fall into five broad categories.

1 General sedatives and tranquillizers
2 Diuretics
3 Drugs which specifically interfere with some aspect of adrenergic neuronal transmission
   (a) by actions on the central nervous system
   (b) by inhibitory actions at adrenergic nerve terminals
   (c) by competitive antagonism of adrenergic transmitters at alpha and beta receptor sites
   (d) by competitive inhibition at autonomic ganglia
4 Drugs acting directly on vascular smooth muscle
5 Drugs acting to inhibit the function of the renin–angiotensin–aldosterone system

The possibilities for drug interaction, both in the course of antihypertensive therapy and during the course of anaesthesia, are considerable. The following review of the pharmacology of antihypertensive therapy emphasizes those aspects of special interest to the anaesthetist.

General sedatives and tranquillizers

Many patients with hypertension receive drugs whose actions are primarily designed to decrease anxiety, and to slow down their general activity. While most of these drugs cannot be considered to be specific antihypertensive agents, their pharmacological actions may under conditions of anaesthesia be additive or synergistic with those of the specific antihypertensive agents, and the drugs in the maintenance of anaesthesia. The commonly used drugs in this category are barbiturates, phenothiazines and benzodiazepines. Rauwolfia alkaloids, and methyldopa, also have powerful sedative effects in addition to their antihypertensive action, but may cause severe depression.

Diuretics

The combination of a diuretic with other antihypertensive agents has greatly simplified the management of hypertensive patients enabling a reduction to be made in the dosage of potent agents which decrease adrenergic vasometer activity. It is estimated that diuretics, either alone or in combination with other drugs, are used in approximately 70 per cent of treated hypertensive patients.

The hypotensive mechanism of action of the diuretics is still controversial but most of the evidence favours a predominant effect related to natriuresis, although reduced systemic vascular resistance and volume depletion contribute a time-dependent effect. In the early stages of diuretic therapy the depletion of blood volume predominates, whereas with prolonged therapy a sustained decrease of systemic vascular resistance can be observed [48].

Diuretics may conveniently be divided into those which encourage excretion of potassium (benzothiadiazide derivatives, chlorthalidone, frusemide, bumetanide and ethacrynic acid) and those which have an action on the distal convoluted tubule (spironolactone, amiloride, triamterene which are potassium sparing. The degree to which the proximally acting drugs decrease the plasma potassium concentration varies according to whether the patients have pre-existing oedema, the cause of their hypertension, and whether there is renal insufficiency. Potassium supplementation by means of slow release potassium chloride preparations is widely used to ameliorate the potassium loss induced by many of the thiazide diuretics. The anaesthetist should always check the plasma potassium concentrations of any patient on diuretic therapy before embarking on anaesthesia for major surgery. A plasma concentration below $3 \cdot 5$ mmol l^{-1} should be regarded as potentially dangerous, and a specific contra-indication to artificial ventilation to a degree which may decrease the Pa,co_2 below 30 mmHg. This degree of alkalosis may enhance a hypokalaemic state in a patient with a low plasma potassium concentration [9].

Benzothiadiazide diuretics. These have direct effects in increasing the renal excretion of sodium and chloride ions unrelated to carbonic anhydrase inactivation, and these drugs initially decrease extracellular fluid and plasma volumes, cardiac output and exchangeable sodium and potassium in hypertensive patients. After several months of therapy, plasma volume and total body water and sodium levels return towards normal, whereas systemic vascular resistance remains reduced.

Diazoxide is a thiazide derivative closely related to chlorothiazide, which when administered intravenously causes a rapid fall of blood pressure related to a marked decrease in systemic vascular resistance and an increase in cardiac output. This agent is largely used for the acute control of malignant hypertension. Patients receiving thiazide diuretics usually receive a supplement of potassium given as a slow-release capsule. It is important to assess the serum potassium levels in patients receiving long term diuretic therapy as hypokalaemia is one of the main problems in these patients.

Furosemide acts directly on the renal tubule inhibiting sodium reabsorption in the ascending loop of Henle and causing a simultaneous loss of chloride and some potassium.

Sprinolactone is a competitive antagonist of aldosterone used in the treatment of hypertension in order to decrease the potassium loss secondary to the use of thiazide diuretics. In renal hypertension, aldosterone secretion increases as a result of the high plasma renin activity, and spironolactone is frequently used to reduce the high level of sodium retention in these patients. Spironolactone is specifically indicated in the initial therapy of patients with primary hyperaldosteronism (Conn's Syndrome), and those patients who have secondary hyperaldosteronism related to renal hypertension.

Amiloride, Triamterene. These drugs block the exchange of sodium for potassium in the distal convoluted tubule and can cause hyperkalaemia [48], and their combination with proximal tubule diuretics can cause complex problems in patients with renal insufficiency.

Drugs acting to decrease adrenergic vasomotor activity

Rauwolfia alkaloids. Extracts of the whole root of rauwolfia *serpentina* have been used since ancient times in Hindu medicine for the treatment of a wide variety of conditions including hypertension.

Reserpine is the prototype of purified rauwolfia alkaloids, and was until recently one of the commonest drugs used in antihypertensive therapy. The cardiovascular effects of reserpine are primarily related to its action in depleting stores of catecholamines and of 5-hydroxytryptamine in brain, heart, blood vessels and adrenal medulla. The effects of reserpine are complex and involve at least three mechanisms. Reserpine competitively antagonizes the uptake of noradrenaline into chromaffin granules in adrenergic nerve endings, and inhibits noradrenaline synthesis as it blocks the uptake of dopamine by the storage granules which contain the hydroxylating enzymes. The clinical effects of reserpine doses of 0.25 to 0.5 mg per day are unlikely to be entirely related to catecholamine depletion; significant impairment of adrenergic nerve function does not occur until catecholamine stores are reduced at least to 30 per cent below normal levels. Cardiovascular reflexes are only slightly inhibited by reserpine in man. The effects of reserpine and similar drugs are cumulative and following withdrawal tissue catecholamine levels are restored slowly over a period of two to three weeks.

Methyldopa. This drug is a powerful inhibitor of the enzyme dopa decarboxylase which is involved in the synthesis of adrenaline and noradrenaline from tyrosine, and which specifically catalyses the conversion of dopa to dopamine. Methyldopa reduces tissue concentrations of dopamine and noradrenaline in the central nervous system, in most peripheral tissues, but not in the adrenal medulla. Dopamine is replaced in the tissues by α-methyl dopamine and noradrenaline is replaced by α-methyl noradrenaline, the latter being released by nerve stimulation and by indirectly acting sympathomimetic amines, thus satisfying the criteria for a 'false transmitter'. The mode of action of methyldopa is commonly ascribed to its effect in generating such a false transmitter, but the pressor activity of α-methyl noradrenaline is only slightly less than that of noradrenaline, and this false transmitter is readily released to adrenergic nerve terminals. Furthermore, the tissue concentration of α-methyl noradrenaline declines more slowly than the hypotensive effect after withdrawal of methyldopa therapy. Current opinion regards the central nervous effects of methyldopa [30] (cf. those of clonidine) as being the main mechanism in reducing blood pressure. Methyldopa oral doses of 250 mg to 3 g daily, are usually given in three or four divided doses. This dose range does not greatly inhibit cardiovascular reflexes and the hypotensive effect is due to reduction of both cardiac output and of systemic vascular resistance.

Adrenergic neurone blockers derived from guanidine

Guanethidine may be regarded as the prototype of this series, of which bethanidine, debrisoquine, guanclor, guancydine are the analogues. The membrane pump in adrenergic neurone terminals, which terminates the action of noradrenaline by causing its uptake into storage granules, is a promiscuous one which is also capable of taking up guanidine analogues. The uptake of noradrenaline into granules is inhibited by concentration of guanidine drugs at this site, causing a progressive depletion of noradrenaline in these stores and a decreased release of noradrenaline in response to adrenergic nerve stimulation. Guanethidine, bethanidine and debrisoquine are taken up into cardiac muscle cells against a concentration gradient, and their effects both in the heart and other tissues are antagonized by tricyclic antidepressant drugs which competitively inhibit the uptake of the guanidine compounds.

Guanethidine is one of the more popular guanidine derivatives, normally administered orally in doses of 10 to 100 mg per day. It has a long duration of action and the effects of a constant dose may increase over a period of weeks. Systemic vascular resistance progressively falls with chronic administration, and when a persistent hypotensive action has been achieved, vascular reflexes are depressed, and the ability of the myocardium to respond to stress is said to be depressed.

Bethanidine has been extensively used in the management of hypertension since 1963, and has a more rapid onset (1–2 hours), and a shorter duration of action (1–12 hours) than guanethidine. It causes as much postural hypotension as guanethidine but does not exert an initial sympathomimetic effect.

Debrisoquine, and other guanethidine derivatives have actions similar to those of guanethidine and bethanidine.

Competitive antagonists of adrenergic transmission at α and β receptors

The concept that two types of cellular receptive sites exist, which respond to stimulation by sympathomimetic amines, was introduced by Ahlquist [1]. Ahlquist's differentiation of α- and β-receptors was based on the observation that two types of response to sympathomimetic drugs could be ascribed according to different *rank orders of potency* of these drugs at various sites in the mammalian body. He defined α-receptors as those whose response to adrenaline > noradrenaline > phenylephrine > isoprenaline, whereas β-receptors were defined as those whose response to isoprenaline > adrenaline > noradrenaline > phenylephrine. While no major counter proposals to Ahlquist's schema have developed, further developments in the classification of β-receptors have occurred.

Adrenergic α-receptor blocking agents

These agents are not widely used in the treatment of hypertension since β-adrenergic receptors are not blocked and reflex tachycardia in response to falling blood pressure is undesirable. Two adrenergic α-receptor blockers may be useful in the management of patients with phaeochromocytoma.

Phenoxybenzamine is a haloalkylamine which produces a type of competitive blockade at α-receptors known as a nonequilibrium blockade, because stable attachment of phenoxybenzamine to the receptor site precludes the mass-action equilibrium between agonist and antagonist which is characteristic of true competitive blockade.

Phentolamine is an imidazoline compound exerting a true competitive blockade of α-receptors, and has a rapid onset and short duration of action.

Adrenergic β-receptor antagonists

These drugs have become widely popular in the management of patients with high blood pressure, angina pectoris and other manifestations of ischaemic heart disease. A β-receptor antagonist is defined as a competitive specific antagonist at any β-receptor site; that is, it moves the dose-response curve for agonist/antagonist interaction to the right without altering its slope. This relationship emphasizes that there is no such state as complete irreversible β-receptor blockade and that an increase in the dose of the agonist (e.g. isoprenaline) will induce an appropriate response.

In addition to their specific antagonism at β-receptors, these drugs may exhibit some or all of the following characteristics [38]:

Tissue selectivity. They may exhibit a selectivity or specificity for one tissue or receptive site. Such specificity reflects that β-receptors antagonists exhibit different *rank orders of potency* at any specific receptive site and for any agonist. For instance propranolol is approximately twice as specific for peripheral β_2 receptors (e.g. bronchial smooth muscle, uterine muscle, vascular smooth muscle) as it is for cardiac receptors, whereas practolol is about 100 times less effective in blocking these β_2 receptors than the cardiac β_1 receptors.

Intrinsic sympathomimetic activity. In addition to occupying receptors and causing competitive antagonism, some of these drugs also act as partial agonists, and are described as having intrinsic sympathomimetic activity.

Local anaesthetic activity. Many but not all β-receptor antagonists are capable of acting as local anaesthetics when applied to surface membranes or intact nerves. It has been clearly established that this local anaesthetic activity is quite independent of their β-receptor antagonism. Associated with this membrane stabilizing activity are other actions on excitable tissues in the heart, causing increased A-V conduction time and direct impairment of the intrinsic myocardial contractile state. It must be emphasized that these effects become important only when large doses of β-receptor antagonists are used, and that in most clinical situations where doses of propranolol of less than 500 mg per day are being administered, it is most unlikely that any direct impairment of myocardial contractility will occur. However, with patients being treated with up to 2 g of propranolol per day, it is possible that this action related to local anaesthetic activity may be of importance [40].

A number of drugs which also exert local anaesthetic effects on surface membranes and nerves (quinidine, diphenylhydantoin, procainamide, lignocaine) also exhibit characteristic effects on the voltage/time relationships of intracellularly recorded potentials in automatic and other excitable tissues in the heart. By altering the maximum rate of depolarization of pacemaker and cardiac muscle cells, these effectively increase the refractory period and decrease the tendency of the cell to undergo either spontaneous or propagated depolarization. This is the basic mechanism underlying the antidysrhythmic activity of drugs 'quinidine-like' properties.

β-receptor antagonists in the treatment of hypertension

Although β-receptor antagonists have been used empirically in the management of hypertension, the mechanism of their antihypertensive actions is complex and the influence of the varied mechanisms differs according to the many types of hypertension. The following mechanisms have been proposed to explain the hypotensive actions of the many β-receptor antagonists which are clinically available.

1 β-receptor blockade—causing a <u>decrease of cardiac output, heart rate and myocardial contractility</u>
2 <u>Suppression of renin</u> activity
3 Suppression of <u>central nervous sympathetic activity</u> by a specific β-receptor antagonism

Choice of β-receptor antagonist in the treatment of hypertension is now determined largely by the fact that most β-receptor antagonists are equi-effective as hypotensive agents, and are as potent as other antihypertensive medications, though the side-effects are less important. The dose range for most agents is now considered to be fairly narrow and the dose-response above a given limit is relatively flat [30]. Thus for propranolol or oxprenolol (non-cardioselective) the daily dose lies between 80 and 320 mg per day, whereas atenolol (cardioselective, having no local anaesthetic or partial agonist activity) can be given in a single daily dose of 50–100 mg. Pre-existing disease or other unpredictable side-effects may also determine the choice of β-receptor antagonist. Cardioselective antagonists should be used in patients with asthma or chronic obstructive airways disease, in diabetics, and in patients who exhibit Raynaud's phenomenon or evidence of peripheral limb ischaemia [30]. Very large doses of β-receptor antagonists have been used in patients with refractory hypertension, but this regime has been largely superseded by combination therapies.

Labetalol. This agent has <u>strong β-receptor and weak α-receptor antagonistic properties</u>, and has been widely used in the treatment of hypertension [37]. Unlike previous <u>attempts</u> to combine α- and β-receptor blocking properties, labetalol therapy is not associated with an unacceptable degree of postural hypotension.

Drugs acting directly on <u>arterial smooth muscle</u>

Hydrallazine. In common with other phthalazine derivatives, hydrallazine causes a reduction of arterial pressure by a <u>direct action on vascular smooth muscle</u>, especially that of <u>renal arterioles</u>. The fall in arterial pressure associated with hydrallazine therapy is accompanied by an <u>increase in heart rate</u>, reflexly induced through barostatic mechanisms, though hydrallazine does appear to have a minor effect on the central nervous system to induce tachycardia. It is now common to find patients with hypertension of renal origin treated with a combination of hydrallazine and β-receptor blockers. Hydrallazine is particularly useful in the acute management of accelerated hypertension, and for the management of <u>acute hypertension arising in the post-operative period.</u> For these purposes it may be administered either intramuscularly or intravenously in doses of 5–10 mg at a time.

Prazosin. This drug has recently been introduced as an antihypertensive agent having a <u>direct effect of relaxation of vascular smooth muscle.</u> In this respect its effects are similar to those of hydrallazine and the drugs may be used in combination with β-receptor blockers in patients with renal vascular disease. Recent evidence shows prazosin to also have α-blocking effects. The average dose is between 3 and 7·5 mg per day.

Minoxidil. This potent long-acting oral vasodilator has found a limited place in the management of hypertension, particularly in those patients with refractory hypertension, with severely impaired and deteriorating renal function. Hypertrichosis is very common; the combination of tachycardia and fluid retention usually requires the careful titration of a diuretic and a β-receptor antagonist to achieve the best results with this drug.

Sodium nitroprusside is generally used in the acute management of malignant hypertension or hypertension occurring in the postoperative period. It is administered by continuous intravenous infusion of a solution of 0·01 per cent sodium nitroprusside.

Drugs acting on the <u>central nervous system</u>

Clonidine. Clonidine is an imidazoline derivative which exerts an antihypertensive effect by <u>reduction of heart rate and cardiac output.</u> Its site of action is predominately in the <u>central nervous system</u> though peripheral vascular effects have also been demonstrated. Unlike most other antihypertensive agents, sudden withdrawal of clonidine therapy may be associated with <u>overshoot</u> of blood pressure associated with other withdrawal symptoms such as restlessness, tremor, headaches and nausea [30, 41]. These effects may be relieved by administration of propranolol and phentolamine to provide combined α- and β-receptor blockade, or by intravenous or intramuscular administration of clonidine. An acute episode of rebound hypertension can be rapidly controlled by the use of an infusion of sodium nitroprusside.

ANAESTHESIA AND THE HYPERTENSIVE PATIENT

The attitudes of anaesthetists to hypertensive patients have changed very considerably over the past four decades. Up to 1930, hypertension and ischaemic heart disease were regarded as strong contraindications to general anaesthesia and surgery, and the inherent mortality during and after operation was very high. In the thirties, the surgical management of hypertension was in its heyday, and the standard of anaesthesia for these procedures was associated with a remarkably low mortality in the centres where such surgery was performed. With the advent of antihypertensive drug therapy, anaesthetists began to express concern about the disturbance of circulatory homeostasis in hypertensive patients during anaesthesia and surgery [8, 11, 21, 36]. The initial concern about the possible interactions between rauwolfia alkaloids and anaesthesia was extended with the advent of more potent antihypertensive agents, and more recently a controversy has centred around possible interactions between β-receptor blockers and anaesthesia [38]. Most adverse effects due to drug interaction between antihypertensive and anaesthetic agents can be predicted and thus prevented to a large extent by consideration of their appropriate pharmacological properties. Studies of anaesthesia in hypertensive patients have made it increasingly clear that the main problem in these patients is the association of hypertension with either ischaemic heart disease or cerebral vascular disease, rather than pharmacological interaction between antihypertensive drugs and anaesthetic agent. Because of the cardiovascular instability observed in untreated hypertensive patients, and the increased risk of cardiovascular accidents in these patients, effective antihypertensive therapy has been recommended before elective surgery is contemplated [11, 41].

There has been recent controversy [39] concerning the management of the patient who is found to be hypertensive before anaesthesia and surgery. A recent study [18], of patients with mild untreated hypertension (diastolic pressure < 110 mmHg) or well controlled hypertension, concluded that such patients were at no greater risk during anaesthesia and surgery than were normotensive control patients. This contrasts with evidence that patients with severe untreated hypertension (diastolic pressure > 120 mmHg) are at substantially greater risk of developing myocardial ischaemia than their normotensive counterparts [43, 44, 45]. It would seem prudent to delay anaesthesia and elective major surgery in patients with severe hypertension defined as a sustained diastolic pressure greater than 110 mmHg, although such a decision clearly cannot be a generalization. Each patient should be assessed independently taking account of the duration and severity of the hypertension, the existence of signs or symptoms of left ventricular hypertrophy or failure, or of myocardial ischaemia, and the scope of the projected surgery. Perhaps the most important considerations should be the experience of the anaesthetist and the availability of adequate monitoring and postoperative intensive care facility.

Pre-existing antihypertensive drug therapy should be maintained up to and including the morning (or afternoon) of surgery, and provision should be made for adequate therapy to be maintained throughout the postoperative period. Existing therapy should certainly not be withheld because the patient's blood pressure is found to be normal in the preoperative period.

In dealing with the hypertensive patient, the anaesthetist must bear in mind, not only those aspects of the pathophysiology and treatment of the condition but also the predictable behaviour of hypertensive patients during anaesthesia and surgery [43, 45]. To this end, the problems encountered during anaesthesia may be considered under the following headings:

1   Excessive hypotension in response to what might be considered a reasonable dose of an induction agent (barbiturate, steroid or eugenol derivative). This response is usually a reflection of the greater degree of arteriolar dilatation induced in hypertensive patients whose blood vessels behave according to Fig. 2.1. Hypertensive patients treated with drugs which decrease arterial pressure by causing arterial dilatation do not become normal in terms of their vascular reactivity. Such patients show responses which are characteristic of the untreated hypertensive patient [44], thus their responses can still be typified by line H in Fig. 2.1. The effect of antihypertensive therapy is to reduce their arteriolar flow resistance to a normal value (approximately 5 units in Fig. 2.1) by decreasing the percentage vascular smooth muscle shortening. In response to a constrictor stimulus, the flow resistance increases according to curve H rather than curve N. Thus the pressure responses to a constrictor stimulus are still

exaggerated in a similar way to those observed in untreated hypertensive patients [44]. For these reasons, hypertensive patients should be given drugs slowly and in reduced dosage, anticipating such effects. The author's present preference is to induce anaesthesia in these patients with fentanyl (300–500 μg), given in divided doses over a period of 5 minutes, while the inhaled gas mixture is changed from 100 per cent oxygen to 50 per cent nitrous oxide and 50 per cent oxygen after 2–3 minutes. A very small dose of an induction agent (thiopentone 50–75 mg; Althesin 12–15 mg) may then be used to hasten the loss of consciousness without the risk of precipitate hypotension.

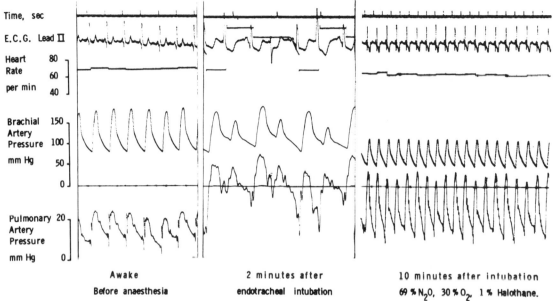

Fig. 2.3. Bidirectional junctional tachycardia and hypertension following laryngoscopy and intubation in a treated hypertensive patient. Myocardial ischaemia, indicated by ST segment depression and T wave inversion (right-hand panel), persisted during the subsequent maintenance anaesthesia despite the cessation of dysrhythmia. (From Prys-Roberts, Greene, Meloche & Foëx 1971; with permission of the *British Journal of Anaesthesia*.)

2   Excessive hypertension, tachycardia, cardiac dysrhythmia and evidence of myocardial ischaemia during and following endotracheal intubation (Fig. 2.3) and certain surgical stimuli, are perhaps the main cause for concern on the part of the anaesthetist [44]. These responses represent an exaggeration of what occurs in most healthy patients, and while there is little evidence that transient hypertension *per se* is likely to cause permanent injury, it is the associated evidence of myocardial ischaemia which gives the greatest cause for concern. Whatever the stimulus, tachycardia and hypertension are associated with a sudden increase in myocardial wall tension and work and consequently of myocardial oxygen uptake. If the condition of the coronary circulation is such as to allow a major increase in blood flow with appropriate distribution to all areas of the myocardium, then it is probable that no harm will arise in these circumstances. However, for the patient with coronary artery disease, whether or not related to or caused by hypertension, such an increase in myocardial oxygen demand may not be adequately met and the electrocardiographic evidence of ischaemia will commonly ensue. While these responses are certainly attenuated by deep anaesthesia or by thorough topical anaesthesia, they are by no means stopped; with deep anaesthesia

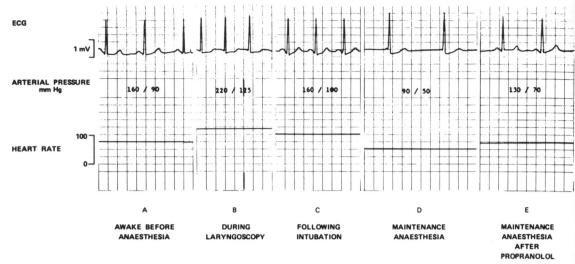

Fig. 2.4. Myocardial ischaemia related to fast and slow junctional dysrhythmia in a treated hypertensive patient. Following laryngoscopy and intubation (Panels B and C) a junctional tachycardia was associated with severe hypertension and led to marked ST segment depression which slowly resolved as heart rate and blood pressure returned towards normal levels and normal sinus rhythm was re-established. During maintenance anaesthesia (nitrous oxide, enflurane (1·2 per cent inspired) and oxygen: Panel D) a slow A-V junctional rhythm became established causing a marked reduction of arterial pressure which led to further ST segment depression. Following 2·5 mg propranolol i.v., normal sinus rhythm with an acceptable arterial pressure was sustained for the duration of the anaesthesia and surgery, and was not associated with further evidence of myocardial ischaemia.

there is a greater incidence of ischaemia due to hypotension associated with junctional rhythm (Fig. 2.4).

Pretreatment with a β-receptor blocking drug has been shown to be very effective in attenuating the responses to endotracheal intubation [42], and maintenance of pre-existing β-receptor blockade in patients with either hypertension or ischaemic heart disease is to be recommended [40, 41].

3   Recent advances [24] in understanding the morphology and functioning of the coronary vasculature have given prominence to the role of the subendocardial collateral network (Fig. 2.5). This collateral system becomes of great importance to the patient whose epicardial or intramural coronary arteries may be occluded by atheromatous disease. The subendocardium is the region of the myocardium where wall tension during contraction is highest; this region also has the lowest Po_2 of any organ of the body and also has the highest oxygen uptake. Where intramural vessels are occluded, the subendocardial collateral system distributes blood flow to the occluded area, but this system may also be subject to occlusion by high intracavitary left ventricular diastolic pressures. Such high pressures usually occur when the left ventricle is in a state of acute failure as a result of an increase in systemic vascular resistance, a situation which is particularly common in the patient with severe hypertension. In such patients, monitoring by a Swan-Ganz balloon catheter in the pulmonary artery can give a good indication of sudden increases in left ventricular and atrial pressures [27, 53], and allow steps to be taken to reduce the ventricular afterload [49].

4   Problems may arise due to induction and maintenance of anaesthesia in patients

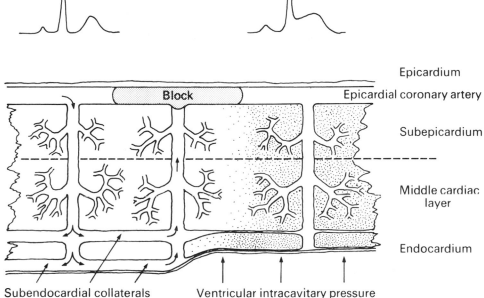

Epicardium

Epicardial coronary artery

Subepicardium

Middle cardiac layer

Endocardium

Subendocardial collaterals   Ventricular intracavitary pressure

Fig. 2.5. Subendocardial collateral system and its importance in ischaemic heart disease. The diagram represents the cross-section of the ventricular myocardium, showing the branching and perforating subsidiaries from the main epicardial coronary artery. The only collateral circulation occurs in the subendocardial region, and becomes of considerable importance when atherosclerosis affects the epicardial vessel to cause a block. The subendocardial collateral vessels are thin-walled and in a state of chronic dilatation due to the low Po_2 of surrounding tissue. They are susceptible to compression by high diastolic intracavitary pressures within the ventricle, leading to subendocardial ischaemia (dotted area) and the corresponding ST segment depression or elevation depending on the ECG lead placement. (Modified from Holsinger & Eliot 1972; with the permission of *Heart and Lung*.)

with hypokalaemia secondary to prolonged diuretic therapy. Hypokalaemia is less likely to occur in the future due to the increasing use of either spironolactone or potassium supplements with diuretics, but in any case it should be recognized and averted by preoperative assessment of the patient's electrolyte status. Hyperventilation which decreases the Pa,co_2 to less than 30 mmHg should be avoided to prevent excessive hypokalaemia [10].

A similar problem may be encountered in patients with renal hypertension who have undergone a recent period of haemodialysis. The author has observed a number of such patients who, despite an acceptable response to induction of anaesthesia, have demonstrated a progressive reduction of both arterial and central venous pressure during the first 15–20 mintues of maintenance anaesthesia. Up to two litres of fluid may be needed to restore both central venous and pulmonary arterial 'wedge' pressures and arterial pressures.

5 During maintenance anaesthesia the commonest cause of acute arterial hypotension is a transition from sinus to A-V junctional rhythm (Fig. 2.4) [41]. Junctional rhythm implies that atrial contraction occurs more or less simultaneously with ventricular contraction, thus the atrial contribution to ventricular filling is lost. In the hypertensive patient who has decreased diastolic compliance secondary to muscle hypertrophy, the loss of the atrial kick is particularly important, and causes a marked decrease of cardiac output and arterial pressure. The resulting impairment of coronary

perfusion may lead to severe myocardial ischaemia. No consistently successful method for the restoration of junctional rhythm to sinus rhythm has been devised but a number of methods have been proposed

(*a*)   small doses of succinylcholine [15]
(*b*)   atropine (0·6 to 1·2 mg) to increase heart rate [40]
(*c*)   calcium chloride 250 mg to improve atrial fibre conduction [40]
(*d*) β-receptor antagonists [38, 42]
(*e*)   decrease concentration of any volatile hydrocarbon anaesthetics
(*f*)   resolve any existing hypocapnia and maintain Pa,CO_2 in the normal range [40, 43]

6   Rebound hypertension during recovery from anaesthesia is a troublesome complication in a few patients. If the diastolic pressure exceeds 110 mmHg, active therapy should be commenced using drugs which decrease arteriolar tone. Diazoxide or sodium nitroprusside may be used as continuous intravenous infusions, but a means of controlling the infusion and monitoring arterial pressure is essential. Hydrallazine is a very satisfactory alternative and can be given in 5–10 mg increments at 10-minute intervals until the desired reduction of arterial pressure is achieved. If there is severe systolic hypertension (250 mmHg), with or without tachycardia (>100 beats per minute), 10 mg labetalol or some other β-receptor antagonist should be given intravenously and repeated until control of systolic pressure and heart rate are achieved [41].

Maintenance of antihypertensive therapy into the postoperative period may be difficult if the patient is unable to absorb drugs by mouth. The combination of hydrallazine and labetalol is particularly effective in this respect as these drugs can be given as a continuous intravenous infusion. The dose can be estimated according to the bioavailability of the normal daily oral requirement [41].

7   Pressor agents, whether administered by the anaesthetist or surgeon, should be used with considerable caution in hypertensive patients. Patients receiving antihypertensive drugs which deplete noradrenaline storage at sympathetic nerve endings are particularly sensitive to the effects of exogenous noradrenaline or any other pressor agent having direct α-receptor stimulating properties. Infiltration of the surgical field with solutions containing adrenaline or noradrenaline should be discouraged.

ATHEROMATOUS VASCULAR DISEASE

Atheromatous arterial disease affecting segments other than the coronary circulation can exist separately or in association with hypertension. A patient with atheromatous disease in any part of his circulation must be considered to have generalized disease and in particular to be at risk from coronary atheromatous disease. Lack of symptoms of angina, or of a history of a previous myocardial infarct, does not preclude serious coronary atheromatous disease, nor the potential for episodes of myocardial ischaemia.

Carotid arterial disease

Atheroma of the extracranial carotid arterial system is a major cause (40–50 per cent) of cerebrovascular insufficiency which may manifest itself as a major stroke. More than 75 per cent of patients who develop strokes have warning symptoms in the form of transient ischaemic attacks (TIA) consisting of transient, often unilateral, blindness or fleeting focal neurological dysfunction lasting minutes or hours. Many patients present with symptomless bruits of the carotid arterial system.

The predominant lesion (91 per cent) associated with such events is an atheromatous plaque which occludes the internal carotid artery at the bifurcation of the common carotid artery. Similar symptoms may result from atheromatous occlusion of the common carotid arteries anywhere between their origins at the aortic arch or innominate artery and the bifurcation (7·5 per cent).

Diagnosis of the lesions has traditionally been based on selective carotid arteriography, which is an invasive, uncomfortable and potentially hazardous technique requiring hospital admission. Recent developments in the use of ultrasound have become more popular as means of identifying and quantifying the lesions of the carotid system. Either high-frequency (10 MHz) 'B' mode ultrasonic scanning, or a pulsed-Doppler scanner (MAVIS—Mobile Artery and Vein Image System) can be used in three orthogonal directions to give anterior-posterior, lateral and cross-sectional projections of the arteries. Using a duplex scanning system, the blood velocity can also be measured at range-gated sites in the arterial system (Fig. 2.6) to give a full range of information on the imaging and flow characteristics of a vascular occlusion.

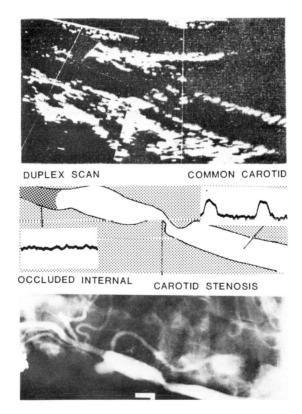

Fig. 2.6. Comparison of three methods for defining carotid arterial occlusion. The upper diagram shows a duplex ultrasonic scan in which a pulse-echo B-scan display is coupled with a range-gated 5 MHz Doppler flow-meter. The former gives the graphic display of the blood vessels and any occlusive formation while the latter (indicated by the vertical and horizontal thin white beams) makes it possible to measure the blood velocity pattern at the preselected site (insets in the centre panel). The ultrasonic displays are contrasted with the standard arteriogram display in the lower panel. (Courtesy of R. J. Lusby, FRACS, FRCS, Department of Surgery, University of Bristol.)

Carotid endarterectomy is the surgical procedure of choice in dealing with these atheromatous lesions [55], and carries a good prognosis of long-term success (70–94 per cent) and a low operative morbidity and mortality (1–4 per cent). Monitoring of general anaesthesia for carotid endarterectomy or carotid bypass grafting should include electroencephalography to identify episodes of cerebral ischaemia and to indicate the requirement for a Javed shunt. Reliance on measuring the internal carotid stump pressure above clamps occluding both the common and external carotid arteries, thus supposedly reflecting the perfusion pressure transmitted through the Circle of Willis, is at best arbitrary and takes no account of regional cerebral perfusion. It has been proposed that carotid endarterectomy should be performed under the influence of cervical plexus block so that the patient's consciousness and motor control may be used to identify unacceptable ischaemia [10].

Aorto-iliac disease

Patients with aorto-iliac and peripheral atheromatous disease in the femoral and popliteal arteries usually present with the symptom of intermittent claudication, either in the gluteal region or in the calves. Frequently these patients also present with peripheral ischaemia in the feet and with gangrenous changes. The advances in replacement of the atheromatous vessels with dacron grafts, autologous saphenous vein grafts or preserved umbilical vein grafts have meant a major increase of surgery in patients with concurrent hypertension or coronary artery disease. The risks associated with major surgery in these patients with severe cardiovascular disease are considerable, and a points scoring system such as that described by Goldman and colleagues [19] has greater merit in identifying specific risk factors than the older ASA system. Diagnostic arteriography under general anaesthesia can be a hazardous procedure and should not be treated lightly. Preoperative drug therapy should be maintained up to and including the day of the procedure and electrocardiographic monitoring (CM_5 or V_5 lead) should be standard [5].

Definitive surgery of aorto-iliac disease is often accompanied by major blood loss and direct measurement of arterial and central venous pressures should be standard in addition to the ECG. The use of a Swan-Ganz catheter to monitor pulmonary arterial and capillary wedge pressures should be considered in those patients with a history of left ventricular failure either secondary to coronary artery disease or to severe hypertension. Cross-clamping of the aorta during a graft procedure normally causes a marked but transient increase of arterial pressure as a result of the increase in systemic vascular resistance. This response is least marked in those patients with almost complete aortic occlusion, and most marked in those patients who have a small symptomless aneurysm. The increased impedance to left ventricular injection caused by aortic cross-clamping may provoke acute left ventricular failure in those patients with borderline failure secondary to severe hypertension.

Patients who suffer from severe coronary artery disease may show evidence of myocardial ischaemia during the period of aortic cross-clamping [4, 33]. In either case the solution to the problem is to unload the ventricle by producing arteriolar dilatation, in that part of the arterial circulation system which is above the aortic clamp. This is done through the use of sodium nitroprusside or nitroglycerin. It is important to use a drug which has an evanescent effect on the arterioles in order that profound hypotension does not occur when the aorta is unclamped at the end of the graft procedure.

Renal artery disease

Occlusion of a renal artery by atheroma causes unilateral renal ischaemia which is usually manifest as severe hypertension, often refractory to standard therapy. These patients require careful diagnosis by a combination of arteriography, selective renal vein catheterization for estimation of plasma renin activity, intravenous pyelography and biochemical estimations of renal function. It is important to lateralize the occlusive lesion in order to assess the probability of improving either renal function or the severe hypertension by surgery to bypass the occlusion. These patients are often receiving very high doses of β-receptor antagonists in addition to other antihypertensive drugs, and they frequently have severe anaemia, left ventricular hypertrophy and failure, and poor renal function [40, 52].

ISCHAEMIC HEART DISEASE

Coronary artery disease may co-exist with hypertension and almost certainly does co-exist with other manifestations of atheromatous disease. While this subject is covered in detail in Chapter 1, certain aspects relevant to this co-existence are dealt with here. While patients may present with a history of angina pectoris or a previous myocardial infarct, most have no symptoms or signs of their underlying disease until the first attack of angina or coronary occlusion, which may occur during or shortly after anaesthesia.

Angina pectoris

Approximately 5 per cent of all patients over the age of 35 may be expected to have symptomless ischaemic heart disease [31], whereas those who present with angina usually have extensive disease involving at least two major coronary vessels [29]. Attitudes to the risk of anaesthesia and surgery in patients with angina have changed dramatically over the past few years with the advent of procedures to revascularize the myocardium, or to bypass occluded coronary vessels. It is important to differentiate between the risks of anaesthesia for a patient with severe angina undergoing coronary artery bypass, in whom the operation is designed to improve coronary circulation, and on the other hand a similar patient whose surgery is incidental to the disease. In the latter case, the operative mortality is higher [3, 61].

A high percentage (25–50 per cent) of patients with angina may exhibit a normal resting electrocardiogram, but may develop an abnormal electrocardiogram during exercise [31]. However, there is a high incidence of false negative results in exercise ECG testing in patients with angiographically demonstrable lesions, and a high incidence of false positive results in patients with normal coronary arteriograms [6].

Myocardial infarction

The effect of previous myocardial infarction on the risk of anaesthesia and surgery has been the subject of extensive enquiry. Current opinion is largely based on the survey by Topkins and Artusio [56], and more recent studies and reviews have not altered their basic conclusions [3, 32, 51, 54, 56].

The risk of further myocardial infarction occurring during or after operation is

10 times greater in patients over the age of 50 having a previous myocardial infarct, than in those who have no demonstrable cardiovascular disease, and the mortality as a result of such a postoperative myocardial infarct is very high. The interval between surgery and the previous infarct is very important as the risk diminishes considerably as the interval increases. Surgery performed within three to six months of a previous myocardial infarct carries a particularly high risk; the reinfarction rate in the first three months may be of the order of 40 per cent with a high mortality [51, 56]. Between three and six months after previous infarction, the chances of further infarction after surgery decline, and between six months and one year the risks are no different from those in an otherwise healthy group of elderly patients.

These retrospective statistical approaches, while useful in defining the serious danger period after previous infarction, do little to indicate the best course of management for these patients. Since the advent of surgery for coronary arterial disease, the experiences of anaesthetists in this field have enabled the factors which may precipitate further myocardial infarction during or after anaesthesia to be more clearly defined. These may be conveniently classified under two headings; those factors which increase myocardial work and oxygen requirement out of proportion to available coronary blood flow, and conversely, factors which tend to reduce coronary blood flow out of proportion to the existing myocardial work.

It has been stated that patients with ischaemic heart disease do not tolerate arterial hypotension [61] though the evidence used to support this statement was relevant to hypotension and cardiogenic shock as a complication of myocardial infarction, rather than hypotension during anaesthesia. Fig. 2.7 shows that in certain patients, a decrease of either systolic or diastolic pressure can lead to severe but reversible myocardial ischaemia which can be identified on the CM_5 lead electrocardiogram. It is the author's experience that moderate degrees of hypotension are rather better tolerated by patients with ischaemic heart disease than comparable degrees of hypertension. Hypertension reflects an increase in systemic vascular resistance and consequently an increase in myocardial work. Combined with tachycardia, which shortens diastole and therefore the time available for coronary flow, hypertension represents the greater threat to adequate myocardial perfusion in these patients. It is believed that permanent

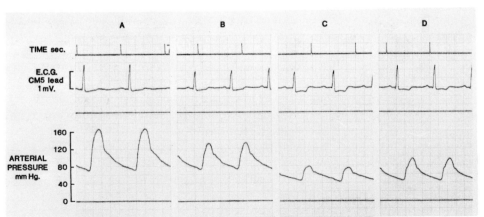

Fig. 2.7. Progressive deterioration of ST segment depression in relation to decreasing arterial pressure in a treated hypertensive patient with pre-existing coronary arterial disease. The arterial hypotension occurred during elective hypotension for parotid surgery. Note particularly the increased PR interval in panel C associated with the ischaemic response, and the resolution of both the PR interval and the ST segment with the increase in arterial pressure (Panel D).

changes in myocardial cells may occur after 5–10 minutes of myocardial under-perfusion, and may lead to infarction [50]. The factors which precipitate such ischaemia can be defined and steps to eliminate these factors should be taken. Hypertension and tachycardia are usually associated with noxious stimuli such as laryngoscopy and intubation, and surgical interventions. The cardiovascular responses to these noxious stimuli can be markedly attenuated by adrenergic β-receptor blockade [38, 40, 42]. Current experience suggests that patients receiving β-receptor blockers for the treatment of ischaemic heart disease should not have these drugs withdrawn precipitously before surgery [2, 7, 34, 38]. It may be judicious, however, to reduce the dosage and substitute coronary vasodilator drugs in those patients receiving very high doses of β-receptor blockers (more than 1 g/day of propranolol, or its equivalent) [40].

One of the commonest causes of hypotension complicated by myocardial ischaemia in these patients is a persistent supraventricular dysrhythmia, such as A-V junctional rhythm or atrial extrasystolic rhythm [41].

PREOPERATIVE ASSESSMENT

All patients with cardiovascular disease require careful preoperative assessment, as only by recognizing and correcting problems beforehand can the patient and the anaesthetist be adequately prepared for all eventualities. Perhaps the most important feature, frequently neglected, of the preparation of these patients, is a discussion of the previous medical care with the patient's physician. When a physician has spent months assessing and treating a complex disease state and has achieved a satisfactory result, it is nothing short of presumptuous for a surgeon or anaesthetist to summarily change or discontinue the patient's medication. Acute withdrawal of β-receptor blockers may precipitate severe angina and myocardial infarction [3, 7, 30, 34, 38].

Both the history and clinical examination should be thorough, with emphasis on a search for specific symptoms and signs which will indicate problems of direct interest during anaesthesia. The multifactorial risk index of Goldman *et al* [19] is particularly useful in identifying cardiac risk factors, although for some inexplicable reason hypertension does not feature in the classification of risk factors. A subsequent paper identified some problems in patients with mild or moderate untreated hypertension, and those whose hypertension had been adequately treated.

History and examination

Care should be taken to elicit the pattern of drug taking, its effect, and factors which have necessitated changes in therapy, particularly of any increasing drug requirement in the weeks leading up to the operation.

Symptoms (orthopnoea, paroxysmal nocturnal dyspnoea) and signs (gallop rhythm, pulsus alternans, basal crepitations in the lung fields) of left ventricular failure are important to elicit as they indicate the degree to which the left ventricle can cope with increased loads. Evidence of left ventricular hypertrophy should be sought from the chest radiograph and from the 12 lead electrocardiograph. By summing the amplitude of the S wave in lead V_1 and that of the R wave in V_5, an index is obtained which indicates hypertrophy if the summated value exceeds 35 mm (3·5 mV).

Evidence of angina pectoris, the factors such as exercise or emotional stress which precipitate attacks, and the response to coronary vasodilators or β-receptor blockers

[28], are all indicators of the severity of ischaemic heart disease, whether related to hypertension or not.

The electrocardiogram is the main recordable index of the state of the patient's heart in these conditions and should be examined in detail for evidence of previous myocardial infarction, both old and recent. Ischaemic changes are notoriously difficult to interpret, and the author has found the classification of Punsar, Pyorala & Siltanen [46] to be the most useful means of identifying positive indices of ischaemia both in the resting and exercising patient. Opinions are still divided as to the value of electrocardiographic recording during exercises as a means of assessment before operation [6, 28, 31, 46]. Many patients with ischaemic heart disease can tolerate exercise well but are much less tolerant of emotional stresses [28].

Evidence of severe intraventricular conduction defects must be sought with particular reference to trifascicular block. It is advisable in all, and mandatory in some cases with severe conduction defects, to consult with a cardiologist with a view to insert a pacing catheter prior to anaesthesia.

Monitoring during and after anaesthesia

To provide proper care for patients with cardiovascular disease, the anaesthetist needs to supplement his basic skills with continuous information from electronic monitors. The electrocardiograph is essential in order to recognize the onset and patterns of dysrhythmia and to detect evidence of myocardial ischaemia in the form of ST segment depression. While the standard 12 leads of the diagnostic electrocardiogram are invaluable for preoperative assessment, it is usual to display only one lead for continuous monitoring. Leads I, II or III, the most commonly used for this purpose, are not particularly suited for intra-operative monitoring. The bipolar lead designated CM_5 (reference electrode over the manubrium sterni, exploring electrode in the V_5 position—anterior axillary line in the 5th intercostal space) provides the best single lead identification of ST segment changes and provides good visualization of the P wave and a tall QRS complex [5, 11, 41].

Direct arterial pressure recording provides instantaneous indication of the dramatic changes of pressure which may be observed in these patients. Central venous pressure measurement is neither more nor less useful than in any other group of patients and is indicated when major changes of blood volume may be expected. Measurement of balloon-occluded 'wedge' pressure in the pulmonary artery using one of the varieties of Swan-Ganz catheters [27, 53] is specifically indicated in patients with evidence of left ventricular failure, or patients receiving high doses of β-receptor blocking drugs, especially during any form of surgery where major blood loss may be expected [40].

REFERENCES

1 AHLQUIST RP. Study of the adrenotropic receptors. *Am J Physiol* 1948; **153**: 586–600.

2 ALDERMAN EL, COLTART DJ, WETTACH GE, HARRISON DC. Coronary artery syndromes after sudden propranolol withdrawal. *Ann Intern Med* 1974; **81**: 625–7.

3 ARKINS R, SMESSAERT AA, HICKS RG. Mortality and morbidity in surgical patients with coronary artery disease. *JAMA* 1964; **190**: 485–8.

4 ATTIA RR, MURPHY JD, SNIDER M, LAPPAS DG, DARLING RC, LOWENSTEIN E. Myocardial ischemia due to infrarenal aortic cross-clamping during aortic surgery in patients with severe coronary artery disease. *Circulation*, 1976; **53**: 961–5.

5 BLACKBURN H, TAYLOR HL, OKOMOTO N, RAUTAHARJU P, MITCHELL PL, KERKHOF AC. Standardization of the exercise electrocardiogram. A systematic comparison of chest lead configurations

employed for monitoring during exercise. In: Karvonen MJ, Barry AJ, eds. *Physical activity and the heart.* Springfield: CC Thomas. 1967: 101.

6 BORER JS, BRENSIKE JF, REDWOOD DR, *et al.* Limitations of the electrocardiographic response to exercise in predicting coronary-artery disease. *New Engl J Med* 1975; **293**: 367–71.

7 CARALPS JM, MULET J, WIENKE HR, MORAN JM, PIFARRE R. Results of coronary artery surgery in patients receiving propranolol. *J. Thorac Cardiovasc Surg* 1974; **67**: 526–9.

8 DINGLE HR. Antihypertensive drugs and anaesthesia. *Anaesthesia* 1966; **21**: 151–72.

9 EDWARDS R, WINNIE AP, RAMAMURTHY S. Acute hypocapneic hypokalemia: an iatrogenic anesthetic complication. *Anesth Analg* 1977; **56**: 786–92.

10 ERWIN D, PICK MJ, TAYLOR GW. Anaesthesia for carotid artery surgery. *Anaesthesia* 1980; **35**: 246–9.

11 FOËX P, PRYS-ROBERTS C. Anaesthesia and the hypertensive patient. *Br J Anaesth* 1974; **45**: 575–88.

12 FOLKOW B. The haemodynamic consequences of adaptive structural changes of the resistance vessels in hypertension. *Clin Sci* 1971; **41**: 1–12.

13 FOLKOW B. Cardiovascular structural adaptation; its role in the initiation and maintenance of primary hypertension. *Clin Sci Mol Med* 1978; **55**: 3s–22s.

14 FROHLICH ED, TARAZI RC, DUSTAN HP. Re-examination of the hemodynamics of hypertension. *Am J Med Sci* 1969; **257**: 9–23.

15 GALINDO A, WYTE SR, WETHERHOLD JW. Junctional rhythm induced by halothane anesthesia— treatment with succinylcholine. *Anesthesiology* 1972; **37**: 261–2.

16 GOLDBY FS. The pathology of hypertension. In: Marshall AJ, Barritt DW, eds. *The hypertensive patient.* Tunbridge Wells: Pitman Medical, 1980: 266–92.

17 GOLDBY FS, BEILIN LJ. How an acute rise in arterial pressure damages arterioles. Electron microscopic changes following angiotensin infusion. *Cardiovasc Res* 1972; **6**: 569–84.

18 GOLDMAN L, CALDERA DL. Risks of general anesthesia and elective operation in the hypertensive patient. *Anesthesiology* 1979; **50**: 285–92.

19 GOLDMAN L, CALDERA DL, NUSSBAUM SR, *et al.* Multifactorial index of cardiac risk in noncardiac surgical procedures. *New Engl J Med* 1977; **297**: 845–50.

20 GUYTON AC. An overall analysis of cardiovascular regulation. *Anesth Analg* 1977; **56**: 761–8.

21 HICKLER RB, VANDAM LD. Hypertension. *Anesthesiology* 1970; **33**: 214–28.

22 HODGE JV, SMIRK FH. (1967) The effect of drug treatment of hypertension on the distribution of deaths from various causes. *Am Heart J* 1967; **73**: 441–52.

23 HOLLANDER WB. Hypertension, antihypertensive drugs and atherosclerosis. *Circulation* 1973; **48**: 1112–27.

24 HOLSINGER JW, ELIOT RS (1972) The potential role of the subendocardium in the pathogenesis of myocardial infarction. *Heart Lung* **1**, 356.

25 KANNEL WD, SCHWARTZ MJ, McNAMARA PM. Blood pressure and risk of coronary heart disease: the Framingham Study. *Dis Chest* 1969; **56**: 43–52.

26 KAPLAN N. *Clinical hypertension.* New York: Medcom Press, 1973.

27 LAPPAS D, LELL WA, GABEL JC, CIVETTA JM, LOWENSTEIN E. Indirect measurement of left-atrial pressure in surgical patients—pulmonary-capillary wedge and pulmonary-artery diastolic pressures compared with left-atrial pressure. *Anesthesiology* 1973; **38**: 394–7.

28 LESCH M, GORLIN R. Pharmacological therapy of angina pectoris. *Mod Concepts Cardiovasc Dis* 1973; **42**: 5–10.

29 LIKOFF W, KASPARIAN H, SEGAL BL, NOVACK P, LEHMAN JS, Clinical correlation of coronary arteriography. *Am J Cardiol* 1965; **16**: 159–64.

30 MARSHALL AJ. Methyldopa, clonidine and rauwolfia derivatives. In: Marshall AJ, Barritt DW, eds. *The hypertensive patient.* Tunbridge Wells: Pitman Medical, 1980: 441–63.

31 MASTER AM, GELLER AJ. The extent of completely asymptomatic coronary artery disease. *Am J Cardiol* 1969; **23**: 173–9.

32 MAUNEY FM Jr, EBERT PA, SABISTON DC Jr. Postoperative myocardial infarction: a study of predisposing factors, diagnosis and mortality in a high risk group of surgical patients. *Ann Surg* 1970; **172**: 497–503.

33 MELOCHE R, POTTECHER T, AUDET J, DUFRESNE O, LEPAGE C. Haemodynamic changes due to clamping of the abdominal aorta. *Can Anaesth Soc J* 1977; **24**: 20–34.

34 MILLER PR, OLSON HG, AMSTERDAM EA, MASON DT. Propranolol—withdrawal rebound phenomenon. *New Engl J Med* 1975; **293**: 416–18.

35 MITCHELL JR, SCHWARTZ CJ. Relationship between arterial disease in different sites. A study of the aorta, coronary, carotid and iliac arteries. *Br Med J* 1962; **1**: 1293–301.

36 PICKERING GW. *High blood pressure*. 2nd ed. London: Churchill Livingstone, 1968.

37 PRICHARD BNC, RICHARDS DA. The combination of alpha and beta adrenoceptor blockade. In: Marshall AJ, Barritt DW, eds. *The hypertensive patient*. Tunbridge Wells: Pitman Medical, 1980: 433–40.

38 PRYS-ROBERTS C. Beta-receptor blockade and anaesthesia. In: Grahame-Smith DG, ed. *Drug interactions*. London: Macmillan, 1977: 265–74.

39 PRYS-ROBERTS C. Hypertension and anesthesia—fifty years on. *Anesthesiology* 1979; **50**: 281–4.

40 PRYS-ROBERTS C. Hemodynamic effects of anesthesia and surgery in renal hypertensive patients receiving large doses of receptor antagonists. *Anesthesiology* 1979; **51**: S122.

41 PRYS-ROBERTS C. Management of anaesthesia in the hypertensive patient. In: Marshall AJ, Barritt DW, eds. *The hypertensive patient*. Tunbridge Wells: Pitman Medical, 1980: 369–86.

42 PRYS-ROBERTS C, FOËX P, BIRO GP, ROBERTS JG. Studies of anaesthesia in relation to hypertension V: adrenergic beta-receptor blockade. *Br J Anaesth* 1973; **45**: 671–81.

43 PRYS-ROBERTS C, FOËX P, GREENE LT, WATERHOUSE TD. Studies of anaesthesia in relation to hypertension IV: the effects of artificial ventilation on the circulation and pulmonary gas exchanges. *Br J Anaesth* 1972; **44**: 335–49.

44 PRYS-ROBERTS C, GREENE LT, MELOCHE R, FOEX P. Studies of anaesthesia in relation to hypertension II. Haemodynamic consequences of induction and endotracheal intubation. *Br J Anaesth* 1971; **43**: 531–47.

45 PRYS-ROBERTS C, MELOCHE R, FOËX P. Studies of anaesthesia in relation to hypertension I. Cardiovascular responses of treated and uncreated patients. *Br J Anaesth* 1971; **43**: 122–37.

46 PUNSAR S, PYORALA K, SILTANEN P. Classification of electrocardiographic S-T segment changes in epidemiological studies of coronary artery disease. *Ann Med Intern Fenn* 1968; **57**: 53–63.

47 INTER-SOCIETY COMMISSION FOR HEART DISEASE RESOURCES. Guidelines for the detection, diagnosis and mangement of hypertensive populations. *Circulation* 1971; **44**: A–263–72.

48 ROBERTS CJC. Diuretics. In: Marshall AJ, Barritt DW, eds. *The hypertensive patient*. Tunbridge Wells: Pitman Medical, 1980: 389–409.

49 SHELL WE, SOBEL BE. Protection of jeopardized ischemic myocardium by reduced ventricular afterload. *New Engl J Med* 1974; **291**: 481–6.

50 SOBEL BE (1974) Biochemical and morphological changes in infarcting myocardium. In: Braunwald E, ed. *The myocardium: failure and infarction*. New York: HP Publishing, 1974: 247.

51 STEEN PA, TINKER JH, TARHAN S. Myocardial reinfarction after anesthesia and surgery. *JAMA* 1978; **239**: 2566–70.

52 SWALES JD. Pathogenesis: the kidney, adrenal cortex and sodium regulation. In: Marshall AJ, Barritt DW, eds. *The hypertensive patient*. Tunbridge Wells: Pitman Medical, 1980: 113–55.

53 SWAN HJC, GANZ W, FORRESTER J, MARCUS H, DIAMOND G, CHONETTE D. Catheterization of the heart in man with use of a flow-directed balloon-tipped catheter. *New Engl J Med* 1970; **283**: 447–51.

54 TARHAN S, MOFFITT EA, TAYLOR WF, GIULIANI ER. Myocardial infarction after general anesthesia. *JAMA* 1973; **220**: 1451–4.

55 THOMPSON JE, GARRETT WV. Peripheral-arterial surgery. *New Engl J Med* 1980; **302**: 491–503.

56 TOPKINS MJ, ARTUSIO JF Jr. Myocardial infarction and surgery: a five year study. *Anesth Analg* 1964; **43**: 716–20.

57 VETERANS ADMINISTRATION COOPERATIVE STUDY GROUP ON ANTIHYPERTENSIVE AGENTS. Effects of treatment on morbidity in hypertension: results in patients with diastolic blood pressures averaging 115 through 129 mmHg. *JAMA* **202**: 1028–34.

58 VETERANS ADMINISTRATION COOPERATIVE STUDY GROUP ON ANTIHYPERTENSIVE AGENTS. Effects of treatment on morbidity in hypertension: II results in patients with diastolic blood pressure averaging 90 through 114 mmHg. *JAMA* 1970; **213**: 1143–52.

59 VETERANS ADMINISTRATION COOPERATIVE STUDY GROUP ON ANTIHYPERTENSIVE AGENTS. Effects of treatment on morbidity in hypertension: III influence of age, diastolic pressure and prior cardiovascular disease; further analysis of side effects. *Circulation* 1972; **45**: 991–1004.

60 VOLHARD F, FAHR T. *Die Brightsche Nierenkrankheit. Klinik, Pathologie und Atlas*. Berlin: Springer, 1914.

61 WYNANDS JE, SHERIDAN CA, BATRA MS, PALMER WH, SHANKS J. Coronary artery disease. *Anesthesiology* 33, 260–81.

Chapter 3
Lung Disease

M. A. BRANTHWAITE

The preservation of adequate gas exchange is essential for safe anaesthetic management and this requirement must be fulfilled in spite of abnormalities of ventilatory function imposed by disease, surgery, anaesthetic drugs or technique. Lung function is therefore of greater importance to the anaesthetist than either anatomy or pathology, and this concept has determined the approach to pulmonary disease which has been adopted in this chapter.

CLINICAL ASSESSMENT

THE HISTORY

The cardinal symptoms of lung disease are dyspnoea, cough and the production of sputum, although these symptoms, alone or in combination, may also indicate disorders of other systems.

The subjective sensation of dyspnoea often correlates poorly with the results of objective tests of respiratory or cardiac function but, in practical terms, it is helpful to know the extent to which physical activity is limited. It is wise to ask specific questions to determine the degree of disability because the limitation imposed by dyspnoea, especially when it is slowly progressive, may be accepted by the patient as 'normal' [52]. The other important feature of dyspnoea is its temporal pattern—the time scale of its onset and progression and, above all, whether or not it is variable in severity. Variable dyspnoea is commonly caused by reversible airways obstruction and the anaesthetic significance of this lies in the ease with which a number of drugs and manoeuvres (e.g. *d*-tubocurarine or endotracheal intubation) can provoke severe bronchoconstriction in patients with this propensity. Many of these patients show considerable lability of bronchial tone throughout the day, and an early morning accentuation of symptoms is common [33]. Paroxysms of severe nocturnal dyspnoea occur in some cases and, although it may be difficult to exclude cardiac disease on the history alone, careful questioning generally reveals that postural changes are not the provoking factor.

Cough and the expectoration of sputum commonly occur together, but non-productive coughing is also important because it represents either bronchial irritation, congestion (e.g. early left ventricular failure) or, occasionally, distortion of the trachea or bronchi. If the cough is productive, it is useful to know whether it is persistent, what volume of sputum is produced daily and whether the sputum is purulent or mucoid. This information enables a realistic optimum condition to be defined for each patient.

An evaluation of these three symptoms—dyspnoea, cough and the production of sputum, provides much useful information about pulmonary function, but additional symptoms warrant discussion in specific conditions, e.g. bone pain or muscle weakness in malignant disease, or general malaise, fever and weight loss in tuberculosis. In addition, all patients should be asked about smoking, past experience of general anaesthesia and recent drug therapy.

PHYSICAL EXAMINATION

While the history is being elicited, the build and colour of the patient and the quality of the voice can be noted, audible wheeze detected, and dyspnoea recognized when the free flow of speech is interrupted because of the need to pause for breath. It is sometimes informative to ask the patient to cough. This sounds ineffective if the vital capacity is very small or if the vocal cords are damaged. A 'fruity' cough indicates loose sputum within the bronchial tree, although it may be located too deeply for immediate expectoration.

During physical examination, particular attention should be paid to the pattern, excursion and symmetry of respiratory movements. Localized pulmonary disease may result in gross displacement of the mediastinum and the position of the trachea should be determined with care.

Added sounds may be detected during auscultation in patients who have little or no history of respiratory disease, and the presence of rhonchi on forced expiration provides a warning that the bronchial calibre is abnormal. Râles or 'crackles' are caused by the sudden opening of collapsed air spaces. They occur early in inspiration in patients with generalized airways obstruction and late in inspiration if associated with restrictive lung diseases [49].

Some manifestations of pulmonary disease are detected during the examination of other systems. Use of the accessory muscles and tracheal tug are features of severe dyspnoea, anxiety and restlessness may be caused by hypoxia, and systolic hypertension, sweating, peripheral vasodilatation and drowsiness occur in patients with acute carbon dioxide retention. Tachycardia and pulsus paradoxus are important features of airways obstruction, and there is good correlation between the degree of paradox and the severity of the airways obstruction until the patient is exhausted [38]. 10 mmHg of paradox (a pressure difference of 10 mmHg between systolic blood pressure in inspiration and expiration) is common in patients with asthma, and values of 35–40 mmHg may be reached when the obstruction is very severe.

Chronic hypercapnia is associated with sodium retention and an inability to handle a water load [75] so that peripheral oedema occurs and the jugular venous pressure is elevated. Hypoxia and acidosis both cause pulmonary hypertension [4] which may ultimately be irreversible. Examination will then reveal a parasternal heave, accentuation of the pulmonary second sound, and a third and/or fourth heart sound, often best heard in the epigastrium, just below the xiphisternum (see page 61).

ADDITIONAL INVESTIGATIONS

A chest X-ray is commonly regarded as a routine investigation in all patients admitted to hospital [14] and is certainly required in those with pulmonary disease. Features of particular importance to the anaesthetist are whether or not the trachea is deviated or distorted, whether there is any deformity of the thoracic cage, and whether there is any localized disease of the lungs or pleura which was missed on physical examination. The criteria of normality in a standard six foot postero-anterior chest film are:

1 the right dome of the diaphragm is at the level of the 5th–7th rib and is 1–2·5 cm higher than the left dome;

2 the transverse diameter of the heart is less than 50 per cent of the transverse diameter of the chest;

3 the shadow of the left hilum is slightly smaller than the right and lies 0·5–1·5 cm higher;

4 the horizontal fissure meets the sixth rib in the axilla;

5 the vascular markings are roughly symmetrical and are larger in the lower than in the upper half of the lung fields.

Although important as a means of locating and defining pulmonary disorders, the chest X-ray is often a poor reflection of functional impairment (Fig. 3.1). Cor

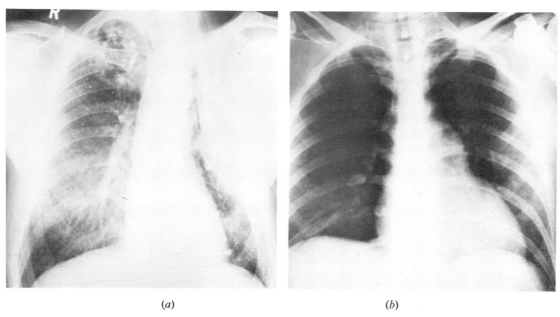

(a)   (b)

Fig. 3.1. (a) Chest X-ray of symptom-free, athletic 40-year old male. Pulmonary tuberculosis treated by thoracoplasty more than 20 years previously. (b) Chest X-ray of shocked, 37-year-old female suffering from acute amniotic fluid embolism. Pao$_2$ 6·7 kPa while breathing oxygen (6 l/min; MC mask).

pulmonale secondary to chronic lung disease may be recognized if there is cardiomegaly, prominent hilar vessels and loss of peripheral vascular markings, although there is sometimes radiological evidence of pulmonary vascular engorgement during acute exacerbations. This may represent either primary left ventricular disease, perhaps accentuated by hypoxia, or left ventricular dysfunction secondary to chronic lung disease [15]; alternatively it may merely reflect an increase and/or redistribution of extracellular fluid [45]. Tomography is helpful when opacities are ill-defined or overlap other structures, and computerized axial tomography is being used increasingly to detect disease which is inapparent on the routine radiograph.

An ECG is of value in patients with advanced pulmonary disease (Fig. 3.2). A tall peaked P wave in standard lead II (P pulmonale) indicates right atrial hypertrophy and a dominant R wave in leads V_1–V_4 and in standard lead III occurs in right ventricular hypertrophy. Rhythm disorders are relatively uncommon in chronic lung disease, although right bundle branch block may occur if there is pulmonary hypertension and tricuspid incompetence.

Assessment is incomplete without an estimation of haemoglobin and haematocrit to detect either anaemia, or polycythaemia secondary to chronic hypoxia; both can contribute to dyspnoea and to tissue hypoxia [31]. Other haematological and biochemical investigations may be appropriate in some circumstances.

Examination of the sputum is essential. Microscopy is required to confirm the presence of pus cells and to distinguish 'purulent' sputum caused by eosinophils in certain types of allergic lung disease. It is sometimes necessary to stain fresh sputum to identify micro-organisms as quickly as possible, and acid-fast bacilli, fungi and malignant cells can also be identified in this way. All sputum should be cultured on appropriate media and the sensitivity to antibiotics of any organisms which are isolated should be determined.

Fibreoptic bronchoscopy, usually carried out under local anaesthesia, provides access to the bronchial tree as far as subsegmental level [68]. Biopsies or 'brush biopsies' can be obtained from the bronchial walls, and cells lying free in the alveoli can be removed by bronchial lavage [27]. Tiny fragments of pulmonary tissue can be removed during fibreoptic bronchoscopy by transbronchial biopsy which should be carried out under radiological control to avoid puncturing the pleura. Lung tissue can also be obtained by needle or trephine biopsy through the chest wall [59]. Rigid bronchoscopy is used diagnostically for examination of the proximal bronchial tree, often as a prelude to surgery, and is performed under general anaesthesia in the majority of cases.

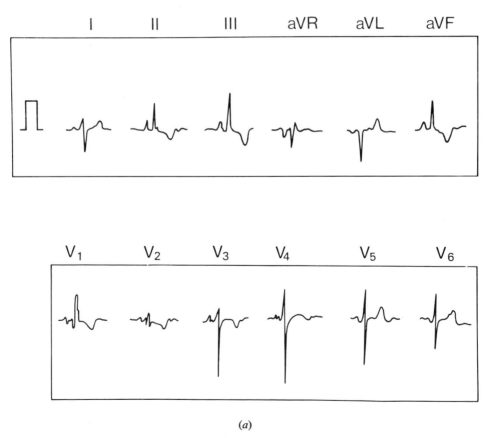

(*a*)

Fig. 3.2. (*a*) ECG recorded from a 36-year-old man with cor pulmonale. There is evidence of right axis deviation, P pulmonale and right ventricular hypertrophy and strain.

LUNG FUNCTION TESTS

Formal tests of lung function [19] are used to supplement, not to replace, clinical assessment. They are indicated when there is a need:

1 to determine the nature of the pulmonary disorder, particularly in circumstances where several abnormalities may be contributing to disability, e.g. chronic bronchitis associated with mitral stenosis;

2 to quantitate the degree of impairment, often as a baseline for therapy;

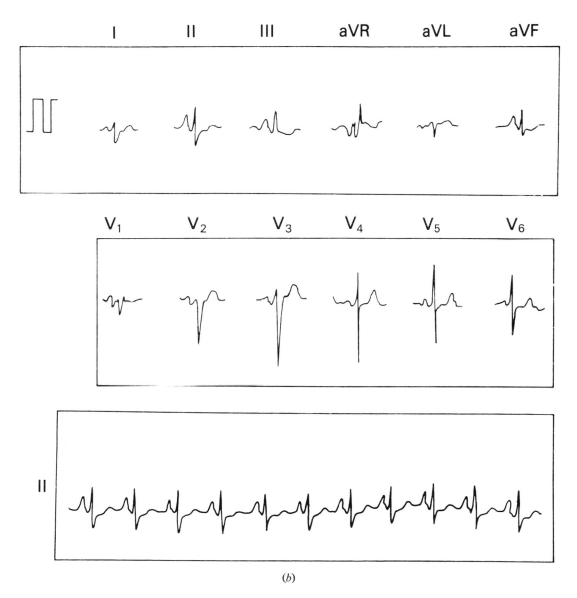

(*b*)

Fig. 3.2. (*b*) ECG recorded from 50-year-old man with pulmonary hypertension caused by chronic airways obstruction with emphysema. Downward displacement of the heart and diaphragm commonly obscures the dominant R wave in right precordial leads and an rS pattern, often accompanied by inverted T waves, is seen throughout the precordial leads.

3   to further the understanding of pathological physiology.

The tests vary considerably in complexity; some are time consuming to perform, and some methods are based on theoretical assumptions which may not be fulfilled in practice. The results vary both within and between normal individuals [67], and the deviation from the predicted value for subjects of comparable age, sex and height should exceed 20 per cent before a value is declared 'abnormal'. In addition, the reliability of the predicted values is questionable, particularly at the extremes of age, either because few studies have been carried out or because 'normality' is difficult to define (e.g. in the elderly). All these limitations should be borne in mind when the tests are requested and the findings are interpreted.

TESTS INVOLVING NO INSTRUMENTATION

These provide minimal information about overall respiratory function and are sometimes recommended as screening tests to determine 'fitness for operation'. They include the ability to walk up one or two flights of stairs while maintaining a conversation without distress, the ability to blow out a lighted match held at a distance of six inches in front of the open mouth (Snider match test), and the ability to breath hold for more than thirty seconds. Failure to extinguish the match in the Snider test is said to indicate a one-second forced expiratory volume of less than a litre.

MEASUREMENTS OF LUNG VOLUME

The tidal volume, vital capacity (VC) and its subdivisions, and the one-second forced expiratory volume (FEV_1) can all be determined at the bedside using a simple wet or dry spirometer incorporating a timing device.

Reduction in the vital capacity is a nonspecific feature common to both obstructive and restrictive pulmonary disease. A proportionately greater decrease in the FEV_1 indicates airways obstruction and, if this is detected, the test should be repeated 5–10 minutes after the supervised administration of a broncho-dilator aerosol.

Serial measurements of vital capacity are a useful index of progress in restrictive lung disease, and in paralytic disorders (e.g. poliomyelitis, myasthenia gravis) or in patients with crushed chest injuries. Generalized airways obstruction is monitored using either the ratio of FEV_1 to FVC, or using the peak expiratory flow rate (PEFR). A number of robust, simple and inexpensive meters are available for this purpose.

The determination of functional residual capacity (FRC), residual volume (RV) and total lung capacity (TLC) is more difficult. Helium dilution or nitrogen washout can be used if the lungs are normal, but plethysmography is required if gas mixing within the lungs is abnormal. Plethysmography provides a measurement of thoracic gas volume which includes air spaces which are not communicating freely with the airway, and the figure may therefore differ considerably from FRC measured by helium dilution or nitrogen washout.

The TLC is decreased in restrictive lung disease, but the residual volume may be relatively normal so that the ratio of RV to TLC is increased. The RV/TLC ratio is also increased when there is generalized airways obstruction. In these circumstances, both RV and TLC are increased, but the change in RV is proportionately greater than the increase in TLC because airway closure occurs prematurely during expiration. Closure of peripheral airways is one of the factors preventing lung deflation beyond residual volume in both health and disease [10]; it occurs when the force maintaining patency (elastic recoil) is less than the force favouring closure (the excess of intrapleural pressure over airway pressure). Premature closure occurs either if the calibre of the airways is decreased, or if there is loss of elastic recoil. Airway closure occurs even earlier in expiration if the intrapleural pressure is increased voluntarily (forced expiratory effort) or if the airway pressure is decreased by the use of a negative expiratory pressure during artificial ventilation.

The effects of generalized airways obstruction on lung volumes are compared with those of restrictive pulmonary disease in Table 3.1.

Table 3.1. Summary of the common physiological findings in obstructive and restrictive ventilatory defects.

	Obstructive	Restrictive
FEV$_1$	Low	Low
FVC	Low (often < VC)	Low
FEV$_1$/FVC	Low	Normal or high
VC	Low	Low
FRC	High	Low
TLC	High	Low
RV/TLC	High	Normal or high
Airway resistance	High	Normal for lung vol.
	May improve with bronchodilators	

MEASUREMENTS OF THE MECHANICAL PROPERTIES OF THE
LUNGS AND AIRWAYS

The previous section describes how indirect indices can be used to detect and monitor changes in airway resistance. These tests are partly dependent upon effort, whereas absolute measurements of airway resistance require patient cooperation but are otherwise independent of voluntary effort. Simultaneous observation of gas flow rate, atmospheric and alveolar pressure, is required for the measurement of airway resistance, and these variables can be determined by incorporating a pneumotachometer into the airway circuit used during plethysmography. Airway resistance is calculated from the following formula.

$$\text{resistance} = \frac{\text{atmospheric—alveolar pressure}}{\text{volume flow rate}}$$

There is a hyperbolic relationship between lung volume and airway resistance but the airway conductance, or reciprocal of resistance, is linearly related to lung volume. The best comparative figure is therefore specific airway conductance (sGaw), or the conductance per unit lung volume, which is generally determined at FRC.

Another method used to characterize and quantitate airway resistance is the flow-volume curve [64]. Instantaneous expiratory air flow in litres per second is plotted against lung volume during a forced vital capacity manoeuvre (Fig. 3.3). Tidal ventilation occurs well below TLC in the normal subject and the instantaneous expiratory flow rate is trivial by comparison with the maximum reached during forced expiration. Tidal ventilation occurs much nearer to TLC when there is generalized intra-thoracic airways obstruction, and expiratory flow rates during quiet breathing

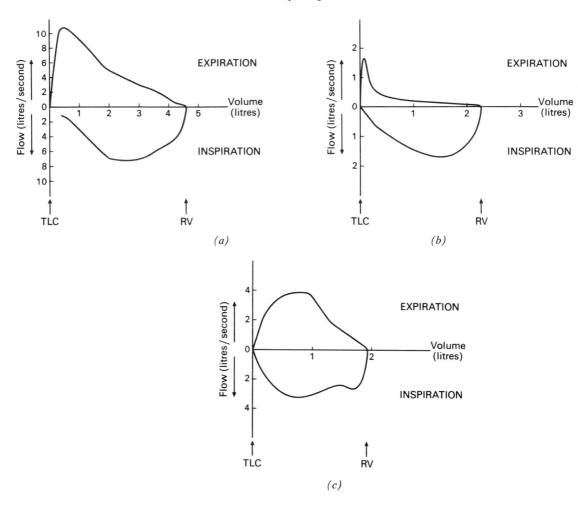

Fig. 3.3. Flow-volume curves (*a*) normal. (*b*) chronic obstructive airways disease. (*c*) upper respiratory tract obstruction (laryngeal sarcoid).

approximate to the maximum possible. In extrathoracic obstruction, e.g. laryngeal or upper tracheal disease, there is a greater reduction in expiratory flow rate near TLC than lower in the vital capacity, where the flow rate can be normal provided sufficient expiratory force can be maintained. In addition, inspiratory flow rates are preferentially decreased by extrathoracic obstruction and so the contour of the flow-volume loop differs from either the normal, or the pattern seen with generalized intrathoracic airways obstruction. Another spirometric approach to the quantitation of generalized intrathoracic airways obstruction is to measure the mean transit time of forced expiration [65]. The area under the plot of expired volume against time is determined and divided by the vital capacity. Mean transit time is prolonged when there are many lung units emptying slowly and appears to be a more sensitive method for detecting peripheral airways obstruction than either the flow-volume curve or measurements of forced expiratory volume or peak flow rate.

Compliance, or ease of distensibility, may refer to the lungs alone or to the combination of lungs and chest wall. It is determined by relating changes in lung

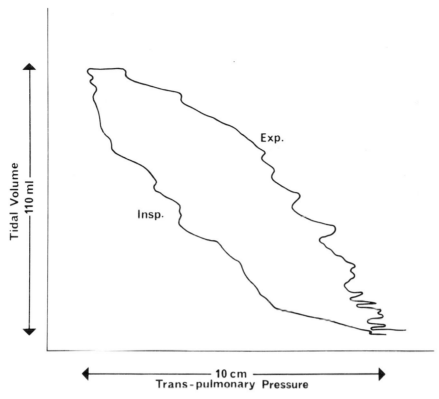

Fig. 3.4. Pressure-volume loop recorded from a 2½-year-old, 10·7-kg child following repair of the tetralogy of Fallot. The child was breathing spontaneously with a continuous positive airway pressure of 2 cm H_2O (0·2 kPa).

volume to the corresponding changes in either transpulmonary, or transthoracic pressure at points of 'no flow' in the respiratory cycle. Unfortunately, air flow from atmosphere to alveoli may be incomplete during the short inspiratory time available during ventilation at normal respiratory frequencies, especially if there is any degree of generalized airway disease. Under these circumstances, values for dynamic compliance (derived by relating pressure changes to volume achieved during a series of tidal volumes of increasing depth), are likely to be significantly smaller than figures for static compliance which relate pressure and volume changes during 2–3 second periods of apnoea at each volume. Indeed, the extent to which dynamic compliance varies with respiratory frequency can be used as an index of airways obstruction [64].

It is sometimes important to differentiate pulmonary compliance from thoracic cage compliance but this requires the measurement of transpulmonary pressure. Characteristically, pulmonary compliance is decreased in restrictive disease of the lung, normal when the restriction is imposed by disease of the thoracic cage, and increased in emphysema because of alveolar wall destruction.

The relationship between pressure and lung volume can be expressed graphically as a 'pressure-volume loop' (Fig. 3.4). The work of breathing (pressure × volume) is indicated by the area within the loop and it is possible to subdivide this into work required to overcome elastic forces (compliance), and that required to overcome non-elastic forces (airway resistance). Reliable results are difficult to obtain, the usual source of error being inaccuracies in the measurement of intrathoracic pressure with the oesophageal balloon, and the tests have no routine application.

MEASUREMENTS OF GAS EXCHANGE

The arterial blood gas tensions provide useful information about the effectiveness of gas exchange and facilities for blood gas analysis are widely available. Unfortunately, the accuracy of the results depends upon the care with which the sample is collected and stored, whether this be arterial or arterialized capillary blood, and faulty handling and maintenance of the equipment are other common sources of error. A good estimate of arterial carbon dioxide tension (Pa,co_2) can be obtained without blood sampling by the rebreathing method, although this is difficult to carry out in patients who fail to co-operate [28]. Methods for monitoring arterial blood gas tensions on a continuous basis have been developed, using intravascular or transcutaneous electrodes [69, 70] for oxygen tension, and analysis of end-tidal gas concentrations for an approximate estimation of arterial carbon dioxide tension [30].

An increase in Pa,co_2 indicates hypoventilation. This may be due to a decrease in minute volume, or to a reduction in effective alveolar ventilation caused by an increase in dead space while the minute volume remains normal. It is important to remember that anaesthetic apparatus can contribute significantly to the total dead space.

Arterial hypoxaemia can exist without significant desaturation because of the shape of the haemoglobin dissociation curve, and measurements of oxygen tension are therefore of more value in assessing respiratory function than either saturation or content. In the absence of intracardiac shunts, arterial hypoxaemia while breathing air is caused by:

1 a reduction in alveolar ventilation which is always accompanied by hypercapnia except following a period of prolonged passive hyperventilation;

2 the passage of blood through lung tissue which is either totally unventilated (intra-pulmonary shunting) or underventilated relative to pulmonary blood flow in the same area (ventilation/perfusion mismatch);

3 possibly by defective diffusion across the alveolar membrane.

The effects of defective diffusion and ventilation/perfusion mismatch can be overcome by the inhalation of high inspired oxygen concentrations.

It has proved difficult to devise methods for separating the influence of the various factors which can contribute to defective oxygen uptake and there is often poor correlation between the results obtained with different techniques. The simplest tests in common use are measurements of the alveolar-arterial oxygen gradient (A-a)Do_2 and of the 'diffusing capacity' or 'transfer factor' for carbon monoxide (T_1co). The (A-a)Do_2 depends in part upon the mixed venous oxygen tension and may therefore be high in the absence of pulmonary disease, e.g. if the cardiac output is low [35].

The diffusing capacity or transfer factor can be measured either for oxygen or, more simply, for carbon monoxide which behaves similarly because it too combines avidly with haemoglobin. The test is carried out either as a single breath or as a steady state manoeuvre and the values obtained depend upon the method employed. The test cannot distinguish between defects caused by diffusion and those due to ventilation/perfusion imbalance and the results are also influenced by the volume of pulmonary blood exposed to the gas. Gas transfer may even be higher than normal if there is an increase in pulmonary blood volume as in left to right shunts or early mitral stenosis (Table 3.2). Measurements of gas transfer are also increased if there is an abnormal

Table 3.2. Pulmonary function in a 58-year-old male with partial anomalous pulmonary venous drainage (causing pulmonary plethora). There is evidence of a mild restrictive defect but gas transfer corrected for lung tolume (K_{CO}) is greater than predicted.

	Predicted	Result
FEV_1 (ml)	1900	1100
FVC (ml)	2730	1540
FEV_1/FVC (%)	69·5	71·4
T_1CO (mmol min^{-1} kPa^{-1})	4·9	4·7
V_A (litres)		2·6
K_{CO} (mmol min^{-1} kPa^{-1} l^{-1})	1·41	1·80

volume of blood in the lungs because of recent pulmonary haemorrhage [50] and resolution or renewal of bleeding can be demonstrated with serial tests.

Another factor influencing gas transfer is the volume of lung to which the carbon monoxide gains access during the study, and interpretation of the results of the single breath test is facilitated by relating gas transfer to the alveolar volume determined simultaneously by helium dilution: the transfer coefficient or K_{CO} is gas transfer per unit of lung volume. Similarly, measurements of gas transfer made by the rebreathing technique depend upon the minute volume during the test and this should be quoted when the results are compared with predicted figures. Serial measurements of gas transfer are particularly useful when following diseases which interfere with oxygen uptake at alveolar level (Table 3.3).

Table 3.3. Progressive improvement in pulmonary function, particularly in gas transfer, during the resolution of pulmonary sarcoidosis (treated with corticosteroids) in a female of 38.

	Predicted	7.11.73	18.2.74	19.6.74	4.9.74	13.11.74
VC (ml)	3500	2350	2950	2800	2800	2950
T_1CO (mmol min^{-1} kPa^{-1}) single breath	7·56	4·32	5·00	5·37	6·0	6·87
K_{CO} (mmol min^{-1} kPa^{-1} l^{-1})	1·73	1·08	1·21	1·37	1·51	1·52

The regional distribution of pulmonary blood flow can be investigated either by pulmonary angiography or by external scanning over the lung fields after the intravenous injection of macro-aggregated radio-iodinated human serum albumin. Quantitative investigations of the distribution of both ventilation and perfusion require scanning following the inhalation or intravenous injection of radioactive gases. Although studies with radioactive gases are complex and their use largely restricted to specialized centres, valuable clinical information has been obtained [1]. A finding of particular interest to anaesthetists is the demonstration that during expiration from TLC to RV, there is a point (the closing volume) where the small airways in the dependent parts of the lungs start to close. The closing volume is near to residual volume in health but may approach FRC or even lie within the range of tidal ventilation when the lungs are abnormal [10]. Closure of small airways during tidal ventilation favours hypoxaemia because pulmonary blood flow continues without interruption to these inadequately ventilated areas. The reduction in FRC which accompanies general anaesthesia brings the closing volume closer to the range of tidal ventilation and is one factor contributing to postoperative hypoxaemia.

Another way in which ventilation and perfusion can be studied simultaneously is by following the disappearance of a mixture of soluble and insoluble gases either during rebreathing or during a single slow exhalation after inspiring from residual volume to total lung capacity. An insoluble gas, e.g. argon or helium equilibrates with the residual gas in the lungs and its concentration reaches a plateau. The concentration of a soluble gas, e.g. freon-22 or dimethyl ether, falls as it dissolves into and is carried away by the pulmonary blood. Equilibration of the insoluble gas provides a means of measuring residual volume, whereas clearance of the soluble

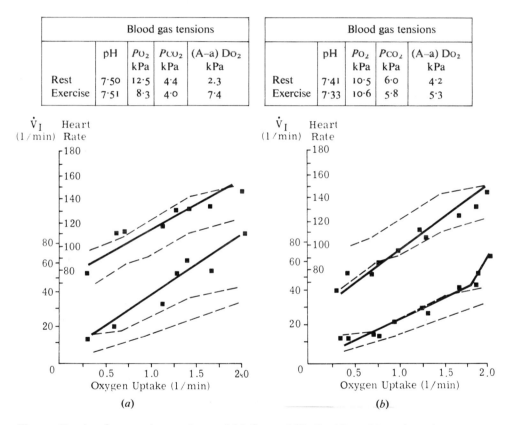

Blood gas tensions						Blood gas tensions				
	pH	P_{O_2} kPa	P_{CO_2} kPa	(A–a) D_{O_2} kPa			pH	P_{O_2} kPa	P_{CO_2} kPa	(A–a) D_{O_2} kPa
Rest	7·50	12·5	4·4	2.3		Rest	7·41	10·5	6·0	4·2
Exercise	7·51	8·3	4·0	7·4		Exercise	7·33	10·6	5·8	5·3

(a)   (b)

Fig. 3.5. Results of progressive exercise test (*a*) before and (*b*) after bilateral broncho-pulmonary lavage, undertaken for the treatment of alveolar proteinosis.

In each record, heart rate (upper panel) and minute volume (lower panel) are plotted against oxygen uptake during progressive exercise at a work rate which is increased each minute. The dotted lines indicate the normal range, and the solid squares are values obtained at each work load when the patient exercised. The solid lines are regression equations through the squares.

Before treatment, ventilation is excessive for the oxygen uptake achieved although the heart rate is within normal limits. After treatment, both ventilation and heart rate remain normal until a high rate of oxygen uptake is reached. During the first study, arterial hypoxaemia and widening of the alveolar-arterial oxygen tension gradient occurred (the exercise values for blood gas tensions being collected during the last minute of the study); after treatment, the arterial oxygen tension did not fall on exercise but the (A-a)D_{O_2} remained abnormal throughout.

gas indicates the rate of blood flow [62]. These tests can be carried out on both lungs simultaneously by following the concentration of the gases at the mouth, or they can be used to investigate regional lung function by catheterizing segmental bronchi with a fibre-optic bronchoscope through which a balloon-tipped sampling catheter is introduced [77].

EXERCISE STUDIES

Exercise requires a simultaneous increase in cardiac output and alveolar ventilation, and both cardiovascular and respiratory disorders diminish exercise tolerance. The extent of this limitation can be studied [71] by relating heart rate and minute ventilation to oxygen uptake while undertaking increasing work loads on a cycle ergometer. The relationship between oxygen uptake and both heart rate and minute volume is approximately linear in normal subjects but either the absolute values or the rate of change of one or other of these variables is abnormal when there is cardiovascular or respiratory disease. Exercise tests are particularly valuable in the investigation and serial assessment of patients with fairly minimal disease (Fig. 3.5), and also as a means of evaluating patients in whom symptoms appear to be out of proportion to their disability as judged by other measurable criteria.

The availability of such a wide range of lung function tests can be a source of confusion. In practical terms, the following are the most useful:

1   the FEV_1/FVC ratio or PEFR for the study of generalized airways obstruction;
2   serial measurements of VC in restrictive, paralytic and traumatic conditions;
3   arterial blood gas tensions as an estimate of whether or not overall ventilatory function is adequate;
4   measurements of the transfer factor for carbon monoxide or the transfer coefficient as an index of progress in disease at alveolar level.

GENERALIZED AIRWAYS OBSTRUCTION

This section deals with disorders which are characterized by a varying degree of narrowing of peripheral parts of the bronchial tree caused by constriction of bronchial muscle, mucosal oedema, or the presence of plugs of inspissated mucus. Lung function tests reveal a reduction in vital capacity and in the FEV_1/FVC ratio, and an increase in airway resistance. The lungs are hyperinflated but gas transfer is normal, at least in uncomplicated cases of asthma. The condition is said to be reversible when there is an improvement by 20 per cent or more in at least one index of obstruction following bronchodilator therapy. In the early stages of asthma, paroxysms of airway narrowing occur with return to normal lung function between attacks, whereas many patients with advanced asthma or chronic bronchitis suffer from persistent airways obstruction with little or no reversibility.

ASTHMA

It is customary to classify asthma into 'extrinsic' and 'intrinsic'. Extrinsic asthma occurs predominantly in atopic subjects, often developing at a young age following eczema in infancy. Hypersensitivity to one or more allergens can be demonstrated by skin testing, and eosinophilia in both blood and sputum is common. Extrinsic asthma also occurs in non-atopic subjects who become sensitized to a specific substance such as an industrial chemical, or an avian or fungal antigen. Intrinsic asthma is the term used to describe reversible airways obstruction in a non-atopic subject, in whom a provocating factor cannot be identified. The onset tends to occur at a later age and the disease is often more resistant to treatment. Blood and sputum eosinophilia are common and the disorder sometimes represents an early or isolated manifestation of polyarteritis nodosa. Fleeting infiltrations may appear on the chest X-ray in association with eosinophilia, e.g. in polyarteritis nodosa and in bronchopulmonary aspergillosis.

There are three aspects of asthma which are of particular importance to the anaesthetist. The first is that many patients require continuous bronchodilator therapy which may include corticosteroid drugs. Secondly, bronchial tone is labile and bronchoconstriction can be provoked during anaesthesia and, finally, a few patients in status asthmaticus require treatment by mechanical ventilation or possibly bronchopulmonary lavage.

Drugs used in the management of asthma [72, 73] include theophylline derivatives (aminophylline, choline theophyllinate), β-sympathomimetic stimulants (salbutamol, orciprenaline, terbutaline, ephedrine, etc.), atropine and related compounds, disodium cromoglycate and corticosteroids. These drugs act in a number of different ways [57] and there is some evidence that combinations of drugs act synergistically. The β-sympathomimetic stimulants are thought to augment levels of cyclic AMP within bronchial tissue and they differ from one another in their degree of β-specificity. The theophylline derivatives are phosphodiesterase inhibitors and retard the breakdown of cyclic AMP. Vagal stimulation causes bronchoconstriction which can be blocked with atropine, while corticosteroids act in many ways, probably augmenting intracellular cyclic AMP, restoring sensitivity to β-adrenergic receptors and suppressing inflammation. Corticosteroids in large doses partially suppress the development of immune responses and interfere with their unwanted consequences, but the immediate allergic component of bronchial asthma is often controlled equally effectively by disodium cromoglycate. This drug prevents the release of histamine following the combination of allergen and immunoglobulin E and therefore acts as a prophylactic agent. It is most important that patients using disodium cromoglycate are taught that it will not relieve an acute attack, whereas increased doses of other drugs are likely to be effective.

Systemic corticosteroid therapy is given either as injections of ACTH or using an oral steroid, commonly prednisone; some patients are maintained on topical steroids given by inhalation, e.g. beclomethasone dipropionate ('Becotide' 200–800 µg/day). Topical steroids are effective without causing systemic side-effects and without suppressing endogenous adrenal function [44]. However, they predispose to oral moniliasis and, although invasion of the lower respiratory tract is unlikely, it would be wise to treat moniliasis with amphotericin lozenges before anaesthesia and intubation.

Short courses of corticosteroids lasting a few weeks or months are often prescribed in asthma. A retrospective history of drug treatment is therefore as important as knowledge of current medication. Additional doses of a systemic corticosteroid may be needed preoperatively if there is any doubt about adrenal responsiveness, and steroids may also be required later if airways obstruction is precipitated by anaesthesia or by postoperative pulmonary infection. This is particularly likely in patients maintained regularly on inhaled drugs because the therapeutic effect will be diminished if bronchial secretions interfere with drug deposition and absorption. Theophylline or atropine derivatives and sympathomimetic agents can be continued throughout the operative period as required, and patients who use a bronchodilator aerosol regularly should be advised to take a dose about 15 minutes before induction of anaesthesia. Patients who are known to have labile bronchial tone should be anaesthetized with particular caution: it is wise to avoid opiates, barbiturates, *d*-tubocurarine, cyclopropane or *β*-sympathomimetic blocking agents and, if possible, to spray the cords and trachea with local anaesthetic before intubation.

Severe bronchoconstriction during general anaesthesia occurs most commonly immediately after induction and intubation, and virtually complete respiratory obstruction can result. Intravenous aminophylline 4–6 mg/kg given over 10 minutes is the drug of choice when this happens, and hydrocortisone is usually given at the same time although it has no immediate effect. If spontaneous ventilation is present, it may be possible to give 1 or 2 'puffs' (100–200 μg) from a pressurized aerosol containing salbutamol but it is difficult to administer the drug by this route to an apnoeic patient in such a way that it is carried into the trachea effectively. Salbutamol can be given intravenously, either as a bolus (0·2 mg over 5 minutes) or by infusion (5 μg per minute). Anaesthetic agents which sensitize the myocardium to adrenergic drugs should probably be withheld if salbutamol is used. It is important to avoid vigorous intermittent positive pressure ventilation because of the risk of air trapping; the possibility of an unsuspected pneumothorax should be considered if cyanosis and a high inflation pressure persist in spite of suction, a high inspired oxygen concentration, gentle controlled ventilation and treatment with aminophylline, hydrocortisone and salbutamol. Ether is still used very occasionally to relieve intractable bronchoconstriction.

Most patients admitted to hospital with severe, acute asthma ('status asthmaticus') respond to reassurance, oxygen, and bronchodilator drugs given intravenously and by inhalation [5, 6, 11, 16]. Corticosteroids are used in most cases and antibiotics are often given too although the infective origin of many attacks of asthma is questionable [18]. Serial measurements of peak expiratory flow rate, heart rate and the degree of arterial paradox provide good evidence of progress, supplemented if necessary by measurements of arterial blood gas tensions. Hypoxaemia and a normal or low arterial carbon dioxide tension are the usual findings in acute asthma but the Pa,co_2 increases in severe cases as the patient becomes exhausted and the degree of arterial paradox decreases at the same time. 'Exhaustion' or a rising Pa,co_2 are the common indications for mechanical ventilation in severe acute asthma, but a raised arterial carbon dioxide tension on admission to hospital should not be used as the sole criterion for instituting ventilatory support because it will often fall rapidly if the patient responds promptly to treatment.

The chief hazards of mechanical ventilation during an acute attack of asthma are right heart failure caused by gross over-inflation of the lungs (Fig. 3.6) and lung rupture leading to a pneumothorax which is often under tension and rapidly fatal. High inflation pressures result if the inspiratory period is curtailed unduly to permit prolonged expiration and this increases the risk of pneumothorax. A slow respiratory rate should be used, preferably with inspiration and expiration approximately equal in duration; an end-inspiratory pause allows the inspired gas to reach slowly-filling lung units and improves carbon dioxide elimination. It may be necessary to accept an elevated carbon dioxide tension at first, but this is preferable to increasing the minute volume to the point where over-distension occurs and heart failure is inevitable.

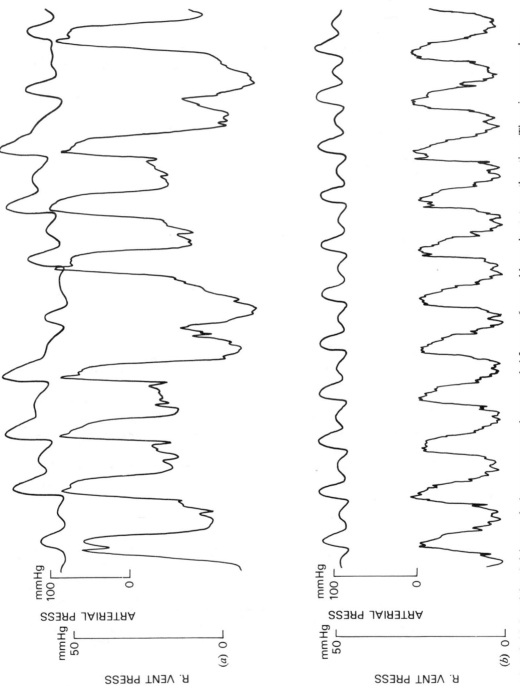

Fig. 3.6. (a) Arterial and right ventricular pressure tracings recorded from a 26-year-old man in status asthmaticus. There is a gross pulsus paradoxus; $Pa,_{CO_2}$ 15·0 kPa. (b) 30 minutes later, established on intermittent positive pressure ventilation.

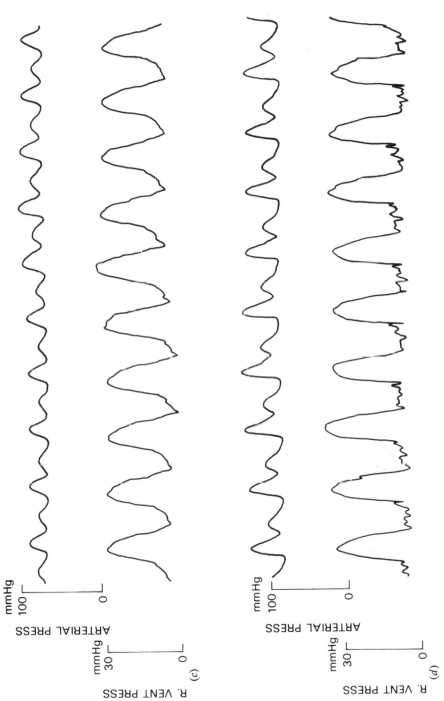

Fig. 3.6. (*c*) After 1 hour on IPPV with a minute volume of 9 litres. Acute right ventricular failure caused by further over-distension of the lungs. Pa,CO_2 9·9 kPa. (*d*) After a further 30 minutes. Minute volume reduced to 7 litres and chest circumference had decreased by 1·5 cm. Pa,CO_2 10·3 kPa.

Subsequent recovery in this patient was uneventful.

Some authors advocate a negative pressure during expiration to assist deflation but this accentuates air trapping. Positive end-expiratory pressure is contraindicated because it too accentuates overdistension. An expiratory flow choke which allows the airway pressure to reach atmospheric at the end of expiration is a more logical choice, if it is felt that maintaining a positive pressure in the airway during expiration will diminish premature airway closure. However, the effect of the expiratory flow choke is to create a positive pressure at the end of expiration if the expired volume is not exhaled completely in the time available and it is usually wiser to allow expiration to occur without hindrance [8].

Patients who fail to respond to conventional bronchodilator treatment and require mechanical ventilation are likely to be suffering from airway obstruction caused by plugs of inspissated mucus. Various techniques for removing these plugs by mechanical means have been described: fibreoptic bronchoscopy and limited lavage, or the repeated instillation of small volumes of normal saline (2 ml every 15 minutes) down the endotracheal tube are the methods usually favoured today.

CHRONIC BRONCHITIS

Chronic bronchitis is said to be present when a patient complains of persistent cough and sputum for more than three months in two successive years, but has no evidence of localized pulmonary disease [53]. The symptoms vary in severity from the mild cough and slight sputum production of the chronic smoker to complete disablement with respiratory failure and cor pulmonale. Bronchial mucus is secreted in excess in all forms of the disease [12] and there is generally evidence of airways obstruction which is at least partly reversible in the early stages. Recurrent bronchial infection occurs, often with increasing frequency as the years go by [26], and emphysema is a common but by no means inevitable accompaniment.

Numerically, chronic bronchitis accounts for most of the pulmonary disease which is seen in association with general surgical practice [54]. The anaesthetic problems which it imposes are, again, threefold in number:

1 the presence of excess bronchial mucus predisposes to infection; atelectasis and bronchopneumonia occur if the secretions are not expectorated;
2 airways obstruction is present and is commonly irreversible;
3 carbon dioxide unresponsiveness develops in some cases so that ventilatory drive is largely dependent upon hypoxia.

Good preoperative preparation is invaluable when surgery is required in patients with chronic bronchitis, but all too often this is either neglected or is impossible because of the need for immediate surgical treatment. Ideally, preparation should start when the decision to operate is taken. Exhortations to stop smoking and to lose weight if necessary are worthwhile, although often unsuccessful unless supervised at frequent intervals. The sputum should be examined and antibiotics prescribed if it is purulent. The most common pathogens causing an exacerbation of chronic bronchitis are *S. pneumoniae* and *H. influenzae* and, if treatment is started before the results of sputum culture are available, or if no pathogens are isolated, it is reasonable to prescribe on the assumption that infection is caused by these two organisms [47, 58]. Tetracyclines are used commonly but, although effective *in vitro*, they are not bactericidal and it is preferable to use co-trimoxazole (2 tablets b.d.), ampicillin (500 mg q.d.s.) or amoxy-cillin (250 mg t.d.s.). The latter has a similar antibiotic spectrum to ampicillin but blood levels are virtually independent of the timing of the dose in relation to meals, and there is some evidence which suggests that amoxycillin penetrates sputum more effectively than ampicillin. Unfortunately, co-trimoxazole, ampicillin and amoxycillin are all expensive. In hospitalized patients, injections of penicillin (1 million units q.d.s.) and streptomycin (0·5 g b.d.) for five days are usually effective, but care is needed to avoid streptomycin ototoxicity in these often elderly patients. Other antibiotic combinations may be indicated according to the results of sputum culture.

Most patients with chronic bronchitis of a severity sufficient to cause dyspnoea suffer from demonstrable airways obstruction. This usually improves if sputum production is lessened by the elimination of infection but specific bronchodilator therapy should always be tried [73]. The selective β-sympathomimetic agent salbutamol is probably the drug of first choice. It is best given by inhalation (2 'puffs' (200 μg) from a pressurized aerosol every 4–6 hours); the oral preparation (2–4 mg q.d.s.) is less effective and side-effects are more common. Some patients respond well to inhaled atropine and can be managed conveniently with 'Atrovent', an aerosol preparation of ipratropium bromide, 20–40 μg q.d.s. The combination of salbutamol and atropine is often most effective, although some patients become resistant to atropine or its derivatives after a few weeks. Theophylline preparations and corticosteroids are useful sometimes but the latter should never be prescribed unless the response to treatment can be evaluated carefully because many patients with chronic obstructive bronchitis derive no benefit from them but are reluctant to discontinue medication which creates a sense of euphoria.

It is customary to prescribe 'physiotherapy' when patients with chronic bronchitis are admitted to hospital [42]. Breathing exercises are the simplest form of treatment and are designed to improve voluntary control of the respiratory muscles and coordinate respiration with other activities. In addition, some physicians advocate intermittent positive pressure breathing (IPPB) with the 'Bird' ventilator for periods of 10 to 30 minutes several times each day. Bronchodilator drugs (e.g. 2·5–10 mg salbutamol) can be administered conveniently through the nebulizer, some patients finding it easier to inhale the drug this way than by using a pressurized aerosol. However, it is doubtful whether the therapeutic effect is any greater when the drug is given with IPPB than when the pressurized aerosol or Wright's nebulizer are used [43], even though the patterns of drug absorption and excretion *do* differ according to the method of administration. IPPB with or without a bronchodilator provokes coughing in many patients and therefore it is also recommended as a means of mobilizing secretions. Unfortunately, it is very difficult to confirm its efficacy and, indeed, measurements of arterial blood gas tensions may show deterioration rather than improvement after treatment, especially if therapy is prolonged until the patient is tired [29]. It is important to realize, however, that measurements of arterial blood gas tensions are not the sole criterion of progress. Even if treatment with IPPB is not available, regular visits from the physiotherapist will focus the patient's attention on the need to cough. It may be possible to assist expectoration by percussing and shaking the chest but this is likely to do more harm than good if there is little or no sputum.

Controlled oxygen therapy is often required during acute exacerbations of chronic bronchitis [46] and may also be of value as a long-term measure in patients with severe pulmonary hypertension or secondary polycythaemia complicating chronic hypoxia [13]. Diuretics are indicated if there is evidence of fluid retention, although over-enthusiastic dehydration is undesirable because the sputum becomes viscid and difficult to expectorate. The role of digitalis is controversial [60] but it should not be withheld if signs of heart failure persist in spite of oxygen and diuretic therapy, though the incidence of side effects is increased in hypoxaemic patients.

Drugs or techniques which interfere with respiration, either centrally or peripherally, should be avoided during operation if possible. Local anaesthesia frequently creates good operating conditions and extradural anaesthesia is particularly useful for lower abdominal surgery. Bronchodilatation is often a valuable feature of spontaneous ventilation during procedures carried out under extradural anaesthesia. Insertion of an epidural catheter allows analgesia to be prolonged into the postoperative period, so improving ventilation and the ability to cough.

Patients with chronic bronchitis who require general anaesthesia often ventilate inadequately if allowed to breathe spontaneously. It is often prudent to control ventilation electively and to continue this for some hours postoperatively, at least until the circulation is stable and the action of relaxant and other drugs has worn off completely. Use of a mixture of nitrous oxide and oxygen for a few hours enables artificial ventilation to be continued while long-acting drugs are excreted, and extubation can then be performed at a time when respiratory depression is minimal. The risks of marrow depression are negligible if nitrous oxide is only used for short periods [48].

Postoperative hypoxia is a particular problem in these patients, whatever anaesthetic technique is employed. It cannot always be relieved by increasing the inspired oxygen concentration because this results in unacceptable respiratory depression. The optimum oxygen concentration for each individual can only be determined by trial and error and it is often necessary to adopt a compromise between hypoxaemia and respiratory depression. The desired concentration can only be achieved reliably using a high flow delivery mask based on the Venturi principle.

EMPHYSEMA, BRONCHIECTASIS AND PRIMARY HYPOVENTILATION

The purist may object to the inclusion of these disorders in a section entitled 'generalized airways obstruction' but in terms of functional derangement they are most appropriately considered here.

Bronchiectasis

Production of purulent sputum over prolonged periods of time from dilated disorganized bronchi is the characteristic feature of bronchiectasis. The disease can be localized or diffuse and severe bronchiectasis is the typical pulmonary manifestation of cystic fibrosis, a congenital defect in exocrine secretion. Airways obstruction is often present too although the lung volumes are smaller than normal if there is extensive alveolar destruction and fibrosis. Bronchodilator drugs provide little help for many patients and the most important aspect of management is postural drainage [21], combined when necessary with antibiotic treatment. Percussion of the chest after lying for 20–30 minutes in the position which favours drainage from the affected segment must be carried out regularly by a physiotherapist or by a relative at home. Forced expiration [66], a cough simulated by the patient compressing his own chest while exhaling forcibly through a widely open glottis, is an effective alternative. Eventually the volume of sputum produced each day will decrease and then infection is easier to control. Unlike infection in chronic bronchitis, the pathogens present in bronchiectatic cavities are unpredictable and change rapidly in response to treatment. Frequent sputum culture is essential and antibiotics should be given at the first sigh of renewed infection. Tetracycline, amoxycillin, cloxacillin or co-trimoxazole are effective in many patients but some require potentially toxic antibiotics such as the aminoglycosides or lincomycin. Anaerobic infections predominate in some patients but can usually be cleared, at least temporarily, by metronidazole. Patients being prepared for operation should be given appropriate antibiotics according to the results of sputum culture, and potentially toxic agents should be included if necessary.

Bronchiectasis is one of the conditions where regular treatment by the physiotherapist is invaluable and admission to hospital a week or more before elective surgery should be arranged if possible. Ideally, the patient should be segregated to minimize the risks of cross-infection.

Emphysema

The pathology of emphysema is destruction of alveolar walls leading to loss of gas exchanging surface, loss of elastic recoil and overdistension of remaining lung tissue. It occurs in isolation in the elderly, and also as a primary condition in patients suffering from the familial disease, α_{-1} antitrypsin deficiency in which the lungs are damaged because of a failure to inactivate proteolytic enzymes. Most commonly, however, emphysema co-exists with chronic bronchitis. Lung function tests indicate airways obstruction, resulting primarily from loss of elastic recoil, and there is gross overdistension with a high static compliance, and a significant reduction in gas transfer (Table 3.4). The cardinal symptom is dyspnoea, although cough, sputum and 'wheeze' are notable when chronic bronchitis is present as well. Hypoxia and hypercapnia are late features by comparison with chronic bronchitis, hence the distinction between 'pink puffers' (emphysema) and 'blue boaters' (chronic bronchitis with cor pulmonale). Post mortem studies show that this clinical distinction is not reflected in differences in pathology, and central disturbances in the control of respiration [23] are probably responsible for the contrast between the somnolent blue boater and the dyspnoeic pink puffer.

Treatment is unrewarding in patients with emphysema unless there is reversible airways obstruction, or profuse secretions which are infected or difficult to expectorate. In particular, physiotherapeutic manoeuvres other than breathing exercises are probably contraindicated.

Patients with emphysema and airways obstruction are always difficult to manage during general anaesthesia. Loss of active expiratory effort hinders deflation of the lungs and a negative expiratory pressure accentuates overdistension by facilitating early closure of intrathoracic airways. Local anaesthesia is often preferable, provided the posture required during surgery does not embarrass spontaneous ventilation. Paradoxically, patients with pure emphysema and little airways obstruction are often easy to ventilate mechanically but it is still difficult to re-establish spontaneous ventilation successfully.

Primary hypoventilation

Patients with normal lungs occasionally underventilate and so become hypoxic, hypercapnic, and eventually develop cor pulmonale. Many are obese and somnolent ('Pickwick syndrome'). They show a defective ventilatory response to the inhalation of

Table 3.4. (*a*) Pulmonary function in a 58-year-old male with chronic bronchitis and asthma. There is evidence of airways obstruction and hyperinflation, but gas transfer is well preserved.

	Predicted	Result
FEV_1 (ml)	2710	850
FVC (ml)	3900	2300
FEV_1/FVC (%)	69·5	36·9
VC (ml)	3900	2450
FRC (ml)	3610	5190
TLC (ml)	6150	6840
RV/TLC (%)	36·5	64·0
*T_1co (mmol min^{-1} kPa^{-1})	7·57	7·77
V_A (litres)		4·36
K_{co} (mmol min^{-1} kPa^{-1} l^{-1})	1·4	1·78

Table 3.4. (*b*) Pulmonary function in a 36-year-old man with primary emphysema. There is evidence of airways obstruction and gross hyperinflation, and gas transfer is severely impaired.

	Predicted	Result
FEV_1 (ml)	3840	950
FVC (ml)	4980	4450
FEV_1/FVC (%)	77·0	21·3
FRC (ml)	3990	8240
TLC (ml)	7150	10590
RV/TLC (%)	30·4	66·0
*T_1co (mmol min^{-1} kPa^{-1})	10·7	2·67
V_A (litres)		5·69
K_{co} (mmol min^{-1} kPa^{-1} l^{-1})	1·67	0·47

* Measurements of gas transfer were carried out by the single breath method.

carbon dioxide and in some cases at least, the site of the primary lesion is in the brain stem. The importance of the condition to the anaesthetist is the extreme sensitivity of these patients to all forms of respiratory depressant drugs. Controlled ventilation with nitrous oxide oxygen, relaxants and minimal sedation is probably the technique of choice if anaesthesia is required (see page 404).

RESTRICTIVE LUNG DISEASES

Pulmonary restriction can be caused by lung disease, or by lesions of the thoracic cage (e.g. kyphoscoliosis; ankylosing spondylitis), the soft tissues (e.g. dermatomyositis; scleroderma), neuromuscular disorders (Chapter 7) or the pleura (effusion, fibrosis, neoplasm). Some apparently severe deformities (e.g. pectus excavatus) cause virtually no impairment of ventilatory function.

It is important to distinguish between pulmonary and extrapulmonary restriction because the defect in extrapulmonary disease is often purely mechanical, whereas pulmonary disorders generally cause considerable interference with gas exchange as

Table 3.5. (*a*) Pulmonary function in a 56-year-old female with a mesothelioma of the left pleural cavity. There is a restrictive defect but well-preserved gas transfer.

	Predicted	Result
FEV$_1$ (ml)	2600	1930
FVC (ml)	3400	2430
FEV$_1$/FVC (%)	76·5	79·4
VC (ml)	3400	2430
FRC (ml)	3140	2153
TLC (ml)	5310	3803
RV/TLC (%)	36·0	36·1
*T$_1$co (moll min^{-1} kPa^{-1})	6·50	6·61
V$_A$ (litres)		3·49
K$_{co}$ (moll min^{-1} kPa^{-1} l^{-1})	1·68	1·9

Table 3.5. (*b*) Pulmonary function in a 56-year-old male suffering from fibrosing alveolitis. There is a restrictive ventilatory defect and gas transfer is impaired.

	Predicted	Result
FEV$_1$ (ml)	3260	2300
FVC (ml)	4700	2700
FEV$_1$/FVC (%)	69·5	85·2
VC (ml)	4700	2450
FRC (ml)	4250	2947
TLC (ml)	7320	4747
RV/TLC (%)	35·8	48·3
*T$_1$co (moll min^{-1} kPa^{-1})	9·47	3·43
V$_A$ (litres)		3·75
K$_{co}$ (moll min^{-1} kPa^{-1} l^{-1})	1·46	0·92

* Measurements of gas transfer were made by the single breath method.

well (Table 3.5). The distinction is not absolute however, because gross distortion of the thoracic viscera (e.g. kyphoscoliosis) predisposes to bronchopulmonary infection and consequent pulmonary damage.

The significance of extrapulmonary restriction for the anaesthetist is twofold—total compliance (i.e. chest wall and lung) is poor so that considerable effort is required to inflate the lungs, whether this effort is expended by the patient, the anaesthetist or a machine; secondly, a serious reduction in lung volume impedes the ability to cough effectively. Unless the vital capacity is more than about twice the tidal volume, coughing is ineffective and secretions provoked during anaesthesia may accumulate and cause atelectasis. The reduction in lung volume also favours hypoxaemia because the closing volume approximates to, or lies within, the range of tidal ventilation. There is however little risk of carbon dioxide retention in these patients until their disability is extreme, and a high inspired oxygen concentration can generally be given if necessary. The most important requirement during anaesthesia is to avoid drugs causing prolonged respiratory depression, and to minimize any additional mechanical embarrassment such as tight bandages, pneumoperitoneum or abdominal distension.

The same considerations apply to patients with pulmonary disease causing restriction but, in addition, there are often abnormalities in the distribution of both ventilation and perfusion, and sputum production is excessive in some patients. Sometimes the disturbances of ventilation and perfusion are so well matched that the arterial blood gas tensions are normal, at least while the patient is at rest. More often there is hypoxaemia and a reduction in $Paco_2$: the effects of the increase in physiological dead space are obscured by hyperventilation while the excess of perfusion relative to ventilation causes a shunt effect which is difficult or even sometimes impossible to correct with high inspired oxygen concentrations. Unlike patients with variable airways obstruction, there is generally little change during anaesthesia, and even severely hypoxic patients often tolerate the procedure well provided ventilation is controlled and further hypoxia is avoided. It is in the postoperative period, when the ability to breathe and cough is impaired by pain or analgesic drugs, and pulmonary function is compromised further by the sequelae of anaesthesia, surgery, blood transfusion, recumbency, etc., that hypoxia, and sometimes even carbon dioxide retention are a particular hazard. A period of postoperative ventilatory support may be necessary but is usually easy to discontinue after the acute episode is over, even though lung function is severely curtailed. This again is in marked contrast to the difficulty associated with controlled ventilation in patients with generalized airways obstruction.

Additional problems are imposed by specific conditions. For example, corticosteroid and immunosuppressant drugs are used to treat some types of pulmonary fibrosis, so steroid supplements may be necessary during the operative period and particular care is needed to avoid infection. Occasionally, pulmonary fibrosis is associated with chronic airways obstruction (e.g. in the late stages of sarcoidosis), although extreme lability of bronchial calibre is uncommon. Finally, there is a high incidence of pneumothorax in some disorders, e.g. eosinophilic granuloma, and air leaks are often very persistent.

PULMONARY INFECTION, INFARCTION AND NEOPLASM

INFECTION

The advent of antibiotics has changed the behaviour and importance of many pulmonary infections. In patients with previously healthy lungs, pneumonias caused by *Klebsiella pneumoniae*, virulent staphylococci or *Mycoplasma pneumoniae* are now cause for greater concern than pneumococcal pneumonia [24]. Viral infection of the lungs can also prove rapidly fatal, especially if complicated by staphylococcal super-infection. In patients receiving long-term corticosteroid or immunosuppressive therapy, opportunistic organisms such as *Pneumocystis carinii*, *Candida albicans* or *Nocardia asteroides* can invade the respiratory tract and cause a pneumonia which is difficult both to identify and to treat [76].

Pulmonary tuberculosis is now a much smaller cause of morbidity and mortality than in pre-antibiotic days. Mechanical therapy such as collapse, plombage or thoraco-plasty is rarely required, but a few patients subjected to these manoeuvres in the past still present for surgery, some with chronic respiratory disability. Active pulmonary tuberculosis is also important, largely because it can 'flare up' and spread rapidly following anaesthesia rather than because it causes severe functional impairment; significant nonpulmonary tuberculosis may also be present (e.g. of the renal tract). Symptoms which might suggest the presence of active tuberculosis are often non-specific and easily overlooked. Weight loss, lethargy and night sweats are common if there is extensive disease, but in many patients the systemic manifestations are not prominent. Chronic cough in the elderly bronchitic may represent co-existent, active tuberculosis whereas younger patients present more commonly with an isolated haemoptysis, pleural effusion or with symptomless disease which is only apparent on the chest X-ray. When pulmonary tuberculosis is active, cross-infection can occur via anaesthetic apparatus and all ventilatory equipment used for tuberculous patients should be sterilized immediately after use.

INFARCTION

Acute massive pulmonary embolism presents as a cardiovascular crisis [55] although dyspnoea and disturbances of ventilatory function occur too. Chronic pulmonary thrombo-embolic disease presents with dyspnoea, often with signs of pulmonary hypertension and right heart failure. The physiological dead space is increased but hyperventilation is usual and the arterial carbon dioxide tension is low. Mismatch of ventilation and perfusion results in arterial hypoxaemia in spite of the high minute volume. Additional hypoxia is dangerous because it causes a further increase in pulmonary vascular resistance and can precipitate cardiac arrest; similarly, anaesthetic agents which cause pulmonary vasoconstriction should be avoided (Fig. 3.7).

NEOPLASM

Primary tumours of the lung are common and the majority are malignant. The five-year survival figures for all forms of treatment of bronchial carcinoma are poor, but resection is regarded as the treatment of choice in something like 20–25 per cent of cases. These patients can be difficult to manage during anaesthesia either because of the functional state of the rest of the lungs or because of the nature and site of the tumour. The association between cigarette smoking and pollution and both chronic bronchitis and carcinoma of the bronchus [17] means that many patients submitted to surgery already have extensive pulmonary disease, and some are inoperable solely on the grounds of respiratory disability. Formal tests of lung function are often disappointingly unhelpful as a means of selecting those who will withstand resection, perhaps because it is impossible to determine how much the abnormal findings are caused by the tumour-bearing area. Regional tests of ventilation and perfusion may help to determine suitability for resection; for example, defective ventilation caused by bronchial obstruction and diminution of pulmonary blood flow to the nonventilated segment may mean that the diseased area is not contributing to pulmonary function at all.

Tumours lying centrally (within a proximal to a segmental bronchus) are most likely to interfere with pulmonary function by causing partial or complete obstruction of a bronchus. They can also invade adjacent structures such as the pericardium or even the heart, and tumour sometimes grows along the pulmonary veins into the left atrium so that radical removal involves intrapericardial resection. Peripheral tumours are less likely to interfere with pulmonary function but they sometimes infiltrate the chest wall and attempts at resection result in severe haemorrhage. Some malignant tumours

5*

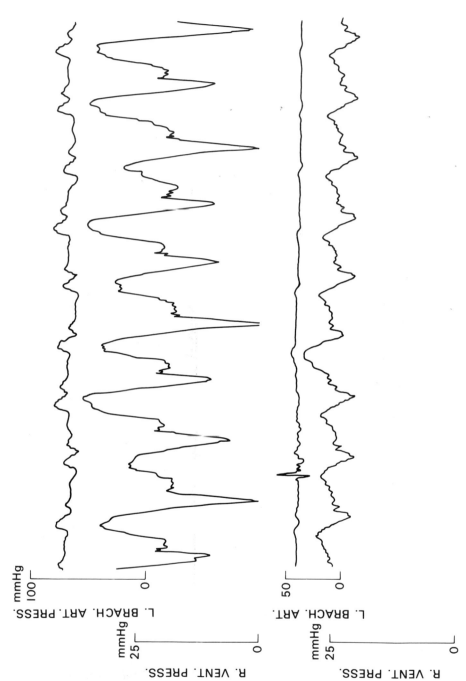

Fig. 3.7. (*a*). Arterial and right ventricular pressure records obtained from a man of late middle age suffering from acute pulmonary embolism. Cardiac arrest occurred during induction of anaesthesia, (*b*) probably because of further increase in the pulmonary vascular resistance caused by cyclopropane. External cardiac massage emptied the right ventricle (*c*) and spontaneous ejection from the heart returned (*d*). In spite of resuscitation, the patient succumbed to right ventricular failure two days later.

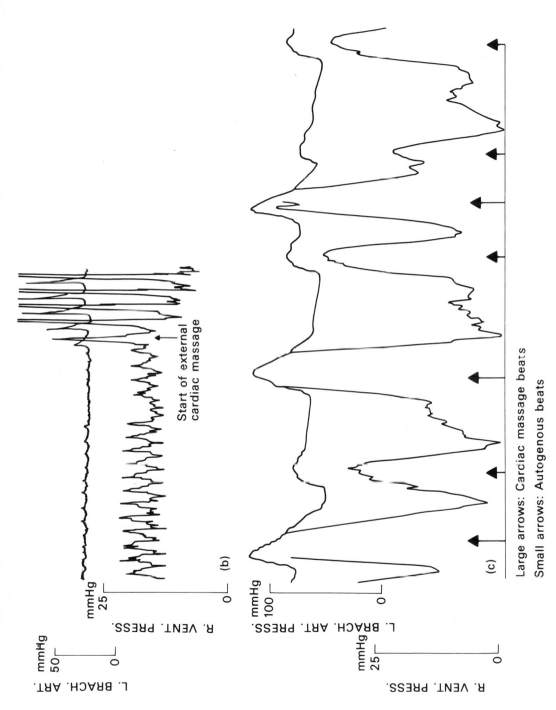

Large arrows: Cardiac massage beats
Small arrows: Autogenous beats

Fig. 3·7. (*c*) and (*d*).

secrete hormones which mimic or augment the actions of endocrine glands [2] while others are associated with peripheral neuropathy, myopathy or cerebellar degeneration [32]. In a very small percentage of cases, the neuromuscular disorder causes an abnormal response to muscle relaxant drugs.

Bronchial adenocarcinoma and alveolar cell carcinoma are neoplasms which either form solitary nodules or spread within the lung by growing along the alveolar walls. A similar diffuse infiltration occurs if secondary carcinoma spreads by permeating the pulmonary lymphatics (lymphangitis carcinomatosis). These patients present with progressive dyspnoea and open lung biopsy is required occasionally to confirm the diagnosis; tests of lung function indicate hypoxia and hyperventilation with a picture of restrictive ventilatory defect.

Benign tumours of the lung are relatively uncommon. Bronchial adenomata are generally benign and are usually vascular tumours which present with haemoptysis or with recurrent episodes of distal collapse and infection; sometimes they consist of secreting carcinoid tissue.

The resection of bronchial tumours is facilitated if the operated lung is allowed to collapse once the chest is open. This can be achieved by endobronchial intubation of the contralateral lung or by the use of a double lumen tube. Carbon dioxide elimination is easy to achieve during one-lung anaesthesia but arterial hypoxaemia is common, largely because some percentage of the pulmonary blood flow continues to pass through the unventilated lung [36, 37]. Oxygen can be insufflated into the collapsed lung during prolonged one-lung procedures (e.g. oesophageal resection) to promote diffusion oxygenation of the blood flowing through that lung [56].

Malignant disease in the superior mediastinum, or occasionally benign fibrosis, can cause superior vena caval obstruction, sometimes associated with compression of the trachea or oesophagus. In superior caval obstruction, the action of intravenous agents given in the usual site may be delayed and intravenous infusions are best established in the lower limbs. Hypoxia, coughing or straining increase the already elevated intracranial pressure so causing petechial haemorrhages in the conjunctiva and probably within the brain, and minor trauma to the respiratory tract can cause prolonged bleeding. Intubation, controlled ventilation and a slight head up tilt help to minimize the cardiovascular sequelae.

PLEURAL DISEASE, PNEUMOTHORAX AND LUNG CYSTS, BRONCHOPLEURAL FISTULA

Pleural effusions impede ventilation by causing compression (restriction) of the lung and are commonly associated with underlying pulmonary disease such as pneumonia or pulmonary infarction. Unless the effusion is small, it is wise to aspirate or drain the fluid before embarking on general anaesthesia for all but the most minor procedures. Chronic effusions cause fibrous thickening of the visceral pleura and decortication may be required to free the lung. Chronic empyemata, often tuberculous in origin, may need similar management although in these cases the function of the underlying lung is often very limited. The chief operative hazard is haemorrhage.

An acute empyema requires drainage to cure the infection and to prevent subsequent pulmonary restriction. Insertion of a wide bore intercostal tube is needed to allow thick purulent material to drain freely, and this often necessitates resection of a short length of rib. This is a minor procedure which should be carried out under local anaesthesia with the patient sitting upright so that inadvertent damage to the lung, which is ill-protected by fibrous tissue in the acute stage, does not result in 'spillage' of infected pleural fluid into the bronchial tree.

A certain amount of air in the pleural cavity can be tolerated without discomfort or respiratory distress, provided overall lung function is good and the air is not under tension. Symptoms are probable if more than 50 per cent of one lung is collapsed, especially if this occurs suddenly, or if there is sufficient tension to cause mediastinal displacement, or if the pneumothorax is associated with lung disease or thoracic trauma. Immediate relief follows the introduction of an intercostal drain which, in most cases, is best inserted in the mid-axillary line and threaded upwards towards the apex of the pleural cavity. Suction may be needed to keep the lung expanded, especially if there is a large air leak.

The presence of a pneumothorax is a considerable hazard during general anaesthesia for at least three reasons. Coughing, straining or the use of controlled ventilation accentuates the air leak and leads to a rapid increase in intrathoracic pressure which prevents adequate ventilation and causes cardiovascular collapse. Alternatively, the tension in the pleural cavity rises so high that air escapes into the mediastinum and subcutaneous tissues and even the pericardial cavity. Finally, and much more insidiously, the tension in the pleural space increases gradually during the early stages of anaesthesia with nitrous oxide because this gas diffuses rapidly out of the blood into the air-filled space, and nitrogen is only reabsorbed slowly [74]. All these hazards are eliminated if the pleural cavity is drained. Chest drains are often clamped while patients are being moved, and it is important to confirm that the drain is both patent and connected to the underwater seal before anaesthesia is induced.

Comparable hazards surround the management of patients with lung cysts [22]. These can be congenital (Fig. 3.8) or they develop in later life, generally in association

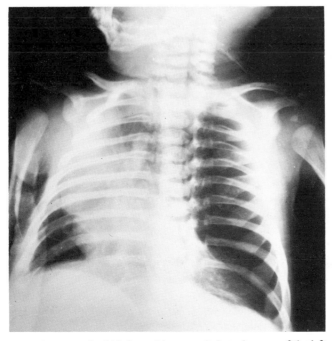

Fig. 3.8. Chest X-ray of a 3-month-old infant with congenital emphysema of the left upper lobe. Resection of the lobe was followed by complete recovery.

with emphysema. The fact that the cyst remains inflated means that there must be some sort of communication with the bronchial tree, but this may be intermittent or 'valvular'. To avoid the risks of overdistension and rupture during anaesthesia, it is preferable to isolate the affected lobe or lung with an appropriate endobronchial tube or blocker, even in patients in whom the cyst is symptomless. If this proves impossible and either respiratory or cardiovascular disturbances occur, the cyst should be drained with any needle, cannula or tube which is available. This will probably result in a broncho-pleuro-cutaneous fistula, but unless the air leak is enormous, it is generally possible to maintain effective alveolar ventilation by using a large minute volume.

Occasional patients appear with a chronic bronchopleural fistula, with or without a communication to the skin. The fistulous communication is fibrous and anaesthesia is often surprisingly uneventful, especially if spontaneous ventilation can be retained.

An acute bronchopleural fistula is a much more hazardous condition. The magnitude of the air leak varies, depending on the size of the fistula and changes in airway and intrapleural pressure. In addition, there is often an accumulation of pleural fluid or blood which can flood the rest of the bronchial tree if the fluid level rises above the level of the fistula. Insertion of a chest drain relieves tension and facilitates evacuation of pleural fluid. If there is a large effusion, e.g. following pneumonectomy, the patient should be nursed and subsequently anaesthetized sitting bolt upright, but slightly tilted so that the affected side is dependent. Isolation of the fistula with an endobronchial or double lumen tube must precede artificial ventilation or any change of posture.

RESPIRATORY FAILURE

Respiratory failure [9, 25] is defined as an inability to maintain normal arterial blood gas tensions in the absence of an intracardiac shunt while breathing air at sea level. In chronic airways obstruction, hypercapnia and hypoxia commonly occur together whereas in restrictive disorders, and in pulmonary vascular disease, hypoxia is the prominent feature and hypercapnia is a late or even terminal event. Renal retention of bicarbonate results in a normal or near normal pH when carbon dioxide retention is chronic. Any deterioration in ventilatory efficiency causes a further increase in Pa,CO_2 and fall in pH, and the pH may also fall because of a coincident metabolic acidosis caused by tissue hypoxia. Cor pulmonale is a frequent concomitant of chronic respiratory failure, and electrolyte derangements due to disease or diuretic therapy are also common. Treatment is largely directed towards management of the underlying disease, but controlled oxygen therapy, diuretics, correction of electrolyte abnormalities, respiratory stimulants or artificial ventilation may all be required. Many of these patients have such severe disease that heroic measures are best withheld unless there is an acute and potentially reversible component to their condition.

Artificial ventilation in particular is associated with both hazard and discomfort and the benefits which it might confer must be weighed against the disadvantages. The availability and quality of hospital resources and the patient's domestic circumstances are also factors which should be considered carefully before subjecting those with chronic disease to prolonged ventilatory support. In general, patients with chronic bronchitis have a far better prognosis than those with emphysema, bronchiectasis or pulmonary fibrosis, especially if the need for mechanical ventilation is precipitated by a severe infection [61].

A more optimistic approach can be adopted in the management of acute respiratory failure. The treatment of severe acute asthma has been described already, but there are also a number of disorders which affect the lungs at alveolar level which can result in respiratory failure [7]. Fulminating pneumonia, oedema caused by the inhalation or aspiration of noxious substances, embolism of fat or amniotic fluid, and the nebulous conditions of 'shock lung' and 'post-perfusion' or 'pump lung' all lead to similar functional derangements. Complete recovery is possible if the patient can be supported through the acute stage of the illness [63].

The pathogenesis of many of these disorders is incompletely understood and there are probably vascular, inflammatory and possibly immunological mechanisms operating in the lungs. A self-perpetuating process of pulmonary damage can occur if vasoactive peptides and enzymes are liberated from the aggregates of platelets and white cells which often develop intravascularly in these disorders and which are then filtered by the pulmonary capillaries.

The physiological sequelae consist of atelectasis and pulmonary oedema, resulting in a gross reduction in compliance and severe mismatch of ventilation and perfusion, generally with considerable intrapulmonary shunting as well. The oedema is interstitial rather than intra-alveolar at first and is caused by vascular damage rather than by an increase in pulmonary hydrostatic pressure.

Characteristically, these patients hyperventilate with a minute volume far in excess of normal. The arterial carbon dioxide tension is normal or low and the arterial oxygen tension remains very low in spite of oxygen enrichment [41]. Metabolic acidosis is common, and hypoxia and the effort of hyperventilation combine to precipitate hypotension, a rising jugular venous pressure and peripheral circulatory failure. Hypercapnia commonly occurs at this stage when the patient is too exhausted to sustain the degree of hyperventilation required to offset the increase in physiological dead space. Bronchoconstriction is a prominent feature in a few instances, especially following the inhalation of gastric juice or other irritants. This adds to the mechanical difficulty of sustaining a high minute volume. The principles of treatment are:

1 to relieve hypoxia;
2 to eliminate the work of breathing and the associated metabolic demand for oxygen;
3 to prevent further pulmonary damage.

Intermittent positive pressure ventilation increases the intra-alveolar pressure so helping to suppress the formation of oedema, and to re-expand atelectatic areas. Recruitment of alveoli with a long time constant is favoured by the use of a slow respiratory rate with a large tidal volume, end-inspiratory plateau and a positive end-expiratory pressure (e.g. + 10 cm of water) (Fig. 3.9). High inspired oxygen tensions should be avoided to prevent further pulmonary damage [78]. Ideally, the inspired oxygen concentration should not exceed 40 per cent although this recommendation should be balanced against the arterial oxygen tension which results, and the effects of varying the inspired gas mixture. An 'acceptable' figure for Pa,O_2 cannot be defined because tissue oxygen requirements vary enormously, depending on cardiac output, the oxygen carrying capacity of the blood, the level of metabolic demand and the state of other crucial organs such as the brain or kidneys. The risks of oxygen-induced pulmonary damage must therefore be weighed against those of either continued arterial hypoxaemia or alternative forms of treatment, for each individual patient.

Heavy sedation is needed to control restlessness and to suppress ventilatory drive, but even if normal arterial blood gas tension are achieved, many patients still 'fight the ventilator' and require muscular paralysis. If an adequate oxygen tension cannot

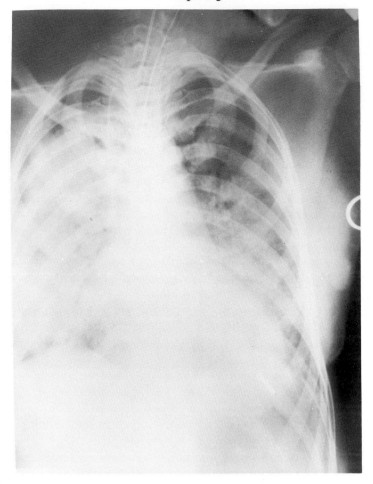

Fig. 3.9. Chest X-ray of a 30-year-old female. Six years after double valve replacement (aortic and mitral), anaesthesia for the removal of a retained placenta was complicated by the inhalation of gastric acid. The X-ray was taken between 6 and 8 hours later.

Table 3.6. Serial measurements of arterial blood gas tensions showing the influence of a changing pattern of ventilation. The first values relate to the time when the chest X-ray in Fig. 3.9 was taken, and a positive end-expiratory pressure of 10 cm H_2O (1·0 kPa) was in use throughout the entire period.

	P_{O_2} (kPa)	P_{CO_2} (kPa)	F_1O_2 (%)	$\dot{V}$ l/min	R breaths/min
12.8.73	5·8	10·1	68	10	20
	7·1	9·5	100	10	20
	7·3	6·1	77	14	20
	13·1	5·2	73	12	14
13.8.73	18.5	3.9	73	12	14
14.8.73	14·8	5·3	60	10	13

be achieved by these means, further manoeuvres to decrease metabolic demand or raise the mixed venous oxygen tension by increasing the cardiac output may help (e.g. mild hypothermia or possibly infusion of an inotropic agent). Extracorporeal support with a membrane oxygenator may occasionally tide the patient over the acute phase of the illness, but this is a highly specialized technique with many complications [34].

Diuretic therapy is probably of little value unless incautious transfusion has been employed in an attempt to support a failing circulation. Transfusion should be restricted to the volume required to maintain a normal cardiac filling pressure and other measures should be employed if circulatory failure persists. There is some evidence in favour of high dose corticosteroid therapy [39, 51], started as soon as possible after the initiating event but only continued for 12 to 24 or 36 hours. This treatment has few side effects, other than in patients with acute head injuries who show in increased incidence of gastrointestinal bleeding; prolonged treatment with corticosteroids is disadvantageous because of the increased risk of infection and hence the greater chance of irreversible pulmonary damage [20]. Methyl prednisolone sodium succinate is the preparation advocated most widely at present, part of its beneficial effect being attributed to the large anion which is taken up by biological membranes and is thought to inhibit cell and lysosomal destruction [79].

A number of patients with acute respiratory failure which might otherwise prove fatal can be treated successfully by these vigorous measures, and aggressive therapy is justified because many of them are young and previously healthy. Long-term follow-up is advisable in case tracheal damage has resulted from prolonged intubation or tracheostomy [3], and to observe whether pulmonary function returns to normal (Table 3.7) [40].

Table 3.7. Serial lung function tests from the patient described in the caption to Fig. 3.9. Initially, there is a restrictive defect with impaired gas transfer, but one year later there is only slight restriction and gas transfer is normal.

	Predicted	August 1973	December 1973	June 1974
FEV$_1$ (ml)	3330	2255	2420	2550
FVC (ml)	3940	2460	2600	3000
TLC (ml)	5610	3950	—	4290
T$_1$co (mmol min^{-1} kPa^{-1})	9·2	5·5	7·1	7·1

CONCLUSION

Pulmonary disorders impose many burdens on the anaesthetist and a number of conditions are disappointingly chronic and irreversible. It is encouraging to realize that pulmonary disease also offers the anaesthetist opportunity to supplement technical skill with clinical judgment and knowledge which, in some cases, can make all the difference between success and failure.

REFERENCES

1 ACKERY DM, STIRLING GM. Radio-isotopes in the study of pulmonary function and disease. In: Stretton TB, ed. *Recent advances in respiratory medicine*, No. 1. London: Churchill Livingstone, 1976: 1–38.

2 ANDERSON EG. Non-metastatic syndromes associated with carcinoma of the bronchus: 1 endo-crine disorders. *Hosp Med* 1966; **1**: 11–14.

3 ANDREWS MJ, PEARSON FG. Incidence and pathogenesis of tracheal injury following cuffed tube tracheostomy with assisted ventilation: analysis of a two-year prospective study. *Ann Surg* 1971; **173**: 249–63.

4 BARER GR, HOWARD P, SHAW JW. Stimulus-response curves of the pulmonary vascular bed to hypoxia and hypercapnia. *J Physiol* 1970; **211**: 139–55.

5 BLOOMFIELD P, CARMICHAEL J, PETRIE GR, JEWELL NP, CROMPTON GK. Comparison of sal-butamol given intravenously and by intermittent positive-pressure breathing in life-threatening asthma. *Br Med J* 1979; **1**: 848–50.

6 BRANTHWAITE MA. The management of severe asthma. In: Baderman J, ed. *Management o f medical emergencies*. Tunbridge Wells: Pitman Medical, 1978: 48–56.

7 BRANTHWAITE MA. Adult respiratory distress syndrome. In: Besser GM, ed. *Advanced medicine* 13. Tunbridge Wells: Pitman Medical, 1977: 289–302.

8 BRANTHWAITE MA. *Artificial ventilation for pulmonary disease*. Tunbridge Wells: Pitman Medi-cal, 1978.

9 BREWIS RAL. Diseases of the respiratory system. Respiratory failure. *Br Med J* 1978; **1**: 898–900.

10 *British Medical Journal* Leading article. 'First in, last out' in the lung. *Br Med J* 1973; **3**: 119–20.

11 *British Medical Journal* Leading article. Management of severe acute asthma. *Br Med J* 1978; **1**: 873–4.

12 *British Medical Journal* Leading article. Bronchial secretions. *Br Med J* 1975; **2**: 51–2.

13 *British Medical Journal* Leading article. Domiciliary oxygen. *Br Med J* 1977; **2**: 77–8.

14 *British Medical Journal* Leading article. Clinical audit in diagnostic radiology. *Br Med J* 1977; **2**: 479–80.

15 BURROWS B, KETTEL LJ, NIDEN AH, RABINOWITZ M, DIENER CF. Patterns of cardiovascular dysfunction in chronic obstructive lung disease. *N Engl J Med* 1972; **286**: 912–18.

16 CAMPBELL IA, HILL A, MIDDLETON H, MOMEN M, PRESCOTT RJ. Intermittent positive-pressure breathing. *Br Med J* 1978; **1**: 1186.

17 CAPLIN M, FESTENSTEIN F. Relation between lung cancer, chronic bronchitis, and airways obstruc-tion. *Br Med J* 1975; **3**: 678–80.

18 CLARKE CW. Relationship of bacterial and viral infections to exacerbations of asthma. *Thorax* 1979; **34**: 344–7.

19 CLARKE S. Respiratory function tests. *Br J Hosp Med* 1976; **15**: 137–53.

20 CLOWES GHA Jr, HIRSCH MFE, WILLIAMS L, *et al*. Septic lung and shock lung in man. *Ann Surg* 1975; **181**: 681–92.

21 COCHRANE GM, WEBBER BA, CLARKE SW. Effects of sputum on pulmonary function. *Br Med J* 1977; **2**: 1181–3.

22 CULLUM AR, ENGLISH ICW, BRANTHWAITE MA. Endobronchial intubation in infancy. *Anaes-thesia* 1973; **28**: 66–70.

23 DOUGLAS NJ, LEGGETT RJE, CALVERLEY PMA, BRASH HM, FLENLEY DC, BREZINOVA V. Tran-sient hypoxaemia during sleep in chronic bronchitis and emphysema. *Lancet* 1979; **1**: 1–4.

24 FEKETY FR Jr, CALDWELL J, GUMP D, *et al*. Bacteria, viruses, and mycoplasmas in acute pneu-monia in adults. *Am Rev Respir Dis* 1971; **104**: 499–507.

25 FLENLEY DC. Clinical hypoxia: causes, consequences and correction. *Lancet* 1978; **1**: 542–6.

26 FLETCHER C, PETO R. The natural history of chronic airflow obstruction. *Br Med J* 1977; **1**: 1645–8.

27 GEE JBL, FLICK RB Jr. Bronchoalveolar lavage. *Thorax* 1980; **35**: 1–8.

28 GODFREY S. Improving the reliability of the rebreathing method of measuring mixed venous P_{CO_2}. *Br Med J* 1965; **1**: 1163–5.

29 GORMEZANO J, BRANTHWAITE MA. Pulmonary physiotherapy with assisted ventilation. *Anaes-thesia* 1972; **27**: 249–57.

30 GOTHARD JWW, BUSST CM, BRANTHWAITE MA, DAVIES NJH, DENISON DM. Applications of respiratory mass spectrometry to intensive care. *Anaesthesia* 1980 **35**: 890–5.

31 HARRISON BDW. Polycythaemia in a selected group of patients with chronic airways obstruction. *Clin Sci* 1973; **44**: 563–70.

32 HERON JR. Non-metastatic syndromes associated with carcinoma of the bronchus: neuromuscular disorders. *Hosp Med* 1966; **1**: 106.

33 HETZEL MR, CLARK TJH, BRANTHWAITE MA. Asthma: analysis of sudden deaths and ventilatory arrests in hospital. *Br Med J* 1977; **1**: 808–11.

34 HILL JD, RATLIFF JL, PARROTT JCW, *et al.* Pulmonary pathology in acute respiratory insufficiency: lung biopsy as a diagnostic tool. *J Thorac Cardiovasc Surg* 1976; **71**: 64–71.

35 KELMAN GR, NUNN JF, PRYS-RORERTS C, GREENBAUM R. The influence of cardiac output on arterial oxygenation: a theoretical study. *Br J Anaesth* 1967; **39**: 450–8.

36 KERR JH, CRAMPTON-SMITH A, PRYS-RORERTS C, MELOCHE R, FOËX P. Observations during endobronchial anaesthesia. II. Oxygenation. *Br J Anaesth* 1974; **46**: 84–92.

37 KHANAM T, BRANTHWAITE MA. Arterial oxygenation during one-lung anaesthesia I & II. *Anaesthesia* 1973; **28**: 132–8 & 280–90.

38 KNOWLES GK, CLARK TJH. Pulsus paradoxus as a valuable sign indicating severity of asthma. *Lancet* 1973; **2**: 1356–9.

39 KUSAJIMA K, WAX SD, WEBB WR. Effects of methyl prednisolone on pulmonary microcirculation. *Surg Gynecol Obstet* 1974; **139**: 1–5.

40 LAKSHMINARYAN S, STANDFORD RE, PETTY TL. Prognosis after recovery from adult respiratory distress syndrome. *Am Rev Respir Dis* 1976; **113**: 7–16.

41 LAMY M, FALLAT RJ, KOENIGER E, *et al.* Pathologic features and mechanisms of hypoxaemia in adult respiratory distress syndrome. *Am Rev Respir Dis* 1976; **114**: 267–84.

42 *Lancet* Leading article. Chest physiotherapy under scrutiny. *Lancet* 1978; **2**: 1241.

43 *Lancet* Leading article. Wet or dry inhalers? *Lancet* 1978; **1**: 79–80.

44 *Lancet* Leading article. Are steroid inhalers safer than tablets? *Lancet* 1979; **1**: 589–90.

45 *Lancet* Leading article. Oedema in cor pulmonale. *Lancet* 1975; **2**: 1289–90.

46 *Lancet* Leading article. Oxygen in acute-on-chronic respiratory failure. *Lancet* 1979; **1**: 1172–3.

47 *Lancet* Leading article. Antimicrobial treatment of chronic bronchitis. *Lancet* 1975; **1**: 505–6.

48 *Lancet* Leading article. Nitrous oxide and the bone-marrow. *Lancet* 1978; **2**: 613–14.

49 *Lancet* Leading article. Inspiratory crackles. *Lancet* 1974; **1**: 969–70.

50 *Lancet* Leading article. Carbon monoxide as a test for lung haemorrhage. *Lancet* 1977; **1**: 407–8.

51 LOZMAN J, DUTTON RE, ENGLISH M, POWERS SR Jr. Cardiopulmonary adjustments following single high dosage administration of methylprednisolone in traumatized man. *Ann Surg* 1975; **181**: 317–24.

52 MCGAVIN CR, ARTVINLI M, NAOE H, MCHARDY GJ. Dyspnoea, disability and distance walked: comparison of estimates of exercise performance in respiratory disease. *Br Med J* 1978; **2**: 241–3.

53 Medical Research Council. Definition and classification of chronic bronchitis for clinical and epidemiological purposes. *Lancet* 1965; **1**: 775–9.

54 MILLEDGE JS, NUNN JF. Criteria of fitness for anaesthesia in patients with chronic obstructive lung disease. *Br Med J* 1975; **3**: 670–3.

55 MILLER GAH. The management of acute pulmonary embolism. *Br J Hosp Med* 1977; **18**: 26–31.

56 O'SHEA PJ, SAVAGE TM, WALLON B. Effect of oxygen insufflation during one-lung anaesthesia. *Proc R Soc Med* 1975; **68**: 772–3.

57 PATEL KR. Role of adrenoceptors in bronchial asthma. *J R Coll Physicians Lond* 1979; **13**: 165–71.

58 PATERSON IC, PETRIE GR, CROMPTON GK, RORERTSON JR. Chronic bronchitis: is bacteriological examination of sputum necessary? *Br Med J* 1978; **2**: 537–8.

59 PAYNE CR, STOVIN PGI, BARKER V, MCVITTIE S, STARK JE. Diagnostic accuracy of cytology and biopsy in primary bronchial carcinoma. *Thorax* 1979; **34**: 294–9.

60 PETCH MC. Digoxin for heart failure in sinus rhythm. *Thorax* 1979; **34**: 147–9.

61 PETHERAM IS, BRANTHWAITE MA. Mechanical ventilation for pulmonary disease. *Anaesthesia* 1980; **35**: 467–73.

62 PETRINI MF, PETERSON BT, HYDE RW. Lung tissue volume and blood flow by rebreathing: theory. *J Appl Physiol* 1978; **44**: 795–802.

63 PONTOPPIDAN H, WILSON RS, RIE MA, SCHNEIDER RC. Respiratory intensive care. *Anesthesiology* 1977; **47**: 96–116.

64 PRIDE NB. The assessment of airflow obstruction. *Br J Dis Chest* 1971; **65**: 135–69.

65 PRIDE NB. Analysis of forced expiration—a return to the recording spirometer? *Thorax* 1979; **34**: 144–7.

66 PRYOR JA, WEBBER BA, HODSON ME, BATTEN JC. Evaluation of the forced expiration technique as an adjunct to postural drainage in treatment of cystic fibrosis. *Br Med J* 1979; **2**: 417–18.

67 RURY JH, BUTLER J. Variability of routine pulmonary function tests. *Thorax* 1975; **30**: 548–53.

68 SACKNER MA. Bronchofiberscopy. *Am Rev Respir Dis* 1975; **111**: 62–88.

69 SKEATES SJ. The noninvasive measurement of arterial oxygen. *Br J Clin Equip* 1978; **3**: 63–70.

70 SOUTTER LP, CONWAY MJ, PARKER D. A system for monitoring arterial oxygen tension in sick newborn babies. *Biomed Eng* 1975; **10**: 257–60.

71 Spiro SG, Hahn HL, Edwards RHT, Pride NB. An analysis of the physiological strain of submaximal exercise in patients with chronic obstructive bronchitis. *Thorax* 1975; **30**: 415–24.

72 Sterling GM. Asthma. *Br Med J* 1978; **1**: 1259–62.

73 Tattersfield AE. Airway pharmacology. *Br J Anaesth* 1979; **51**: 681–91.

74 Webb SJS, Nunn JF. A comparison between the effect of nitrous oxide and nitrogen on arterial P_{O_2}. *Anaesthesia* 1967; **22**: 69–81.

75 White RJ, Woodings DF. Impaired water handling in chronic obstructive airways disease. *Br Med J* 1971; **2**: 561–3.

76 Williams DM, Krick JA, Remington JS. Pulmonary infection in the compromised host. I & II. *Am Rev Respir Dis* 1976; **114**: 359–94 & 593–627.

77 Williams SJ, Pierce RJ, Davies NJH, Denison DM. Methods of studying lobar and segmental function of the lung in man. *Br J Dis Chest* 1979; **73**: 97–112.

78 Winter PM, Smith G. The toxicity of oxygen. *Anesthesiology* 1972; **37**: 210–41.

79 Wilson JW. Cellular localization of ^{3}H-labeled corticosteroids by electron microscopic auto-radiography after hemorrhagic shock. In: Glenn TM ed. *Steroids and shock*. Baltimore, London & Tokyo: University Park Press, 1974: 275–99.

FURTHER READING

Cotes JE. *Lung Function: assessment and application in medicine*. 4th ed. Oxford: Blackwell Scientific Publications, 1979.

Flenley DC, Lane DJ, eds. *Respiratory Disorders. Medicine (Oxford)* 1979. 3rd series, volumes 22–4.

Kaper ER, ed. Anesthesia and respiratory function. *International Anesthesiology Clinics* **15** (2). Boston: Little, Brown & Co., 1977.

ACKNOWLEDGMENTS

I am indebted to the following for permission to reproduce clinical and physiological details:

Dr I. Dowdeswell for Figs 3.3 and 3.5, Tables 3.2, 3.3, 3.4, 3.5 and 3.7

Dr R. D. Bradley for Figs 3.6 and 3.7

Dr J. Pfitzner for Fig. 3.4.

Fig. 3.8 is reproduced from *Anaesthesia* 1973 **28**, 66–70 by permission of the Editor.

I am grateful to Professor T. J. H. Clark, MD, FRCP, for reading and commenting on the manuscript.

Chapter 4
Renal Disease

L. STRUNIN AND K. W. PETTINGALE

STRUCTURE AND FUNCTIONS OF THE KIDNEY

Normal man has two kidneys which receive a total blood flow of about 1300 ml/min which is equal to about 25 per cent of the resting cardiac output. Within the kidney the renal artery rapidly subdivides into very small vessels which supply each functional unit of the kidney—the nephron. Each human kidney contains about 1 million nephrons which drain via collecting tubules into the renal pelvis and thence to the ureter. The nephron consists of two parts, Bowman's capsule and the renal tubule proper. Bowman's capsule contains the artery supplying the nephron as a tuft of capillary vessels known as the glomerulus. The renal tubule consists of a proximal convoluted tubule, the loop of Henle, the distal convoluted tubule and a collecting tubule. The loops of Henle and the collecting tubules lie in the renal medulla; the remaining parts of the nephrons lie in the cortex. The length of the human renal tubule is about 3 cm and as there are approximately a million nephrons in each kidney, the total tubule length is about 40 miles.

The major function of the kidney is to secrete urine thereby controlling the *milieu interieur*. From the large blood supply the renal glomeruli filter 170–200 litres/24 hr of protein free fluid from the blood, or some 50–60 times the plasma volume. This filtrate, which has the same crystalloid composition as the plasma, is extensively reabsorbed by the renal tubules. Most of the water is reabsorbed so that the normal daily urine output is some 1500 ml. Water reabsorption may be varied to compensate for change in plasma volume. Nearly all the sodium and chloride presented to the tubules is reabsorbed. Potassium and hydrogen ions may be actively secreted into the urine and, in addition, the kidney tubules manufacture ammonia which removes hydrogen ions in the urine as ammonium ions. By these mechanisms the kidney can control the osmolality of the plasma and its acid–base balance.

Glucose is completely reabsorbed by the renal tubules provided the plasma level does not exceed 10–11 mmol/l (180–200 mg/100 ml). Under normal circumstances proteins do not appear in the urine. The kidney is the only route of elimination for the breakdown products of protein metabolism and in particular, urea and creatinine are found in the urine. In addition, the urine is the major source of excretion of water soluble drugs and their metabolites, usually as conjugates. Although most drug metabolism takes place in the liver, the kidney cells also contain microsomes with an oxidase enzyme system, and some drug metabolism can occur within the kidney.

RENAL BLOOD FLOW (RBF)

Renal blood flow is controlled in two ways, by intrinsic autoregulation and as a result of extrinsic, autonomic and hormonal regulation.

Autoregulation of RBF occurs over a range of changes in mean arterial pressure of

80–180 mmHg. This autoregulation occurs within the kidney itself, since it is also seen in the denervated perfused isolated organ. Glomerular filtration rate (GFR) is also autoregulated, and it has been suggested that there are cells which are sensitive to changes in perfusion pressure, located in capillaries close to the glomerulus (juxtaglomerular cells). During general anaesthesia autoregulation of RBF is abolished and decreased RBF occurs with even moderate decreases in arterial blood pressure. If arterial blood pressure falls to low values, renal blood flow may decrease to the point where urine flow stops. It is well recognized that acute renal failure may then ensue, but the mechanism is not clear. It is believed that increased renin-angiotensin activity initiated by the decrease in RBF is responsible for the changes seen in acute renal failure. Supporting evidence is the fact that renal biopsies taken early in acute renal failure, under these circumstances, rarely show any change in glomerular structure.

When small or moderate amounts of catecholamines are administered intravenously, a decrease occurs both in RBF and GFR. In addition a decrease in RBF, from whatever cause, will initiate renin release from the juxtaglomerular cells. An α-globulin in plasma converts renin to angiotensin I, which is converted to angiotensin II, a potent pressor and renal vasoconstricting substance. Furthermore, angiotensin II controls the release of aldosterone. The effects of angiotensin are similar to those seen following adrenaline infusions; thus small amounts reduce RBF without affecting GFR, but increasing quantities decrease both RBF and GFR. The reduction in RBF seen during haemorrhagic hypotension is the result of increased concentrations of circulating angiotensin, aldosterone and catecholamines. The prostaglandins probably balance the effects of activation of the renin-angiotensin system. When prostaglandins are infused intravenously there is an increased blood flow to the outer nephrons, which have short loops of Henle, resulting in a diuresis and loss of sodium; the increased blood flow to the juxtamedullary nephrons with their long loops of Henle, however, results in sodium retention. As a further complicating factor antidiuretic hormone (ADH), which is secreted from the posterior lobe of the pituitary, exerts a tonic effect on water reabsorption in the distal convoluted tubule. ADH secretion is mainly responsive to change in tonicity of the plasma and extracellular fluid. However, morphine and probably most of the inhalational agents will also stimulate ADH secretion. Therefore, urine flow may not be related to either RBF or GFR during anaesthesia. The interrelation, therefore, between the various hormones, arterial blood pressure and the effects of general anaesthesia on renal blood flow is not clearly established.

RBF may be measured by observing the clearance from the plasma of an indicator such as p-aminohippuric acid (PAH), which is completely, or almost completely, extracted from the blood during each passage through the kidney. Measurement of GFR depends on the clearance of inulin which is filtered out by the glomeruli in the same concentration as in the plasma, that is to say inulin is neither reabsorbed nor excreted in the tubules.

RENAL FUNCTION TESTS

Table 4.1 shows some commonly used renal function tests with their reference values. As with disease of most organs of the body, there is no single comprehensive test of renal function and most of the following tests should be undertaken and interpreted in the light of the history and examination of the patient.

Table 4.1. Renal function tests.

Test	Normal range
Plasma	
Electrolytes	
Sodium (Na)$^+$	135–148 mmol/litre
Potassium (K)$^+$	3·8–5 mmol/litre
Chloride (Cl)$^-$	95–105 mmol/litre
Bicarbonate (HCO$_3$)$^-$	21–25 mmol/litre
Calcium total (Ca)$^{++}$	2·1–2·7 mmol/litre
Magnesium (Mg)$^{++}$	0·7–1·0 mmol/litre
Osmolality	280–295 mosmol/kg
Urea	2·5–6·5 mmol/litre
Creatinine	45–120 μmol/litre
Uric acid	0·1–0·4 mmol/litre
Urine	
Volume/24 hr	1–2 litres
Electrolytes/24 hr	
Sodium	50–200 mmol
Potassium	30–100 mmol
Chloride	100–300 mmol
Specific Gravity	1003–1030
Osmolality	300 1000 mosmol/kg
Creatinine/24 hr	8·8–17·7 mmol
Creatinine clearance	110–130 ml/min
Urea clearance	60–95 ml/min
Glomerular filtration rate (GFR)	105–140 ml/min

SPECIFIC GRAVITY

This is an easy ward test to perform but is not very helpful when large molecules, such as proteins, are present in the urine. In patients with a low urine output a low specific gravity may indicate failure of the kidney to concentrate and excrete electrolytes.

OSMOLALITY

This is a more useful measurement than the specific gravity since it measures the number of particles in the urine and is not greatly influenced by substances such as urea, glucose or protein which have large molecules. It is, therefore, essentially a measurement of the number of ions in the urine. If plasma osmolality, or the actual individual plasma electrolytes are measured at the same time, then the ratio of urine to plasma osmolality may be determined. Under normal circumstances, and depending on the patient's diet, urine osmolality should exceed plasma osmolality. If urine and plasma osmolality are similar, or urine osmolality is less than the plasma, then renal failure may be occurring. Osmolality is easily measured by the depression of the freezing point (Osmometer).

PLASMA ELECTROLYTES

Since the concentration of plasma electrolytes is determined primarily by urine output, changes in plasma sodium, potassium and bicarbonate and chloride may be indications of renal function. The water content of the plasma is also important and is also controlled by the kidney. Individual plasma measurement of electrolytes may, therefore, be misleading when water balance is not taken into account. For example, in the intensive care situation the commonest cause of a low plasma sodium is water overload and not depletion of sodium. Measurement of plasma potassium is obviously important and in renal failure levels may exceed the threshold for cardiac irregularities (above 6 mmol/l). If sodium and bicarbonate are retained as may be seen in the severely ill patient, then plasma chloride level may be low. Metabolic acidosis due to failure to secrete hydrogen ions results in a low plasma bicarbonate and may be evidence of renal failure.

UREA

Urea is the main breakdown product of normal protein metabolism and is usually excreted in the urine. In renal failure, urea will be retained, and a plasma urea concentration which increases by more than 6·6 mmol (40 mg) per day is an indication of serious renal impairment. In the dehydrated patient urea concentration may also rise but may not necessarily reflect irreversible change in renal function. As the liver is the main site of urea production, urea concentration may fall in liver failure and is not necessarily related to a change in renal function.

CREATININE

This is also a breakdown product of protein metabolism and is a more useful test of renal function than urea since it is not so adversely affected by extrinsic factors. A plasma creatinine concentration in excess of 177 μmol/l (2 mg/100 ml) indicates renal failure. Creatinine is normally excreted almost entirely by glomerular filtration and since its production is constant there is normally a very steady blood level. Creatinine clearance is therefore a convenient way of measuring GFR requiring only one determination of blood and urine concentration within 24 hr. However, the chemical reaction for creatinine measures other chromogens, and when there is advanced renal disease creatinine is also secreted by the tubules. The effect of both these changes is to overestimate the GFR in severe renal failure when the true GFR is less than 10 ml/min.

URIC ACID

Uric acid is normally excreted by the distal tubules and in renal failure this substance is retained. It is of interest that in renal failure associated with methoxyflurane anaesthesia, where high volumes of urine are secreted but there is retention of nitrogenous compounds, uric acid is also retained, indicating that the site of damage may be the distal tubule. This is consistent with fluoride, a normal metabolite of methoxyflurane, being the cause of the renal damage.

URINARY PROTEIN AND DEPOSITS

Glomerular filtrate contains appreciable quantities of protein which is normally reabsorbed by the tubules. Proteinuria of greater than 100 mg in 24 hr indicates renal damage, usually to the glomeruli.

Microscopic examination of the urine may be helpful. Red and white blood cells and hyaline casts may be found occasionally in normal urine, but increased numbers indicate renal disease. Casts are mixtures of precipitated proteins and polysaccharides with red cells or degenerate tubule cells. Blood and granular casts come from the renal parenchyma and usually indicate glomerular disease.

URINE VOLUME

Under normal circumstances urine volume is dependent on fluid intake. However, in renal failure there is usually a fall in urine volume and daily urine volumes of less than 1 litre in a patient with a normal water intake should lead to some doubt about renal function. If this is combined with a rise in blood urea concentration and other signs of renal failure then appropriate steps should be taken. However, increased urine volumes are also consistent with renal failure. High output failure (so called) may be seen, for example, in patients with pituitary damage where there is failure of ADH secretion. Urine volume alone, therefore, may not necessarily be a good guide to renal function.

URINARY CONCENTRATION TEST

This is a valuable overall test of tubular function. Urine osmolality (or specific gravity) is tested after fluid deprivation for 24 hr. The kidney should be able to produce urine approximately three times the osmolality of plasma, e.g. 800–1000 mosmol/kg (S.G. above 1022). An alternative method, which avoids the discomfort of fluid deprivation is intramuscular injection of 5 units pitressin tannate followed by a 24-hr urine collection.

The urine dilution test is of no value in assessing renal function.

RENAL FAILURE

Renal failure is arbitrarily divided into acute and chronic. Acute renal failure is usually taken to indicate that the failure is potentially reversible and the result of some rapidly occurring process. Chronic renal failure indicates that the renal failure is not reversible and is usually due to some inherent disease of the kidneys themselves. There is obviously overlap between these two conditions as one may lead to the other, or acute renal failure may occur in a patient with pre-existing renal damage.

ACUTE RENAL FAILURE

A progressive rise in blood urea and creatinine concentrations is the most reliable indication of acute renal failure. Urine volume, osmolality or composition are not such useful measurements. A urine volume of less than 300 ml per day, is a commonly quoted diagnostic criteria but it should be remembered that patients may have 'normal' or increased urine volume and still have renal failure. The reason for this paradox may be a failure to secrete ADH. Alternatively, the remaining functioning nephrons are doing their best to excrete the load of solute presented to them and therefore secrete a reasonable volume; even so, they cannot excrete the total load required of them and retention of substances is still occurring. Terminology such as pre-renal failure, functional renal failure, acute tubular necrosis or other synonyms should be avoided and the term acute renal failure used to cover all eventualities [3].

The causes of acute renal failure include acute-on-chronic renal failure, nephrotoxic drugs, obstructive lesions of the urinary tract and conditions associated with reduced renal blood flow (Table 4.2). The association of acute renal failure with

Table 4.2. Causes of acute renal failure. (After Robson 1975) [3].

Primary renal disease
Urinary tract obstruction
Nephrotoxic drugs and poisons
Renal ischaemia

(*a*) Medical origin:	respiratory infection and failure
	septicaemia
	cardiac failure
	viral hepatitis
(*b*) Surgical origin:	trauma and burns
	shock and infection after cardiovascular surgery
	after surgery in the jaundiced patient
	haemorrhage
(*c*) Obstetric origin:	post-partum and accidental haemorrhage abortion
	disseminated intravascular coagulation

jaundice and anaesthesia and surgery is also referred to in Chapter 5. Acute renal failure occurs following surgical operations on jaundiced patients more commonly than it does after comparable operations on non-jaundiced patients. The fall in renal blood flow associated with anaesthesia tubules and the role of infection are important factors in determining whether renal failure occurs.

CHRONIC RENAL FAILURE

In chronic progressive renal failure the functioning nephrons are gradually reduced in number, and there is a consequent fall in GFR. Since the same solutes present themselves for excretion as before, each functioning nephron is in a continuous state of osmotic diuresis, resulting in polyuria (most noticeable at night), failure of urine concentration, and diminished ability of the distal tubules to conserve cations, acidify or form ammonia. Most of the clinical manifestations result from this disturbance in

Table 4.3. Causes of chronic renal failure.

Renal destruction due to an immunological process
    e.g. glomerulonephritis
        periarteritis nodosa
        rheumatoid arthritis
        systemic lupus erythematosus
Infection
    e.g. pyelonephritis
Urinary tract obstruction
Congenital lesions
    e.g. polycystic disease
Hypertension and arterial disease
    e.g. gout
        diabetes mellitus

water and electrolyte balance with added metabolic acidosis. The retention of substances such as urea and phosphate produces little clinical effect until very advanced renal failure has developed.

The common causes of chronic renal failure may be grouped under five main headings: renal destruction due to an immunological process, urinary tract infection, urinary tract obstruction, congenital lesions and hypertension. Some examples are listed in Table 4.3.

CLINICAL PICTURE OF RENAL FAILURE

The clinical and biochemical features of acute or chronic renal failure are similar, although the time course may vary. The two conditions can, therefore, be considered from these points of view.

BIOCHEMICAL FEATURES

An inability to control water excretion in renal failure may be reflected in water overload with the development of oedema. This may manifest itself, for example, as pulmonary or cerebral oedema. Similarly, fluid restriction may lead to dehydration in the patient who is still capable of secreting some urine as the kidney attempts to excrete the high solute load.

The derangement in sodium metabolism may lead to hypertension as a result of retention of sodium and thus concomitant water. In certain forms of renal failure there may be a sodium leak and the net result will be hypotension. Measurement of plasma sodium may be misleading and is only really helpful as some guide to the patient's stage of hydration.

Potassium metabolism is altered and in general potassium is retained within the body. Plasma potassium concentrations in excess of 6 mmol/litre are associated with cardiac irregularities. A common cause of death in renal failure is cardiac arrest associated with high plasma potassium concentration.

The normal urinary excretion of hydrogen ions is equivalent to some 40–60 mmol per day. In renal failure, this does not occur and results in retention of hydrogen ions with a low plasma pH and a low plasma bicarbonate. In addition, the kidneys' inability to metabolize parathyroid hormone leads to a loss of bicarbonate in the urine thus reducing the buffering capacity of the plasma. Phosphate is also retained, further limiting the kidneys' ability to excrete hydrogen ions.

A common phenomenon in the seriously ill patient, usually seen in the intensive care unit and often associated with major surgery, is a combination of metabolic alkalosis, potassium deficiency and paradoxical acid urine. Although not strictly speaking a form of renal failure, the kidney is of course relevant in this situation. The probable initiating cause of the sequence is pre-existing potassium depletion, inability of the kidneys to excrete sodium as a result of catecholamine and corticosteroid secretion associated with stress. Therefore the kidney is forced to retain hydrogen ions in an attempt to buffer a metabolic alkalosis due to potassium deficiency and inability to secrete sodium and bicarbonate. Nevertheless, some hydrogen ions are excreted and so the urine is acid whereas the plasma which is alkaline, and the urinary potassium concentration is very high. In this situation up to 100 mmol of potassium may be lost per day. If this potassium excretion is not balanced by potassium administration, cardiac irregularities may occur extremely suddenly, even though the plasma potassium concentration may be in the normal range. This is because intracellular potassium has been depleted. The treatment of this condition consists of administering potassium chloride intravenously, monitoring plasma and urinary potassium concentrations. A sign that things are improving is the appearance of sodium in the urine along with bicarbonate. It is possible to encourage the kidney to excrete bicarbonate by administering a carbonic anhydrase inhibitor (acetazolamide) although this should be administered cautiously as it may lead to further potassium loss in the urine.

Renal failure is associated with several derangements in calcium metabolism and symptomatic bone disease is most likely to occur either when renal disease is slowly progressive or in children when bone growth is very active. Plasma calcium is usually low in renal failure, due to a number of factors. Elevation of plasma phosphate depresses the calcium level due to their reciprocal relationship. Renal tubular reabsorption of calcium is reduced, mainly due to acidosis. Finally calcium absorption is reduced due to deficiency of vitamin D. The kidney normally converts intermediate metabolites of vitamin D formed in the liver (25-hydroxycholecalciferol) to 1,25-dihydroxycholecalciferol, which is the active metabolite of vitamin D. Deficiency of this substance eventually leads to compensatory overproduction of parathormone with hypertrophy of the parathyroid glands (secondary hyperparathyroidism—see Chapter 16). Such hypertrophy may result in autonomous nodules developing (tertiary hyperparathyroidism). The bone disease resulting from renal failure is thus osteomalacia with the superimposed effects of hyperparathyroidism, e.g. osteosis fibrosa. Soft tissue or metastatic calcification complicates the picture when there is gross hyperparathyroidism.

Magnesium metabolism is also deranged. Magnesium is handled by the kidney by the same mechanism as for potassium and therefore excretion is impaired although plasma levels may be normal.

Cardiac contractility depends on the relationship between sodium, calcium, hydroxyl, potassium, magnesium and hydrogen ions. Since one or all of these ions may be deranged in renal failure it is hardly surprising that cardiac problems occur commonly in patients with renal failure.

RETENTION OF SUBSTANCES

Urea, uric acid, creatinine, amines and urochromogen are retained in the plasma as a result of renal failure. Excess uric acid retention may lead to gout; amines are thought to be associated with the lassitude and nausea which are characteristic of acute renal failure. Urochromogen is responsible for the sallow yellow skin colour which is also characteristic of renal failure.

HAEMATOLOGICAL FEATURES

Anaemia is extremely common in renal failure. One cause is depression of erythropoiesis because of failure of the body to manufacture erythropoietin. The manufacture of this substance seems to be related to the blood urea concentration: the higher the blood urea the less erythropoietin is manufactured. Gastrointestinal bleeding is also common in renal failure and may contribute to anaemia. Furthermore, cell survival is reduced as a result of the red cell damage within the kidneys; haemochalysis may also contribute to the red cell damage.

Haemoglobin concentration in patients with renal failure may be of the order of 5 g/100 ml. However, certain compensations take place which include an increase in cardiac output, an increase in the concentration of 2,3 diphosphoglycerate (2,3 DPG) which enables the patient's red blood cells to give up their oxygen more easily; the patient's blood volume may be normal and the viscosity of the blood is decreased. In addition, metabolic acidosis shifts the oxygen dissociation curve to a more favourable position for the anaemic patient. Blood transfusion should be avoided in patients with renal failure except where there are symptoms associated with the anaemia; not too much notice should be taken of the actual haemoglobin value. Patients should be given iron or folic acid if necessary and other causes of anaemia should be excluded. If blood transfusion is essential then the blood should be screened for hepatitis B antigen (HBsAg) and, if possible, washed red blood cells (where the white blood cells have been removed) should be used. Blood transfusion has no long-term beneficial effect in renal failure, and, indeed, bone marrow depression may be temporarily increased. The potassium, sodium and water load of a blood transfusion may have adverse effects and there is always the risk of viral hepatitis. In addition, transfusion may provoke an antibody response either to red or white blood cells and this may prejudice a future renal transplant. Repeated blood transfusion is expensive and the iron load may lead to haemosiderosis.

CLINICAL FEATURES

As a result of the changes outlined above, the characteristic clinical picture of a patient with renal failure is one of deterioration. The speed of the deterioration will depend on the cause of the renal failure. Lassitude and nausea with increasing anaemia are often the first signs. Water retention may lead to oedema manifest as pulmonary oedema, pleural or pericardial effusion. Hypertensive vascular disease secondary to chronic renal failure may give rise to cerebral haemorrhage or other cardiovascular symptoms. Without treatment patients eventually lapse into uraemic coma. This is associated with electrolyte disturbances, metabolic acidosis and raised blood urea; death usually occurs from either cardiac or respiratory failure. The correlation between the clinical picture and the associated biochemical findings is summarized in Table 4.4.

Table 4.4. Summary of clinical features of renal failure.

Clinical manifestation	Biochemical basis
1 Thirst, polyuria, nocturia (3–4 litres/24 hr)	Osmotic diuresis. Loss of concentrating power
2 Acidosis; Kussmaul respiration	Inability to excrete hydrogen ions
3 Cramps, tetany, convulsions	Hypocalcaemia. Phosphate retention. Failure to activate vitamin D
4 Anaemia	Bone marrow depression. Deficient erythropoietin. Reduced RBC survival
5 Anorexia, nausea, vomiting, hiccough, foetor, Haematemesis/melaena, diarrhoea (uraemic colitis)	Unknown. ? Retention of substances
6 Headache, lassitude, malaise, tremor, insomnia, depression, confusion, coma	Unknown. ? Retention of substances
7 Hypertension and sequelae	Multi-factorial. Renin-angiotensin production
8 Pericarditis with/without effusion. Tamponade	Unknown
9 Uraemic lung on chest X-ray	Unknown. ? Pulmonary oedema
10 Skin pigmentation, purpura, pruritis	Unknown. ? Retention of substances

TREATMENT OF RENAL FAILURE

Many patients with chronic renal failure may be adequately treated over many years by fluid restriction and a low protein diet. The management of such patients is rarely of concern to the anaesthetist and the problems they present for general anaesthesia are covered below. However, patients with acute renal failure or chronic renal failure where conservative measures have failed may be encountered by the anaesthetist in the Intensive Care Unit or may present for anaesthesia and surgery. Treatment can be divided into immediate and long-term, control of electrolyte and acid–base balance, nutrition, anaemia and infection, dialysis and possibly eventual transplantation.

DIURETIC DRUGS

The use of diuretic drugs such as mannitol, frusemide and ethacrynic acid is controversial. It is common practice to administer these drugs, often in large doses, to patients in the early stages of acute renal failure. Certainly mannitol may help in the prevention of renal failure if given, for example, pre- and perioperatively to the jaundiced patient or to patients undergoing aneurysm surgery. However, whether mannitol is of any value once renal failure is established is still a matter for debate. There is an obvious risk of circulatory overload if large doses of mannitol are administered and an increase in urine flow does not occur.

Frusemide and ethacrynic acid in large doses cause renal vasodilatation and normally prevent the re-absorption of sodium and chloride in the ascending loop of Henle. Therefore, sodium and chloride become osmotically active as diuretics. However, it has been shown that both drugs increase circulating renin concentrations and activation of the renin-angiotensin system may be relevant in the aetiology of renal failure (see above). Furthermore, large doses of frusemide may lead to eighth nerve damage and deafness. It remains to be established that either of these diuretic drugs is of real value once renal damage has occurred.

ADRENERGIC BLOCKING AGENTS

In the shocked patient with low arterial blood pressure, renal blood flow is also low and urine output is poor. This situation may lead to acute renal failure. Adequate fluid replacement may be all that is necessary. However, if arterial blood pressure is not improved by infusion of appropriate fluid alone the use of adrenergic blocking agents is commonly employed in an attempt to cause renal vasodilatation. The renal vasculature is predominantly controlled by α-receptors and therefore α-adrenergic blocking agents such as phentolamine and phenoxybenzamine have been used. Although in individual cases the administration of these drugs may be associated with an increased urine output and apparent reversal of potential renal problems, it remains to be established, as with diuretic drugs, that adrenergic blocking agents can reverse acute renal failure.

HYPERKALAEMIA

Retention of potassium and a rise in the plasma potassium concentration above 6 mmol/litre may lead to cardiac arrest. In acute renal failure there may not be time to institute dialysis to lower plasma potassium concentration to a safe level and immediate treatment may be required. Intravenous calcium gluconate will offset the effects of a raised plasma potassium concentration: sodium bicarbonate and insulin will both cause potassium to move into cells. If insulin is administered then dextrose should be given concomitantly to avoid a fall in blood sugar level. None of these measures removes potassium from the body and therefore in the long term dialysis is the only effective method. As an intermediate treatment calcium resonium enemas may also be used; these remove potassium from the body but are rather unpleasant for the patient.

DIALYSIS

Two forms of dialysis are available—peritoneal and haemodialysis. The relative advantages and disadvantages of these two forms of treatment are shown in Table 4.5.

Table 4.5. Peritoneal dialysis *v* Haemodialysis: Advantages and disadvantages.

	Peritoneal dialysis	Haemodialysis
Cost	Low	High
Effectiveness	Slow	Rapid
Setting-up	Rapid	Slow
Shunt needed	No	Yes
Apparatus	Minimal	Large and needs special facilities
Infection	Yes, peritoneal	Shunt site
Disequilibrium	No	Can occur
Site	Hospital only	Patient can be treated at home
Supervision	Easy—minimal training	Special training required

Peritoneal dialysis consists of passing a catheter through the abdominal wall into the peritoneal cavity. Electrolyte solutions are then infused into the peritoneal cavity, left *in situ* for a cycle of 1–2 hr and then drained. The peritoneum acts as an exchanging membrane so that urea, hydrogen ions and other electrolytes will pass into the dialysate fluid which is drained from the peritoneum. The passage of water is controlled osmotically using glucose added to the dialysate. A high glucose concentration will draw water from the patient whereas a low glucose allows water to pass into the patient. Filling the peritoneal cavity with fluid may cause respiratory embarrassment and it may be necessary to ventilate patients artificially whilst peritoneal dialysis is taking place. Respiratory embarrassment is minimized by shortening the dialysis cycle and by sitting the patient up when the peritoneum is filled with fluid. Drugs which depress respiration should be avoided whilst dialysis is in progress. In general, peritoneal dialysis is preferred where recovery of renal function is likely, metabolic changes are relatively slow or there is serious cardiovascular instability. It is not suitable for the long-term treatment of chronic failure. Where catabolism is rapid (as evidenced by rapidly rising urea and creatinine levels in the blood) haemodialysis may be necessary to treat acute renal failure.

Haemodialysis has revolutionized the treatment of chronic renal failure. Indeed, patients may lead a relatively normal life and carry out treatment themselves at home. Dialysis may only be necessary on a few occasions per week and patients may be maintained for many years with such treatment. However, there are obvious inconveniences, the necessity for a shunt or fistula and the geographical attachment to a dialysis machine. Many types of haemodialysis machines are available. In essence, arterial blood is removed from the patient and passed through one side of a coiled membrane and then returned intravenously. On the other side of the membrane dialysis fluid is circulated from a bath. The membrane is permeable to water, electrolytes and glucose but not to proteins or red blood cells. By suitable adjustment of the dialysis fluid, the patients' water balance, urea and electrolytes and acid–base balance may be corrected to normal. The priming volume of a modern haemodialysis machine is very small and blood transfusion is not usually necessary. Safety devices are incorporated to check for membrane leaks and the presence of air bubbles.

The prime objective of dialysis is to provide time for the patient's own kidneys to recover. If renal failure is irreversible then an alternative to long-term haemodialysis is transplantation. The decision to carry out a transplant is a difficult one. The long-term results of haemodialysis and transplantation are currently very similar. A successful transplant, however, means that the patient does not have to rely on geographical proximity to a dialysis machine and the quality of life may be good. Furthermore, the cost of haemodialysis is avoided. If transplantation fails, as for example when the transplanted kidney is rejected, then it may be possible to re-establish the patient on haemodialysis and subsequently carry out another transplant. Currently the result of second or subsequent transplants are not as good as on the first occasion. Another factor is the shortfall of donor kidneys compared with patients awaiting transplantation. Although theoretically there are sufficient donor kidneys available, in practice the problems of approaching relatives for permission to remove a patient's kidneys have often proved insuperable.

SHUNTS AND FISTULAE

For successful haemodialysis, access is required to both the venous and arterial sides of the circulation. Two methods are in common use. Firstly, a Scribner shunt made of Teflon may be inserted between an artery and a vein usually in one of the patient's upper limbs. Although the initial placement of such a shunt may be straightforward they are, unfortunately, prone to clotting and infection and subsequent exploration of the limb may be necessary for insertion of further shunts. These surgical procedures may be very lengthy and are not always readily done under local infiltration. Nerve blocks of the upper and lower limbs have the advantage that sympathetic blockade may assist the surgeon in finding suitable vessels. General anaesthesia has also been used and others have described the use of stellate ganglion block with general anaesthesia to improve the visualization of vessels of the upper limbs [1, 4, 5]. Scribner shunts need protection when not in use if the patient is to go about his day-to-day occupation a further problem is the constant risk of the shunt coming apart causing haemorrhage.

As an alternative an arterio-venous fistula may be constructed, either directly or using a Gortex graft. This is known as a Cimeno fistula and has the advantage that it does not require external protection between use. The fistula is usually established in the upper limb since fistulae in the lower limb may create too large a shunt for the patient's cardiovascular system to tolerate. The limb swells and the veins become 'arterialized'. In order to haemodialyse the patient, percutaneous cannulation of the vessels is required. However, even a Cimeno fistula is prone to infection, and on occasion even in the upper limb the shunt may be so great as to cause unacceptable embarrassment to the cardiovascular system. Since the patient with renal failure may depend for his life on his superficial veins and peripheral arteries it is obviously incumbent on the anaesthetist not to damage them. It is also not advisable to use a shunt or fistula for the injection of drugs. Where possible for minor procedures under anaesthesia either local or inhalational general anaesthesia should be employed. For more major procedures, the vessels in the neck may be utilized for central venous pressure measurement and intravenous infusion.

DISEQUILIBRIUM

This is a phenomenon which can occur in patients with very high blood concentrations of urea and sodium, or severe metabolic acidosis. If such patients are haemodialysed then it is possible to lower the plasma concentrations of these substances rapidly. However, urea, sodium and hydrogen ions will have crossed the blood/brain barrier and will be present in the CSF and cerebral cells. Rapid lowering of plasma levels is not accompanied by an equally rapid lowering of the level in the CSF and the brain itself. As a result of this disequilibrium water is drawn into the brain causing cerebral oedema, which may have fatal results. It is important, therefore, that when plasma levels of urea, sodium and hydrogen ions are high, patients are dialysed slowly.

NUTRITION

Although careful fluid balance and protein restriction are indicated in the early stages of renal failure and may be part of the general management, patients still require an adequate calorie intake. This may be provided by carbohydrates or fats. In the early recovery phase of acute renal failure protein may be administered in small quantities so as to prevent catabolism of the patient's own muscle proteins. Even in chronic renal failure some protein must be allowed in the diet for the same reason. The correct amount is determined on the basis of serial measurements of blood urea and creatinine.

ANAEMIA

The management of anaemia has been discussed above. Gastrointestinal haemorrhage, so called uraemic bleeding, is also a common occurrence. Such bleeding is often the cause of death in a patient with renal failure.

INFECTION

Patients with renal disease are very prone to infection. Carefully planned antibiotic therapy is part of the general treatment. However, most antibiotics are excreted in the urine and blood levels may reach toxic concentrations in patients with renal failure. Blood assays may be helpful if potentially toxic antibiotics are necessary. Bizarre fungal and viral infections may be seen in the patient who has undergone renal transplantation and has received immunosuppressive treatment. All anaesthetic equipment, therefore, should be sterile and care should be taken not to introduce infection into the respiratory tract. Many patients with renal failure develop concomitant respiratory problems. Intermittent positive pressure ventilation (IPPV) may then be necessary.

The risk of lung infection when IPPV is instituted is obviously high and is a major intensive care problem in managing such patients.

Hypertension is common in patients with renal disease. It may be the initiating cause of renal damage or it may be secondary to release of renin from kidneys which have been damaged by some other mechanism. Hypertension can usually be controlled by dialysis and drug therapy. In patients with no urine output where release of renin is thought to be contributing to hypertension bilateral nephrectomy may be helpful. Bilateral nephrectomy may also be indicated if there is infection of the urinary tract, haematuria, or large polycystic kidneys which may interfere with subsequent transplantation. The anaesthetic problems in such patients are essentially similar to those for renal transplantation [2].

POSTOPERATIVE RENAL FAILURE

A situation which may confront the anaesthetist with regard to renal function is the patient whose urine output falls postoperatively. This is usually associated with major surgery and in the majority of instances is also associated with hypovolaemia. The only true anaesthetic cause of postoperative renal failure is probably methoxyflurane to which reference has already been made. Postoperative oliguria usually responds to appropriate infusion of either crystalloids or blood, urine output then increases and all is well. However, if adequate fluid replacement is not effective, diuretics such as mannitol or frusemide may be considered. The relevant arguments as to the use of these drugs have already been covered. At this stage it is important to measure urea, electrolytes, and acid–base parameters in order to establish whether these are initially abnormal and to provide a baseline with which to compare subsequent measurements. If the blood urea, or creatinine or plasma potassium continue to rise even if urine volume is relatively normal, consideration should be given to early dialysis. Peritoneal dialysis may be all that is required and even patients who have undergone abdominal surgery may also undergo peritoneal dialysis quite satisfactorily. Indeed, peritoneal dialysis is sometimes used in the treatment of peritoneal infection, not in this instance for treating renal failure but in order to 'wash out' the infection. It is wise to consult a nephrologist at this stage rather than when the situation is beyond control.

ANAESTHESIA FOR PATIENTS WITH
ESTABLISHED CHRONIC RENAL DISEASE

Apart from the nature of the surgical procedure contemplated, information is required regarding the patient's electrolyte and acid–base status, haemoglobin, current drug therapy and current treatment for renal failure. Signs of water overload, a plasma potassium in excess of 6 mmol/litre or serious acid–base derangement are indications for preoperative dialysis. Anaemia will only require treatment if the patient has symptoms. If major surgical procedures are contemplated then blood should be cross-matched and be available at the time of surgery. This blood should be screened for HBsAg and if renal transplantation is likely in the future then the red blood cells should be washed if possible. Drug therapy likely to cause problems during anaesthesia includes β-blockers and other hypotensive drugs. At the preoperative visit, the patient should be carefully examined for any signs of infection and the presence of arteriovenous shunts or fistulae.

ANAESTHETIC PROBLEMS

In general, patients with chronic renal disease are underweight and thin. They are, therefore, much more prone to pressure injuries and peripheral nerve damage during surgical procedures and extra care should be taken in positioning the patient on the operating table. The patient's weight should be measured and due allowance made for any oedema when calculating drug doses. The patient's reduced oxygen carrying capacity should be borne in mind with premedication and during general anaesthetic techniques. Atropine is perhaps best avoided because the tachycardia which it produces may not be beneficial in the anaemic patient. The special risk of infection requires that all anaesthetic apparatus should be sterile and appropriate precautions employed during its use. If blood transfusion is required, particular care should be paid to using blood which has been screened for HBsAg.

Local analgesic techniques, particularly nerve blocks, may be used with advantage in patients with chronic renal disease. Spinal and epidural analgesia should be viewed with some caution in view of the risk of infection, although epidural analgesia has been used successfully for renal transplantation. The weight of the patient should be borne in mind when calculating the dose of a local analgesic drug.

All the commonly employed general anaesthetic techniques have been used successfully in patients with chronic renal disease. Drugs which are primarily excreted in the urine should be avoided. The major problem of drug administration in patients with chronic renal disease relates to the altered volumes of distribution of such drugs. This may lead to a prolonged half life of the activity of drugs in the body and may be followed by prolonged activity. In order to avoid such problems modest doses of drugs should be employed and particular attention should be paid to the weight of the patient so that excess amounts of drugs are not administered. Studies of blood levels of drugs such as nondepolarizing muscle relaxants show that there is considerable variation in the decay of such compounds in plasma as compared with normal patients. The variation is such that it is very difficult to predict, for the individual patient, how long drugs will persist in an active form in the body fluids. Therefore drugs such as nondepolarizing muscle relaxants or respiratory depressants should be given with caution to patients with chronic renal disease and it should be anticipated that on occasion their actions will be prolonged even following modest dosing.

Neuromuscular blocking drugs

Suxamethonium causes fasciculation prior to the onset of paralysis. During fasciculation, potassium is released from the muscles and there is a rise in plasma potassium concentration. Normally this rise is of the order of 0·5 mmol/litre and is not of great consequence. However, in patients with chronic renal disease whose plasma potassium concentration may already be raised, any further rise may be detrimental. If the plasma [K] is high, approaching 6 mmol/litre, any further rise may precipitate cardiac dysrhythmia. The decision to use suxamethonium entails balancing the advantages of rapid paralysis for intubation in an emergency situation against the risk of using a slower onset nondepolarizing relaxant, or deciding that surgery can be delayed until dialysis can be employed to lower the plasma potassium concentration to a safe level. In any event the electrocardiogram should be monitored in patients with chronic renal disease when suxamethonium is used. The maximum rise in plasma potassium concentration may not necessarily occur immediately after administration of suxamethonium but may be seen up to 30 min later. If changes occur in the electrocardiogram suggesting a rise in plasma potassium, measurement is essential and, if a rise has occurred, then the measures already outlined above to lower plasma potassium concentration should be taken immediately.

Pancuronium and d-tubocurarine are excreted in significant amounts in the urine. They do not give rise to changes in plasma potassium concentration. They have both been used successfully in patients with chronic renal failure and during renal transplantation. It is likely that their action at the motor-end plate is terminated by redistribution rather than as a result of excretion from the body. If the renal pathway is denied to these drugs then they are probably eventually excreted in the bile. Nevertheless, in patients with poor renal function caution should be exercised in the use of these drugs and as small a dose as possible employed.

Gallamine presents a somewhat more complex picture. Individual cases have been reported of patients given gallamine during surgery, who later developed acute renal failure. It was apparently not possible to reverse the effects of the gallamine for some time. Gallamine is excreted in the urine, appearing within some 2 hr of administration, and in this it is similar to *d*-tubocurarine and pancuronium. It is therefore difficult to see why these latter drugs are not usually associated with prolonged action even in the anephric patient. However, since alternatives to gallamine exist it would seem preferable to avoid its use in the patient with renal problems.

Inhalational agents

All the inhalational agents will reduce renal blood flow (RBF), glomerular filtration rate (GFR) and urine output. These changes are due to release of ADH, catecholamine secretion and/or a fall in arterial blood pressure. During general anaesthesia autoregulation of the renal circulation is diminished and renal blood flow is proportional to changes in blood pressure. Additional factors such as hypoxia or hypercarbia also increase secretion of catecholamines and diminish RBF. In the normal kidney and even in the damaged one it is unlikely that any of these effects will lead to further renal damage unless excessive changes occur. However, metabolism of some volatile anaesthetic agents gives rise to inorganic fluoride. Inorganic fluoride in excess of 50 mmol/litre will cause renal damage. Of the currently available agents methoxyflurane is the only one likely to be associated with problems. Exposure of patients to prolonged deep methoxyflurane anaesthesia may be followed by renal failure characteristic of fluoride intoxication. Most patients will eventually recover but some will go on to develop permanent renal damage. If other potentially nephrotoxic drugs are given at the same time as methoxyflurane anaesthesia then the likelihood of renal damage is increased. The tetracyclines have come under suspicion in this regard. It therefore seems sensible to avoid methoxyflurane in patients who already have renal damage and to limit its dose in those with normal renal function.

Halothane is probably the most commonly used volatile anaesthetic in patients with renal disease and provided that the dosage is limited to prevent undue cardiovascular effects then renal function will not be disturbed to any great extent. There is some evidence that halothane causes ADH secretion which may reduce urine output during anaesthesia. Nitrous oxide seems to have little effect on renal haemodynamics or urine output. Adequate oxygenation, nitrous oxide and modest amounts of halothane constitute a straightforward inhalation anaesthetic technique for patients with renal damage.

Enflurane and its isomer, isoflurane, are fluorinated hydrocarbons which undergo some metabolism in the body to inorganic fluoride. However the amount of inorganic fluoride produced as a result of such metabolism is small and blood levels are unlikely to approach those associated with renal damage. Nevertheless some caution should be exercised in the use of fluorinated hydrocarbons in patients with established renal disease.

Sedatives and analgesics

All the commonly used analgesics and sedatives undergo metabolism by the liver and eventual excretion in the urine. In chronic renal disease the half life of removal of such drugs from the plasma may be increased and this may lead to prolongation of the action of the drug concerned. Since it is usually non-active compounds that are excreted in the urine the impaired renal excretion is not likely to lead to additional problems in the termination of action of a drug. Therefore, care in dosage should be exercised and it should be anticipated that on occasion even modest dosing of sedatives and analgesics may be followed by prolonged action in patients with chronic renal disease.

POSTOPERATIVE PROBLEMS

The severity of postoperative complications will be related, of course, to the surgery carried out. Where minor procedures have been undertaken the patient should be returned as rapidly as possible to his preoperative regime as far as to renal function is concerned. After major surgery immediate dialysis may be necessary in order to readjust the patient's electrolyte, water and acid–base balances to normal. During surgery no sodium containing fluids should have been administered, but if blood transfusion was necessary then the water and sodium load may need to be removed by dialysis. In patients with poor renal function a short period of postoperative dialysis may help them to get over the stress of anaesthesia and surgery and return to their preoperative condition.

Pulmonary infection is common in patients with chronic renal disease. Deep breathing exercises and general physiotherapy should be started as soon as possible and excessive doses of respiratory depressant analgesic drugs should be avoided. If muscle relaxant drugs have been used and there is any doubt as to whether they have been reversed adequately, the patient should be artificially ventilated. This should be for as short a period as possible in order to avoid introducing infection into the lungs. If antibiotics are needed in the postoperative period they should only be administered on culture and sensitivity tests, dosage being monitored by blood levels to minimize the risk of toxicity.

RENAL TRANSPLANTATION

Renal transplantation is an alternative to long-term haemodialysis in patients with end-stage chronic renal disease. This technique uses a kidney from another human being, either an unrelated cadaver donor or an unrelated or related live donor. These are all examples of homotransplants. Patients between 15 and 50 years of age are considered as suitable recipients providing they do not have other generalized systemic disease, chronic extrarenal infection, chronic peptic ulceration or an acute active immunological renal lesion.

The first renal transplants performed were between identical twins. Here the transplant came from a living donor and there were obviously no immunological problems. However, most patients with chronic renal disease are not one of a pair of identical twins and both immunological problems and the availability of suitable donor kidneys have to be considered.

The majority of renal transplants utilize kidneys obtained from cadaver donors. Here the kidney is removed as soon as possible after death and may then be preserved either by cooling or by perfusion for up to 12 hr or even, under some circumstances, up to 24 hr. This allows time first of all to assess the function of the kidney and also to allow for matching of the kidney to a suitable recipient. There has been much argument as to how well kidneys need to be matched. Clearly, absolute matching is not possible except between identical twins. In general, ABO blood grouping is perfectly feasible and more complicated matching of white cell antibodies is sometimes possible. A better way of obtaining a close match is to use a live donor, especially a member of the patient's own family. This also avoids prolonged ischaemia time between removal of the kidney and its reimplantation. Emotional and ethical difficulties may arise when a doctor who has a patient with end-stage renal failure is approached by the patient's relatives or friends offering to donate a kidney for transplantation. This is a difficult situation and one which has not been entirely resolved. The success rate for live donors is somewhat better than that for cadaver donors, but even so the difference between the two is not thought by some to justify extensive use of live donors. The chief advantages of using a live donor are that the transplant can be a planned procedure, and because both donor and recipient can be operated on simultaneously in adjoining theatres, the ischaemia time can be very short. Transplantation using a cadaver donor is frequently an emergency procedure and may be associated with a prolonged ischaemia time.

ANAESTHESIA FOR RENAL TRANSPLANTATION

Anaesthesia for renal transplantation is now a relatively simple and straightforward procedure. Patients awaiting transplantation should be well controlled by haemodialysis and in general most of the initial problems have been overcome. Nevertheless, the procedure may still be an emergency one, often in the middle of the night, and particular attention should be paid to getting all the equipment ready and observing a number of straightforward precautions. Firstly, the patient may have a full stomach and induction of anaesthesia should be such as to avoid the risk of vomiting and inhalation. A 'crash induction' using thiopentone and suxamethonium may be necessary. The patient's plasma potassium concentration must be known to be in the safe range if suxamethonium is to be used. The risk of introducing infection into the renal transplant patient is high. Following the transplant, the patient will be put onto immunosuppressive drugs and steroids and any infection introduced at the time of surgery may be serious. The anaesthetic equipment should be sterile and special care should be taken when putting up infusions, etc.

Many anaesthetic agents and techniques have been used for renal transplantation and there is no evidence to show that any of them is particularly preferable. The operation itself is extraperitoneal, the kidney being located usually in the right iliac fossa, and the operating time is relatively short. However, if bilateral nephrectomy is performed simultaneously, surgery may be prolonged and muscle relaxation is essential. The most important criterion is maintenance of the blood pressure so that the new kidney will be adequately perfused as soon as it has been implanted. Techniques ranging from neurolept-anaesthesia to epidural analgesia and from cyclo-propane to halothane and even methoxyflurane have been recommended for renal transplantation by various authors. The authors' present technique involves induction of anaesthesia with thiopentone, followed by suxamethonium if necessary for rapid intubation, pancuronium bromide for neuromuscular block (using the lowest possible dose) oxygen, nitrous oxide and small increments of analgesics. IPPV is used attempting to maintain normocapnia. Halothane may also be used, but the dose is kept to a minimum to avoid hypotension. Once the various vascular connections are completed mannitol is given to stimulate a diuresis, and, hydrocortisone and azathioprine (Immuran) are given to start immunosuppressant therpay. If all has gone well the kidney should begin to secrete urine immediately. Postoperatively, patients are allowed to breathe spontaneously and only ventilated artificially if there is doubt about reversal of the neuromuscular blocking drugs used.

ANAESTHESIA FOR THE PATIENT WITH A RENAL TRANSPLANT

Such patients may of course present for any form of surgery and it is important not to damage their transplant. After a careful history and examination transplant function should be assessed. If the patient has still got a working fistula or shunt this may be useful either for a preoperative dialysis if necessary, or for postoperative use. As with all patients with renal disease, the anaesthetist should avoid damaging veins if possible. For minor procedures, inhalation or local anaesthesia may be preferable. These patients are particularly at risk from infection because of immunosuppression and sterile equipment and sterile techniques must be used. Osteoporosis is common and extra care must be taken when lifting or positioning the patients on the operating table. Gastrointestinal bleeding may occur as the result of steroid therapy and the additional stress of further anaesthesia and surgery; antacids may be indicated. Extra steroids should be given with the premedication and one should be certain that the patient returns to their previous steroid therapy as soon as possible postoperatively. Clearly any nephrotoxic drugs should be avoided as should anaesthetic techniques which may adversely affect renal function.

REFERENCES

1 GALIZIA EJ, LAHIRI SK. Anaesthesia for arteriovenous fistulae: a modified stellate ganglion block. *Anaesthesia* 1974; **29**: 362–5.
2 JENKINS LC, MALONEY PJ, CYR W. Anaesthesia for simultaneous bilateral nephrectomy. *Can Anaesth Soc J* 1973; **20**: 259–73.

3 ROBSON JS. Acute renal failure. In: Walker WF, Taylor DEM, eds. *Intensive care.* Proceedings eighth Pfizer international symposium. Edinburgh: Churchill Livingstone, 1975; 144–59.
4 SAMUEL JR, POWELL D. Renal transplantation: anaesthetic experience of 100 cases. *Anaesthesia* 1970; **25**: 165–76.
5 SAVEGE TM, STRUNIN L. Regional blockade with bupivicaine (Marcain) for the insertion of Scribner shunts. *Anaesthesia* 1971; **26**: 498–500.

RECOMMENDED GENERAL READING

BEVAN DR. *Renal function in anaesthesia and surgery.* London: Academic Press; New York: Grune & Stratton, 1980.

Chapter 5
Liver Disease

L. STRUNIN AND K. W. PETTINGALE

BASIC PRINCIPLES

ANATOMY AND PHYSIOLOGY

The liver is the largest organ in the body weighing, in the adult, about 1500 g. Seventy per cent of the blood supply comes from the portal vein and 30 per cent from the hepatic artery. Within the liver these vessels branch and, accompanied by a bile duct, form a network of sinusoids which terminate in the hepatic veins draining the liver. The network of sinusoids is usually described as lobules, but these are difficult to distinguish in man although they are easily seen in animal livers. More recently, a functional unit called an acinus has been defined by studying the distribution of Indian ink after injection into the portal vein. The acinus consists of a group of sinusoids running between a terminal portal tract (a bile duct, portal vein and hepatic artery within a fibrous sheath) and two or more terminal hepatic venules. These intersect at approximately right angles and each half acinus is therefore basically a tetrahedral structure. Liver cells adjacent to the hepatic venules are functionally different from those near the portal tracts as they receive blood which has already lost oxygen during its passage through the central parts of the acinus. These cells therefore are especially susceptible to hypoxic conditions and account for so called 'centrilobular necrosis' associated with shock. It is of interest that primary or secondary hepatic tumours obtain their blood supply almost entirely from the hepatic artery. Therefore ligation and/or infusion of cytotoxic drugs into the hepatic artery will cause tumour necrosis preferentially.

Two types of cells are found within the liver—the hepatocyte and the Kupffer cell. Within the cytoplasm of the hepatocyte many different components are found which are collectively called organelles. Mitochondria are concerned with energy supply and the rough endoplasmic reticulum, consisting of parallel membranes and granular particles called ribosomes, is the site of protein synthesis. The smooth endoplasmic reticulum, which lacks ribosomes forms, vesicles called microsomes if liver cells are mechanically disrupted. The smooth endoplasmic reticulum is the site of bilirubin conjugation, bile salt synthesis, and the major area for drug detoxication. Enzymes concerned in these reactions are collectively called microsomal enzymes. Bile cannaliculi are formed by the cell membranes of adjacent hepatocytes. These connect with bile ductules in the portal tracts and eventually drain into the biliary tree. The Kupffer cell is phagocytic and is particularly concerned with taking up bacteria which enter the portal vein from the intestine. The liver produces one litre of bile per day which is released into the duodenum during digestion. At other times bile passes into the gall bladder where it is concentrated to about one fifth of its volume. Bile normally contains electrolytes, protein, bilirubin, lipids, and bile salts. In addition many drugs are excreted in the bile although they may be subsequently reabsorbed, i.e. they undergo enterohepatic circulation.

Bilirubin comes mainly from the breakdown of haem released during destruction of old erythrocytes. Further small amounts arise within the hepatocyte itself and from the bone marrow. Bilirubin is insoluble and is tightly bound to plasma albumin. It is rapidly taken up from the blood by hepatocytes via an uptake mechanism which probably involves two bilirubin binding proteins called Y and Z. The majority of bilirubin is conjugated within the liver with glucuronic acid by the microsomal enzyme glucuronyl transferase, although other conjugates occur. Conjugated bilirubin is then excreted in the bile and may also be excreted in the urine. In the intestine bilirubin conjugates are reduced by bacteria and compounds such as stercobilins and urobilinogen are produced. This latter undergoes enterohepatic circulation and is in part excreted in the urine.

Most plasma proteins are synthesized by the liver with the exception of the immunoglobulins and antihaemophilic factor (factor VIII). Plasma albumin concentration usually falls in chronic liver disease and most patients with cirrhosis have low albumin synthesis rates and a small albumin pool. Plasma globulin concentrations are frequently increased. This may represent the response to bacteria which are not removed by the Kupffer cells and then have access to the systemic circulation. In patients with autoimmune liver disease hyperglobulinaemia may be part of the disease process. Ammonia is produced by the deamination of amino acids and other nitrogenous substances and is very toxic. It is rapidly converted into urea by the liver. In liver failure, blood ammonia increases and blood urea concentration is often low. However, the severity of hepatic encephalopathy bears little relation to the blood ammonia concentration. There are about 20 amino acids in plasma and the liver is capable of regulating the blood concentration of each with a precision comparable to that of blood glucose control. In liver failure amino acid metabolism becomes abnormal and these changes may be relevant to the pathogenesis of hepatic encephalopathy.

The hepatocyte cell membrane is unusually permeable to glucose which is removed from the blood for storage as glycogen, or for oxidation. Glucose homeostasis is maintained either from glycogen hydrolysis or from the conversion of protein and fats to glucose by gluconeogenesis. Potassium is also released from the liver in proportion to the glucose secreted. Insulin stimulates glycolysis and glycogen synthesis but inhibits gluconeogenesis. Insulin seems to act directly on the hepatic enzymes and not by its more usual method of altering membrane permeability. Adrenaline and glucagon act in opposition to insulin. It should be remembered that the liver actively removes insulin from the blood. This results in about one third of the insulin produced by the pancreas being removed from the portal blood before it reaches the systemic circulation. Glucose tolerance is impaired in patients with liver disease and patients may present a clinical picture of maturity onset diabetes. Ketosis is rare. In fulminant hepatic failure, however, although the initial changes are similar, hypoglycaemia may supervene.

LIVER FUNCTION TESTS

Although the liver is involved in most of the important metabolic functions of the body it is remarkable how few of these are upset by liver disease. The regenerative capacity of the liver enables many of its functions to continue satisfactorily. Regrettably, therefore, no satisfactory single test of liver function exists. A series of tests may be made which will examine various aspects of liver function but it should be remembered that

Table 5.1. Liver function tests.

Test	Normal range
Sodium	130–145 mmol/l
Potassium	3·5–5 mmol/l
Bicarbonate	20–28 mmol/l
Urea	3·3–6·7 mmol/l
Glucose	2·8–5 mmol/l
Creatinine	0·044–0·1 mmol/l
Total Protein	60–80 g/l
Albumin	35–50 g/l
Globulin	25–30 g/l
Bilirubin	3–20 μ mol/l
Prothrombin time	12–13 seconds
Alkaline phosphatase (ALP)	30–85 iu/l
Aspartate aminotransferase (AST)	10–50 iu/l
Alanine aminotransferase (ALT)	10–45 iu/l
Lactate dehydrogenase (LDH)	90–300 iu/l
Hydroxybutyrate dehydrogenase (HBD)	100–250 iu/l
Gamma glutamyl transferase (GGT)	5–34 iu/l

Note:
(i) The term transaminases is used to cover aspartate (AST) and alanine aminotransferase (ALT). AST is usually the only one measured.
(ii) Serum glutamate-oxalacetate transaminase (SGOT) is equivalent to AST and serum glutamate-pyruvate transaminase (SPGT) is equivalent to alanine aminotransferase (ALT).

these are crude and somewhat inaccurate measurements. It is possible to have severe derangement of liver function, which may become manifest after anaesthesia and surgery, and yet was accompanied by perfectly normal preoperative 'liver function tests'. The biochemical tests available should not be considered in isolation, but should accompany a careful history and clinical examination of the patient. Particularly, the appearance and 'fitness' of the patient may be more relevant than the figures obtained from biochemical testing. Table 5.1 gives a list of common liver function tests with their normal range. The relevance of changes in these tests will be found in the appropriate section in this chapter. Haematological measurements and blood gas measurements, although not strictly speaking liver function tests, are obviously relevant since bleeding and alterations in ventilation are common accompaniments of liver disease. Too much reliance should not be placed on single estimations of any of these tests and where possible serial measurements should be made so that any trend may be detected as this is often more relevant in diagnosis.

JAUNDICE

Although it is traditional to classify the causes of jaundice according to mechanism, e.g. increased bile pigment production, defective uptake and transport within the hepatocyte, defective conjugation or defective excretion, in practice it may be difficult to attribute jaundice to any one mechanism in a given patient. For example, hepatocellular damage may result in jaundice by all four mechanisms.

Increase in bile pigment load to liver cell

The capacity of the liver to handle bile pigment may increase considerably, so that even in chronic haemolytic states the serum bilirubin is rarely raised above 50 micro-moles per litre. Higher levels usually indicate additional hepato-cellular dysfunction.

Defective bilirubin transport

The best example of this is Gilbert's disease, which is the commonest variety of familial unconjugated, non-haemolytic hyperbilirubinaemia although the defect may also occur in patients with resolving virus hepatitis. Serum bilirubin is not raised above 50 micromoles per litre and is unaffected by steroid therapy.

Defective conjugation by hepatic microsomes

This defect may result from two mechanisms: *enzyme deficiency* such as is found in neonatal or 'physiological' jaundice and in the very rare, usually fatal, Crigler-Najar hyperbilirubinaemia; and *enzyme inhibition*, a factor in maternal serum, probably a pregestational steroid which may inhibit glycuronyl transferase and cause neonatal jaundice. Bilirubin is unconjugated in both and so does not appear in the urine.

Defective excretion

Here the defect may be either within the bile canaliculi and small ducts within the liver, i.e. intrahepatic cholestasis, or in the main bile ducts between the liver and the duodenum, i.e. extrahepatic obstruction.

Intrahepatic cholestasis. This may occur as a result of widespread hepato-cellular damage, such as in virus or alcoholic hepatitis or macronodular cirrhosis, and in these instances serum bilirubin may be dramatically reduced by steroid therapy. A chole-static picture may be seen in patients with the Dubin–Johnson syndrome (familial conjugated hyperbilirubinaemia) which may be enhanced by ictogenic steroids (such as methyltestosterone or norethanalone). Cellular reactions around the ductules and intralobular ducts may occur as a result of drug sensitivity due, for example, to the phenothiazine group of drugs. Inflammatory reactions around the intralobular and septal bile ducts occur in primary biliary cirrhosis and biliary atresia; and similar reactions around still larger ducts occur in ascending cholangitis.

Extra-hepatic obstruction Large bile duct obstruction may result from gallstones, strictures, carcinomas of the bile duct, and carcinoma of the head of the pancreas. Hyperbilirubinaemia in both the intra- and extrahepatic obstructive type is predominantly conjugated and is accompanied by bile in the urine. Unconjugated hyperbilirubinaemia may occur later: firstly because there is invariably a decrease in red cell survival in obstructive jaundice and also because conjugation becomes defective.

CLASSIFICATION OF LIVER DISEASE

Table 5.2 illustrates a classification of liver disease relevant for the anaesthetist contemplating anaesthetizing patients with hepatic dysfunction. It is not intended that this classification should replace the classical ones found in text books devoted to the liver, but it may be of more use in narrowing down the field of problems and investigations required before undertaking anaesthesia for surgical procedures in such patients.

Table 5.2. Classification of liver disease.

	Measurements	Comment
Biliary obstruction	Raised: bilirubin ALP AST Prolonged: Prothrombin time	Response to vitamin K ? Renal function
Chronic liver disease (*a*) No gastro-intestinal bleeding (*b*) With gastrointestinal bleeding	Raised: bilirubin transaminases ALP Albumin low: Globulin high As above +low: Hb, PCV, platelets, other clotting factors	Response to vitamin K ? Renal function ? Grading ? Response to transfusion
Acute liver disease	Raised: bilirubin transaminases Prolonged: prothrombin time Low: albumin, platelets	(1) Response to sedatives (2) Evidence of bleeding
Viral hepatitis	Positive: HBsAg	Precautions against cross-infection particularly staff
Liver tumours	Ultrasound scintiscanning and computerized axial tomography (CAT) scan	Alpha fetoprotein raised in primary hepatoma

In conjunction with the table a series of questions must be asked.
1   Is the patient jaundiced and what is the bilirubin level?
2   What is the prothrombin time; does it respond to vitamin K?
3   To establish chronic liver disease, are serial measurement of proteins and transaminases abnormal?
4   Is the patient bleeding from the gastrointestinal tract? If so has this altered the patient's level of consciousness other than that associated with hypotension. If so, then the patient's liver disease is severe and hepatic coma may be occurring.
5   Has the patient received any sedative drugs? If so, what was their effect?
6   Has the patient been screened for markers of infection with viral hepatitis B, such as HBsAg, or e antigen, or is there evidence of other virus infection?
7   Has renal function been assessed?
Other liver function changes, such as alkaline phosphate (ALP) raised in biliary obstruction, are well recorded in the literature, but are not overhelpful to the anaesthetist.

VIRAL HEPATITIS

Hepatitis may result from infection with a number of viruses, most commonly either virus hepatitis A (HAV) or virus hepatitis B (HBV); less commonly cytomegalovirus, herpes simplex virus or Epstein-Barr virus (infectious mononucleosis) may be responsible. Hepatitis A is endemic in all parts of the world. The infection is not normally transmitted by blood transfusion; and although severe and sometimes fatal hepatitis may result, in most cases recovery is complete and there is no progression to either chronic liver disease or a carrier state. In contrast, hepatitis B is commonly transmitted parenterally and, in addition to occasionally causing fulminant hepatic failure, may be associated with the development of both chronic liver disease and a symptomless carrier state. This is more likely to happen in patients with liver and kidney disease, a history of drug abuse, after tattooing, and persons coming from countries with a high endemic rate of infection with hepatitis B. The carrier state may be quantified and characterized serologically by the finding of hepatitis B surface antigen (HBsAg) and the absence of surface antibody. In some carriers hepatitis B DNA polymerase activity is present and another antigen, the e antigen, may also be detected. The presence of both HBsAg and e antigens indicates a highly infectious individual.

The application of serological testing to the blood transfusion service has dramatically reduced the risk of transfusion hepatitis. However such hepatitis still occurs even in the absence of detectable infection with either virus A or B or other viruses which are known to cause hepatitis. The description non-A non-B hepatitis is now used for such occurrences, and is the major cause of transfusion hepatitis in countries where screening for hepatitis A and B is carried out. Although the virus of non-A non-B hepatitis has not been characterized there is some evidence that a chronic carrier state exists and that in some patients chronic liver disease may occur.

The risk of infection to anaesthetic personnel by viral hepatitis is a recognized hazard. However, simple measures are effective in preventing infection being transmitted from patients to staff. Awareness of the problem is important and implies that patients should be screened for the presence of HBsAg and if possible e antigen; but even if these facilities are not available, patients in the high risk categories should be regarded as antigen positive until proved otherwise. Most cases of hepatitis among anaesthetists follow accidental inoculation, and present casual attitudes to the spillage of blood should be tempered with restraint. The wearing of gloves, a disposable gown and mask, the use of disposable anaesthetic equipment where appropriate and safe disposal of such equipment afterwards, are obvious precautions. Hepatitis B virus is susceptible to heat, ethylene oxide, aqueous formaldehyde (10 per cent), glutaraldehyde (2 per cent) and most proprietary bleach solutions. Sterilization of equipment, therefore, should not be a problem.

Despite precautions inadvertent inoculation of potentially infected material may occur. Subjects should be screened for hepatitis B surface antibodies, since if these are present, there is little risk of infection occurring. In all other subjects, provided it is clear that infected material was indeed inoculated, then a dose of specific anti-HBs immunoglobulin should be administered. This form of immunoglobulin is recommended for the treatment of hepatitis B infection. Human normal immunoglobulin (gammaglobulin) is effective in preventing hepatitis A infection but is not effective in the treatment of hepatitis B infection, although it does appear to have a beneficial effect in preventing non-A non-B hepatitis. Immunoglobulin confers only passive immunity and as yet there is no vaccine available to provide active immunity against viral hepatitis.

The advent of specific serological diagnosis of viral hepatitis [8] means that there is now additional help in determining the cause of jaundice both before and after surgery. This should help to eliminate patients who have viral hepatitis undergoing unnecessary and potentially hazardous surgery as well as helping to elucidate the cause of some cases of unexplained postoperative jaundice or hepatitis.

CHRONIC LIVER DISEASE (HEPATIC CIRRHOSIS)

Chronic liver disease often produces little alteration in liver function and may be clinically and biochemically undetectable. Only when some additional insult, often iatrogenic, produces further deterioration in liver function, does the underlying chronic liver disease become clinically obvious as jaundice, ascites or encephalopathy. Therefore the natural history of chronic liver disease is not necessarily one of progressive deterioration and with careful management, avoiding the precipitation of complications, patients may be kept well for many years.

PATHOLOGY

There are some 1400 deaths each year in England and Wales certified as due to cirrhosis. Cirrhosis, however, is not a single entity and the characteristic pathological changes of necrosis, fibrosis, and regeneration nodules may result from many aetiological factors. In addition there may be histological features specific for certain diseases. The major causes of cirrhosis are listed in Tables 5.3 and 5.4.

Table 5.3. Genetic causes of cirrhosis.

Haemochromatosis	Nieman–Pick disease
Wilson's disease	Cystinosis
Galactosaemia	Gaucher's disease
Fructosaemia	Hurler's disease
Glycogen storage disease (Type 4)	Hepatic porphyria
Alpha-l-antitrypsin deficiency	Sickle cell disease
Mucoviscidosis	Thalassaemia

Table 5.4. Non-genetic causes of cirrhosis.

Alcoholic
Chronic active hepatitis (HBsAg positive and negative and non-A, non-B)
Post hepatic (viral, toxin or radiation damage)
Primary biliary cirrhosis
Secondary biliary cirrhosis (following any longstanding biliary obstruction)
Ulcerative colitis
Passive venous congestion
Veno-occlusive disease

The size of the liver is very variable, ranging from shrunken to very large and may change during the course of the disease. However, there is always an increased resistance to the flow of blood in the portal venous system, resulting eventually in congestive splenomegaly and colateral venous channels. This picture is usually described as portal hypertension. Another late complication of cirrhosis is the development of primary liver cell carcinoma (hepatoma).

CLINICAL FEATURES

Compensated cirrhosis is compatible with a complete feeling of well-being and when symptoms do occur they are usually vague; such as malaise, dyspepsia, weight loss, loss of libido and menstrual disturbances. Physical signs are also often absent and many of the skin changes described in cirrhosis, such as white spots, paper money skin, white nails and palmar erythema have little diagnostic value. Finger clubbing and cyanosis are occasionally seen, but are non-specific. Generalized pigmentation may indicate haemochromatosis or primary biliary cirrhosis. One of the most useful physical signs of cirrhosis is the presence of spider naevi on the skin of the face, arms and upper torso. They may occur transiently in pregnancy and viral hepatitis, but are particularly florid in alcoholic cirrhosis and chronic active hepatitis.

Chronic liver disease characteristically produces evidence of a high output circulatory state, with flushed extremities, dilated veins, capillary pulsation and a collapsing pulse. Although arterio-venous fistulae in the lungs have been demonstrated in liver disease which may account for some of the changes, e.g. finger clubbing, the more likely explanation is that a vasodilator substance is either produced by, or not inactivated by, the damaged liver.

In cirrhosis, the proportion of blood supply derived from the portal vein diminishes gradually and there is a relative increase from the hepatic artery. Thus the effects of portacaval anastomosis on the blood supply to the liver is less marked in the cirrhotic patient, but the effects of systemic hypotension and hypoxaemia are more marked. Since the regeneration nodules are mainly supplied by arterial blood, systemic hypoxaemia may result in severe liver necrosis. These regeneration nodules progressively distort the portal venous system with consequent rise in portal venous pressure, development of collateral channels bypassing the liver, splenomegaly and hypersplenism.

A palpably enlarged liver is mainly associated with alcoholic cirrhosis or haemochromatosis, whereas a shrunken liver is more likely with cryptogenic cirrhosis. The cirrhotic liver is firm and it may be possible to detect irregularities on the surface in the macronodular type. Splenomegaly and venous collaterals on the abdominal wall are good indicators of portal hypertension.

In the later stages of chronic liver disease there may be progressive water retention, hyponatraemia, azotaemia and oliguria due to reduced renal plasma flow, leading to 'hepato-renal failure'.

Signs which suggest that chronic liver disease has become decompensated include jaundice, oedema, ascites, a flapping tremor and other signs of impending hepatic coma. A change in size or shape of the liver may indicate a hepatoma. Clinical features of specific types of cirrhosis are shown in Table 5.5.

Table 5.5. Clinical features of specific types of cirrhosis.

Type	Histological factors	Clinical features
Alcoholic	Micronodular Fat if drinking Focal necrosis with neutrophil infiltration Mallory's hyalin Centrilobular fibrosis Siderosis	Florid spider naevi Anorexia and vomiting Obesity and nutritional deficiencies Muscle wasting, impotence Abdominal pain, diarrhoea Fever, hypoglycaemia Hyperlipidaemia
Chronic active hepatitis	Portal infiltration with mononuclear and plasma cells 'Piecemeal' necrosis Rosette formation	
(a) HBsantigen negative		Young female, recurrent jaundice, amenorrhoea, striae, acne, fever, polyarthritis, thyroiditis, skin lesions, ulcerative colitis, renal tubular acidosis, pleurisy
(b) HBsantigen positive		Male, primary hepatoma commonly develops
(c) Drug induced		Oxyphenisatin, methyldopa, isoniazid
Haemochromatosis	Iron deposition in hepatocytes, Kupffer cells, portal tracts and septa	Skin pigmentation, diabetes mellitus, cardiac abnormalities, arthropathy, testicular atrophy, impotence, abdominal pain
Wilson's disease	Chronic aggressive hepatitis Glycogen vacuolation Fatty infiltration	Young person Kayser–Fleischer rings Neurological or psychiatric abnormality Haemolytic anaemic Bone lesions
Primary biliary cirrhosis	Damaged bile ducts Portal infiltration Lymphoid follicles, granulomas, duct proliferation Portal fibrosis Cirrhosis late	Early pruritis, skin pigmentation, xanthelasma and xanthomas 'Autoimmune' diseases Steatorrhoea, bone thinning and pathological fractures
Secondary biliary cirrhosis	Broad serpiginous bands of connective tissue Duct proliferation Oedema at junction of parenchyma and septa Polymorph infiltration	Long history of obstructive jaundice
α-$_1$-antitrypsin deficiency	Bile duct proliferation PAS positive globules in parenchymal cells Periportal fibrosis Cholestatic picture	Attacks of neonatal hepatitis Later development of cirrhosis rarely associated with pulmonary form of disease

MAJOR COMPLICATIONS

ENCEPHALOPATHY

Three types are described:

Acute. This follows fulminant hepatic necrosis, for example by viral hepatitis or drug toxicity, e.g. paracetamol. Mortality for this type is over 50 per cent.

Acute on chronic. This is usually seen in patients with cirrhosis, when episodes of encephalopathy may be precipitated by a number of factors such as gastrointestinal bleeding, electrolyte disturbance, infection, constipation, sedative and other drugs, alcohol ingestion, anaesthesia and surgery, and paracentesis. If treatment of the precipitating factor is possible, complete recovery usually follows.

Chronic. This type is uncommon, but may follow a portasystemic shunt, e.g. portacaval anastomosis. The majority of patients with chronic encephalopathy present a neurological or psychiatric problem rather than an hepatic one, and usually have well-compensated inactive cirrhosis. Mortality is low, but morbidity is often high.

Clinical features

These may be divided into defects of cortical, extrapyramidal and pyramidal function. *Cortical features* consist of disturbed consciousness, personality changes such as irritability, lethargy and apathy; intellectual deterioration; visiospatial apraxia and psychiatric abnormalities, such as paranoia and aggression. *Extra-pyramidal features* consist of dysarthria, apraxia (flapping tremor) and cogwheel rigidity. *Pyramidal features* consist of spasticity, hyperreflexia, clonus and intermittent extensor plantar responses.

Acute encephalopathy is characterized mainly by disturbed behaviour and loss of consciousness, and the deepest grades of coma are seen in this type. Patients with viral hepatitis who become apathetic, lethargic, drowsy or irritable should be observed carefully for other neurological signs of encephalopathy such as flapping tremor, and treatment instituted if encephalopathy is suspected. An electroencephalogram (EEG) may be helpful in deciding on the diagnosis. Acute-on-chronic encephalopathy differs clinically from the acute type only in the respect that the degree of coma seen is rarely as deep and the rate of progression of the coma is much slower—often taking several days rather than hours. Patients will also usually have other features of chronic liver disease determined from their history or physical examination.

Chronic encephalopathy presents quite a different clinical picture. The patient shows mainly personality and behaviour changes with some impairment of intellect; disturbances of consciousness are not seen, and the extra-pyramidal and pyramidal signs are less commonly found.

Patient assessment

Ascertain the presence of liver disease. Patients with chronic encephalopathy may have few features of liver disease and are often misdiagnosed. The diagnostic, clinical and biochemical features of liver disease have already been described.

Exclude precipitating factors: Elimination of these is crucial to the successful management of the acute and chronic variety of encephalopathy.

Psychometric and neurological assessment: Such assessments will not only determine the severity of encephalopathy but when performed sequentially, will monitor the response to therapy. Since visiospatial apraxia is a well-recognized feature of encephalopathy, the most popular methods of assessment are constructing a five-pointed star and a handwriting chart. However, very sophisticated tests of motor and cognitive function may detect evidence of encephalopathy before other clinical or electroencephalographic evidence appears. Such testing is likely to be valuable only in the chronic form of encephalopathy.

Electroencephalography (EEG): This is a valuable test in assessing both the occurrence and severity of encephalopathy and determining the likelihood of survival. The EEG changes are not specific to liver failure but may occur in other metabolic conditions such as renal failure. As the patient becomes progressively more comatose the EEG wave forms pass through certain characteristic changes. The normal dominant EEG frequency of 8–13 Hz gradually slows, then increases in amplitude, with triphasic waves and then decreases until the record becomes flat. The appearance of triphasic waves, followed by progressive decrease in amplitude and flattening indicates that recovery is unlikely. EEG changes are used in conjunction with various physical signs to grade hepatic coma (see Table 5.6).

Table 5.6. Grading of hepatic coma [3, 5].

Mental state		EEG
Grade 1	Confusion/euphoria	Normal
Grade 2	Drowsy	Generalized slowing
Grade 3	Sleeping but rousable	Delta activity
Grade 4	Comatose—respond to pain	Triphasics
Grade 5	Comatose—no response	Flat

Note: Grades 4 and 5 are sometimes combined

Treatment

Avoidance and correction of precipitating factors. Occasionally patients may respond after correction of such factors alone. However, chronic encephalopathy will not have any precipitating factors.

Protein restriction. Complete protein restriction is indicated in severe acute encephalopathy whereas moderate restriction (30–50 g daily) is indicated in the more chronic, less severe forms.

Purgation. This alone may induce a partial remission. The usually recommended method is magnesium sulphate enemas once or twice daily.

Antibiotics. Poorly-absorbed antibiotics, such as neomycin, have been shown to benefit encephalopathy, probably by diminishing bacterial urease activity and reducing ammonia production. Neomycin should only be used for short periods because of its toxicity to the eighth nerve, kidneys and gastrointestinal tract.

Lactulose. This is a synthetic disaccharide which is not hydrolysed or absorbed in the small bowel but metabolized to lactic and acetic acid by bacterial action in the colon, thus increasing faecal acidity. The exact mechanism of action of lactulose is not known but the alteration of faecal acidity seems essential. Lactulose causes diarrhoea and the dose should therefore be adjusted so that the patient produces one to two soft stools daily. Lactulose is probably most useful in the treatment of patients with chronic encephalopathy.

L-dopa. This drug has been successfully used in both acute and chronic encephalopathy.

Other methods. Numerous methods have been tried in order to remove 'coma factors'. These have varied from exchange blood transfusion, steroids, temporary liver support with a variety of animal livers, charcoal haemoperfusion, and more recently haemodialysis using membranes which are permeable to large molecules. Most of these methods have been assessed in patients with acute encephalopathy. Although individual patient successes have been recorded with all the methods outlined above, none has proved entirely satisfactory. Much work is still in progress and it remains to be seen whether a satisfactory 'artificial liver support system' is a practical possibility.

ASCITES

Ascitic fluid is in dynamic equilibrium with plasma although the volume exchange between the two compartments is small, amounting to about 500 ml in 24 hr. Many factors contribute towards the formation of ascites including reduction in albumin concentration, increase in portal venous pressure and lymphatic congestion, but the major factor is excess sodium retention by the kidney. The reason for this sodium retention is not fully understood. A reduced glomerular filtration rate always results in sodium retention by the tubules and patients with ascites often show such a reduction. A second factor may be increased secretion of aldosterone and elevated levels of renin and aldosterone have been observed in some patients with ascites, due possibly to the failure of the diseased liver to metabolize aldosterone. However, the increase in extracellular volume which results from hyperaldosteronism normally triggers a third or naturetic factor which reduces aldosterone secretion and leads to sodium loss. In cirrhotic patients with ascites this 'third factor' is not released and sodium retention persists. The nature of 'third factor' is unknown but may be the result of pressure changes in the peritubular vessels, redistribution of blood to deeper more salt-retaining nephrons by cortical vasoconstriction, or the action of a chemical substance, such as renin, bradykininogen, or prostaglandin.

The management of ascites is important, since many patients experience little or no symptoms from their enlarged abdomen, but 'treatment' may produce marked deterioration. It is possible to classify patients with ascites into three main types by measuring glomerular filtration rate, and urinary and sodium water excretion in response to a water load.

Water and salt excretors. In these patients renal function is only mildly affected. Glomerular filtration rate is normal and patients are able to excrete both salt and water after a water load. In this instance the increased sodium reabsorption which leads to ascites is probably taking place in the collecting ducts due to either the action of aldosterone or third factor. Bedrest and salt-restricted diet usually results in a spontaneous diuresis, although occasionally a diuretic drug is needed. (A normal British diet contains about 100 mmol sodium per day—no added salt reduces the intake to 50 mmol per day).

Water excretors and salt retainers. These patients also have a normal glomerular filtration rate and can excrete water normally after a water load, but excrete much less salt. Here, increased sodium reabsorption is taking place in the distal tubule or the ascending loop of Henle. These patients invariably respond to diuretic drugs acting on the distal tubule, such as spironolactone 100–150 mg per day, or triampterene 150–300 mg per day, or amiloride 15–30 mg per day. Failure to respond to a 'distal' diuretic usually means that insufficient sodium is reaching the distal tubule because of increased absorption in the ascending loop of Henle, and an additional diuretic acting at this site, e.g. thiazides, frusemide, or ethacrynic acid is needed.

Water and salt retainers. Patients in this group have a significantly impaired glomerular filtration rate and are unable to excrete salt or water after a water load. This means that there is insufficient sodium reaching the loop of Henle to generate free water and the site of increased sodium absorption is proximal. Thus diuretics acting on the ascending loop of Henle will not increase sodium excretion. Here the basis of treatment is to improve renal perfusion and nephron filtration and expand the extracellular volume in order to reduce proximal tubular reabsorption via the 'third factor' effect.

Many therapies have been tried, for example, mannitol, high dose steroids, noradrenaline, angiotensin II, dopamine, L-dopa, prostaglandin A1, plasma, salt free albumin and large doses of frusemide. The last may be effective by its action in increasing renal blood flow. Although many of the above agents may have temporary success, many patients are refractory. Persistent use of diuretics may precipitate progressive renal failure. Finally, in patients with resistant ascites the use of ascitic fluid transfusion may be indicated. Ascitic fluid is withdrawn through a pump, ultra-filtered so that fluid and small crystalloids are removed, and then reinfused into a vein thus retaining the protein content.

INFECTION

There is a high incidence of Gram-negative bacteraemia in cirrhosis associated with a high mortality rate. The features are often atypical unexplained deterioration, hypotension and encephalopathy. Peritoneal infection is also common.

SEVERE JAUNDICE

This is usually a result of hepatocellular dysfunction, such as superimposed hepatitis in alcoholics or relapsing chronic active hepatitis. In addition cirrhosis may produce an intrahepatic cholestatic picture. Extra-hepatic biliary obstruction is very rare and surgery should not be considered until cholangiography—preferably retrograde via an endoscope, has been performed.

VITAMIN DEFICIENCY

In the absence of biliary obstruction specific deficiencies do not occur as a result of chronic liver disease but are due to associated malnutrition or malabsorption. Serum B_{12} may be elevated when there is considerable hepatic cell necrosis as stored B_{12} in the liver is released. With chronic biliary obstruction there will be deficiencies of fat soluble vitamins, A, D, E and K. This later vitamin is of course essential for the manufacture of prothrombin by the liver.

DIAGNOSTIC INVESTIGATIONS

Routine 'liver function tests' are of little value. They are usually normal in compensated cirrhosis, and although they may be useful in distinguishing liver disease from other causes of jaundice, there is no specific pattern which indicates cirrhosis.

In the established cirrhotic patient, the most useful tests with which to monitor hepatocellular function are bilirubin and plasma albumin levels, along with a measurement of prothrombin activity. Table 5.7 lists investigations which may be valuable in distinguishing between different types of cirrhosis.

Table 5.7. Investigations useful for distinguishing between specific types of cirrhosis.

Type	Investigation
Alcoholic	Red cell and serum folate
	Red cell transketolase (for thiamine deficiency)
Chronic active hepatitis	Serum immunoglobulins
(*a*) HBsantigen negative	Leucopenia and thrombocytopenia
	High titre of antinuclear, smooth muscle and antomitochondrial autoantibodies
(*b*) HBsantigen positive	HBsantigen, α foeto-protein
Haemochromatosis	Serum iron and iron binding capacity
	Haemosiderosis
	Desferrioxamine test
Wilson's disease	Serum, hepatic and urinary copper
	Serum caeruloplasmin
Primary biliary	Mitochondrial autoantibody
	Serum IsM Skeletal survey
Secondary biliary	Retrograde or percutaneous cholangiography
α-$_1$-antitrypsin deficiency	Serum α-$_1$-antitrypsin

Liver biopsy

The critical diagnostic test for cirrhosis is liver biopsy. Although needle biopsy is subject to sampling errors—for instance when taken from very large regenerative nodules—it should allow a firm diagnosis of cirrhosis to be made, and may indicate the underlying aetiology. The biopsy may also be used to assess the extent of necrosis or inflammatory reaction, and for instance, in chronic active hepatitis, may determine the type of treatment. The response to treatment may be monitored by biopsy, for example in haemochromatosis and in Wilson's disease, and the diagnosis of hepatoma may also be determined. If a needle biopsy is equivocal, laparoscopy and wedge biopsy may be indicated.

Bromsulphthalein retention test

The main use of this test is in the diagnosis of the Dubin–Johnson syndrome when a prolonged test is performed and the 2-hr retention is greater than at 45 min. The test is not helpful in the routine assessment of liver function and although abnormalities do occur in the immediate postoperative period, the changes are nonspecific.

Liver scanning

This investigation is particularly useful in detecting primary or secondary malignant lesions in the liver. Radionuclides bound to colloid, such as [^{99}Tc^m] technectium sulphur colloid, are taken up by the Kupffer cells in the liver and areas of defective uptake may be detected by a gamma camera and indicate that the liver structure is infiltrated by tumour. In cirrhosis, uptake of radionuclides is generally reduced and patchy throughout the liver, but there is increased uptake in the area of an enlarged spleen. Selenium labelled methionine is taken up preferentially by the hepatocytes and areas of increased uptake will be seen when there is a primary liver cell tumour.

Non-invasive scanning of the liver may be carried out using both ultrasound and computerized axial tomography (CAT).

Barium swallow—oesophagoscopy—gastroscopy

Gastrointestinal bleeding is a common precipitating factor of hepatic coma in patients with chronic liver disease. Bleeding may occur either from oesophageal varices or from erosions in the gastric mucosa. A barium swallow, oesophagoscopy and gastroscopy may be necessary to locate the source of bleeding.

Portal venography and hepatic venous catherization

In cases where the diagnosis of portal hypertension is difficult to establish these investigations are indicated to demonstrate whether the cause is intra- or extrahepatic.

General management

Since nothing can reverse the pathological changes of cirrhosis the main aims of management are to prevent further damage, detect and treat complications (such as encephalopathy and ascites) and avoid making hepatocellular function worse. In addition, drugs that induce liver damage such as isoniazid, methyldopa, or oxyphenisatin (a laxative) should be stopped. If alcoholic patients can be persuaded to abstain there may be an improvement in their life expectancy, although the cirrhotic process is only modified and does not reverse. Patients with haemochromotosis can have their outlook improved by venesection and those with Wilson's disease may have their disease process halted by a low copper diet and penicillamine therapy. Cirrhosis due to active chronic hepatitis may be improved by corticosteroids and immunosuppressive agents such as azathioprine. This later drug is also on trial as a treatment for primary biliary cirrhosis.

ANAESTHESIA

Preoperative assessment

Patients with chronic liver disease may obviously present for any surgical procedure but commonly anaesthesia is required for surgery related to chronic liver disease.

Table 5.8. Surgical procedures for chronic liver disease.

Oesophagoscopy
Gastroscopy
Laparoscopy
Injection of oesophageal varices
Transection of the oesophagus
Boerema button insertion
Portacaval shunt
Lieno-renal shunt
Mesenterico-caval jump graft

Table 5.8 lists some of the common surgical procedures undertaken. A careful history and examination is of more value than rigid attention to small changes in liver function tests. Nevertheless, it is useful to assess liver function using a scale system (Table 5.9) as this gives an indication of the likely prognosis of the patient.

This system makes use of weighting whereby one, two, or three points are scored for increasing abnormality of each of the five parameters shown in Table 5.9. Thus, in

Table 5.9. Grading of severity of liver disease [4].

Clinical and biochemical measurements	Points scored for increasing abnormality		
	1	2	3
Encephalopathy (grade) (see Table 5.6)	None	1 and 2	3, 4 or 5
Ascites	Absent	Slight	Moderate
Bilirubin μmol/100 ml	up to 25	25–40	> 40
Albumin g/litre	35	28–35	< 28
Prothrombin time (seconds prolonged)	1–4	4–6	> 6

Patient scores 1, 2, or 3 for each of five factors. Patients scoring 5 or 6 are regarded as good risks; patients scoring 7, 8 or 9 are regarded as moderate risks; those scoring 10 or more are poor risks.

patients with good hepatic function the total score is five points whereas patients with poor hepatic reserve have scores of up to fifteen points. Those patients whose score totals five or six are considered to be good operative risks, seven, eight or nine moderate risks, and patients with ten to fifteen poor operative risks. Allowance should be made in the grading for patients with primary biliary cirrhosis in whom the level of bilirubin is usually out of proportion to other evidence of hepatic failure. Only patients classified as good or moderate risks should be subjected to anaesthesia and surgery except in a dire emergency.

Premedication

In the acutely ill patient premedication is omitted. In the well-compensated patient the normal premedicant drugs are well tolerated. It should be remembered that there has to be significant liver damage before metabolism of drugs is materially affected. The major problem in administering sedative and analgesic drugs to patients with liver disease is the effect of these drugs on the central nervous system, and this is not necessarily related to the liver's lack of ability to metabolize them. It is useful to administer an analgesic drug as part of the premedication to assess the patient's response as this may give useful information as to the dosage of drugs required for postoperative pain relief and sedation. It has been the authors' experience that pethidine and promethazine are useful in this respect and are not normally accompanied by excessive prolongation of action or untoward affects. Diazepam is useful for endoscopic investigations, bearing in mind that it is a highly protein-bound drug and in patients with grossly raised globulin levels the drug may have a prolonged effect.

Anaesthesia

All general, regional and spinal anaesthetic techniques will lower splanchnic blood flow. Under normal circumstances this does not seem harmful, but in patients with chronic liver disease further liver damage may ensue. The basic principle therefore of any an aesthetic technique used in patients with chronic liver disease should be to ensure that splanchnic blood flow is interfered with as little as possible. To this end, careful attention should be paid to oxygenation, avoidance of hypotension and the maintenance of arterial P_{CO_2} within the normal range. Avoidance of drugs which are primarily metabolized by the liver and adjustment of the dosage in accordance with the 'fitness' of the patient are sensible precautions. Drugs which are highly protein-bound should also be treated with caution since many patients will have raised globulin levels. Increased dosage of such drugs will be required, for example d-tubocurarine or pancuronium, and there may then be difficulties in reversing the effects of such drugs. Halothane is not contraindicated in patients with chronic liver disease but the dose should be kept to a minimum so as to avoid undue hypotension resulting in reduction of splanchnic blood flow. Volatile agents which directly affect the splanchnic circulation such as cyclopropane, diethylether and methoxyflurane are best avoided.

A satisfactory sequence, which may be recommended for major surgery [6] is the induction of anaesthesia with a short-acting barbiturate or Althesin (note that increased doses may be required because of protein binding), maintenance of anaesthesia with oxygen, nitrous oxide, intermittent positive pressure ventilation to maintain normocapnia, muscle relaxation by means of pancuronium bromide and increments of analgesic agents such as pethidine or its synthetic derivatives.

Postoperative management

Patients who have undergone extensive abdominal or intrathoracic surgery may require postoperative intermittent positive pressure ventilation until the effects of anaesthesia and surgery have worn off. Such periods of artificial ventilation should be kept to a minimum to avoid introducing unnecessary infection and where possible patients should be allowed to breathe spontaneously. Analgesic drugs should be administered with caution and the patient should have been observed as to the effect of the premedication. Depression of liver function is common after surgery and anaesthesia and relates to the extent of the surgery. Obviously in patients with pre-existing liver disease this depression may produce changes in liver function tests. A reduction in protein synthesis, increased jaundice and raised transaminases may be seen. These changes should normally revert to the preoperative state within five to ten days.

MANAGEMENT OF LIVER PROBLEMS
REQUIRING ANAESTHESIA AND SURGERY

DIAGNOSIS OF JAUNDICE

Mechanical obstruction of the biliary tree by, for example, stones, stenosis or neoplasm, is often amenable to surgical treatment. It is very important to establish the site of block of the biliary tree and an intravenous cholangiogram may not be effective in the presence of severe jaundice. Therefore percutaneous cholangiography may be necessary. For this procedure a needle is passed blindly through the abdominal wall into the liver until bile is aspirated and then the contrast medium is injected and a radiograph taken. This procedure is usually carried out with the patient conscious, but sedated, commonly, with diazepam. Percutaneous cholangiography is not without risk. Haemorrhage, biliary peritonitis and septicaemia may occur. This latter arises since, in the presence of longstanding biliary obstruction, the bile is usually infected; in addition, endotoxin may be released into the circulation during the percutaneous puncture. It is therefore advisable that the procedure should not be embarked on until, firstly, an adequate intravenous infusion is established and, secondly, provisions made for the patient to come straight to the operating theatre for a laparotomy immediately following the percutaneous cholangiogram. The site of a biliary obstruction may also be assessed by ultrasound and by gastroscopy. In the latter instance the gastroscope is passed into the duodenum and radiopaque contrast medium may be injected directly into the biliary tree through the ampulla of Vater and in addition, some obstructive lesions may be dealt with directly. A further manoeuvre that may be helpful in patients with biliary obstructive lesions that require surgery is preliminary drainage of the distended gallbladder by a percutaneously inserted catheter. This will lower bilirubin concentration and lessen the risk of postoperative renal failure.

Apart from a general assessment of the patient's condition prior to surgery the anaesthetist should obtain some additional information before anaesthetizing the jaundiced patient. If the prothrombin time is abnormal the response to vitamin K should be noted and if necessary additional vitamin K given preoperatively. All jaundiced patients should have their urine output monitored during surgery by means of an indwelling urinary catheter. If bilirubin concentration is above 200 μmol/litre (11.5 mg per 100 ml) urine output should be maintained pre-, per- and postoperatively by infusion of either 5 or 10 per cent mannitol. Urine output should be at least 50 ml per hour. In patients undergoing major surgery, central venous pressure (CVP) should be monitored both for fluid replacement and in order to prevent overload with mannitol. Frusemide is not as suitable as mannitol since with the former it is difficult to maintain a steady diuresis. Maintenance of a diuresis in the jaundiced patient will avoid postoperative renal failure due to concentration of bilirubin, and possibly endotoxin, in the tubules of the kidneys as a result of the fall in renal blood flow associated with anaesthesia. The use of mannitol as described above will prevent postoperative renal damage in the severely jaundiced patient undergoing anaesthesia and surgery.

TREATMENT OF BLEEDING

Haemorrhage, usually from the upper gastrointestinal tract is a frequent complication of severe liver disease. In acute liver failure and after liver transplantation, bleeding may result from haemorrhagic diathesis due to a combination of defects, There may be failure to synthesize factors such as prothrombin complex (factors II, VII, IX and X), and increased consumption of factors such as fibrinogen and platelets either in the spleen or areas of necrosis and intravascular coagulation. Increased gastric acidity may also be a factor.

In chronic liver disease the usual source of gastrointestinal bleeding is from oesophageal varices, although a bleeding peptic ulcer, gastric erosion or even a ruptured oesophagus must always be considered especially in the alcoholic patient with cirrhosis.

The most useful investigation in the diagnosis of upper gastrointestinal bleeding is fibreoptic endoscopy. In the severely ill patient this may be performed without any sedation or anaesthesia. Under more reasonable circumstances, diazepam is useful or occasionally a general anaesthetic may be indicated. Care should be taken to avoid inhalation of blood or vomit during the procedure. Emergency barium studies are not helpful, but if the bleeding can be controlled then a barium study should be performed later when the patient has recovered sufficiently to attend the radiology department.

The general principles of management are directed towards resuscitation, control of haemorrhage, preventing hepatic encephalopathy and finally assessing the degree of portal hypertension with a view to elective surgery. In chronic liver disease, of course, it is portal hypertension which is responsible for the haemorrhage arising in the upper gastrointestinal tract.

Blood loss should be replaced with fresh blood, where possible, and clotting factors by fresh-frozen plasma. Assessment of the adequacy of resuscitation should be by measurement of the patient's pulse, blood pressure and CVP. Prothrombin time and platelets are the most useful measurements to determine whether the patient's own liver is coping with the extra load on his clotting factors. A nasogastric tube should be passed and drained by gravity in order to make some assessment of blood loss. A careful fluid intake and output chart should be kept. Neomycin 1 g 6-hourly and magnesium sulphate 30 ml 25 per cent 8-hourly should be administered via the nasogastric tube in an attempt to sterilize and empty the bowel. The colon should be emptied by enemas using 10 per cent dextrose. Dietary protein should be withheld and all analgesic and sedative drugs avoided. If it is clear that there is no risk of the patient lapsing into hepatic coma then small doses of diazepam may be permitted. However, if there is any doubt concerning the patient's conscious level, sedative drugs should be avoided and where necessary the patient restrained by physical means. Intramuscular vitamin K should be administered for at least 3 days. Blood should be warmed prior to transfusion and remembering the liver's difficulty in dealing with citrate, calcium gluconate should be administered (1 g approximately for each litre of blood given). Antacids and histamine (H$_2$) receptor antagonists may be given to reduce gastric acidity.

Intravenous vasopressin

Intravenous vasopressin controls bleeding from oesophageal varices in about 50 per cent of patients, due to its action of reducing portal venous pressure. This, however, also reduces hepatic blood flow and may impair hepatic function to the extent that encephalopathy may be precipitated. Despite this, vasopressin is simple to use and often effective and is generally regarded as the initial agent of choice. Vasopressin (Pitressin) 20 units diluted with 200 ml of 5 per cent dextrose and infused over 20 min. Portal pressure falls within 3 min of the injection, it is maximal 10–15 min after injection and the action is maintained for about 1 hr. Where necessary the infusion may be repeated, approximately every 2 hr, but its efficiency diminishes with time. Vasopressin produces abdominal colic, evacuation of the bowel and facial pallor as side-effects. If these are not observed the batch of vasopressin should be considered inactive and replaced.

Selective infusion of vasopressin into the superior mesenteric artery has been used, as this technique spares the blood flow through the hepatic artery and may avoid further damage to liver function and also the distressing side-effects of the drug. However, the success rate is not as high as with intravenous infusion and intra-arterial infusion should probably only be considered when intravenous infusion has failed to control haemorrhage, or in patients with ischaemic heart disease in whom intravenous vasopressin is contraindicated.

Balloon Tamponard (Sengstaken–Blakemore Tube)

The Sengstaken–Blakemore tube is passed by mouth down the oesophagus and into the stomach. The tube has attached to it two balloons, a gastric and an oesophageal. The gastric balloon is inflated initially with 80–100 ml of air and the tube pulled up to the cardia. The oesophageal balloon is then inflated to a pressure of 40 mmHg and if possible a radiograph is taken to verify the position of the tube. The addition of a fourth lumen with an oesophageal opening for suction (Boyce modification) reduces the risk of pulmonary aspiration of saliva. The principle of the tube is that the oesophageal balloon compresses the varices and traction on the tube pulls the cardia of the stomach up towards the mouth thereby further reducing blood flow in the oesophagus. The tube itself is hollow to allow gastric aspiration. A new tube should be selected for each patient and tested for leaks prior to insertion. If all goes well the oesophageal balloon is deflated after 24 hr, and if the gastric aspirate remains clear the gastric balloon may also be deflated but the tube should be left *in situ* for a further 24 hr as re-bleeding can usually be controlled during this time by reflating the balloons. Balloon tamponard successfully controls haemorrhage in over 90 per cent of patients with upper gastrointestinal bleeding associated with liver disease.

There are, however, some serious hazards associated with balloon tamponard. These include pulmonary aspiration, particularly during insertion of the tube, and mucosal ulceration from balloon pressure.

Injection of varices

In patients where balloon tamponard and vasopressin have failed to control haemorrhage, direct injection of bleeding oesophageal varices may be effective. The technique consists of oesophagoscoping the patient with either a rigid or fibreoptic oesophagoscope, visualizing the varices and with a long needle injecting directly into the varix 2–3 ml of sclerosant fluid. Usually this procedure has to be carried out under general anaesthesia.

It should be remembered that patients requiring injection of oesophageal varices may have a risk score over 9 [4] and therefore be bad risks. Further haemorrhage from the varices is an obvious hazard. It is therefore essential that an adequate infusion line is established, and adequate supplies of fresh blood are available before injection is contemplated. Anaesthesia for such patients should be with the minimum of drugs which require the liver for their metabolism or excretion. A suitable technique has been suggested [7] and consists of induction with either thiopentone or Althesin, suxamethonium for intubation and increments if necessary to maintain paralysis, and intermittent positive pressure ventilation with oxygen and nitrous oxide. If a prolonged procedure is anticipated then pancuronium may be used. Although cholinesterase levels may be reduced in patients with acute or chronic liver disease, the action of suxamethonium does not appear to be unduly prolonged in such patients. Suxamethonium is, of course, essential in order to be certain that intubation is rapid and inhalation of blood or vomit avoided. After injection is completed, if there is any further bleeding, a fresh Sengstaken–Blakemore tube should be inserted before the endotracheal tube has been removed. Otherwise patients should be allowed to recover consciousness, and turned on their side before being extubated.

Devascularization procedures

These include oesophageal transection, gastric transection, oesophagogastrectomy, gastric devascularization and splenectomy. Of these, only transthoracic oesophageal transection is commonly employed. This is a major procedure on a patient who may well be in the bad risk category (score 10–15, Table 5.9). Anaesthetic considerations are similar to those already outlined. A double lumen endotracheal tube is not necessary and should be avoided lest bronchial bleeding be incurred. A nasogastric tube should not be passed prior to opening the chest and exposing the oesophagus, but should then be passed and checked by the surgeon for its final position before being secured by the anaesthetist at the nose end. Postoperatively it may be necessary to draw the attention of the nursing staff to the chest drain which may appear unusual for patients undergoing 'liver surgery'.

Portasystemic shunts

The object of the portasystemic shunt is to reduce portal hypertension and therefore the risk of bleeding from the upper gastrointestinal tract. The most commonly performed shunt is an end-to-side portacaval shunt but this of course removes some 70 per cent of the liver's blood supply. Alternatively, a lienorenal shunt, or a mesenteric caval jump graft (using a Dacron tube) may be performed. The latter shunts have the theoretical advantage that they do not divert such a large amount of blood away from the liver as does the portacaval shunt and this may reduce the incidence of chronic encephalopathy.

Haemorrhage from the upper gastrointestinal tract associated with liver disease is often a dramatic event. It is only to be expected therefore that many procedures have been tried and claims made for their success. However, the natural history of the underlying liver disease is extremely relevant in terms of the actual outcome following an episode of bleeding. Although surgical procedures involving direct attack on varices or the shunting away of blood would appear useful it has yet to be shown that such procedures prolong the patient's life.

LIVER TUMOURS

Primary or secondary tumours of the liver may be amenable to surgical removal, for example by partial hepatectomy. The major anaesthetic and surgical problem associated with such operations is haemorrhage. In addition there may be interference with the venous return from the inferior vena cava during certain parts of the surgical procedure. Adequate intravenous infusion lines, adequate blood available and careful monitoring of blood loss are clear requisites. All blood administered should be warmed and the CVP and blood pressure carefully monitored. Tumours which are not amenable to surgical resection may be treated by hepatic artery ligation and/or infusion of cytotoxic agents. An infusion of glucose and insulin should be given prior to ligation of the hepatic artery in order to minimize any subsequent liver damage. Postoperatively severe deterioration in liver function may occur particularly when cytotoxic agents are infused.

TRANSPLANTATION

Liver transplantation is a rare procedure, with only some hundreds of transplants having been performed worldwide and about 150 in the United Kingdom. The indications for transplantation are primary hepatoma or other hepatic tumour without extrahepatic spread, end-stage cirrhosis and biliary atresia. Evidence of viral infection is usually considered a contraindication. However, the recent availability of highly specific immunoglobulin has enabled at least one transplant to be carried out in a patient who was HBsAg positive. The virus itself, of course, resides in the liver and therefore total hepatectomy is curative. Circulating antigen may be 'neutralized' by infusing highly specific immunoglobulin during the anhepatic period.

Anaesthesia for liver transplantation has been well reviewed in the literature [1, 2] and the reader is referred to the specialized papers for detailed anaesthetic management. The problems to be contended with include severe haemorrhage, hypotension, obstruction of the inferior vena cava, hypothermia and severe acid–base and electrolyte changes.

ACUTE HEPATIC FAILURE

Fulminant hepatic failure may be defined as coma developing within eight weeks of the onset of symptoms in patients where liver function prior to their illness was presumed to be normal. Viral hepatitis is the commonest cause of fulminant hepatic failure. Many drugs can cause liver damage and rarely acute liver failure is seen following general anaesthesia and surgery. More rarely, known hepatotoxins, such as the death cap fungus, are ingested accidentally. The phrase 'acute liver failure' is often used to cover both fulminant hepatic failure and severe encephalopathy secondary to chronic liver disease. Fulminant hepatic failure is fortunately a rare event, nevertheless world wide mortality remains about 80 per cent for a condition which often affects the young and previously healthy individual, with some 300 deaths per year in the United Kingdom. Treatment of such patients, therefore, is a serious challenge and should best be carried out in an intensive care area equipped to deal with such patients. The clinical manifestations of liver failure are multiple and as well as those directly related to hepatic damage, include neurological, acid–base, cardiac, renal, metabolic and haematological disturbances. Foetor hepaticus may be present and the liver is often small to percussion. Clinical jaundice develops over a few days and in most acute cases is preceded by signs of encephalopathy.

Neurological disturbance

Deterioration in conscious level is progressive through euphoria, mild confusion, and drowsiness to coma. Decerebrate rigidity and convulsions are common. The cause of hepatic encephalopathy is probably multifactorial. Coma factors such as ammonia, mercaptans, free fatty acids and biogenic amines have all been implicated, but as yet no clear picture has emerged as to which if any of these compounds is responsible. Secondary factors of particular importance because they may be preventable by correct management, include hypoxia, hypoglycaemia, hypovolaemia and hypotension. The administration of sedatives for control of restlessness during the early stages of encephalopathy may be responsible for deterioration in conscious level. If liver function does return to normal and irreversible brain damage, due, for example, to hypoxia, has not occurred during the comatose period, the brain can also recover completely.

Cerebral oedema is a major problem. Papilloedema is seldom present and brady-cardia and pyrexia are rarely seen, even though gross tentorial herniation may be found at post mortem. Sudden apnoea, cardiac arrest and hypothermia commonly occur and may be central in orgin.

Acid-base disturbance

Hyperventilation is a constant feature during the early stages of coma. It is probable that ammonia toxicity is responsible for the respiratory stimulation. Alkalosis (both respiratory and metabolic) is common. Hypokalaemia, failure to alkalinize urine and continuous gastric aspiration are contributory factors.

Respiratory alkalosis is associated with impaired oxygen dissociation, reduced cerebral and peripheral perfusion and reduced cerebral oxygen consumption. In addition, respiratory alkalosis may result in neurological and EEG changes which are similar in some respects to those of experimental ammonia toxicity and may be potentiated by co-existent metabolic alkalosis. Correction of respiratory alkalosis by either inhalation of carbon dioxide or by infusing the carbonic anhydrase inhibitor acetazolamide produces further clinical and biochemical deterioration, whereas intra-venous administration of sodium bicarbonate produces improvement, correlating well with increased cerebral blood flow and oxygen consumption. However, this improve-ment is only temporary and is limited by the adverse effect of a large sodium load.

Hypoxia is a frequent finding and may be due to pulmonary infection or oedema, or elevation of the diaphragm by ascites or peritoneal dialysis. It is likely that pul-monary capillary permeability is abnormal in acute liver failure and results in inter-stitial and alveolar oedema.

Cardiac disturbance

Cardiac output is high and reflects low peripheral resistance and increased arterio-venous shunting. Cardiac irregularities are common, probably reflecting change in oxygenation, arterial $P\text{CO}_2$, plasma potassium or intracranial pressure. Hypotension, often associated with haemorrhage, is also frequently seen.

Renal disturbance

Renal impairment often progressing to renal failure is common in Grade 3 and 4 coma.

This impairment may be classified into one of three groups: pre-renal uraemia due to dehydration or absorption of nitrogenous compounds from the gut after gastro-intestinal haemorrhage; functional renal failure as a result of diversion of blood flow from the kidney; or be precipitated by an episode of hypotension. Renal failure is a poor prognostic sign.

Metabolic disturbance

Of particular importance is hypoglycaemia which can develop rapidly and may lead to irreversible brain damage unless treated by parenteral glucose administration. Great care must be taken not to overlook hypoglycaemia as the cause of a deteriorating level of consciousness. Oral feeding is not usually possible because of coma or gastro-intestinal bleeding, and the provision of adequate calories may be difficult. Amino acid solutions are contraindicated, fat emulsions and alcohols may further damage the liver, and the metabolic pathway for fructose may be so deranged that acute lactic acidosis occurs. In addition, solutions containing sodium should be avoided because of the inability of these patients to excrete sodium. In practice, therefore, only glucose infusions are used. Solutions stronger than 10 per cent induce an unexceptable osmotic diuresis, and even when combined with insulin may also produce lactic acidosis.

Haematological disturbance

As liver function deteriorates, synthesis of clotting factors declines and disorders of coagulation are invariable. This is manifest as a prolongation of prothrombin time, depression of circulating levels of fibrinogen and factors II, VII, IX and X. In addition thrombocytopenia occurs.

The usual sites of bleeding are the nasopharynx, oesophagus, stomach, gastro-intestinal tract, retroperitoneal space and the bronchial tree. Administration of antacids or histamine (H_2) antagonists may be helpful in reducing haemorrhage from the gastrointestinal tract.

Management

Patients with acute liver failure obviously require general supportive measures aimed at the management of the severely ill and unconscious patient. Regrettably there is no specific treatment and all measures are aimed at keeping patients alive in order to gain time for natural regeneration of the liver to occur.

A major problem is protection of the patient's airway from the risk of aspiration of blood or stomach contents. As the level of consciousness may fluctuate from moment to moment it is very tempting to administer sedative drugs; this should be avoided at all costs. Preferably, patients should be intubated, if necessary using suxamethonium as a short-acting muscle relaxant, in order to protect the airway. The position of the endotracheal tube should be checked by a chest radiograph after insertion. Where possible the patients should be allowed to ventilate spontaneously with, if necessary, added oxygen. The indications for instituting IPPV are apnoea and persistent hypo-ventilation with hypoxia. Avoidance of hypoxia during grand mal fits is a third indication. Pancuronium is the neuromuscular blocking drug of choice for patients requiring prolonged IPPV.

Renal failure should preferably be treated by peritoneal dialysis because of the risks of hypotension during haemodialysis. The value of attempts to replace deficient clotting factors by the administration of fresh blood, platelet concentrates, or fresh-frozen plasma is by no means proven.

Cerebral oedema is the single most common cause of death and as yet there is no effective means of treatment or prevention. Haemorrhage, infection, respiratory and cardiovascular complications are also important.

As already discussed under *Encephalopathy*, specific artificial liver support systems are under intensive investigation. At present, however, none has proved entirely satisfactory.

POSTOPERATIVE LIVER DYSFUNCTION

It is probable that all forms of anaesthesia and surgery are followed by detrimental changes in liver function. In the vast majority of cases, these changes are minimal and give rise to no concern. Furthermore, these changes in liver function can be related to the severity of surgery, minor surface surgery being followed by minimal upsets whereas major procedures, for example, vascular or cardiovascular surgery, are commonly followed by a rise in bilirubin and elevation of transaminases. Patients with pre-existing liver damage may undergo further deterioration postoperatively. There-fore the majority of cases of 'postoperative jaundice' are readily explicable and usually reversible. However, on rare occasions an apparently uncomplicated surgical pro-cedure with no obvious anaesthetic mishaps is followed by jaundice and then a rapid deterioration in liver function and death. This is obviously a matter for concern. Such cases have been reported over the years following all forms of general anaesthesia, spinal and epidural anaesthesia and in association with all forms of surgery. However, in the past twenty years attention has focused primarily on halothane. This is hardly surprising since this agent is one of the most commonly used anaesthetics.

Retrospective, prospective and extensive patient investigations have been carried out in an attempt to establish whether 'halothane hepatitis' is a true entity. The consensus of opinion seems to be that on rare occasions uneventful surgery under halothane anaesthesia may be followed by liver damage. This is not to say that the problem is exclusive to halothane and, indeed, well-reported cases under similar circumstances have occurred with most of the other anaesthetic agents in common use today. A major feature of most studies has been the relationship of liver damage to repeated exposure of halothane. The majority of cases have occurred following exposures at short intervals of time. However, no study has been able to establish the incidence of halothane hepatitis or indeed to compare its frequency with hepatitis following nonhalothane anaesthesia. Hepatitis in this context is usually taken to mean jaundice with changes in transaminases. Jaundice alone following anaesthesia is common and is usually due to obvious causes.

The relationship of liver damage to repeated exposure to halothane has led to the suggestion that this may be a hypersensitivity phenomenon. Indeed eosinophilia has been commonly reported although other stigmata of hypersensitivity have been absent. Numerous workers have carried out immunological testing both on patients believed to have halothane hepatitis, and anaesthetists who believe themselves to be sensitive to the drug. Halothane and complexes of halothane metabolites with large molecules have been used as test antigens. So far all tests have been negative. The fact, however, that these immunological tests are negative does not necessarily rule out a hyper-

7

sensitivity response. It may merely mean that the correct test has not yet been used or that the antigens are incorrect.

Halothane in common with many other volatile anaesthetics undergoes metabolism in the body. Some 10–20 per cent of the inhaled dose is metabolized by the liver to nonvolatile metabolites. Oxidation is the major metabolic pathway but reductive metabolism also occurs. Such metabolism may be enhanced in experimental animals by the use of enzyme induction and hypoxia. In some animal species this leads to hepatic damage. It is however not clear whether these animal models are indicative of what may happen in man when liver damage follows halothane anaesthesia. An alternative mechanism for liver damage may be that one of the metabolites of halothane binds with a protein or other large molecule in the body and acts as a hapten in an immunological reaction. Such a mechanism has also not been demonstrated in man, although there is some evidence to support the concept from experimental animals.

Direct hepatoxicity by halothane is most unlikely. Cases of halothane hepatitis are not commonly associated with prolonged exposure to the agent, nor has any liver toxicity been demonstrated in experimental animals, which one would expect if halothane were a classical hepatotoxin.

The real halothane dilemma therefore is that one of the most useful, most commonly used volatile anaesthetics may on rare occasions, if given repeatedly at short intervals, cause liver damage. For the individual patient this may turn out to be a tragedy. A sense of perspective, however, must be maintained in that alternative anaesthetics may carry a greater risk overall, and may also cause liver damage. Factual data in support of the previous statement is not available. Therefore, anaesthetists have found themselves in difficulties when considering administering halothane repeatedly. What should be done?

Firstly any patient who develops unexplained hepatitis following halothane (that is jaundice and change in transaminases or other liver function tests) and who requires a further anaesthetic should not receive further halothane if suitable alternative agents are available. Such cases are rare. Much more common is the situation where the patient has received halothane on one occasion, uneventfully, and then requires a second anaesthetic shortly afterwards. Should halothane be used again? In this situation the only advice that can be given is that the anaesthetist should be familiar with the patient, his medical history and the surgical procedure planned and should then decide according to the circumstances which anaesthetic agent to employ. The most likely outcome, of course, is that nothing will happen whatever agent is used. Even in patients who have had unexplained hepatitis following halothane and then been exposed subsequently, sometimes hepatitis has recurred and sometimes not. Even when a nonhalothane technique has been used hepatitis has occurred on occasion and at other times has not. It is therefore impossible to predict what the outcome will be when repeated anaesthetics are given close together. A little clearer advice can be given where anaesthesia is required for a patient who has active unexplained hepatitis. If possible anaesthesia and surgery should be delayed until there is evidence that the hepatitis is resolving. If the surgical procedure is such that delay cannot be countenanced then the anaesthetist should appreciate the risk of anaesthetizing such patients in that further deterioration in liver function is probably inevitable. The minimum of drugs should be used and any agents which may adversely affect liver blood flow should be avoided. The technique recommended by the authors would be, induction of anaesthesia by thiopentone, suxamethonium or pancuronium as the muscle relaxants for short or long procedures respectively and ventilation of the patient with oxygen and nitrous oxide with IPPV if necessary. For analgesia, increments of pethidine or one of its synthetic derivatives may be given and no other drugs should be used. Particular attention should be paid to maintaining the arterial Pco_2 within the normal range. These same strictures apply to anaesthetizing patients who are known to be in the early stages of viral hepatitis. Patients with viral hepatitis who are subjected to any stress such as anaesthesia and surgery are known to suffer more damage to their liver than those patients who rest quietly.

Because most cases of postoperative jaundice have a clear explanation it is essential that all cases should be carefully investigated. It is still very common for the non-anaesthetist to see a patient with postoperative jaundice, enquire whether halothane was used as the anaesthetic and automatically write in the patient's notes—halothane hepatitis. Anaesthetists will be all too familiar with this state of affairs. It is clearly most important that patients are not labelled as 'sensitive' to any drug unless it is actually the case. Halothane is still one of the most useful volatile anaesthetic agents and to prevent its use by default is not in the patient's best interest. Equally, it is relevant that the anaesthetist should keep proper anaesthetic records so that it is possible to establish subsequently the drugs used, and also that patients should be seen pre-operatively to establish whether there is any history of liver dysfunction following anaesthesia as this may reduce the risk of inadvertently causing further damage.

DRUGS IN PATIENTS WITH LIVER DISEASE

One of the principle functions of the liver is to detoxify drugs by converting lipid soluble compounds to more water soluble ones which can then be excreted in the urine or bile. This metabolism is carried out by the microsomal enzymes within the endoplasmic reticulum of the hepatocyte. Most drugs undergo an initial step, such as oxidation or reduction and are then conjugated with glucuronic or sulphuric acid. The microsomal enzyme system employs molecular oxygen and cytochromes and the whole system is often referred to as the mixed function oxidase enzyme system.

In chronic liver disease the number of liver cells is reduced and therefore the amount of drug presented to each individual cell for metabolism is increased. This overload actually increases the number of enzymes within the cell and this is called substrate enzyme induction. Therefore it is only when there is very severe hepatic damage that there is an overall alteration in drug metabolism. There is no evidence that patients with liver disease are likely to develop side effects from potentially hepatotoxic drugs if the mechanism of toxicity is hypersensitivity. However, if the toxicity is dose-related this principle does not hold true, for example cirrhotic patients are more likely to sustain liver damage from a drug such as pyrazinamide.

Centrally acting analgesic and sedative drugs may have prolonged actions in patients with liver disease. This is not necessarily a reflection of any altered metabolism by the liver but reflects the fact that brain metabolism is abnormal in such patients. This is of course particularly true in patients with acute liver failure and here all analgesic and sedative drugs should be avoided.

The following additional factors which should be borne in mind.

1 Coagulation factors are synthesized within the liver and therefore liver disease increases the risk in using anti-coagulant drugs.

2 Fluid and sodium retention are common features of liver disease and therefore drugs which contain sodium or have a sodium retaining effect should if possible be

Table 5.10. Drug problems in liver disease.

Drug	Category of use	Problem
Antacids	Anti-peptic ulcer	Contain sodium. Enhances fluid retention
Carbenoxolone		Enhances sodium retention
Phenothiazines	Anti-emetic	Excess sedative effect
Antihistamines		
Opium derivatives	Anti-diarrhoeals	May precipitate coma
Lomotil		
Senna *etc*	Laxatives	Causes potassium loss
Liquid paraffin		May cause malabsorption of fats
Oxyphenisatin		Causes chronic active hepatitis
Digoxin	Cardiac glycoside	75 per cent excreted by liver Accumulates and increases toxicity
Thiazides	Diuretic	May provoke encephalopathy via potassium loss
Frusemide		
Lignocaine	Anti-arrhythmic	Breakdown delayed in liver disease. Duration of action prolonged
Methyldopa	Hypotensive	Can cause chronic active hepatitis
Hydrallazine		95 per cent metabolized by liver Duration of action may be prolonged
Aspirin	Analgesics	Causes gastric irritation
Phenylbutazone		Causes fluid retention and gastric irritation
Indomethicin		Causes gastric irritation
Colchicine		Causes gastric irritation
Morphine	Narcotic analgesics	All provoke encephalopathy
Pethidine (any derivative)		
Pentazocine		
Amitriptyline	Tricyclic	May cause drowsiness and cholestatic jaundice
Nortriptyline	Anti-depressants	
Imipramine		
Ipromiazid	Monoamine oxidase inhibitor	Cause liver cell damage
Phenytoin	Anticonvulsant	May accumulate in liver disease
Benzodiazepines	Tranquillizers	Prolonged action, may provoke encephalopathy
Tolbutamide	Hypoglycaemic	May accumulate since it is mainly metabolized by the liver
Chlorpropamide		May cause cholestasis
Tetracyclines	Antibiotics	Cause liver damage and gastric irritation
Erythromycin		Estolate salt may cause cholestasis May accumulate with toxicity
Chloramphenicol		Toxicity increased
Nitrofurantoin		Causes liver damage
Rifampicin	Antituberculous therapy	Causes liver damage
Isoniazid		Causes liver damage
Pyrazinamide		Causes liver damage
Suxamethonium	Muscle relaxant	Low cholinesterase theoretically prolongs action
d-Tubocurarine	Muscle relaxants	Increased dosage, protein binding, sequestration in liver and spleen, increased volume of distribution
Pancuronium		

avoided, for example, carbenoxolone and phenylbutazone. During surgery intravenous fluids containing sodium should be avoided and 5 per cent dextrose should be the routine infusion fluid.

3 Protein abnormalities (low serum albumin and high globulin) may result in abnormal binding of drugs and may be responsible, for example, for the increased evidence of steroid side-effects in patients with liver disease. Nondepolarizing relaxants are protein bound and it has been suggested that the increased amount of these drugs required reflects this binding. However it is more likely that such drugs are sequestered in the liver and spleen rather than that the protein binding is a major factor.

4 Where there is biliary obstruction, drugs which are usually excreted in the bile may either accumulate or cause toxicity. In addition, drugs which normally act on the biliary tree will fail to reach their site of action.

In summary, in the patient with liver disease, drugs which are known to be hepatotoxic should obviously be avoided. Drugs which rarely cause hypersensitivity type of damage are acceptable if required. Where possible, drugs which are normally excreted unchanged via the urine should be preferred. Drugs which have an effect on the central nervous system or blood coagulation should be treated with caution and if necessary one should start with low doses and observe the patient for ill effects. Table 5.10 shows some commonly used drugs which illustrate these points.

REFERENCES

1 ALDRETE JA, LE VINE DS, GINGRICH TF. Experience in anesthesia for liver transplantation. *Anesth Analg* 1969; **48**: 802–15.
2 FARMAN JV, LINES JG, WILLIAMS RS, *et al.* Liver transplantation in man. Anaesthetic and biochemical management. *Anaesthesia* 1974; **29**: 17–32.
3 KENNEDY J, PARBHOO SP, MACGILLIVRAY B, SHERLOCK S. Effect of extracorporeal liver perfusion on the electroencephalogram of patients in coma due to acute liver failure. *QJ Med* 1973; **42**: 549–61.
4 PUGH RNH, MURRAY-LYON IM, DAWSON JL, PIETRONI MC, WILLIAMS R. Trans-section of the oesophagus for bleeding oesophageal varices. *Br J Surg* 1973; **60**: 646–9.
5 TREY C, BURNS DG, SAUNDERS SJ. Treatment of hepatic coma by exchange blood transfusion. *N Engl J Med* 1966; **274**: 473–81.
6 WARD ME, ADU-GYAMFI Y, STRUNIN L. Althesin and pancuronium in chronic liver disease. *Br J Anaesth* 1975; **47**: 1199–204.
7 WARD ME, DAVIES TDW, STRUNIN L. Anaesthesia for injection of bleeding oesophageal varices. *Ann R Coll Surg Engl* 1976; **58**: 315–17.
8 ZUCKERMAN AJ. Specific serological diagnosis of viral hepatitis. *Br Med J* 1979; **2**: 84–6.

RECOMMENDED GENERAL READING

BROWN BR. *Contemporary anesthesia practise 4. Anesthesia and the patient with liver disease.* Philadelphia: FA Davis, 1981.
SHERLOCK S. Diseases of the liver and biliary system. 5th ed. Oxford: Blackwell Scientific Publications, 1976.
STRUNIN L. *The liver and anaesthesia.* Volume 3 *Major problems in anaesthesia.* Philadelphia: WB Saunders, 1977.

Chapter 6
Medical Diseases in Pregnancy

J. SELWYN CRAWFORD

There are few medical ills which preclude the possibility of pregnancy and a woman is as likely to develop an incidental illness during pregnancy as any nonpregnant woman of childbearing age. This chapter is restricted to the most commonly occurring medical complications, and to those which, although less common, offer a particular challenge to the anaesthetist. Those complications peculiar to pregnancy which are the province more of intensive care, such as severe pre-eclampsia, eclampsia, amniotic fluid embolism, or acute defibrination syndrome related to abruptio, are better discussed in books of a specifically obstetric content.

There are several ways in which the discussion could be presented, but it has been considered most facile to refer to each of the body systems in turn, with, where appropriate, a preliminary brief review of the physiological changes in these systems which occur during pregnancy.

THE CIRCULATORY SYSTEM

Cardiac output

Cardiac output begins to increase during the first 6–8 weeks of pregnancy and the increase continues up to about mid-term. The generally accepted view is that thereafter either the high level is sustained until the end of pregnancy, or there is a slight fall during the final trimester. The results of recent work (Atkins *et al.*, unpublished) throws some doubt on these opinions, suggesting that cardiac output falls throughout the second-half of pregnancy, to reach or even to fall below the pre-pregnancy level by term, but these observations remain to be validated. The rise is a result of increases in both stroke volume and pulse rate, although the relative importance of each contributory factor has not been finally determined. The extent of the ultimate increase in cardiac output varies between patients, but is of the order of 30–50 per cent. During labour, cardiac output increases during a contraction by 15–20 per cent. reflecting the extrusion of blood from the myometrium. Furthermore, there is suggestive evidence that if the pain of labour is poorly relieved, a cumulative rise in cardiac output occurs, which is not seen when analgesia and apprehension are negated. Episodes of markedly reduced cardiac output occur during the second stage of labour, concurrently with the periods of bearing down. There is no published convincing evidence of a regular pattern of change in cardiac output during the immediate postpartum period, although the results of the unpublished investigation referred to suggest that output rises abruptly during the first three days and at a much more gradual rate during the subsequent several weeks or months. The initial increase, if it occurs, is doubtless due to severe reduction in myometrial vascular capacity.

One outstandingly important factor which can influence cardiac output subsequent to the 28th week of pregnancy, is that the uterus is large enough to compress a segment of the inferior vena cava when the patient lies supine. This can occur one or two weeks earlier in cases of multiple pregnancy or hydramnios. Somewhat later in pregnancy this interference with caval blood flow can also occur when the patient lies tilted slightly to the right, and occasionally when the left tilt position is adopted. The extent of caval compression is variable, but complete occlusion of the lumen of the vessel has been demonstrated in some gravida. As a result of caval compression, cardiac output is diminished: the magnitude of the latter effect depends upon the degree by which caval flow has been reduced and upon the effectiveness of the available collateral venous channels, but a reduction of cardiac output by 50 per cent is not uncommon.

Venous and arterial pressures

There is little significant change in central venous pressure associated with pregnancy, labour and delivery, other than variations induced by caval compression, uterine contraction and the Valsalva manoeuvre.

Systemic arterial blood pressure is not influenced systematically by the progress of normal pregnancy; during labour there is a tendency for the pressure to rise if the patient has received inadequate relief from pain and apprehension. Diastolic pressure tends to be slightly reduced during the midtrimester, so that pulse pressure is somewhat increased during this period. The reduction in cardiac output consequent upon caval compression does lead to a dramatic fall in blood pressure in a small proportion of cases: in the remainder, an increased intensity of vasomotor tone sustains the arterial pressure at roughly the normotensive level (although the pulse pressure is likely to be reduced), but this maternal homeostatic mechanism operates to the considerable disadvantage of the fetus.

Blood volume

An increase in whole blood volume starts during the early weeks of pregnancy and continues until 34–36 weeks, after which there is possibly a slight progressive reduction to term. The extent of the increase varies considerably, but there is consistently a greater rise in plasma volume than in red cell volume. The increase in plasma volume is of the order of 40 per cent, that of red cell volume being roughly 20 per cent; the increase in total blood volume is thus $1-1\frac{1}{2}$ litres. The volume of blood lost at vaginal delivery is dependent to a considerable extent upon whether or not an episiotomy has been performed, the method of delivery, and, possibly, whether or not an oxytoxic drug has been given during the delivery process. Blood loss in excess of 500 ml is considered to be excessive, and is designated as 'postpartum haemorrhage'. The volume of blood shed at Caesarean section is, except in cases of an anteriorly lying placenta, less well correlated with the procedure, and although the average loss is approximately one litre some patients might lose less than 300 ml, whilst others, for no obvious reason, lose 3 litres.

Blood components

The profile of levels of serum protein concentration during pregnancy is markedly different from that which is characteristic of the nonpregnant subject: the concentration of serum albumin falls within the first three months to approximately 27 g/l, and thereafter continues to decline at a much slower rate until the final weeks, when the level is of the order of 25 g/l, which is maintained until term. Total serum globulin concentration, on the other hand, rises progressively throughout pregnancy: the β fraction provides the greatest component of this increase, and the α fraction the smallest. It should be noted that although the level of concentration of serum albumin falls during the pregnancy, the mass of circulating albumin remains reasonably stable because of the increase in serum volume; on the other hand, the mass of globulin fractions is almost doubled during the course of pregnancy. The level of concentration of plasma fibrinogen is raised above normal throughout pregnancy, and concurrently there is an increase in the activity of the other factors which promote coagulation. On the other hand, fibrinolytic activity is considerably reduced during pregnancy. This situation of an increased tendency towards coagulation and a diminished facility to promote lysis is reversed within one hour of delivery, by which time the 'normal, non-pregnant' balance is regained.

CARDIAC DISEASE

It will be apparent from this cursory review that pregnancy can present a formidable challenge to the woman with heart disease. However, the therapeutic advances which have been made in cardiology and cardiac surgery during the past decade have reduced the challenge to manageable proportions.

Rheumatic heart disease

The patient with acquired rheumatic heart disease requires to be under closer antenatal supervision than does the uncomplicated patient, but is not to be treated as a delicate invalid. She should be advised to avoid undue exertion, to rest for a short time each day, to restrict her sodium intake lest excessive retention leads to embarrassment, and encouraged—with the provision of sedatives if necessary—to sleep well and long at night. Undoubtedly heart failure can occur in patients in this category and its occurrence is not limited to any specific period between conception and the puerperium. Therapy in such a case is not different from that which is applicable to the non-pregnant patient—up to and including surgical correction of a valve defect: interruption of the pregnancy would serve only to add to the complications and has no place in the treatment of acute heart failure. Indeed termination on medical (nonobstetric) grounds is indicated extremely rarely in patients with rheumatic heart disease.

It is commonly the practice for those patients with symptomatic cardiac disease to be admitted to hospital for the final four weeks of pregnancy. This, coincidentally, provides the opportunity of increased vigilance in the avoidance of thrombophlebitis. One in rather more than each hundred pregnant women develops the latter condition, although the incidence of deep vein thrombosis is of the order of 1 in 500. The occurrence of thrombosis, with its attendant threat of embolism, is obviously of greater moment in the patient with cardiac disease, and specific measures should be applied to guard against it. The regimen applied in cases of established deep vein thrombosis will be discussed later.

Rheumatic heart disease is not itself an indication for delivery by Caesarean section: indeed many authorities would classify it as a contraindication. Certainly, however, when such a patient goes into labour, intensive effort must be made to eliminate pain and exertion. There is little doubt that to this end regional block analgesia is the preferred treatment. The length of the first stage of labour tends to be reduced as a side effect of digitalis therapy, but it can still be long enough for cardiac embarrassment to become excessive in the patient who is unprotected from pain and exertion. Digitalis in clinical dosage has no deleterious effect upon the fetus. It is highly desirable that the patient be spared the effects of bearing down in the second stage, and that she be delivered with the aid of forceps at an obstetrically appropriate time. The inception of cardiac failure in the immediate puerperium is a well-recognized entity. Contributory factors include the autotransfusion of blood (approximately 400 ml) from the uterine vessels, the sudden relief of caval compression consequent upon ill-supervised delivery and the administration of ergometrine. The latter two influences can be avoided: correct positioning of the patient during labour and delivery can ensure that caval compression does not occur. The administration of ergometrine, which can cause a considerable rise in peripheral vascular resistance, can be omitted if necessary in favour of an infusion of oxytocin.

Postpartum deep vein thrombosis is an ever-present hazard, and is of even more ominous import in the case of a patient with cardiac disease. It is possible that this danger is reduced by the provision of an epidural block for labour and delivery, but in all cases of heart disease—and especially in those for whom delivery by Caesarean section is required—intensive physiotherapy should be initiated as soon as is practicable after delivery.

The number of patients with a prosthetic heart valve who present for obstetric care is increasing steadily. If the cardiac surgery had been successful these patients should present few problems in respect to their general care throughout pregnancy, which should be of the order as described in respect to patients with asymptomatic heart disease [1]. Similar remarks apply to the care of these patients during labour, but here there is a complicating feature. It is usual for patients with a valve prosthesis to be on anticoagulant prophylaxis. If this treatment is maintained it is most inadvisable to provide an epidural for labour and delivery. However, if measures are taken to reverse the coagulation defect—and these are proved by laboratory assays to have been successful—either before labour is induced, or early in labour, then an epidural can be initiated, and anticoagulant therapy resumed shortly after delivery [2].

Congenital heart disease

The patient with congenital heart disease poses problems which are different in degree, if not in kind. Among women born with a defect, those whose lesion has been corrected should pose no particular difficulties of management during pregnancy and labour; attention must, however, be directed towards prophylaxis against infective endocarditis in the puerperium. Correction of a lesion by closed cardiac surgery may be undertaken at any time during pregnancy without exposing the mother or fetus to any extra risk. If open-heart surgery is contemplated it should, if possible, be delayed beyond the fifteenth week of pregnancy to avoid the possibility of causing a developmental defect in the infant.

Patients with cyanotic congenital heart disease who survive to childbearing age and become pregnant are relatively few. The tendency is to advise these women against becoming pregnant, because of the associated high mortality rate, but during recent years several reports of the successful outcome of such pregnancies have appeared, and there seems little doubt that if the patient strongly desires to have one child she should not be firmly discouraged if the facilities for appropriate care are available. The major hazards to which a patient in this category is exposed during pregnancy are hypotension

7*

and pulmonary thromboembolism. The former is unlikely to result from caval compression, as the patient avoids the supine position even when not pregnant, but a sudden fall in blood pressure resulting from antepartum haemorrhage could readily bring disaster. Intensive antenatal surveillance will reduce, but will not eliminate, the likelihood of the latter occurrence. Thromboembolism is an associated complication of pregnancy, but measures to guard against this condition by the long-term administration of anticoagulant therapy is not advised in this category of patient because of the danger of inducing haemoptysis from engorged pulmonary capillary loops.

These patients are in the greatest danger during labour and the puerperium. Delivery by Caesarean section in the absence of obstetric indications is inadvisable, because of the threat of hypotension due to haemorrhage. If section is undertaken it is imperative that the patient is not subjected to caval compression. During labour, the potential hazards to which the patient is exposed are: caval compression, exhaustion due to pain and effort, dehydration, appreciable haemorrhage during the third stage. Thus intensive monitoring of systemic blood pressure is required, to ascertain in which lateral position caval compression is not induced; the mother must not be placed in the supine lithotomy position; the pain of labour must be completely relieved, the bearing down reflex obtunded and appropriate oxytocic therapy must be provided to reduce to a minimum the extent of postpartum blood loss. Facilities for the rapid institution of resuscitative measures must be immediately to hand throughout the final weeks of pregnancy (which necessitates that the patient be in hospital during this period), during labour and during puerperium. The considered opinion, as expressed by one recent reviewer [3], is that in respect to at least one of these conditions (Eisenmenger's syndrome), if pregnancy is allowed to continue, it is preferable that delivery should be by the vaginal route, with labour and delivery being conducted under an epidural. The provision of supplemental oxygen in this situation is of advantage, it has been suggested [4], because it leads to a decrease in pulmonary artery pressure.

The risk that thromboembolism will occur is increased during the early puerperium, and to counter this, anticoagulant therapy and early ambulation are advisable. The provision of an epidural block for labour and delivery—a form of therapy which is now advocated by many—possibly has the additional advantage of reducing the likelihood that deep vein thrombosis will develop postnatally.

It is important to bear in mind that although the patient with cyanotic heart disease is at greater risk during pregnancy, the patient with acyanotic congenital heart disease is also at increasing hazard in similar fashion, as pregnancy progresses towards term, and requires equally stringent observation and care.

Hypertension

The incidence of essential hypertension among pregnant patients is the same as that among nonpregnant subjects of similar age group. Moderate hypertension, unattended by specific obstetric complications, is unlikely to pose a serious problem throughout pregnancy up to term. The patient who has hypertension in excess of about 160/100 mmHg (22/13·5 kPa) at the start of pregnancy will require increased vigilance during pregnancy: the advisability of intensifying antihypertensive therapy remains a matter of debate, but certainly if the blood pressure begins to rise, further therapy will be required to avoid heart failure. In many centres it is the practice to induce, or to deliver electively by section at 38 weeks, patients with moderate or severe essential hypertension for the sake of the fetus. Drug therapy might require to be modified when a patient with essential hypertension becomes pregnant. Reserpine and ganglion-blocking agents, if administered late in pregnancy, can have serious effects upon the infant. It has been suggested that the former can upset the neonate's temperature regulation, and ceratinly cases of neonatal nasal obstruction due to mucosal congestion (a dangerous complication in the infant, who is an obligatory nose breather) have been ascribed to transplacentally derived reserpine. Neonatal hypotension and paralytic ileus have been ascribed to ganglion-blocking antihypertensive agents which reached the fetus via the placenta. Recently, a disturbing number of reports have appeared in which acute pancreatitis, occasionally fatal, has been related to a thiazide diuretic administered to a pregnant patient.

The tendency for blood pressure to rise during labour, most notably if pain and apprehension are poorly relieved, stigmatizes this period of pregnancy as the most dangerous in respect to the hypertensive patient. The provision of adequate analgesia and of an appropriate regimen of tranquillizer therapy is mandatory in the proper conduct of labour and delivery in these cases. It should further be noted that the choice of ergometrine in the conduct of the third stage of labour is most unwise, as this oxytocic is likely to cause a marked, and rather sustained, rise in blood pressure. The other available oxytocic agent, Syntocinon, does not induce hypertension (although, if given as an intravenous bolus, it can cause a dramatic fall in blood pressure) and should be used if an oxytocic is considered necessary.

Deep vein thrombosis

The true incidence of deep vein thrombosis (DVT) associated with pregnancy is unknown, but clinically suggestive signs and symptoms are found in roughly 0·2 per cent of pregnancies which are carried beyond the 28th week. It is possible that two-thirds of these cases first become apparent—or are initiated—postpartum. Among the patients who develop antepartum DVT an appreciable proportion will have had a similar condition in a previous pregnancy. The recurrence rate has not been reported but is high enough to encourage the clinician routinely to provide prophylactic anticoagulant therapy in these cases. Therapy (whether active or prophylactic) during the antenatal period consists of induction with heparin and maintenance with an oral anticoagulant. Whilst the former does not traverse the placenta, the oral anticoagulants do so, and thus patients on these drugs should be admitted to hospital before term, and their oral therapy stopped several days before the onset of labour. If haste is required, the coagulation defect is actively reversed. It is customary for heparin therapy then to be re-instituted and continued until the onset of labour, when it is stopped, to be started again 12–24 hours after delivery. At an appropriate time thereafter, oral anticoagulant therapy is recommenced, and is maintained usually for 6–8 weeks; the mother, in this instance, must not breast-feed her infant.

The fact that DVT occurs relatively more frequently postpartum rather than antepartum is in the main a reflection of its close association with operative delivery, especially with those deliveries conducted under general anaesthesia. The incidence subsequent to Caesarean section is some 8–10 times that following vaginal delivery, and this is related to several factors: direct trauma to pelvic veins, unnecessarily prolonged postoperative bed-rest and relative immobility. The higher incidence observed among those vaginally delivered patients who have undergone an operative delivery is likely shortly to be much reduced; it has been a consequence of the fact that operative vaginal delivery has, until recently, been undertaken mainly upon patients who have laboured long, were poorly hydrated, subjected to caval compression during labour and whilst in the lithotomy position, and who lay exhausted for many hours after delivery. Current obstetric management of labour and delivery should greatly reduce the incidence of these provocative factors.

Although the incidence of DVT is related to the several factors noted above, the outstanding correlations are with age and parity, the latter also being at least partly a reflection of maternal age. The slope of a graph of incidence against age begins to rise when the group 31–35 years is reached, and becomes quite steep in respect of mothers aged 36 years or over. Similarly, the incidence amongst mothers who have carried at least four previous pregnancies to viability is relatively high. These data should spur increased vigilance in the care of appropriate patients.

Pulmonary embolism is the commonest cause of maternal death in respect of pregnancies which have been carried beyond 28 weeks. The incidence is approximately 1 : 30,000; the incidence of nonfatal pulmonary embolism is not reported. Twice as many of the fatal cases occur postpartum as occur in the antenatal period, and the incidence following delivery by Caesarean section is approximately 1 : 2,500. Although, as is now well recognized, pulmonary microemboli are an extremely common associate of pre-eclampsia, the clinically intrusive pulmonary embolism is, it appears, almost invariably a resultant of DVT although the presence of the latter is frequently unsuspected prior to the embolic episode.

SICKLE CELL DISEASE

Women with a sickle cell trait who become pregnant pose few problems additional to those associated with pregnancy itself. The pregnant woman with homozygous sickle cell disease is equally as likely to develop a crisis as she was before she became pregnant. The latter observation refers to patients before the 30th week of pregnancy. Manifestly if, subsequent to that gestational period, the patient is encouraged to assume a posture which encourages local venous stasis, she will have been placed at increased risk of going into crisis. Homozygous sickle cell disease characteristically is associated with an increased likelihood of abortion, intrauterine growth retardation, spontaneous onset of premature labour, and perinatal death. Hence these patients, after conception, are very likely to require the care and services of an anaesthetist.

THE RESPIRATORY SYSTEM

The changes which occur in the respiratory system as an accompaniment of pregnancy, although considerable, are of an order which pose relatively little challenge to the anaesthetist in his care of the normal parturient. Engorgement of the mucosa of the upper respiratory tract increases the liability of haemorrhage due to minor abrasions. Vital capacity is unaltered by pregnancy. Tidal volume increases by approximately one-third, a change which is associated with the respiratory alkalosis and metabolic acidosis characteristic of pregnancy throughout gestation. Functional residual capacity decreases significantly, as a result of reduction of both expiratory reserve volume and residual volume.

These changes are rarely of moment in routine obstetric practice, because of the very infrequent occurrence of superimposed respiratory embarrassment. Possibly the condition which will cause concern to the obstetric anaesthetist is kyphoscoliosis. The marked reduction in vital capacity which is a frequent associate of this condition is exacerbated by elevation of the diaphragm caused by the advancing pregnancy. The situation is worse confounded by the fact that many of these patients are unable to be delivered vaginally because of pelvic deformity. Maternal hypoxaemia, reflecting the respiratory embarrassment, is a recognized cause of prematurity or stillbirth related to severe forms of this condition. Manifestly the provision of supplemental oxygen is advisable for those patients who are allowed to labour. The distorted abdominal cavity can make it difficult to gauge the position most appropriate to avoid aortocaval compression, and this must be sought for with care. Labour, if permitted, is best conducted under epidural analgesia, although initiation of this might prove to be impossible because of anatomical difficulties. Centrally-depressant agents should be avoided if possible, because of the danger of supplementing the respiratory embarrassment. If delivery is conducted by Caesarean section the postoperative care of the patient must be of a high order, consideration being given to the fact that relief of the high intra-abdominal pressure will undoubtedly lead to an acute disturbance of pulmonary vascular dynamics.

The course of asthma is uninfluenced by pregnancy. It may be remarked, although it is of doubtful clinical significance, that β-adrenergic bronchodilators, such as salbutamol, are also powerful myometrial relaxants. Of more note, however, is the suggestion that ergometrine may trigger a severe asthmatic attack. Means of relieving bronchospasm should be immediately available for administration to an asthmatic patient in a delivery suite.

The interrelationships between pregnancy and the more unusual types of respiratory disease have recently been admirably reviewed by Fishburne [5].

THE NERVOUS SYSTEM

Very few changes in the functional anatomy of the central and peripheral nervous system are directly associated with pregnancy, labour and delivery. Cerebrospinal fluid (CSF) pressure is unchanged during pregnancy, except in response to caval compression, when it rises; during labour the pressure possibly rises during first stage contractions, and it certainly increases considerably during second stage contractions if the patient bears down. The epidural space—at least in the lower thoracic, lumbar and sacral regions—is considerably encroached upon by distended veins, with the result that the extent of cephalocaudal spread of a solution injected into the space is approximately 50 per cent greater in the pregnant subject than it is in the nonpregnant subject of the same age and height.

Peripheral nerve injuries

During pregnancy, peripheral nerve trunks situated in critical areas can be subjected to compression due to local tissue oedema. More common, is the syndrome of 'obstetrical paralysis' which presents in the early postpartum period and characteristically as a unilateral foot-drop. There is a muscle weakness and loss of skin sensation which most frequently indicate involvement of nerves which receive contributions from the fourth and fifth lumbar roots. Although it was for long considered that this syndrome resulted from trauma to the lumbosacral trunk incurred during a difficult delivery, or as a result of pressure from a malpresenting fetal skull, current opinion holds that the lesion is due to prolapse of one or more lumbar intervertebral discs, and that the frequency of the condition is increased among women who have suffered from low-back pain before pregnancy. The other, more discrete type of obstetric palsy is that due to compression of the peroneal nerve by the inefficient placing of the patient's legs against the lithotomy poles.

Chronic neurological disease

The progress of chronic neurological disease is not systematically affected by pregnancy. If there is a space-occupying lesion, either intracranial or within the spinal canal, then the rise of CSF pressure due either to caval compression or to bearing down could be a complicating factor of significance. Pregnancy in a patient with cerebrovascular disease—specifically with an established history of subarachnoid haemorrhage, or with suspected berry aneurysm—demands no unusual care other than the prevention or control of hypertension, with special attention being paid to the avoidance of those acute episodes of hypertension which can occur during ill-managed labour, delivery and the early puerperium.

Epilepsy and migraine occur with the same frequency among pregnant patients as among nonpregnant women of the same age. However, there is some suggestion that in affected subjects attacks are likely to occur in the early puerperium; this may reflect the extensive shifts in body fluids which characterize this period, but it is equally likely that it reflects the emotional element which contributes to the disease. It may be noted that the antifolate drugs, such as phenytoin, commonly used in the treatment of epilepsy, have been said to be a causative factor in the production of congenital abnormalities, specifically hare lip and cleft palate. Unfortunately, these structural anomalies will have become established by the eighth week of gestation, often before the fact of pregnancy has been appreciated. If it is possible for the epileptic woman to abstain from phenytoin during the early weeks of pregnancy, then it is wiser for her to do so, and to substitute, for example, phenobarbitone as her stable anticonvulsant until the critical period has passed.

MUSCULOSKELETAL SYSTEM

Bone and joint

Despite the nutritional demands made by the fetus, osteomalacia and osteoporosis are rare in pregnancy, at least in Western countries. The most notable change in the musculoskeletal system is a softening and increased distensibility of the interosseous ligaments which permits accentuation of the normal lordosis during late pregnancy and also allows a widening of the space between the adjoining bones which form the symphysis pubis.

The only deleterious effects which disease of the bones and joints are likely to have upon pregnancy, and vice versa, are of a mechanical nature. Abnormalities of the pelvis and hip joints can influence the progress of labour and the mode of delivery; the symptoms of established pathology of the lumbosacral vertebrae can be worsened by the postural changes imposed by the enlarging uterus; the pregnant patient with severe kyphoscoliosis might be caused increasing respiratory embarrassment due to the upward deflection of her diaphragm, although the flaring of the lower thoracic cage which is characteristic of pregnancy could compensate for this.

It is usual for the symptoms of rheumatoid arthritis to be alleviated during pregnancy. This reflects the increased production of corticosteroids, and indeed 25 years ago attempts were made to relieve sufferers from rheumatoid arthritis by the intravenous infusion of blood from appropriately matched pregnant patients.

Muscle

The progress of myopathies is apparently uninfluenced by pregnancy. There has recently been a suggestion, however, that uterine hypotonia, with consequent postpartum haemorrhage, can be a characteristic of the pregnant patient with myotonia dystrophica [6]. The occurrence of malignant hyperpyrexia among pregnant patients has apparently been much more infrequent than was to be expected, considering the number of general anaesthetics to which the parturient population is exposed. The provision of regional analgesia for delivery—vaginal or abdominal—appears to afford the safer prospect for those patients whose family history suggest that they are susceptible in this regard [7]. Myasthenia gravis has been reported to be alleviated, made worse, and unaffected, by the advent and progress of pregnancy, with equal frequency. It has been advised [8] that administration of central depressants be kept to a minimum in the conduct of labour, because of the danger of inducing respiratory depression and the retention of secretions. Exacerbation of the myasthenic symptoms, including the occurrence of crises, is seen with some frequency in the postnatal period, and these patients require to be under close observation for several days postpartum. The infants of myasthenia mothers may exhibit signs of muscle weakness throughout the first 2–3 weeks after delivery. These infants recover spontaneously but are likely to require anticholinesterase therapy to enable them to move and suck vigorously whilst they are affected. Although the level of plasma cholinesterase is relatively low in the pregnant woman, the response to suxamethonium is no different from that of the nonpregnant adult: the frequency of suxamethonium after-pains is, however, much diminished.

ENDOCRINE

Diabetes

The patient with established diabetes is no more likely to be infertile, but possibly has a greater tendency to first trimester abortion, than the nondiabetic woman. Once pregnancy has become established, the diabetic state tends to become more difficult to control than had previously been the case, and increased vigilance is required. Both insulin and oral antidiabetic agents are now considered to be acceptable from the point of view of the welfare of the fetus. Drug therapy may be required by some women previously controlled by diet alone; insulin dose may need to be increased or decreased during the first half of pregnancy, although the tendency in the latter half is for the demand to rise. However, there occurs during normal pregnancy a combination of relative hypoglycaemia and an increased serum concentration of free fatty acids, which has been epitomized by the phrase 'accelerated starvation', and in addition glycosuria, due to a lowered renal threshold to glucose, is quite commonly to be observed during pregnancy. For these reasons, intensive biochemical monitoring of the diabetic patient is necessary, particularly when there are any modifications of drug and diet. From the point of view of the fetus, moderate maternal hyperglycaemia does more harm than does the maintenance of a level of blood glucose concentration slightly below normal. The time of delivery is also dictated by concern for the fetus: most physicians and obstetricians are reluctant to allow pregnancy to continue beyond the 37th completed week because the possibility of intrauterine death increases markedly after that period; however, most paediatricians are reluctant to receive the infant of a diabetic mother delivered before the 34th completed week, because these infants have a delayed maturation of lung surfactant. Thus, increasingly the optimum time of delivery (other things being equal) is being predicated upon the, value of the lecithin-sphingomyelin ratio derived from analysis of liquor obtained from transabdominal amniocentesis. The inclination to deliver the diabetic mother by elective Caesarean section has diminished in many quarters during the past decade, although the presence of any accompanying obstetric pathology usually prompts this line of action. If the mother does require operative delivery, the preoperative regimen is no different from that appropriate to the care of the diabetic patient about to undergo any other surgical procedure (see Chapter 15). The maternal and perinatal consequences of diabetes have been the subjects of a recent review by acknowledged experts in the field [9].

Thyroid disease

One characteristic of pregnancy is the state of 'hypermetabolism', and normally the pregnant patient exhibits a slight enlargement of the thyroid gland, with hyperplasia and an increased uptake of thyroidal iodine. Thus the establishment of a firm diagnosis of thyrotoxicosis during pregnancy requires a skilled and experienced investigator. The thyrotoxic patient who becomes pregnant is not placed at increased risk by so doing; if, however, her endocrine disturbance does appear to be escaping control, there is no contraindication to surgical intervention in the third trimester. The antithyroid drugs cross the placenta with ease and may cause goitre and hypothyroidism in the new born. If the patient can be managed on low doses, with a change to iodine (which also crosses the placenta) during the last trimester the neonate is not placed in jeopardy. Although fertility is reduced as an association of myxoedema, the hypothyroid patient can become pregnant. However, there is an increased incidence of abortion related to this condition, and in efforts to avoid this it is essential that thyroxine therapy be adequately maintained.

Adrenal medulla

A substantial number of cases of phaeochromocytoma diagnosed during, or immediately following, pregnancy have now been recorded. The advent of hypertension, either sustained or labile, without proteinuria or other evidence suggestive of pre-eclampsia, should arouse suspicion of this condition. The choice of therapy is not influenced by the presence of pregnancy.

Pituitary disease

Pituitary necrosis has been classically associated with obstetric shock, although it does undoubtedly occur in the nonparturient. The pituitary enlarges quite considerably during pregnancy; rapid involution of the gland follows delivery and it is possibly because of the latter process that an episode of acute hypotension is peculiarly liable to cause intrapituitary thrombosis during the immediate postpartum period. Hypovolaemia without hypotension is apparently not a provocative factor. The signs and symptoms of hypopituitarism are unlikely to develop unless at least 50 per cent of the active glandular tissue has been destroyed, and there is some reason for supposing that many obstetric patients have incurred a degree of anterior pituitary necrosis without demonstrable effect.

GASTROINTESTINAL

The tone of the physiological gastro-oesophageal sphincter is somewhat diminished during pregnancy, and this plus the increasingly raised intra-abdominal pressure, leads to a high incidence of reflux oesophagitis. A previously unsuspected hiatus hernia may also become manifest during the latter half of pregnancy. Only symptomatic therapy is indicated for these conditions.

Although the rate of secretion of gastric acid is little altered during pregnancy, symptoms of peptic ulceration are considerably relieved throughout pregnancy, and the disease rarely makes its first appearance in the parturient. Perforation of, or bleeding from, a peptic ulcer is most uncommon during pregnancy, but the appearance of either condition demands the prompt application of appropriate therapy.

The pregnant patient commonly suffers from constipation, but this rarely causes more than symptomatic upset. The course of neither ulcerative colitis nor regional ileitis appears to be systematically affected by the advent of pregnancy, and the progress of the pregnancy itself is unaffected by either disease. The incidence of acute appendicitis is no different among parturients than among nonpregnant women of a similar age group. The site of abdominal pain and tenderness is, however, determined by the size of the uterus, and in late pregnancy can be well out into the right flank, or in the right subcostal region. Because of the anatomical distortion, the surgical incision for appendicectomy during the second half of pregnancy should be liberal, and over the site of maximum tenderness.

Haemorrhoids are frequently manifest during late pregnancy, but rarely cause much discomfort before delivery. However, they do contribute considerably to the distress of the puerperal patient. It is possible that the development, or the enlargement, of the haemorrhoidal mass is encouraged by prolonged bearing down at delivery; there is some suggestion that this tendency is increased in those patients whose anal sphincter has been relaxed by regional blockade. Therapy is directed solely to the relief of pain by local application and systemic analgesics. There is no doubt that this condition warrants more intensive investigation to relieve an inordinate amount of unnecessary suffering.

Opinion regarding the effect of labour upon upper gastrointestinal function has changed somewhat in recent years. Earlier it was considered that gastrointestinal motility and the rate of absorption of material from within the stomach and small intestine were depressed when labour became established. It is possible that the depressions observed resulted from narcotic analgesics and were not characteristic of labour. However, there is no doubting that if labour is allowed to become prolonged, and the mother approaches exhaustion, retention of gastrointestinal contents will progressively occur.

URINARY TRACT

Renal function

Renal plasma flow and glomerular filtration rate are each increased by 40–45 per cent throughout the second and third trimester, compared with the prepregnancy values. Dilatation of the extrapelvic portions of the ureters, due mainly to mechanical factors, is initiated towards the end of the first trimester. The renal clearance of many substances such as glucose and aminoacids is increased during pregnancy and this possibly contributes to the establishment of bacterial contamination of the urinary tract which is so common a feature of pregnancy. Proteinuria, indicative of increased glomerular permeability, is a normal concomitant of pregnancy, but the protein concentration in the urine due to this factor alone is very low.

Chronic nephritis

The interreaction between chronic glomerulonephritis and pregnancy depends upon the severity of the renal disease. The greater the hypertension, and the higher the level of blood urea, the less likely it is that the conception will survive; indeed, the more severe the disease, the less fertile the patient. Few well-matched studies have been reported in this area, but several authorities are agreed that if the woman's initial blood pressure is in excess of 150/100 mmHg (20/13·5 kPa), or if her blood urea before conception is over 10 mmol/l, early termination of pregnancy should be seriously considered in view of the maternal risk which continuation would impose. There is, however, a suggestion that intermittent haemodialysis may significantly reduce the risk. Among those less severely affected, about 50 per cent will suffer a permanent deterioration of renal function if pregnancy continues to term.

Nephrotic syndrome

The patient with the nephrotic syndrome who conceives is destined to lose a vast quantity of protein as a result rather of increased glomerular clearance than of deterioration of her renal condition. The loss of serum albumin results in an increased tendency to oedema; the loss of gamma globulins (particularly if accompanied by continued steroid therapy designed to alleviate the renal lesion) renders the patient highly susceptible to infection. Patients thus require a high protein/low salt diet, and may also require diuretic therapy (preferably not with a thiazide derivative—see above). They must also be guarded against infection. Renal function in the nephrotic patient may not deteriorate as a result of pregnancy if standards of care and management are adequate, but increasing hypertension is grave prognostically and if this occurs, termination or early induction of labour is advisable. The fetal outcome is not bad, except in those cases complicated by hypertension, although the birth weight tends to be low.

OPERATIONS FOR NONOBSTETRIC CONDITIONS

The pregnant patient is equally as likely to require operative treatment as is the non-pregnant woman of the same age. There are a few exceptions to this statement, some increasing the likelihood and others diminishing it, but the generalization is a fair one. The natural inclination is to delay the operation if possible until after the pregnancy has been safely concluded. Such an approach is based more upon social and emotional considerations than upon a firm appreciation of the undesirability of operating upon the patient whilst she is pregnant, and it reflects in part at least the unease with which nonobstetric surgeons (and nonobstetric anaesthetists) contemplate a pregnant patient who comes under their care. However irrational the attitude, it is likely to persist. There are occasions, however, when an operation cannot be postponed and pregnant patients may present for general surgical, orthopaedic, neurosurgical, cardiac or gynaecological operations. Discussion of such a circumstance can be divided into two parts, defined by the duration of the pregnancy.

Early pregnancy

There are two major concerns related to nonobstetric operations conducted upon patients who are in the first trimester: the unintentional induction of abortion, and interference with embryonic or fetal development. There is no sound evidence that a patient in the first trimester who is subjected to a surgical procedure, of whatever magnitude, which does not involve the uterus and its appendages is thereby placed at an increased risk of aborting her fetus. A very high percentage of conceptions end in spontaneous abortion before twelve weeks' gestation, and if an abortion does follow the surgical procedure, the patient will be unlikely to view the sequence as coincidental. Thus, purely for this emotional (and possible medico-legal) reason, it is preferable to delay operation until after the twelfth week if at all possible.

Several of the drugs in common use in anaesthesia have been demonstrated to have an effect upon replication and other functions of unicellular organisms. There is also some suggestion that chronic exposure to anaesthetic agents is associated with a relatively high incidence of congenital abnormalities among the progeny of women so exposed during early pregnancy. There is no evidence of an increased incidence of congenital abnormality among the children of mothers who have received an anaesthetic during the early weeks of pregnancy. Teratogenesis is completed with the 16th week of gestation, so that subsequent to that time even this unlikely outcome of a nonobstetric operation no longer requires consideration. The anaesthetist and surgeon who attend a pregnant patient for a nonobstetric operation during her first trimester can take comfort from the fact that over the centuries hundreds of thousands of women have subjected themselves to an amazing range of challenges in order to induce an abortion, almost invariably without success unless they have made a direct attack upon the uterine contents. On the other hand, it must be appreciated that the two factors which can initiate an abortion, or which can, if they occur at a critical moment, impair the orderliness of fetal development, are severe maternal hypoxaemia and hypotension.

Late pregnancy

Between the 16th and 28th weeks, hypoxaemia and hypotension can bring disaster to the fetus, if not to the mother. Subsequent to the 28th week the danger of caval compression must also be borne in mind, and it is advisable to tilt the patient undergoing operation laterally, or displace the uterus away from the inferior vena cava, if the patient must be supine during the procedure. The patient should also be nursed postoperatively in the lateral position until she has recovered sufficiently to recline against a bed-rest or to get out of bed. The basic anaesthetic technique need not be modified from that which the anaesthetist concerned customarily employs for operations of a similar category. Induced hypotension or hypothermia should only be used when the condition of the mother is so critical as to make the accompanying definite risk to the fetus acceptable.

Apparently valid arguments can be adduced both for and against techniques which clearly have a marked effect on the fetal environment. Take, for example, halothane which is a specific relaxant of the myometrium. On the one hand it could be argued that relaxation of uterine tone renders the placental site more susceptible to damage during intra-abdominal surgical manipulation; on the other hand, it could with equal justification be suggested that rendering the uterus hypotonic reduces its threshold of irritability, and hence diminishes the chance that contractions will be induced in the course of the operation. The soundest approach is for the anaesthetist to apply the technique with which he is most at ease, and with which he is least likely inadvertently to induce an episode of hypoxaemia or of hypotension.

Infections

The effects upon the fetus of maternal rubella developing before the 16th week of gestation, and of maternal syphilis, are well known. There is considerable suspicion that other systemic infections, notably viral, to which a patient in early pregnancy becomes subject, can cause either abortion or fetal abnormalities, but the evidence is as yet too tenuous to encourage consideration of therapeutic abortion in such cases. It is, however, considered advisable that the administration of live viral vaccines at any time to a pregnant woman should be avoided if at all possible, but particularly in the first trimester.

DRUGS

Antibacterials

There are several antibacterial drugs which can cause fetal damage, if administered to the pregnant patient. The tetracyclines cause permanent staining of the deciduous teeth, and a reversible depression of bone growth. Streptomycin, kanamycin, gentamycin and vancomycin can cause permanent damage to the eighth cranial nerve of the fetus if administered during pregnancy. Chloroquine can lead to disruption of the fetal cochlea if given during the first trimester, and to retinal damage if administered later in pregnancy. Novobiocin and the sulphonamides displace bilirubin from its binding sites on serum protein; if these drugs are given to the mother shortly before delivery, they can place the neonate at risk of developing kernicterus.

Anticancer drugs

Cytotoxic drugs administered to the mother subsequent to the first trimester are not associated with an increased incidence of fetal abnormality. The relationship between first trimester cytotoxic drug administration and abortion or developmental defects of the fetus is equivocal in respect of most of the currently employed agents; the exception is aminopterin, the use of which has been cited as the cause of abortion and of fetal malformation in an appreciable series of cases. There is some suggestion of a direct association between the administration of cytotoxic drugs during the final two-thirds of pregnancy and low birth weight of the infant.

Although it has been suggested that the patient with leukaemia has a reduced fertility, pregnancy certainly occurs in leukaemic patients. Leukaemia may also be diagnosed for the first time during pregnancy. When leukaemia presents in this way it is more frequently an acute than a chronic variety. The progress of pregnancy is not altered by the disease although the rate of spontaneous abortion is rather high, especially among cases of acute leukaemia. Nor is the progress of the disease affected by the pregnancy. Termination of pregnancy is not indicated, therefore, and can, it is claimed, cause a deterioration of the leukaemia. The principles of treatment include supplementary iron, the avoidance of folic acid, whole blood transfusion as indicated, and either corticosteroids or cytotoxic drugs depending upon the type of leukaemia. Therapy may be withheld altogether throughout pregnancy in a case of slowly progressive chronic leukaemia. Postpartum haemorrhage appears to be more frequent than normal in leukaemic patients, but there is no nonobstetric reason to deliver these patients by Caesarean section.

PRE-ECLAMPSIA

Although this chapter is not intended to cover acute diseases specific to pregnancy, it is appropriate to point out that pre-eclampsia is one of the 'great mimics' in medicine. The diagnosis of pre-eclampsia, based upon hypertension and proteinuria, usually accompanied by nondependent brawny oedema, starting in the second half of pregnancy in a patient (most frequently a primipara) without an antecedent history of renal disease, is reasonably straightforward in the majority of cases. However, the condition can present in any of a number of bizarre fashions, and the difficulty of immediate diagnosis is greatly increased if the patient has not previously attended for antenatal care. The patient may first present with any or several of the following: headache, nausea, vomiting and visual disturbances (with or without a history of migraine), acute abdominal pain (usually central, frequently, but not invariably, indicative of a concealed accidental haemorrhage), purpura (generalized or localized, and can include retinal haemorrhages), acute hepatitis, oliguria, convulsions (with or without a history of epilepsy).

A patient who presents with any of these conditions and who is found also to be in the second half of pregnancy should invariably be first suspected of being pre-eclamptic, and an obstetric opinion must be obtained. Pregnancy is rarely a coincidental finding in these cases, a simple fact which general physicians and surgeons too frequently forget.

REFERENCES

1 TAGUCHI K. Pregnancy in patients with a prosthetic heart valve. *Surg Gynecol Obstet* 1977; **145**: 206-8.
2 GOTHARD JW. Heart disease in pregnancy. The anaesthetic management of a patient with prosthetic heart valves. *Anaesthesia* 1978; **33**: 523-6.
3 GLEICHER N, MIDWALL J, HOCHBERGER D, JAFFIN H. Eisenmenger's syndrome and pregnancy. *Obstet Gynecol Surv* 1979; **34**: 721-41.

4 MIDWALL J, JAFFIN H, HERMAN MV, KUPERSMITH J. Shunt flow and pulmonary hemodynamics during labor and delivery in the Eisenmenger syndrome. *Am J Cardiol* 1978; **42**: 299–303.

5 FISHBURNE JI. Physiology and disease of the respiratory system in pregnancy. A review. *J Reprod Med* 1979; **22**: 177–89.

6 WEBB D, MUIR I, FAULKNER J, JOHNSON G. Myotonia dystrophica: obstetric complications. *Am J Obstet Gynecol* 1978; **132**: 265–70.

7 WILLATTS SM. Malignant hyperthermia susceptibility. Management during pregnancy and labour. *Anaesthesia* 1979; **34**: 41–6.

8 ROLBIN SH, LEVINSON G, SHNIDER SM, WRIGHT RG. Anesthetic considerations for myasthenia gravis and pregnancy. *Anesth Analg* 1978; **57**: 441–7.

9 ROYAL SOCIETY OF MEDICINE. Diabetes in pregnancy: a symposium. *J R Soc Med* 1978; **71**: 202–22.

FURTHER READING

BARNES CG. *Medical disorders in obstetric practice.* 4th ed. Oxford: Blackwell Scientific Publications, 1974.

Chapter 7
Peripheral Nervous Diseases, Neuromuscular Disorders and the Myopathies

PART 1
PERIPHERAL NERVOUS DISEASES, NEUROMUSCULAR DISORDERS AND THE MYOPATHIES

S. A. FELDMAN

Disease of the peripheral nervous system is of particular importance to the anaesthetist if, as a consequence of the disease, the patient is likely to be adversely affected by any of the drugs or techniques used in anaesthetic practice. In some of these diseases, special techniques used by anaesthetists can assist in the diagnosis or management of the disorders.

THE REFLEX ARC AND MUSCLE TONE

The logical starting points for an examination of the diseases of the peripheral nervous system are the reflex arc and muscle tone as these are the physiological basis upon which our concept of disease of this system rests. The reflex arc is affected by many diseases involving both the central and the peripheral nervous system. It is essential therefore that one has an understanding of the interplay of these two levels of nervous system organization, if such fundamental physical signs of peripheral neurological disease as alterations in reflex response and muscle tone are to be correctly interpreted.

REFLEX ARCS

The simplest reflex arc, such as the tendon stretch reflex, consists of a sensory nerve carrying impulses from the periphery to the spinal cord and an efferent motor nerve arising as an axon of a neurone in the anterior horn of the spinal cord and terminating at a myoneural junction.

The activity of the reflex arc is modified by a local self-regulating mechanism which modulates the setting at which any given stimulus triggers a reflex response. This is effected by the muscle spindle system. This regulator is in its turn subjected to finer tuning by impulses from the brain. It is by a combination of this fine and coarse regulation that the tone of the muscles is adjusted and it is for this reason that an examination of muscle tone and reflex response plays an important part in assessment and diagnosis of neurological disease.

In addition to the monosynaptic reflex arc, there are more complex multisynaptic arrangements that are of importance in neurological disease. Monosynaptic reflexes usually involve efferent and afferent pathways utilizing the same peripheral nerve, so that a blow on the patellar tendon causes a sudden increase of tension in the quadriceps femoris muscle and reflex activity that produces contraction of that muscle. The femoral nerve is involved in both the afferent and efferent volley. For this reflex response to occur there must also have been inhibition of the opposing hamstring muscles of the same thigh. This requires a multisynaptic reflex response. The neurological pathways involve interneurones (internuncial neurones), which connect different levels in the spinal cord and result in an alteration in muscle activity. Whereas the monosynaptic reflexes affect extensor muscles, the multisynaptic reflexes involving interneurones, usually affect the flexor muscles. Because of the many synapses involved and the spread through several spinal segments, these reflexes are particularly likely to be affected by drugs and disease. It is this multisynaptic pathway involving the interneurones that is depressed by drugs such as diazepam and other benzodiazepines and is responsible for their 'muscle relaxing' properties.

MUSCLE TONE

Normal muscle tone depends upon the integrity of the stretch reflex and the muscle spindle system. The muscle spindle (Fig. 7.1) consists of an intrafusal fibre activated by the smallest of motor nerves which arise in the anterior horn of the spinal cord (Gamma efferent). Stimulation of these cells produces shortening of the intrafusal fibres of the muscle spindle. As a result of the increased tension in these fibres, a lesser degree of shortening will produce the same stimulation of the large afferent sensory fibre. Thus muscle spindle activity produces an increase in the muscle tone. The intrafusal fibre produces its effect through a cholinergic transmission and is readily affected by muscle relaxant drugs. Muscle tone therefore depends upon the integrity of the muscle spindle

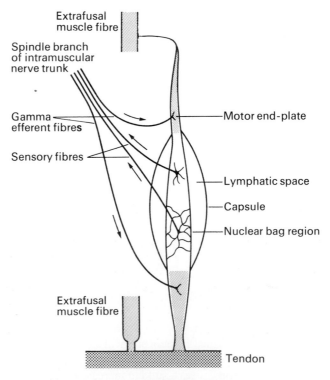

Fig. 7.1. Muscle spindle (highly diagrammatic).

system. Hypertonicity can be produced by loss of the inhibitory influences of the pyramidal and extrapyramidal system upon the motor cells to the intrafusal fibres or by stimulation of this system. Common causes of this are lesions in the internal capsule of the brain which destroy the corticospinal tracts releasing the anterior horn cells from the inhibitory influence of the higher centres and lesions of the midbrain and pons. The hypertonia associated with Parkinson's disease is produced by lesions of the extrapyramidal system, particularly in the region of the substantia nigra.

Hypotonia can be produced by any lesion of the reflex arc or muscle spindle system. This may be due to sensory or motor nerve disease, to disease of the anterior horn cells, to involvement of descending pathways from the higher centres and cerebellum and to lesions of the myoneural junction and muscles. In disease of the peripheral nervous system hypotonia due to lesions of the reflex arc and myoneural junction must be distinguished from causes due to diseases of higher centres and the communicating spinal tracts, producing their effect by alteration in muscle spindle activity. This differentiation can often be achieved by noting the response to active and to passive movements and to reflex activity.

ANAESTHETIC SIGNIFICANCE

Irrespective of the cause of the disease, changes in function are produced by many different lesions of the peripheral neurological system which are of particular significance to anaesthetists. In these conditions anaesthesia itself, or a particular technique of anaesthesia, may carry a special hazard.

Before consideration of the specific diseases that produce these changes in functional activity, the reason for their peculiar significance to anaesthetists will be presented. The changes are:

1 associated with shift of potassium ions;
2 associated with altered innervation of muscles;
3 associated with autonomic disturbances;
4 associated with respiratory impairment;
5 associated with neuromuscular junction dysfunction.

1 Changes associated with changes in potassium ion concentration

The normal resting transmembrane potential of all cells determines the ease with which depolarization of their membrane can occur and hence the electrical excitability of the cell. This is of particular consequence in those cells whose activity depends upon repeated depolarization and repolarization such as occur in the heart, in the brain, in muscle and in the peripheral nervous system. It follows therefore that changes in the resting membrane potential will affect the activity of the neuromuscular system, the heart and the brain. As the cell membrane can be regarded as a semipermeable membrane, the polarity of the resting membrane potential will depend upon the ratio of the concentration on both sides of that membrane of the ion to which the membrane is most permeable. At rest, the most important ion in this respect is potassium.

It can be postulated that the EMF $\propto \dfrac{K_i}{K_o}$

where K_i = potassium conc. inside the cell (150 mmol/litre)
K_o = potassium conc. outside the cell (5 mmol/litre).

Unfortunately only the plasma potassium is readily available for measurement and this can be regarded as the Ko of the heart, nerves and muscle (but not of the brain or the cells of the spinal cord). Changes in this concentration are not uncommon. Provided the degree of change in the plasma potassium is proportional to that inside the cells, the ratio of Ki/Ko will be maintained and it will not then cause changes in the excitability of the heart or changes in neuromuscular transmission. An increase of the Ki/Ko ratio will result in hyperpolarization of the cell membrane and will cause a resistance to critical depolarization of the postsynaptic membrane by acetylcholine. This will reduce the 'margin of safety' of normal neuromuscular transmission [35] and induce a state of sensitivity to nondepolarizing muscle relaxant drugs such as *d*-tubocurarine, and resistance to suxamethonium and decamethonium. When suxamethonium is administered to a patient it causes depolarization of the postsynaptic membrane of the neuromuscular junction with a consequent shift of Na^+ ions into the cells, followed by loss of K^+ ions from within the cell [36]. In the normal patient this potassium flux is barely demonstrable and only produces a measurable change in systemic plasma potassium concentration in particular circumstances although it has been suggested this may be considerably increased after halothane anaesthesia [44]. If the K^+ flux has been of sufficient magnitude it will affect the Ko/Ki ratio and may cause ventricular arrhythmias and cardiac arrest. The effect of a K^+ flux of a given magnitude will depend upon the pre-existing K^+ ion status of the patient. Thus a patient with a total body K^+ ion depletion (i.e. following chronic potassium loss due to ulcerative colitis or liver disease) may have a normal Ko/Ki ratio with plasma values of potassium as low as 2 mmol/litre. The effect of an increase in extracellular potassium of 2 mmol/litre would be to reduce the transmembrane potential to approximately half the normal resting level. The same K^+ flux in a patient with normal potassium reserves and Ko/Ki ratio would be to alter the ratio from 5/150 mmol/litre to 7/150 mmol/litre with far less serious consequences.

2 Changes associated with altered innervation of muscles

Lower motor neurone disease or a lesion of the motor nerve will result in a loss of organization of the motor end-plate, starting within 24 hours and becoming maximal at about 3 weeks. It is evident that the motor nerve exhibits a trophic influence on the myoneural junction. It is possible that this is due to the continuous leakage of acetylcholine from the presynaptic membrane since an artificial end-plate can be induced in a muscle by repeatedly stimulating a motor nerve which is implanted under the epimysium of a muscle. Anatomical changes produced by a denervation are associated with physiological dysfunction. There is a loss of specificity of response to acetylcholine by the postsynaptic membrane of the end-plate and a supersensitivity in the response to acetylcholine and suxamethonium. During the period of degeneration the whole muscle surface appears to alter its permeability in response to depolarizing drugs [27]. As a result K^+ flux is no longer limited to a small area of the muscle surface and its magnitude increases enormously [57]. This change can be detected in animal experiments up to a year after denervation.

Potassium fluxes of this magnitude have also been reported to occur after administration of suxamethonium in patients with upper motor neurone lesion, cord injury, tetanus [42, 43, 47] and in one patient after encephalitis [9]. The mechanism in these patients is obscure as the myoneural junction does not atrophy in these patients. Immobilizing a normal muscle does not cause a major increase in K^+ after suxa-

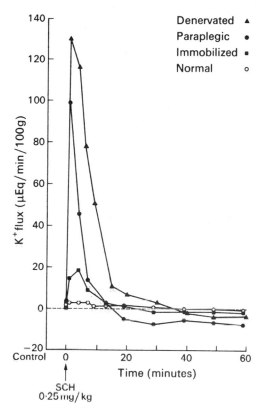

Fig. 7.2. Effect of suxamethonium on potassium concentrations after denervation and immobilization of muscle [21].

methonium if unassociated with muscle trauma [21] (see Fig. 7.2). However, paraplegic muscle shows almost as much efflux of K^+ as denervated muscle in spite of its unaltered sensitivity to acetylcholine and suxamethonium [22] (see Fig. 7.3). Changes in the muscle, whether due to denervation, direct injury, burns, or associated with alterations in muscular activity associated with upper motor neurone disease (and changes which are induced in muscle contraction by halothane and other drugs) increase the K^+ flux which occurs upon administration of suxamethonium. These changes, may be manifest after 24 hours, are maximal at 4–8 days and persist for 6 months or more. These patients are also very sensitive to anticholinesterase drugs.

3 Changes associated with autonomic disturbances

Involvement of the autonomic nervous system by diseases which either affect the cells in the lateral horn of the spinal cord or the efferent sympathetic fibres, may lead to physiological consequences that are of concern to anaesthetists. This is especially likely to occur in the early acute uncompensated state.

Autonomic irritability is common during the initial stages of inflammatory conditions involving the neurones of the autonomic nervous system. This may be clinically manifest as attacks of sweating, hypertension, tachycardia, salivation, loss of pupillary reflexes and sphincter control. Bladder dysfunction and impotence may occur depend-

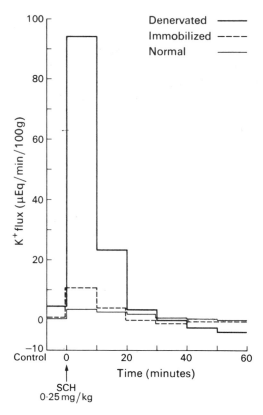

Fig. 7.3. Effect of suxamethonium on total potassium flux after denervation, immobilization, paraplegic and normal muscle [22].

ing upon the spinal level of the disease. During this phase, any drug or anaesthetic technique that excites sympathetic activity, or the injection of exogenous catecholamine may provoke an 'autonomic crisis' due to the denervation sensitivity of the autonomic end organs. This may cause hypertension, ventricular extrasystoles, left ventricular failure, cardiac arrest or cerebral haemorrhage. Light planes of anaesthesia, suxamethonium, pancuronium and catecholamines may be potentially dangerous in these circumstances.

Autonomic irritability progresses eventually to autonomic paralysis. If this is widespread there will be postural hypotension, excessive sensitivity to blood loss and in some patients a marked reduction in cardiac output during IPPV due to a failure of venomotor tone until such times as compensatory mechanisms develop. This may cause prolonged hypotension without a reactionary compensatory phase when the intrathoracic pressure is increased [54] (see Fig. 7.4).

4 Changes associated with respiratory weakness

Many different types of peripheral neurological and muscle disease cause weakness of the muscles of respiration. This may be due to anterior horn cell disease, to motor nerve diseases, to dysfunction of the myoneural junction, or to disease of the muscle itself. All present the anaesthetist with a similar problem as the patient is peculiarly

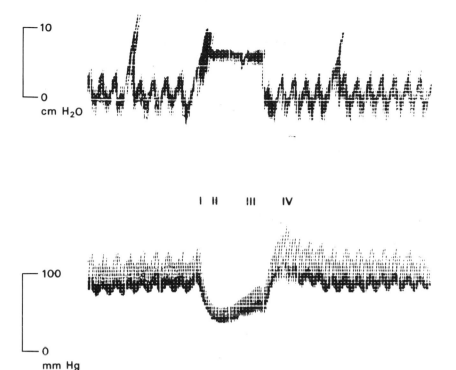

Fig. 7.4. Changes in blood pressure associated with alterations in intrathoracic pressure in a patient during acute stage of autonomic paralysis associated with spinal disease [54]. Upper trace—intrathoracic pressure. Lower trace—blood pressure.

susceptible to any anaesthetic technique that increases the work load on these muscles. An increase in the airway resistance consequent upon intubation with too narrow an endotracheal tube, an anaesthetic circuit with a high internal resistance or the accumulation of bronchial secretion may cause respiratory failure. Drugs which may cause some additional degree of muscle weakness, such as muscle relaxants, volatile anaesthetics and diazepam are contraindicated. Although controlled ventilation obviates many of these hazards it may prove difficult to restore normal ventilation once the normal respiratory drive has been abolished by hyperventilation. These patients present a very difficult anaesthetic problem; wherever possible operations should be performed using a regional block (even then the total dose of local anaesthetic must be reduced). If this is not possible, large doses of muscle relaxants, spontaneous ventilation, a head-down tilt of the operating table, and narrow endotracheal tubes should be avoided.

5 Changes associated with neuromuscular junction dysfunction

The myoneural junction is a weak link in the chain of processes involved in the nervous control of muscle contraction. For muscle contraction to occur there must be sufficient end-plate activity to produce a critical depolarization of the presynaptic (motor nerve) membrane. If the electrolyte balance is normal and acetylcholine production has been adequate, a sufficient quantum of transmitter will then be released to cause a threshold alteration in ionic permeability of the post-synaptic (muscle) membrane, and muscle contraction will result. There is normally a superfluous production of acetylcholine and a surplus of end-plate receptors. This factor provides the margin of safety of this weak link [35]. Providing the transmembrane potential is within normal limits the arrival of acetylcholine at the postsynaptic membrane (end-plate) will cause a depolarization of the end-plate and a propagated action potential producing muscle contraction. It follows that this process can be disturbed by interfering with motor nerve conduction; depression of acetylcholine synthesis; prevention of acetylcholine release; alteration of the transmembrane potential of the postsynaptic membrane; and by alterations in the responsiveness of the muscle adjacent to the end-plate. All these changes will produce muscle weakness, more obvious on exertion, together with the dangers associated with respiratory weakness and difficulty in swallowing (see above). They will also influence the activity of the muscle relaxant drugs and some volatile anaesthetic agents.

Defective nerve conduction and a failure to produce or release a sufficient quantity of acetylcholine will produce muscular weakness with sensitivity to nondepolarizing agents. In motor nerve disease, botulism, and following β-bungarotoxin, insufficient acetylcholine is produced to maintain normal neuromuscular transmission and ultimately atrophic changes will occur in the motor end-plates. If the transmembrane potential is increased above the resting -90mV, a curare-like effect will be produced. Nondepolarizing relaxants will then be potentiated whilst depolarizing agents will be antagonized. The converse is true if a membrane is hypopolarized. Depression of cholinesterase activity as may occur in moderate hypothermia will have little effect on normal neuromuscular transmission but will antagonize nondepolarizing relaxants and may potentiate depolarizing drugs. Potent anticholinesterases such as the organophosphates produce tachycardia, salivation and muscular excitability. Depression of the responsiveness of muscle to threshold depolarization occurs following pethidine, morphine, ether and other volatile anaesthetic agents which have muscle relaxant properties.

DISEASES OF THE PERIPHERAL NERVOUS SYSTEM

Those disease processes that produce the symptoms and pathological changes associated with lower motor neurone loss are included in this chapter. Some of them will result in denervation changes at the myoneural junction, weakness of the muscles of ventilation and autonomic imbalance and may, therefore, present the anaesthetists with hazards which are common to patients with peripheral nerve diseases and indeed their clinical effects may be due to a secondary depression of the reflex arc or due to a functional denervation of muscle.

Many of the symptoms of lower motor neurone disease are extremely difficult to distinguish from diseases affecting the peripheral axonal process itself, or its myelin sheath unless tested by specialized techniques. (See Appendix.) Loss of the myelin sheath is associated with a slowing of nerve conduction due to loss of saltatory conduction. Diseases presenting initially with symptoms limited to the peripheral nerves are discussed in the section 'Peripheral neuritis'.

Abnormalities of myoneural conduction, including myasthenia gravis, myasthenic and myopathic syndromes, are described followed by a brief classification of the muscular dystrophies and myotonias of interest to anaesthetists.

DISEASES OF THE LOWER MOTOR NEURONE

Lower motor neurone disease causes weakness and wasting of the muscles innervated by the affected neurones. During the degeneration of the muscles, fasciculation may occur. This is more common with slowly progressive disease of the neurones themselves than with nerve root involvement. As the efferent pathway of the reflex arc is involved, tendon reflexes will be diminished or absent and there will be muscular hypotonia. The response to muscle relaxants is unaffected unless the nerves to the muscles degenerate. If this occurs a reaction of degeneration will develop with loss of specificity of the end-plate area. Pain is not present unless the sensory nerve is also involved. The lesions and diseases which are most associated with signs and symptoms of lower motor neurone disease are listed in Table 7.1.

Table 7.1. The lesions and diseases which are most associated with signs and symptoms of lower motor neurone disease.

Congenital	Acquired
Spina bifida	Motor neurone disease
Syringomyelia	Poliomyelitis
	Tetanus
	Rabies
	Botulism

Spina bifida

This abnormality is caused by a failure of the embryonic neural groove to close. As a result there is a defect in the spinal cord usually associated with defective closure of the posterior aspect of the vertebral column. It is commonly associated with hydrocephalus. The extent of the defect varies from spina bifida *occulta* to a major defect of the vertebral column and spinal cord usually in the lumbosacral or lumbodorsal area. A sac of meninges, neural tissue and CSF overlie the defect.

The anaesthetist meets these patients when they present in the neonatal period for closure of the myelomeningocoele. Although the legs are usually paretic or paralysed there is thought to be little danger of an excessive K^+ flux with depolarizing relaxants. Closure of the spinal sac may provoke the development of hydrocephalus and necessitate anaesthesia for the insertion of a Spitz-Holter valve. The risk associated with the use of suxamethonium may be increased at this stage if there has been destruction of nerve tissues during closure of a large myelomeningocoele. In spite of this consideration, many hundreds of neonates have received suxamethonium for these operations without ill effects.

Syringomyelia

The aetiology of this disease is unknown. It presents as a slowly progressive weakness with wasting of the muscles of the hand, together with a loss of sensation to pain and temperature due to damage to the decussating fibres of the spinothalamic tract. The sensations of light touch, position and joint sense are retained since they do not cross in this way. This is associated with compression degeneration of the anterior horn cells, producing a lower motor neurone lesion. As the disease progresses the long descending spinal nerve tracts may become involved causing symptoms and signs of upper motor neurone lesions in the lower limb.

These patients may present for surgical operations designed to drain the cystic area of the cord or for cervical decompression. The muscular denervation associated with the disease does not appear to contraindicate the use of suxamethonium, presumably as the rate of functional denervation is very slow in most cases. Should there be a history of rapidly developing paralysis, possibly associated with a tumour producing the syringomyelia, then suxamethonium should be avoided. The dissociated sensory loss dictates that great care must be taken to prevent insensible trauma to the affected limbs.

Motor neurone disease

This is a group of degenerative diseases of the motor system of unknown cause affecting the motor nuclei of the cranial nerves (with the exception of those innervating the extra-ocular muscles), the anterior horn cells of the cord and pyramidal tracts. Not infrequently, all three types present simultaneously. The disease presents in middle life—more often in males than in females. Sensory changes are almost exclusively absent. Syndromes similar in nature and extent also develop after some forms of poisoning and some hereditary and deficiency diseases. Muscle biopsies show clear evidence of denervation degeneration. The three sites of the development of the changes carry with them three main presentations, namely progressive muscular atrophy, amyotrophic lateral sclerosis and bulbar palsy.

Progressive muscular atrophy

This is the commonest form of motor neurone disease and usually presents initially as a weakness of the muscles of the hand and forearm. In the very early stages there may be nothing notable beyond a clumsiness of the fingers leading to inability to fasten buttons. In other cases there is a foot-drop and dragging of the foot is the patient's main complaint.

The muscles of the thenar eminence waste early. Gradually, however, the weakness extends producing wrist drop or even a totally flaccid arm. Fasciculation is often scanty initially though it develops later. The symptoms and signs are asymmetrical at first, but eventually the condition spreads to involve the muscles of all the limbs and the trunk. At this stage there is extensive muscular atrophy and though the pyramidal tracts are almost invariably involved the weakness accompanying the muscle atrophy may lead to a diminution in the activity of the tendon reflexes. Extensor plantar responses can usually be elicited. In general the condition is progressive and ends fatally from two to five years after the initial diagnosis has been made.

Amyotrophic lateral sclerosis

This type of motor neurone disease usually presents with upper motor neurone signs in the lower limbs and lower motor neurone signs in the upper limbs. There is increasing stiffness of a leg which eventually spreads to the other leg. The patient's limbs are weak and the tendon reflexes grossly increased. The plantar responses are extensor, though the abdominal reflexes may be retained. The sphincters of the alimentary and urinary tract are initially intact. Subsequently, muscle fasciculation develops in the muscles of the shoulder girdle and in the thighs. Ultimately, the patient dies of associated bulbar palsy some two to five years from the appearance of the first presenting symptom.

Progressive bulbar palsy

Classically this condition presents as dysphagia and dysarthria. There is often a history of food sticking in the back of the throat or of attacks of choking. Nasal regurgitation of food is also common. The patient's voice is slurred and there may be palatal and pharyngeal paralysis. One characteristic of the former is the inability to pronounce the letter 'B' which is produced like an 'M'. On examination there is paresis of the palate, pharynx and tongue. Profuse fasciculation of the tongue is seen. The jaw jerk is exaggerated. Fasciculation is also observed in the muscles round the shoulder. The condition is progressive and most patients die of the consequences of respiratory tract soiling within a year to 18 months.

Anaesthetic significance

Patients with motor neurone disease may have rapidly progressive denervation of large muscle masses and there is a possibility that there will be a release of myoglobin from degenerating muscle under the influence of suxamethonium. This suggests that it should be avoided in the acute stages of this disease [5]. Sensitivity to nonpolarizing relaxants has also been reported [39]. Neostigmine may cause a tonic response. Patients with progressive bulbar palsy may be at risk during the recovery from an anaesthetic when their depressed swallowing reflexes, together with muscular weakness in the partially denervated tongue, may prove hazardous. These patients should not be extubated until fully conscious and then whenever possible in the lateral position. As with other acute diseases involving the spinal cord, it is advisable to avoid intrathecal and extradural anaesthesia lest the anaesthesia be blamed for increasing the rate of progression of the disease.

Poliomyelitis

This virus infection produces degeneration in the cells of the anterior horn, occasionally affecting those of the lateral horn, producing in addition to loss of motor function a degree of autonomic disturbance. The virus gains access to the body most often via the nasopharynx. By no means all those who are affected, however, develop muscular paralysis. They may simply have a pyrexial illness, or there may be nonspecific signs attributable to the central nervous system, such as headache and neck stiffness. Kernig's sign (limitation of leg extension on the flexed thigh) is often present and there is widespread muscular pain and tenderness in many cases and especially in those who are about to develop muscular paralysis.

Any region of the spinal cord may be affected by the disease, the symptoms produced being largely dependent upon the region involved. Paralysis is typically asymmetrical, but can spread upward after the manner of polyneuritis to induce respiratory paralysis or even bulbar palsy. On the whole, spread of paralysis ceases within 24 hours or at the most two or three days. Thereafter, there is a gradual recovery of much, but usually not of all of the paralysis. Further aspects are discussed in Chapter 8 (page 282).

8

The anaesthetist may become involved in the management of the acutely ill patient because of the need for artificial ventilation. The lack of venomotor control during the initial acute state of this disease may render these patients particularly susceptible to the effects of raised intrathoracic pressure during IPPV [54]. If hypotension occurs it usually responds to infusion of electrolyte solution sufficient to compensate for the increased venous capacity.

Patients who have muscle wasting secondary to the motor nerve involvement may present later for orthopaedic correction of their muscular deformities. The time between the acute disease leading to the muscle denervation and the surgery is usually sufficiently long to ensure that the muscles will not produce an abnormal response to suxamethonium. Patients who have apparently recovered from ventilatory insufficiency due to this disease must be regarded as permanently at risk from the effects of drugs that may produce a reduction of muscle power. After operation it is necessary to monitor the adequacy of ventilation during the postoperative period and to be prepared to ventilate the patient artificially should difficulty ensue. Deep anaesthesia with volatile agents, excessive doses of opiates and narcotics with muscle relaxant properties, the use of interneuronal blocking agents such as diazepam and residual weakness following the use of muscle relaxants may all cause ventilatory problems.

Tetanus

This disease is caused by an exotoxin liberated by *Clostridium tetani*. The water soluble toxin passes along neurovascular bundles to the anterior horn cells of the spinal cord and to the brain stem, causing diffuse neural excitation. The source of the tetanus bacillus is usually animal dung, and the disease most commonly therefore affects agricultural workers who suffer a deep penetrating wound. The first signs of the disease are muscular rigidity and stiffness in the muscles adjacent to the infected wound but soon the infection becomes more generalized and muscle spasms occur. One of the early signs is trismus which gives to the disease its popular name of 'lockjaw'. Spasms of the muscles of the pharynx give rise to dysphagia. The neck is stiff; the facial muscles become involved and produce a horrible fixed grin—'risus sardonicus'. If not treated, the fully established disease causes tonic convulsions to occur. All the muscles of the patient's back contract vigorously to produce a gross arching. There is an incubation period of a few days to a fortnight between the actual infection and the development of symptoms. The longer the incubation period, the better the prognosis.

Tetanus carries a high mortality due to apnoea associated with spasm of the muscles of ventilation occurring at times of high oxygen utilization by the tissues. The ability to control these dangerous spasms has reduced the overall mortality but in spite of this deaths still occur due to antonomic 'storms' associated with sympathetic hyperactivity, from toxic myocarditis and from brain stem lesions.

The neurological nature of the spasms of tetanus is a disturbance of the inhibitor elements involved in reflex activity, especially depression of the activity of the internuncial neurones and the Renshaw cells. Thus a small sensory stimulus which normally produced either no motor response or only a very slight one, gives rise to intense muscular activity over several segments of the spinal cord. The principles of treatment of the disease are now well established. Control of the infection by massive doses of antibiotics is a primary consideration.

Treatment of tetanus

There are two approaches to the drug treatment of the spasms. The more obvious method is to paralyse the patient so that spasms are no longer so disabling, to perform a tracheostomy which will allow the removal of any inhaled foreign material and to feed the patient either by means of small stomach tube or, if necessary, intravenously. The results of this form of treatment when it was first introduced some twenty years ago, were so outstandingly good that they gave a considerable impetus to the developments of units specially directed toward the treatment of tetanus. It is however possible to treat tetanus with drugs which depress the activity of the internuncial neurones of the spinal cord and especially to prevent the wide spread of excitation which causes the spasms. Diazepam and chlorpromazine have both been widely used and the results have been so good that the need for treatment by paralysis and artificial ventilation (which is always a slightly hazardous proceeding, particularly in the neonate) is much less clamant. However, in severe cases, periods of apnoea may occur even without associated spasm of the muscles of ventilation and this indicates the need for more active treatment involving muscle relaxants and artificial ventilation. Curare appears to be the relaxant of choice, although autonomic nervous system involvement may affect the normal venomotor compensation to IPPV and hypotension may result. Gallamine is less suitable as a muscle relaxant due to the tachycardia produced and its marked cumulative properties, especially if renal function is impaired. Pancuronium is contraindicated if any autonomic instability is present as it may trigger off sympathetic discharge causing dangerous hypertension and left ventricular cardiac failure. Episodes of hypotension occurring during the treatment of tetanus are not always the result of therapy; it is now appreciated that a toxic myocarditis, producing changes in the ST segment and T wave of the ECG are not uncommon. If the hypotension is associated with bradycardia, with or without ventilatory depression, it is probable that there is brain stem involvement by the tetanus toxin and the outlook is poor.

Rabies

This virus disease is spread by rabid animals who bite and infect humans with the virus laden saliva which contaminates the wound. Although rare in the U.K., due to strict quarantine regulations for imported animals, it is endemic in many parts of the world. The spread of air travel has resulted in isolated cases occurring in almost every country.

Following infection, the virus passes along the nerve trunks to the brain and spinal cord where it proliferates. The disease causes violent painful spasms and increased reflex excitability. Painful spasms of the muscles of mastication and ventilation occur. For the established disease treatment may necessitate paralysis with a muscle relaxant and artificial ventilation; in spite of therapy there is a high mortality.

Botulism

This very rare disease is the result of infection with the exotoxin of another anaerobic organism *Clostridium botulinum*. It follows the ingestion of infected tinned food. Apart from diarrhoea and vomiting, initial symptoms are related to disturbance of the function of the cranial nerves resulting in ptosis, dysphagia, dysarthria and weakness of the jaw muscles. The toxin affects the motor nerves blocking the release of acetylcholine at the neuromuscular junction, and causing paralysis. Guanidine and the

Veratrum alkaloids, which are believed to act by facilitating the release of acetylcholine may be useful in treatment. An antitoxin is effective if given very early in the condition. Although 4-aminopyridine can be demonstrated to be an effective antidote in experimental botulism, it failed to produce a demonstrable improvement in neuromuscular function in patients suffering from this disease in doses short of those producing convulsions [1].

DISEASES OF PERIPHERAL NERVES

PERIPHERAL NEUROPATHIES

These are disorders of the structure and function of peripheral nerves. The symptoms will depend upon the site and extent of the nerve involvement, rather than the aetiological pathology. Thomas [48] divides the neuropathies into the following.

Symmetrical neuropathy: usually starting distally with loss of vibration and joint sensation, followed by loss of tendon reflexes, weakness and muscle wasting.
Mononeuritis: affecting single and multiple large nerves, i.e. median, ulnar lateral-popliteal neuropathy, Bell's palsy etc.
Autonomic neuropathy: characterized by loss of sweating, fainting attacks associated with hypotension on assuming erect posture, sphincter involvement, urinary symptoms, pupillary abnormalities and impotence.

The neuropathies may be divided into two groups according to the pathological process which predominates.
1 'Dying back' neuropathies, due to primary involvement of the nerve cell, the anterior horn cell in the case of motor nerves and the posterior root ganglion cell in the case of sensory nerves.

Table 7.2. Causes of segmental demyelination and axonal degeneration (after Heathfield [23]).

Causes of segmental demyelination	Causes of axonal degeneration
1 Acute neuropathies (Guillain–Barré)	(*a*) alcoholic neuropathy
2 Subacute and chronic neuropathies	(*b*) diphtheria neuropathy
(*a*) ischaemia or pressure	(*c*) porphyria
(*b*) idiopathic neuritis	(*d*) toxic neuropathies
(*c*) nutritional and metabolic	
diabetes	
alcoholic	
vitamin B_{12} deficiency	
uraemia	
myxoedema	
acromegaly	
liver failure	
amyloid	
(*d*) collagen diseases	
(*e*) carcinoma	
(*f*) peroneal muscular atrophy	

2   Primary disease of the nerve itself usually associated with Schwann cell loss, loss of myelin sheath and segmental demyelination. The Schwann cells are believed to fulfil a trophic function to the nerve in the same way as the glial cells associated with the neurones are believed to play an important role in maintaining the metabolic homeostasis of the neurones. Nerve conduction tests (see Appendix) may be used in order to differentiate between 'dying back' neuropathies and segmental demyelinating neuropathies. Conduction time is little affected by 'dying back' neuropathies but may be considerably prolonged in demyelinating conditions. Heathfield [23] classifies the diseases as being associated with either segmental demyelination or axonal degeneration. The causes of segmental demyelination and anoxal degeneration are listed in Table 7.2.

SEGMENTAL DEMYELINATIONS

ACUTE NEUROPATHY—ACUTE POLYNEURITIS

Guillain–Barré syndrome

This condition often follows a viral infection, commonly by the glandular fever virus, although it may also complicate herpes zoster, infective hepatitis, mumps and cytomegalic virus. It has been suggested that as a result of the virus infection, sensitized lymphocytes destroy the Schwann cells causing segmental degeneration. If there is paralysis of the muscles of respiration and swallowing, urgent tracheostomy and artificial ventilation may be necessary. This syndrome is probably part of a spectrum of disease processes extending from encephalitis, through encephalomyelitis, myelitis, polyradiculitis to some types of peripheral neuritis (discussed in more detail in Chapter 8, page 280). The prognosis is good if management is adequate.

Some cases of acute neuropathy are a manifestation of acute porphyria and the urine and faeces should be examined for porphyrins.

Subacute and chronic neuropathies

Ischaemia and pressure

Ischaemia is probably the commonest cause of chronic or subacute neuropathy involving a major nerve trunk. This may be primary, due to disease of the blood vessels as in diabetes, periarteritis nodosa, or secondary to pressure as with a prolapsed intervertebral disc.

Other common pressure or ischaemic neuropathies include nerve entrapment syndromes, carpal tunnel syndrome and median nerve compression. Systemic diseases, in particular diabetes, increase the vulnerability of peripheral nerves to direct trauma so that pressure neuropathies are more common in these patients. Although often included in this category, Volkmann's ischaemic contracture is more truly an effect of ischaemic changes in the muscle rather than being primarily neuromuscular in origin.

Idiopathic neuropathies

Many cases of transient motor nerve dysfunction and sensory change cannot be readily attributed to any specific aetiological agent. Probably the commonest idiopathic neuropathy is Bell's facial palsy.

Facial nerve palsy can be a symptom of many conditions such as multiple sclerosis, leukaemia, parotid tumour, sarcoid, poliomyelitis and herpes zoster. However, all of these are rare compared to the idiopathic form of Bell's palsy. The onset of symptoms is often preceded by exposure of the face to a draught. Occasionally, it is associated with or preceded by loss of taste on the same side as the palsy. The prognosis for complete recovery is best in those patients who reveal no evidence of depression of nerve conduction following electrical stimulation. Recovery may be delayed for many months and may be incomplete in those more severely affected by the disease. Some authorities advocate treating the condition with steroids if the patient presents within five days of the onset of symptoms; however, the results are equivocal.

NUTRITIONAL NEUROPATHIES

Diabetic neuropathy

This often affects sensory nerves producing diabetic pseudotabes or may affect autonomic nerves when it may present as diabetic atonic bladder, impotence, loss of sweating, loss of pupillary reflexes, loss of cardiac reflexes and altered oesophageal motility (see Chapter 15). The cranial nerves may rarely be affected. It frequently occurs in elderly patients with mild or even undetected diabetes.

Alcoholic neuropathy

This is associated with thiamine deficiency and occurs in spirit rather than beer drinkers (see Chapter 12). Axonal degeneration causing foot drop is common in addition to the symmetrical demyelination. It may be associated with Wernicke's encephalopathy which may cause cranial nerve palsies due to brain stem haemorrhage.

Vitamin B_{12} deficiency

This is associated with pernicious anaemia (see page 341) and subacute combined degeneration of the spinal cord. The combination of cord and peripheral nerve degeneration causes a clinical picture of mixed upper and lower motor neurone loss and is discussed in Chapter 8 (page 284).

Uraemic neuropathy

This commonly occurs in elderly patients. This may be the cause of a lethal shift of potassium ions upon administration of suxamethonium [32].

Myxoedema and acromegaly

These may be associated with a segmental neuropathy.

Liver failure

This is also a very rare cause of neuropathy, as is *amyloid* following chronic infection.

Collagen disease neuropathies

A chronic neuropathy may occur as a complication of polyarteritis nodosa, dermato-myositis and other collagen diseases: polyarteritis nodosa may also cause an ischaemic neuropathy. In these patients the neuritis is secondary to the underlying inflammatory process and the progress of the symptoms of the peripheral nerve disease will be secondary to that of the primary pathological process.

Carcinomatous neuropathies

These may present as either sensory or motor loss. Not infrequently the carcinoma is very small or indeed may only be found on autopsy. It is most commonly reported associated with carcinoma of the bronchus, although it may occur in Hodgkin's disease and in reticuloses, especially when the tumour is largely intrathoracic. The reason for the neuropathy is not clear. It may be due to a nutritional defect but is more likely to be due to an autoimmune response of the lymphocytes to tumour cells. It is suggested that the immunized lymphocytes produce degenerative changes in the Schwann cell causing demyelination.

Peroneal muscular atrophy (Charcot-Marie-Tooth disease)

This is the commonest of a group of familial polyneuritides. It is transmitted as an autosomal dominant characteristic. The course of this and the related muscular atrophies are relatively benign although the foot and leg weaknesses are commonly progressive until shortly after puberty. The disease is almost invariably confined to the distal parts of the limbs. As a consequence the legs look like inverted champagne bottles. These patients frequently present for orthopaedic correction of their malformations and present no special anaesthetic hazard.

AXONAL DEGENERATION (see Table 7.2)

Toxic neuropathies

The list of drugs and toxic substances increases with the prevalent pollution of the environment and the increased usage of potent drugs. The heavy metals have long been known to cause neuropathy. As the result of environmental pollution heavy metal poisoning is becoming increasingly important in the differential diagnosis of epidemics of toxic neuropathies.

Drugs such as phenytoin, isoniazid, thalidomide, methaqualone, nitrofurantoin, vincristine, acrilamide (used as a commercial solvent) and thallium are known to cause toxic neuropathies affecting axons of nerves. Orthocresylphosphates in diesel oil have also caused a minor epidemic of toxic neuropathy.

Diphtheritic neuritis is rare in the western world due to immunization. It frequently affects the cranial and cervical nerves.

Porphyria can cause either a severe neurological defect or a progressive peripheral neuritis. It should be suspected in any acute onset peripheral neuritis, especially if it is associated with autonomic disturbances (see Chapter 9, page 306).

Alcoholic neuritis can involve either the cell bodies causing a 'die back' neuritis, or the nerve itself. It is usually considered as a nutritional neuropathy as it is thought to be secondary to an incomplete dietary intake of the B complex vitamins.

Malformation of nerves

Von Recklinghausen's disease (multiple neurofibromatosis)

This is an inherited condition associated with a Mendelian dominant gene. They may be either sessile or pedunculated pink swellings. When they are sessile they are freely movable on the deep tissues though frequently adherent to skin. The lesions produced are believed to be benign malformations of the neurilemmal sheath in which the Schwann cells and fibroblasts proliferate to form multiple tumours. There is often an accompanying café-au-lait pigmentation of the skin in multiple spots or in larger diffuse areas with an irregular edge. Plexiform enlargement of peripheral nerves some-times occurs, often accompanied by overgrowth of the skin and subcutaneous tissue, to produce a seeming localized elephantiasis. Neurofibromas can also develop in re-lation to spinal nerve roots and are not infrequently intrathecal where they cause spinal cord compression. They may also compress spinal roots in the intervertebral foramina. In the thoracic region particularly, such tumours often have an extraspinal extension which appears as a large shadow in the paravertebral gutter on a chest X-ray. They are often otherwise symptomless. Neurofibromas occasionally develop in the foramen magnum. The acoustic neuroma, so-called, is probably also basically a neurofibroma.

Denervation changes are not common. Should they be present, muscle relaxants should be used with caution. Usually the response to suxamethonium is either normal or diminished. In some cases this resistance to suxamethonium is associated with a marked sensitivity to nondepolarizing muscle relaxants causing a myasthenic type of response. This is probably the result of a reduced production or release of acetylcholine due to the abnormality of the nerve itself [4]. The response must be relatively rare. Yamashita *et al.* [56] have reported both unusual sensitivity and resistance to suxa-methonium. A large number of cases have been anaesthetized without serious incident. (A. R. Hunter, Personal Communication, 1975.)

MYASTHENIA GRAVIS AND MYASTHENIC SYNDROMES

Myasthenia gravis

Myasthenia gravis is a disease associated with a defect of myoneural transmission which is typically alleviated by the use of anticholinesterase drugs. The disease presents as muscle weakness or excessive fatiguability. The presenting symptoms and the pro-gress of the disease in the first five years are so variable that the diagnosis may be difficult and may rest upon the ability to demonstrate the beneficial effect of anti-cholinesterase drugs, a persistent fade at low rates of stimulation (2 Hz), post-tetanic facilitation and tetanic fade on electrical stimulation of motor nerves to affected muscles. The EMG shows a decrease in the height of successsive action potentials produced by motor nerve stimulation (decremental response).

The commonest muscles to be affected by the disease are those of the orbit and mouth, pharynx and shoulder girdle. The levator palpebrae superioris muscle is commonly affected and this produces drooping of the eyelid. Diplopia, difficulty in swallowing and dysarthria are common presenting symptoms. The involvement of the muscles of the hand leading to clumsiness and inability to perform repeated fine movements causes confusion in diagnosing the disease. Characteristically, the weakness, which starts off being transient, becomes more prolonged and frequent. It is typically more noticeable after exercise of a particular group of muscles, thus the dysarthria becomes more pronounced as the patient counts. In advanced cases weakness of muscles of ventilation occurs. Some wasting of muscles may occur but other neurological signs are usually absent and tendon reflexes are intact or brisk. The symptoms and signs of myasthenia closely resemble those produced by an injection of a small dose of curare into a healthy individual.

In view of the depressed margin of safety of neuromuscular transmission in patients with myasthenia gravis it is not surprising that they should be exquisitely sensitive to curare-like drugs and benefit from anticholinesterase drugs. In these patients 1·5 to 3 mg of *d*-tubocurarine may produce complete neuromuscular block of prolonged duration. It has been observed [7] that in addition to this sensitivity to nondepolarizing relaxants, myasthenic patients also exhibit an abnormal response to depolarizing neuromuscular blocking agents, a response that resembles that termed 'dual block' and demonstrated in the chick by Zaimis using tridecamethonium. These patients are resistant to paralysis by depolarizing drugs which produce a phase II block with properties that closely resemble those produced by curare in a normal individual. This observation has been repeatedly confirmed and suggests that the postsynaptic membrane response to depolarizing drugs differs from that of a normal adult.

The symptoms of myasthenia gravis have been ascribed to (a) the presence of 'curare-like' substances in the circulation [45, 46], (b) an abnormality of acetylcholine production or release [12, 17], or (c) a defect of the cholinergic receptors on the post-synaptic membrane [6].

Until 10–15 years ago most of the observations in this disease suggested that it was a primary disease of acetylcholine synthesis or release. The production of transmitter in a releasable form appeared to be insufficient to keep pace with the requirements of rapid rates of motor nerve discharge. In view of the large margin of safety of normal acetylcholine production, this will only become obvious when the available acetylcholine is depressed below 40 per cent of normal. This lack of transmitter would account for the 'train of four' twitch depression [25], the post-tetanic exhaustion phenomena [8] and the reduction of miniature end-plate potentials [11].

Present evidence strongly supports the view that myasthenia gravis is the result of an autoimmune disease in which antibodies are produced against the acetylcholine receptors at the motor end-plate. This accounts for the immediate transferable effects that can be produced in some animals injected with the serum from myasthenic patients. This binding of antibody to receptor sites has been demonstrated in the rat and mouse [3, 29, 50]. Binding of antibody to receptor site would also explain the temporary myasthenic state in babies born to myasthenic mothers. Although anticholinesterase drugs may be required to combat the muscle weakness, the effect usually lasts only 1–12 weeks.

Simpson [41] and Nastuk *et al.* [34] postulated an autoimmune basis for myasthenia gravis on the basis of its similarity with other autoimmune diseases with which it occasionally occurs, the involvement of the thymus and beneficial effects of thymectomy and corticosteroid therapy, and the occurrence of high titres of antibodies in some patients with the disease. This theory has now received widespread experimental support [33]. Although not all patients with myasthenia gravis have antibodies, to striatcl muscle many patients have demonstrable antibodies to α-bungarotoxin receptors (anti-acetylcholine receptor antibodies) [2]. The use of a radio-immunoassay to detect the receptor antibodies in patients with the disease has demonstrated that the titre of antibodies approximately corresponds to the severity of the patient's symptoms and this has become a standard diagnostic test. However, no antibodies have been demonstrated in over 10 per cent of patients with the disease, in particular in those patients with involvement of the ocular muscles alone. Experimental receptor substance antibody prepared by injecting foreign receptor substance into animals as well as the immunoglobulin from patients with a high titre of antibody can cause a decrease in α-bungarotoxin receptor in muscle cultures [13]. It is postulated that there is an increased rate of destruction of these receptors as a result of the receptor antibody activity and that this eventually causes the morphological changes found at the end-plates in patients with this disease. It is possible that in addition to an increased destruction of receptors there may be interference with the usual rapid formation of new receptors at the postsynaptic membrane.

As a result of this process the number of receptor sites available for acetylcholine at the end-plate are diminished and the margin of safety for neuromuscular transmission is consequently reduced.

Because of the very varied presentation and natural history of the disease it is likely that more than one antibody is involved. The varying titre of each antibody in this spectrum determines the predominant type of lesion produced.

The treatment of myasthenia gravis consists of the administration of atropine and anticholinesterase drugs, of which pyridostigmine (Mestinon) 60 mg to 240 mg and neostigmine 15 to 60 mg by mouth are most useful. Atropine is usually required to prevent the bradycardia and to minimize the cramp-like abdominal pains which are more frequently complained of when neostigmine is administered.

Patients whose symptoms are inadequately controlled by anticholinesterase drugs or in whom there is a rapid progression of symptoms should be treated with corticosteroids. It is advisable to initiate the treatment with high doses of prednisolone which may be slowly reduced [24]. Once the treatment is established it is often possible to administer the steroids on alternate days so as to minimize the side effects. Regular anticholinesterase therapy is nearly always required in addition. Should this regime prove inadequate to control the symptoms, or if there is evidence of a tumour of the thymus, thymectomy is advised. Thymectomy followed by radiotherapy is advocated more frequently and earlier than in the past [30] largely due to the reduced incidence of postoperative morbidity, associated with better postoperative care. The operation is indicated if a tumour is present, if the patient is young and the symptoms become rapidly more severe and if conservative measures fail [28]. It is of lesser advantage in the older patients in whom there is little thymic tissue. In patients unsuitable for thymectomy, immunosuppressive therapy may produce an amelioration of the patient's symptoms. Azathioprine has been used with some success in up to 80 per cent of patients treated. However, the side effects of long termed immunosuppressive therapy make it less suitable for the treatment of young patients or mild cases of myasthenia gravis.

Patients on long term anticholinesterase therapy occasionally become increasingly resistant to the drugs, possibly as a result of desensitization of the end-plates. In these patients it is recommended to stop all anticholinesterase drugs for 1–2 weeks. This usually necessitates bed rest and may require tracheostomy to prevent aspiration of secretions and food. In severe cases, artificial ventilation will be required. The use of plasmapheresis during acute exacerbations of the disease or during an anticholinesterase resistant episode occasionally produces a dramatic but temporary improvement in the patient's symptoms [10]. This improvement can often be prolonged by the administration of immunosuppressive drugs [31].

Anaesthetists may be called upon to help in the diagnosis of myasthenia gravis. The increase in twitch height or in the EMG potential of the adductor pollucis muscles to ulnar nerve stimulation following the administration of edrophonium constitutes an unequivocal diagnostic test. Patients with this disease demonstrate poorly maintained tetanic contraction and marked post-tetanic facilitation similar to that seen after the administration of a nondepolarizing relaxant. If the degree of post-tetanic facilitation is less than 25 per cent greater than the pretetanic twitch height then the response to a train of 4 stimuli at 16 ms intervals may be used to demonstrate fatigue [38]. An alternative diagnostic test is to demonstrate exaggerated paralytic response of the isolated arm to an intravenous injection of 0·5 mg of curare in 30 ml of saline [19]. Feldman [18] has demonstrated that the same technique can be used to demonstrate the propensity of myasthenic patients to develop dual block after decamethonium.

Should a myasthenic patient require anaesthesia it is advisable to avoid the use of muscle relaxants whenever possible. However, if thoracotomy for a thymoma is to be carried out, it is usual to ventilate the patient artificially in the postoperative period. Under these circumstances the use of a small dose of nondepolarizing relaxant is permissible (3–5 mg *d*-tubocurarine), although in the author's experience it is seldom required. Should muscle relaxation be required either due to the nature of the operation or in order to effect tracheal intubation, this can usually be obtained by omitting all anticholinsterase drugs for the 4 hours preceding the operation. In these circumstances the patient should be observed carefully for signs of ventilatory inadequacy or difficulty in swallowing during this period. A normal premedication is not contraindicated in these patients and thiopentone may safely be used for induction. A volatile anaesthetic may be used to deepen the anaesthesia sufficiently to allow easy tracheal intubation. There is no contraindication to the use of limited local anaesthetic techniques in patients suffering from this disease although the total safe dose of drugs such as procaine and lignocaine is reduced as these may further depress neuromuscular conduction. Following anaesthesia all myasthenic patients must be observed closely for signs of weakness of the oropharyngeal and respiratory muscles. Atropine 1 mg and pyridostigmine (2·5 mg) i.v. or neostigmine (1–2 mg) i.v. should be given as and when respiratory weakness is evident or when the patient complains of weakness, diplopia or dysarthria.

The myasthenic syndrome

Many patients with malignant disease complain of excessive fatiguability, occasionally but not invariably associated with muscle wasting [16]. The condition is especially frequent in patients with carcinoma of the bronchus but may occur in patients with other forms of malignant disease. It is occasionally associated with motor neuropathy. In a study of myasthenic syndrome patients, it was demonstrated that they differed from patients suffering from myasthenia gravis in that they do not demonstrate fade following low frequency tetanic stimulation, indeed the EMG potential usually increases [55]. There is no evidence of post-tetanic exhaustion as found in patients with myasthenia gravis. The response to muscle relaxants in patients with this condition is sufficiently unpredictable to caution against their use whenever possible. The patients usually respond normally to depolarizing relaxants; however, prolonged paralysis following suxamethonium does occur. There is invariably a prolonged response to nondepolarizing agents which are not easily reversed by anticholinesterase drugs. 4-aminopyridine—a drug which increases calcium flux secondary to its effect on the potassium/sodium pores in the cell membrane—has been shown to improve effectively the EMG response to patients with this disease.

FAMILIAL PERIODIC PARALYSIS

This familial disease, although rare, is of great interest to anaesthetists. It presents in one of two ways [51]. The commoner, which is manifest as bouts of excessive fatiguability and paresis, is associated with a fall in plasma potassium concentration consequent upon a shift of this ion from the extracellular space into the cell. The ensuing hyperpolarization of the cell membrane causes cardiac dysrhythmias and resistance to acetylcholine at the myoneural junction. These patients will exhibit a myasthenic-like sensitivity to nondepolarizing muscle relaxants during an acute episode of the disease. Attacks of muscle weakness frequently occur in the evening, frequently proceeded by a sensation of hunger, sweating, dryness of the mouth, followed by a large carbohydrate meal. It is the subsequent rise in the blood sugar and the release of insulin that is believed to actually produce the shift in potassium causing the paralytic symptoms.

The more unusual form of this disease, hyperkalaemic periodic paralysis, is associated with a shift of potassium from within the cell into the plasma. It is commoner in early childhood and is associated with cramp-like pains on exercise. In extreme cases a depolarizing type of block will occur as a result of the fall in the transmembrane potential. During an attack the patient will be resistant to nondepolarizing relaxants.

MCARDLE'S DISEASE

The rare metabolic myopathy of McArdle's disease (deficient phosphorylase activity) has been reported to sensitize the muscle to the action of suxamethonium causing excessive liberation of myoglobin and the production of myoglobinuria. However, myoglobinuria is probably produced in many patients in subclinical concentrations as the result of exposure to suxamethonium and the finding in McArdle's disease may merely be an exaggeration of a normal response.

MYASTHENIC STATES ASSOCIATED WITH OTHER SYSTEMIC DISEASE

Muscular disease may be associated with thyrotoxicosis and myxoedema. It presents the anaesthetist with the problems of the underlying disease process, together with the problems of a patient with generalized muscle weakness. In the case of thyrotoxic myopathy there may be considerable loss of muscle mass and a myasthenic-like weakness which does not respond to edrophonium. It is possible for the residual weakness that may follow the use of muscle relaxant drugs, to cause ventilatory failure.

A similar myopathy may occur in Cushing's disease or following excessive corticosteroid therapy. In these patients it is possible that a chronic shift in electrolytes due to the effect of the mineralocorticoids might be involved in the abnormal end-plate response.

MYASTHENIC STATES ASSOCIATED WITH IONIC IMBALANCE

Acute shifts or losses of potassium are most important in this context as a chronic potassium depletion is more likely to be equally borne by both the intra- and extracellular stores of this ion. Sudden potassium depletion associated with muscle weakness can occur as the result of massive mucus loss due to mucus secreting tumours of the large bowel and the result of vigorous diuresis induced by frusemide. This is especially likely in the immediate postoperative period when the potassium loss in the urine is exaggerated by the normal response to surgery. Occasionally, severe calcium depletion may produce a similar condition due to the loss of this ion's facilitating effect on acetylcholine release. The administration of magnesium will have a similar effect on neuromuscular transmission to that caused by calcium depletion.

HYPOTHERMIA

Cold has a complex effect on neuromuscular transmission. The initial effect may be a depression of cholinesterase activity and antagonism to the effect of curare-like drugs. Below 30°C the synthesis and release of acetylcholine is impaired in dogs and marked potentiation of the duration of action of nondepolarizing drugs is evident [49]. At these lower temperatures a myasthenic state is induced due to a reduction in the margin of safety of neuromuscular transmission.

PROGRESSIVE MUSCULAR DYSTROPHY AND MYOTONIA

This includes a large variety of diseases, many of which are exceedingly rare. As a result the classification of the muscular dystrophies is difficult. They can be classified on the basis of pathological appearance or, more readily, on the clinical presentations.

Walton [52] defined muscular dystrophy as a 'progressive, genetically determined primary degenerative myopathy'. However, even this definition is open to question. Some forms of the disease are either not progressive or so slowly progressive that they appear to burn themselves out. The evidence that all are genetically determined is uncertain and there is evidence that at least some of the dystrophies are secondary to loss of neurogenic trophic properties.

Walton & Gardner-Medwin's [53] clinical classification is given in Table 7.3.

Table 7.3. Clinical classification of muscular dystrophies [53].

(*a*) X-linked muscular dystrophy	1 Severe (Duchenne type)
	2 Benign
(*b*) Autosomal recessive muscular dystrophy	1 Limb girdle types
	2 Child muscular dystrophy
	3 Congenital muscular dystrophies
(*c*) Fascioscapulohumeral muscular dystrophy	
(*d*) Distal muscular dystrophy	
(*e*) Ocular muscular dystrophy	
(*f*) Oculopharyngeal muscular dystrophy	

X-LINKED MUSCULAR DYSTROPHY (DUCHENNE)

This is exclusively restricted to males, except for the rare occurrence in Turner's syndrome (XO chromosomes, see Chapter 9). It occurs early in life, rarely later than 6 years of age. It affects the muscles of the pelvic girdle followed by shoulder girdle and causes relentlessly progressive weakness, eventually crippling the patient. The cardiac muscle is commonly involved and death occurs due to respiratory weakness or cardiac failure. There is early contracture of muscles and increasing scoliosis. Death usually occurs before the age of 25 years. Neurological examination shows depressed tendon reflexes in upper limbs and knee although ankle jerks remain brisk. The ECG may show tall R waves in the right precordial leads and Q waves in the limb leads due to myocardial involvement. Tachycardia is common. The serum CPK (creatine phosphokinase) is raised.

The rarer form of the more benign disease occurs later in life and is transmitted by affected males through carrier daughters to grandsons. It does not produce severe muscular contractures and deformities and the life span may be essentially normal. The serum CPK is less raised than in the Duchenne type. Cardiac involvement does not occur. A carrier of the disease may be detected by tests including electromyography, muscle biopsy and muscle enzyme studies (the lactic acid dehydrogenase may be abnormal).

AUTOSOMAL RECESSIVE DYSTROPHIES

Limb girdle muscular dystrophy

This can occur in either sex being transmitted as an autosomal recessive trait. The onset of this disease is usually delayed until the second or third decade and in most patients it progresses to become crippling in middle life. The first muscles involved are those of the shoulder or pelvic girdle but it often progresses to involve other muscles.

Childhood muscular dystrophy

This is a rare form of proximal muscular dystrophy occurring in both sexes.

Congenital muscular dystrophy

This is associated with 'floppiness' at birth, occasionally complicated by arthrogryphosis multiplex.

Fascioscapulohumeral muscular dystrophy

This may occur in either sex and may not become obvious until adult development is reached. It appears to be a remitting disease although over a prolonged period of time it is usually progressive. It involves the face and shoulder girdle although it commonly spreads to affect the pelvic girdle. Abortive cases occur and most patients live a normal life.

DISTAL MYOPATHY

This condition is difficult to distinguish from the neuromyopathies as the symptoms are similar to peroneal muscular atrophy, but it is not associated with diminished vibration sense and delayed nerve conduction.

OCULAR MYOPATHY

This is more commonly associated with myotonic dystrophy. In true cases it may be associated with weakness of facial and shoulder girdle muscles. These patients may present for surgery for correction of squints. It has been reported that these patients are usually sensitive to curare-like drugs although their symptoms are unaffected by anticholinesterase drugs [40].

OCULOPHARYNGEAL MYOPATHY

This subdivision of ocular myopathy is unusual in that it also involves the smooth muscle of the pharynx. Most families reported have been of French-Canadian stock.

MYOTONIC DISORDERS

Myotonia is associated with muscular contraction that continues after the termination of a voluntary effort.

The condition is due to disease of the muscle fibres and affects all muscles. The EMG findings demonstrate repetitive after-discharge that occur after nerve block, nerve section and in spite of curarization [11]. Clinically it is associated with inability to loosen the grip of the hand, muscle cramps and stiffness. The condition is hereditary, associated with an autosomal dominant pattern of inheritance. The commonest syndromes are myotonia congenita (Thompson's disease) and dystrophia myotonia. Rarer forms of myotonia may be associated with attacks of muscle spasm brought on by cold and exertion. Myotonia atrophica is associated with atrophy of the muscles.

The symptoms of myotonia congenita usually begin soon after birth and may affect any muscle; they include pain and stiffness in the muscles accentuated by cold. Hypertrophy of muscle masses may occur as the disease progresses. In this condition there is a decremental response of the EMG to repetitive stimulation.

In dystrophia myotonica, the myotonia is associated with muscular atrophy, frontal baldness, cataracts and gonadal atrophy. In some patients cardiac and respiratory impairment may be present adding to the difficulties of anaesthesia. Changes in bone, endocrine function and mental ability may occur. The disease tends to become more severe and its onset earlier in successive generations, although it has been argued that due to an increased awareness of the possibility of the disease occurring in children of affected parents this observation is more apparent than real. Weakness and wasting of the limb muscles, fascial muscles and the muscles of mastication occurs. The disease is progressive and the patient usually becomes bedridden by the early forties.

Sudden cardiac failure, possibly due to ventricular arrhythmias, has been reported.

These patients present special risks during anaesthesia because of frequent occurrence of concomitant heart and respiratory disease, weakness of the jaw muscles and a tendency for prolonged respiratory depression following normal doses of anaesthetic drugs [37].

Abnormal sensitivity to thiopentone associated with respiratory depression has been reported [15, 20] and a normal neuromuscular response following thiopentone has also been found. The reaction to muscle relaxants in these patients is often abnormal.

There have been reports of severe muscle spasm in a patient with this disease after the administration of depolarizing drugs but this is not consistent [26]. Muscle spasms may also be produced during spinal and ether anaesthesia in patients with this disease. It is recommended that suxamethonium should not be used in these patients if at all possible and the minimum dose of thiopentone used to achieve hypnosis. Procainamide, ACTH and potassium depletion by ion exchange resins have been suggested as suitable treatments for dangerous myotonic spasms.

The similarity of the muscle spasms occurring in myotonia following injection of suxamethonium and that occurring in malignant hyperpyrexia suggested a common aetiological pathology. However, it is now believed that patients susceptible to malignant hyperplexia represent a separate genetic myopathy (see below).

ACKNOWLEDGMENT

I would like to acknowledge the invaluable help and advice given by Dr L. J. Findley of the MRC Hearing and Balance Unit, Institute of Neurology, Queen Square, London.

REFERENCES

1 AGOSTON S. Personal communication. 1979.
2 ALMON RR, ANDREW CG, APPEL SH. Serum globulin in myasthenia gravis; inhibition of α-bungarotoxin binding to acetylcholine receptors. *Science* 1974; **186**: 55–7.
3 ANWYL R, APPEL SM, NARAHASHI T. Myasthenia gravis serum reduces acetylcholine sensitivity in cultured rat myotubes. *Nature* 1977; **267**: 262–3.
4 BARAKA A. Myasthenic response to muscle relaxants in von Recklinghausen's disease. *Br J Anaesth* 1974; **46**: 701–3.
5 BEACH TP, STONE WA, HAMELBERG W. Circulatory collapse following succinylcholine: report of a patient with diffuse lower motor neurone disease. *Anesth Analg* 1971; **50**: 431–7.
6 CHURCHILL-DAVIDSON HC, RICHARDSON AT. Motor end plate differences as a determining factor in the mode of action of neuro-muscular blocking substances. *Nature* 1952; **170**: 617–18.
7 CHURCHILL-DAVIDSON HC, RICHARDSON AT. Decamethonium iodide (C10). Some observations using electromyography. *Proc Roy Soc Med* 1953; **45**: 179–86.
8 COOPERMAN LH. Succinylcholine-induced hyperkalemia in neuromuscular disease. *JAMA* 1970; **213**: 1867–71.
9 COGWILL DB, MOSTELLO LA, SHAPIRO HM. Encephalitis and a hyperkalemic response to succinylcholine. *Anesthesiology* 1974; **40**: 409–11.
10 DAU PC, LINDSTROM JM, CASSEL CK, DENYS EH, SHEV EE, SPITLER LE. Plasmapheresis and immunosuppressive drug therapy in myasthenia gravis. *N Engl J Med* 1977; **297**: 1134–40.
11 DENNY-BROWN D, NEVIN S. The phenomenon of myotonia. *Brain* 1941; **64**: 1–18.
12 DESMEDT JE. Bases physiopathologiques du diagnostic de la myasthénie par le test de Jolly. *Rev Neur Par* 1957; **96**: 505–6.
13 DRACHMAN DB, KAE L, ANGUS CW, MURPHY A. Effects of myasthenic immunoglobulin on acetylcholine receptors of cultured muscle. *Ann Neurol* 1977; **1**: 504.
14 DRACHMAN DB. Myasthenia gravis. *N Engl J Med* 1978; **298**: 186–93.
15 DUNDEE JW. Thiopentone in dystrophia myotonica. *Anesth Analg* 1952; **31**: 257–62.
16 EATON LM, LAMBERT EH. Electromyography and electrical stimulation of nerves in diseases of motor unit. Observations on myasthenic syndrome associated with malignant tumours. *JAMA* 1957; **163**: 1117–24.
17 ELMQVIST D. Neuromuscular transmission with special reference to myasthenia gravis. *Acta Physiol Scand* 1965; **64**. Suppl 249: 1–34.
18 FELDMAN SA. Muscle relaxants. London: WB Saunders, 1973.
19 FOLDES FF. Regional intravenous neuromuscular block: a new diagnostic and experimental tool. In: Boulton TB, Bryce-Smith R, Sykes MK, Gillett GB, Revell AL, eds. *Progress in anaesthesiology*.

Proceedings of the fourth world congress of anaesthesiologists. Amsterdam: Excerpta Medica, 1970; 425–30.

20 GILLAM PMS, HEAF PJD, KAUFMAN L, LUCAS BGB. Respiration in dystrophia myotonica. *Thorax* 1964; **19**: 112–20.

21 GRONERT GA, THEYE RA. The effect of succinylcholine on skeletal muscle with immobilization atrophy. *Anesthesiology* 1974; **40**: 268–71.

22 GRONERT GA, THEYE RA. Physiology of hyperkalemia induced by succinylcholine. *Anesthesiology* 1975; **43**: 89–99.

23 HEATHFIELD KWG. Treatment of peripheral neuritis. *Hospital Update* 1975; **1**: 383–9.

24 JENKINS RB. Treatment of myasthenia gravis with prednisone. *Lancet* 1972; **1**: 765–7.

25 KAO I, DRACHMAN DB. Myasthenic immunoglobulin accelerates ACh receptor degradation. *Neurology* 1977; **27**: 364–5.

26 KAUFMAN L. Anaesthesia in dystrophia myotonica: a review of the hazards of anaesthesia. *Proc Roy Soc Med* 1960; **53**: 183–8.

27 KENDIG JJ, BUNKER JP, ENDOW S. Succinylcholine induced hyperkalaemia. *Anesthesiology* 1972; **36**: 132–7.

28 LEGG MA, BRADY WJ. Pathology and clinical behaviour of thymomas: a survey of 51 cases. *Cancer* 1965; **18**: 1131–44.

29 LINDSTROM JM, SEYBOLD ME, LENNON VA, WHITTINGHAM S, DUANE DD. Antibody to acetylcholine receptor in myasthenia gravis; prevalence, clinical correlates and diagnostic value. *Neurology* 1976; **26**: 1054–9.

30 MANN JD, JOHNS TR, CAMPA JF, MULLER WH. Long-term prednisone followed by thymectomy in myasthenia gravis. *Ann NY Acad Sci* 1976; **274**: 608–22.

31 MATELL G, BERGSTROM K, FRANKSSON C, *et al.* Effects of some immunosuppressive procedures on myasthenia gravis. *Ann NY Acad Sci* 1976; **274**: 659–76.

32 MILLER RD, WAY WL, HAMILTON WK, LAYZER RB. Succinylcholine-induced hyperkalemia in patients with renal failure. *Anesthesiology* 1972; **36**: 138–41.

33 NASTUK WL, PLESCIA OJ, OSSERMAN KE. Changes in serum complement activity in patients with myasthenia gravis. *Proc Soc Exp Biol Med* 1960; **105**: 177–84.

34 NASTUK WL, STRAUSS AJL, OSSERMAN KE. Search for a neuromuscular blocking agent in the blood of patients with myasthenia gravis. *Am J Med* 1959; **26**: 394–409.

35 PATON WDM, WAUD DR. The margin of safety of neuromuscular transmission. *J Physiol* 1967; **191**: 59–90.

36 PERRY WCM, ZAIMIS EJ, quoted in Zaimis EJ. Transmission and block at the motor end plate and in autonomic ganglion: the interruption of neuromuscular transmission and some of its problems. *Pharmacol Rev* 1954; **6**: 63–7.

37 RAVIN M, NEWMARK Z, SAVIELLO G. Myotonia dystrophia—an anesthetic hazard: two case reports. *Anesth Analg* 1975; **54**: 216–18.

38 ROBERTS DV, WILSON A. Physiology of neuromuscular transmission. In: Greene R, ed. *Myosthenia gravis*. London: Heinemann, 1969: 14–19.

39 ROSENDAUM KJ, NEIGH JL, STROBEL GE. Sensitivity to non-depolarizing muscle relaxants in amyotrophic lateral sclerosis. A report of two cases. *Anesthesiology* 1971; **35**: 638–41.

40 ROSS RT. Ocular myopathy sensitive to curare. *Brain* 1963; **16**: 67–74.

41 SIMPSON JA. Myasthenia gravis; a new hypothesis. *Scot Med J* 1960; **5**: 419–36.

42 SMITH RB. Hyperkalemia following succinylcholine administration in neurological disorders: a review. *Can Anaesth Soc J* 1971; **18**: 199–201.

43 STONE WA, BEACH TP, HAMELBERG W. Succinylcholine danger in the spinal-cord-injured patient. *Anesthesiology* 1970; **32**: 168–9.

44 STOVNER J, ENDRESEN R, BJELKE E. Suxamethonium hyperkalaemia with different induction agents. *Acta Anaesthesiol Scand* 1972; **16**: 46–50.

45 STRUASS AJL, SEEGAL BC, HSU KC, BURHOLDER PM, NASTUK WL, OSSERMAN KE. Immunofluorescence demonstration of a muscle binding, complement-fixing serum globulin fraction in myasthenia gravis. *Proc Soc Exp Biol Med* 1960; **105**: 184–91.

46 STRUPPLER A. Experimentelle Untersuchungen zur Pathogenase der Myasthenie. *Ztschr ges exper med* 1954; **125**: 224–73.

47 TOBEY RE, JACOBSEN PM, KAHLE CT, CLUBB PJ, DEAN MA. The serum potassium response to muscle relaxants in neural injury. *Anesthesiology* 1972; **37**: 332–71.

48 THOMAS PK. Peripheral neuropathy. *Br Med J* 1970; **1**: 349–52.

49 THORNTON RJ, FELDMAN SA, BLAKENEY C. *Hypothermia and neuromuscular conduction*. Proceedings 6th World Congress of Anaesthesiologists (abstracts), Mexico City. Amsterdam: Excerpta Medica, 1976: 12.

50 TOYKA KV, DRACHMAN DB, PESTRONK A, KAO I. Myasthenia gravis passive transfer from man to mouse. *Science* 1975; **190**: 397–9.

51 VAN'T HOFF W. Familial myotonic periodic paralysis. *QJ Med* 1962; **31**: 385–402.

52 WALTON JN. Muscular dystrophy and its relation to other myopathies. Research Publications Association for Research in Nervous and Mental Diseases 1961; **38**: 378–421.

53 WALTON JN, GARDNER-MEDWIN D. Progressive muscular dystrophy and myotonic disorders. In: Walton JN, ed. *Diseases of voluntary muscle*. London: Churchill-Livingstone, 1974: 561–613.

54 WATSON WE, SMITH AC, SPALDING JMK. Transmural central venous pressure during intermittent positive pressure respiration. *Br J Anaesth* 1962; **34**: 278–86.

55 WISE RP. Muscle disorders and the relaxants. *Br J Anaesth* 1963; **35**: 558–64.

56 YAMASHITA M, MATSUKI A, OYAMA T. Anaesthetic considerations in von Recklinghausen's disease. *Anaesthetist* 1977: **26**: 317–18.

57 ZAIMIS EJ. Transmission and block at the motor end plate and on autonomic ganglia. The interruption of neuromuscular transmission and some of its problems. *Pharmacol Rev* 1954; 53–7.

APPENDIX

SPECIAL INVESTIGATION OF PERIPHERAL NERVE AND NEUROMUSCULAR DAMAGE

Nerve conduction velocity

Normal values depend upon the diameter of the nerve studied but for large myelinated nerves 40–50 m/sec is usual. In demyelinating conditions nerve conduction reduced to 5–30 m/sec.

Terminal latency

This is an unusual delay in establishing a muscle action potential after motor nerve stimulation. This is increased in demyelineating conditions and prolonged in the later stages of axonal degeneration.

Electromyography (compound muscle action potentials)

Muscular degeneration of the Duchenne type may produce fibrillation potentials. In myasthenia gravis there is a typical EMG picture of small action potentials, fade on tetanic stimulation, post-tetanic facilitation for 0·5 to 20 sec and post-tetanic exhaustion which follows a brief period of facilitation—this latter effect differs from a true curare-like neuromuscular block and more closely resembles the effect of hemicholinium [8].

In myotonic diseases repetitive after-discharge occurs following motor nerve stimulation.

Mechanical twitch response

The mechanical response of a muscle (usually the adductor pollucis longus) to direct and indirect stimulation can be used to diagnose neuromuscular disease, such as myasthenia gravis and to demonstrate the response to edrophonium. Like the EMG it only provides information about the nerve and muscle actually tested.

Edrophonium (Tensilon) test

This is a standard test for suspected myasthenia gravis. It involves withholding all drugs for 12 hours and is therefore best performed in the early morning. 10 mg of edrophonium (Tensilon) are injected i.v. and the patient's powers of repetitive muscular action tested. It is useful to record the patient's ability to read aloud before and after the test; this reveals improvement in the ability to focus and to articulate. The response to stimulation of a motor nerve and the recording of muscle twitch response and the improvement in the 1st to 4th twitch response using a 2 Hz supramaximal stimulation should be elicited. An increase of greater than 25 per cent after the administration of edrophonium is a positive response. If the 4th twitch is less than 70 per cent the height of the 1st then myasthenia gravis should be suspect. If the 4th twitch response increases to within 20 per cent of the height of the 1st following edrophonium this also suggests that the patient is suffering from myasthenia gravis.

PART 2 MALIGNANT HYPERPYREXIA

F. R. ELLIS

HISTORICAL

Malignant hyperpyrexia is a pharmacogenetic disease induced by certain drugs used in anaesthetic and psychiatric practice. It is inherited as a Mendelian dominant.

An awareness of the instability of body temperature during anaesthesia dates from the latter part of the last century. Hypothermia was a serious hazard due to the practice of swaddling the patient in disinfectant-drenched drapes. Postoperative heat stroke was described by various authors in the early years of the present century. It was ascribed to uncontrolled environmental conditions during 'heat waves'. With hindsight it is likely that some of these hyperpyrexic patients were suffering from the specific condition now referred to as malignant hyperpyrexia. Also it may be that the patients who react to these adverse circumstances may have an underlying defect in their ability to cope with stress such as has been suggested by Wingard [32].

We owe to Denborough and Lovell [9] the first modern description of malignant hyperpyrexia. They described an Australian family in which multiple deaths had occurred under diethyl ether anaesthesia during which high temperatures had been recorded. They drew attention to the hereditary nature of malignant hyperpyrexia. Since then their findings have been confirmed by others [4, 21].

In the late 1960s various workers [4, 32], detected the presence of a primary muscle abnormality (myopathy) both in patients who had developed malignant hyperpyrexia and in some of their relatives and Harriman *et al.* [17] described this condition as malignant hyperpyrexia myopathy.

A similar but probably not identical condition occurs in pigs. Hall and others [15] reported that pigs developed hyperpyrexia and died during anaesthesia especially when suxamethonium was used, and it is now known that pigs of the Landrace, Poland, China and Pietran strains are all liable to develop malignant hyperpyrexia. One of the features of these strains is the high ratio of their muscle mass to total body mass, and although the histological stigmata of myopathy have not been found in the pig, the human myopathy associated with malignant hyperpyrexia frequently affects young muscular people who have evidence of muscle hypertrophy.

CLINICAL ASSOCIATIONS

Patients with myopathy have a greater chance of congenital musculoskeletal defects. It is commonly found that families with the malignant hyperpyrexia phenotype have greater incidence of squints, [31] inguinal hernias, kyphoscoliosis, subluxation of the patellae, pes cavus, etc. Although these and other musculoskeletal abnormalities cannot be considered to be genetic identifiers, anaesthetic drugs should be administered to these patients with the knowledge that there is a greater probability of malignant hyperprexia than in the general population.

INCIDENCE

An incidence of 1:20,000 has been given for a Canadian population [4], whereas in a ten year survey in the U.K. an incidence of 1:200,000 of the anaesthetized population was found. The difference is difficult to explain as the two populations are ethnically fairly similar. Incidences of between 1:50,000 and 1:100,000 have been quoted for other European communities and as high as 1:6,000 for Japan. However, it is not certain that all cases are either correctly diagnosed or reported. Proof of diagnosis by muscle testing is carried out in only a few centres, and incidence figures in these circumstances must also be treated with a degree of circumspection.

The incidence of patients *susceptible* to malignant hyperpyrexia (MHS) having anaesthesia is probably much greater than for *actual* cases of the acute syndrome. The reasons for this discrepancy are: that anaesthesia even with triggering drugs does not always cause the MH reaction [16]; many anaesthetics are of too short a duration for triggering to occur; the trigger drugs are not always used; and some drugs such as Althesin may protect the patient for a time and delay the development of MH [18].

ACUTE CLINICAL MALIGNANT HYPERPYREXIA

A rise of deep body temperature occurs at a rate of more than 2°C per hour. This is not diagnostic as it can occur in many conditions, for example, acute septicaemia and infusion of pyrogens. The rise in malignant hyperpyrexia is, however, progressive.

Muscle contracture (muscle rigidity, muscle spasm) occurs early in over 75 per cent of cases. Muscle contracture is not invariable and it may develop several hours after the condition has been established. It is likely that the muscle contracture (and even the rise of temperature itself) are both secondary to a more basic disturbance. Hence, its time of development is not necessarily concurrent with the pyrexia.

Tachycardia develops early and may progress to bradycardia, extrasystoles and cardiac arrest which is usually irreversible. An unexplained tachycardia is perhaps the most useful sign to warn anaesthetists of developing MH, and should never be ignored.

Tachypnoea occurs if the patient is breathing spontaneously.

Cyanosis results from the inability of the oxygen transport mechanisms to cope with the metabolic storm.

Capillary oozing sometimes develops and is due to a consumptive coagulopathy.

BIOCHEMICAL CHANGES IN ACUTE MALIGNANT HYPERPYREXIA

Metabolic acidosis due primarily to intense lacticacidaemia is invariable. The major source of lactic acid is the muscle tissue which is metabolically hyperactive. It is possible that at least some of the heat may be produced by the liver reconverting lactate to glucose [8]. Patients have recovered even when a blood pH of less than 7·0 has been recorded during the acute stage.

Respiratory acidosis. When P_{CO_2} has been measured it has always been found to be greatly raised [25]. The increased CO_2 production could be used as an early sign of MH if the expired P_{CO_2} is being monitored continuously, and any unexplained increase in alveolar P_{CO_2} should be investigated.

Hyperkalaemia is usual. The efflux of potassium from cells may be due to primary cell-membrane defect produced by the causative drugs, to severe hypoxia of muscle tissue or as a direct result of the acute acidosis.

Serum enzymes such as serum creatine phosphokinase (CPK), lactic dehydrogenase, transaminases, etc. have all been found to be raised during the acute hyperpyrexia. Serum CPK is often extremely high and in a recent case a level of 80,000 i.u./l was measured (normal < 60 i.u./l). The CPK activity subsides within a day or two but may remain slightly raised indefinitely.

Calcium. It has been demonstrated that the muscle ionic calcium level in the cytoplasm rises from the normal of less than 10^{-7} mol/l to greater than 10^{-5} mol/l during the development of malignant hyperpyrexia. This probably accounts for the muscle contracture because the muscle is unable to relax if ionic calcium continually stimulates the formation of the actin-myosin complexes in the myofilaments.

It is possible that the raised intracellular ionic calcium levels indicate that oxidative phosphorylation of ADP to ATP is uncoupled. The level of ATP in muscle cells falls more rapidly in muscle from susceptible pigs than normal pig muscle in the presence of halothane [20].

Serum calcium levels have been found to be raised in hyperpyrexic pigs and less than normal in hyperpyrexic humans, although the value of the human data could be more suspect due to the uncontrolled nature of the 'experimental' situation.

Many research workers have investigated the calcium-binding properties of sarcoplasmic reticulum taken from susceptible pigs and susceptible humans [24]. The results are conflicting. Both increased and decreased binding have been found by different workers although the calcium metabolism in the pig and the human may differ [3].

Myoglobinuria results from the massive breakdown of muscle during and after the acute hyperpyrexic episode. The first and subsequent specimens of urine should always be examined for myoglobin although the urine is usually very obviously discoloured. Heavy myoglobinuria may lead to acute renal failure.

Plasma thyroid hormone levels were shown to fall rapidly during the development of malignant hyperpyrexia in Pietran pigs and the timely administration of tri-iodothyronine (T_3) has been shown to restore the pigs to an apparently normal metabolic state [26]. This work is at present unconfirmed in other breeds of pig and in humans. In a study of susceptible patients undergoing muscle biopsy under a form of general anaesthesia, we detected no consistent thyroid hormone abnormalities.

DIFFERENTIAL DIAGNOSIS

With increasing awareness by anaesthetists, a provisional diagnosis of malignant hyperpyrexia is more often made at a time when the full syndrome has not developed. Anaesthesia is abandoned if one only of the more characteristic signs are seen.

Positive identification of the early MH proband can only be made using muscle testing. Commoner causes of MH signs should be sought at the time so as to avoid unnecessary invasive screening. The following list is offered to indicate other possible causes.

Infection
Exogenous pyrogens
Blood transfusion reaction
Convulsions
Atropine overdose
Thyroid crisis

Peripheral circulatory failure
Muscle spasm with suxamethonium
Myotonic dystrophy or myopathy
Denervation
Apparent muscle spasm with suxamethonium
Failure to relax— extravascular injection
                 — hydrolysed drug
Instrumentation with light anaesthesia
Fibrosis of jaw muscles or joints
Myoglobinuria
Crush syndrome
Muscle spasm
Familial paroxysmal rhabdomyolysis
McArdle's disease, etc

AETIOLOGY OF MALIGNANT HYPERPYREXIA

No discussion of malignant hyperpyrexia would be satisfying without mention of the aetiology. There are several theories but none has gained general acceptance.

The first question to be answered is whether the disease is due to a central (hypothalamic) defect or a peripheral muscle cellular defect. The evidence of a peripheral abnormality is indisputable. This was first demonstrated when a patient was reported who developed generalized muscle rigidity during an episode of malignant hyperpyrexia: however, one limb in which the blood supply had been occluded in preparation for orthopaedic surgery remained flaccid; a neural mechanism was thus eliminated [29]. Living muscle tissue from susceptible individuals develops contracture *in vitro* when halothane is administered [12]. A similar contracture occurs with all of the inhalational anaesthetic vapours.

Malignant hyperpyrexia must be due to a stimulation of metabolism as it has been calculated that if all heat loss mechanisms failed to operate, the body would only gain $1.3°C$ per hour. In a fulminating case the rate of rise of body temperature can be greater than $6°C$ per hour.

It is now accepted that intracellular calcium levels rise. This may be the link that explains why suxamethonium, which does not enter the cell, and the inhalational anaesthetics, both cause malignant hyperpyrexia, because the anaesthetics affect the calcium binding properties of sarcoplasmic reticulum. Suxamethonium activates the cell membrane and could cause a rise in intracellular calcium by release from the terminal vesicles of the T-tubular system in the muscle cell.

Berman *et al.* [2] showed that the demand for oxygen by the hyperpyrexic pig did not reflect the massive rise in temperature. Their results could only be explained by an anaerobic source of heat but this could not be expected to result in early and severe cyanosis which seems to be common in humans. Since then it has been shown that oxygen consumption does rise to high levels [27].

The stimulation of metabolism may be due to an increased 'normal' metabolism, such as occurs during muscle work; or the metabolic stimulation could result from inefficient metabolism, for example, from uncoupled oxidative phosphorylation. The drugs which cause malignant hyperpyrexia have not been shown to be uncouplers in clinical concentrations. A recent suggestion is that one of the 'futile' glycolytic pathways could be activated. This is an inefficient pathway designed for heat production and occurs normally in some animals such as the bumble bee which is able to keep warm enough to fly on cold days without performing mechanical work. (Wasps which do not use futile metabolism cannot fly on cold days.) As no specific metabolic defect has been demonstrated it is not possible to decide which of these hypothesis is closest to the truth.

The recent studies by Cheah and Cheah [6] have demonstrated a mitochondrial calcium defect in porcine malignant hyperpyrexia muscle. The control of the increased calcium efflux by spermine suggests an abnormality in mitochondrial membrane phospholipase. In the absence of this control, the calcium activated phospholipase would cause liberation of free fatty acids from the mitochondrial membrane, and the fatty acids would cause an increased efflux of calcium from the sarcoplasmic reticulum. No comparable human studies have yet been made.

TREATMENT OF THE ACUTE PHASE

Unfortunately the monitoring of body temperature is exceptional in the type of patient most likely to develop malignant hyperpyrexia. The diagnosis is often made only when the condition is well established and the metabolic derangements are severe. With early diagnosis, for example when suxamethonium produces muscle contracture and the body temperature begins to rise, it is possible to treat the patient adequately by avoiding any further drugs and vigorously cooling the body surface.

General management

Whenever the diagnosis is made, however provisionally, anaesthesia (and therefore surgery) must be terminated and all known causative drugs withdrawn. An intravenous infusion of cold saline should be started and blood must be taken for estimation of electrolytes and blood gases. Surface cooling can be initiated with ice packs on the praecordium, groins and axillae but the patient cools quicker if submerged in water at 20–25°C, or if arteriovenous blood cooling can be established.

The patient's lungs should be ventilated with a high concentration of oxygen and the body temperature recorded, preferably using a rectal probe and an electrical thermometer. An electrocardiogram should be monitored and all events timed and recorded.

Bicarbonate should be given according to the base deficit but an initial 100 mmol could be administered before the blood gas results are available. If the potassium is high, 20 units of insulin can be given together with glucose to avoid hypoglycaemia.

Specific drugs

Dantrolene sodium has been shown to be effective in preventing an MH reaction in susceptible pigs when it is given prophylactically [19], and evidence is accumulating of its efficacy in treating the acute MH reaction in both pigs and humans. Dantrolene must now be considered the drug of first choice for MH. The recommended dosage is 1–2 mg/kg initially and repeat every 5–10 minutes up to 10 mg/kg or until the disease is controlled. Further dantrolene may be required to control the ensuing instability over the succeeding 24–48 hours.

High dosage glucocorticoids have been effective in controlling MH in several patients without further medication, and should be given not only for any specific effects in stabilizing membranes but also for their antishock attributes; they increase cardiac output and increase peripheral blood flow. The recommended dose is 10 mg/kg methylprednisolone, 2 mg/kg dexamethasone or 50 mg/kg hydrocortisone [10].

Procaine has been used successfully to control malignant hyperpyrexia [1]. The dose required is high (30–50 mg/kg) and the myocardium may be so depressed as to require isoprenaline to maintain cardiac output. In some patients it is possible that procaine may activate rather than depress muscle activity [7].

TREATMENT OF THE LATE COMPLICATIONS

The successful acute management of malignant hyperpyrexia results in a patient who, though alive, is severely deranged biochemically.

Acute hypoxia may leave neurological defects and coma has been reported for several days. However, coma in the first days does not necessarily mean that the brain damage is sufficient to cause mental impairment. Dramatic recoveries have been reported.

Renal failure due to myoglobinuria can be avoided by forced diuresis if this is started early enough. The end result of renal failure seems to be good and dialysis is only required for 7–10 days.

The electrolyte imbalance may take several days to correct and most patients require high dosage of potassium to replace the loss during the acute phase.

PREDICTION OF SUSCEPTIBILITY TO MALIGNANT HYPERPYREXIA

The inheritance of the malignant hyperpyrexia gene is dominant and so roughly 50 per cent of close relatives of an indexed case will be affected.

Various tests have been described but the one used by the author is the development of muscle contracture *in vitro* [13, 14]. Muscle specimens are taken across the motor point of the vastus internus and kept alive in a physiological solution. A fascicle is microdissected and attached to a strain gauge which measures muscle tension. When halothane is admitted to the muscle bath the tension increases if the muscle is taken from a susceptible person, and falls if from a normal person. Susceptible muscle is also more sensitive to caffeine than normal muscle [4].

The suggestion that a raised CPK indicates susceptibility to malignant hyperpyrexia [22], has proved unfounded in the author's experience. In fact using the muscle contracture test, there are more susceptible patients with a normal CPK (i.e. < 60 i.u./l) than patients with raised CPK [11]. The use of CPK as a screening test should be abandoned because of the very real danger of false negatives.

DRUGS TO AVOID IN PATIENTS SUSCEPTIBLE TO MALIGNANT HYPERPYREXIA

SUXAMETHONIUM: one third of susceptibles develop immediate muscle contracture.

VOLATILE ANAESTHETIC VAPOURS: all of those in common use have been associated with malignant hyperpyrexia or have been shown to be dangerous *in vitro*.

ANAESTHETIC GASES: both cyclopropane and nitrous oxide [10] have been incriminated.

ATROPINE: atropine premedication is more liable to cause the early development of muscle contracture and a more fulminating hyperpyrexic response [23].

PHENOTHIAZINES: Trimeprazine has caused two proven deaths [28] and chlorpromazine has been thought to be responsible for at least one case.

MOOD ELEVATORS: tricyclic antidepressants, especially in combination with monoamine oxidase inhibitors, have caused death by malignant hyperpyrexia in several patients.

LIGNOCAINE: lignocaine has been used in several fatal cases usually to control extrasystoles and has been shown to activate muscle *in vitro*.

DRUGS TO USE IN PATIENTS SUSCEPTIBLE TO MALIGNANT HYPERPYREXIA

Premedication with small doses of diazepam.
Thiopentone and Althesin (both thought to protect the patient against malignant hyperpyrexia).
Fentanyl and droperidol.
Pancuronium [5].
Most susceptible patients tolerate nitrous oxide, but this agent must be used with great caution with full temperature monitoring.
Procaine is the drug of choice for local anaesthesia. Preliminary results suggest that prilocaine and bupivacaine are also safe.

REFERENCES

1 BELDAYS J, SMALL V, COOPER DA, BRITT BA. Postoperative malignant hyperthermia: a case report. *Can Anaesth Soc J* 1971; **18**: 202–12.
2 BERMAN MC, HARRISON GG, BULL AB, KENCH JE. Changes underlying halothane induced malignant hyperpyrexia in Landrace pigs. *Nature* 1970; **225**: 653–5.
3 BRITT BA, ENDRENYI L, BARCLAY RL, CADMAN DL. Total calcium content of skeletal muscle isolated from humans and pigs susceptible to malignant hyperthermia. *Br J Anaesth* 1975; **47**: 647–53.
4 BRITT BA, LOCHER WG, KALOW W. Hereditary aspects of malignant hyperthermia. *Can Anaesth Soc J* 1969; **16**: 89–98.
5 CAIN PA, ELLIS FR. Anaesthesia for patients susceptible to malignant hyperpyrexia: a study of pancuronium and methylprednisolone. *Br J Anaesth* 1977; **49**: 941–4.
6 CHEAH KS, CHEAH AM. Mitochondrial calcium transport and calcium activated phospholipase in porcine malignant hyperthermia. *Bioch Biophy Acta* 1980 (in press).
7 CLARKE IMC, ELLIS FR. An evaluation of procaine in the treatment of malignant hyperpyrexia. *Br J Anaesth* 1975; **47**: 17–21.
8 DENBOROUGH MA, HIRD FRJ, KING JW, MARGINSON MA, MITCHELSON KR, NAYLOR WG, REX MA, ZAPF P, CONDRON RJ. Mitochondrial and other studies in Australian Landrace pigs affected with malignant hyperthermia. In: Gordon RA, Britt BA, Kalow W, eds. *International symposium on malignant hyperthermia*. Springfield, Illinois: Charles C Thomas, 1973; 229–37.
9 DENBOROUGH MA, LOVELL RRH. Anaesthetic deaths in a family, *Lancet* 1960; **2**: 45.
10 ELLIS FR, CLARKE IMC, APPLEYARD TN, DINSDALE RSW. Malignant hyperpyrexia induced by nitrous oxide and successfully treated with dexamethasone. *Br Med J* 1974; **4**: 270–1.
11 ELLIS FR, CLARKE IMC, MODGILL M, CURRIE S, HARRIMAN DGF. An evaluation of creatinine phosphokinese in screening patients for malignant hyperpyrexia. *Br Med J* 1975; **2**: 511–13.
12 ELLIS FR, HARRIMAN DGF, KEANEY NP, KYEI-MENSAH K, TYRRELL JH. Halothane-induced muscle contracture as a cause of hyperpyrexia. *Br J Anaesth* 1971; **43**: 721–2.
13 ELLIS FR, KEANEY NP, HARRIMAN DGF, *et al*. Screening for malignant hyperpyrexia. *Br MJ* 1972; **3**: 559–61.
14 ELLIS FR, HARRIMAN DGF, CURRIE S, CAIN PA. Screening for malignant hyperthermia in susceptible patients. In: Aldrete JA, Britt BA, eds. *Second international symposium on malignant hyperthermia*. New York: Grune & Stratton, 1977; 273–85.

15 HALL LW, WOOLF N, BRADLEY JWP and JOLLY DW. Unusual reaction to suxamethonium chloride. *Br Med J* 1966; **2**: 1305.

16 HALSALL PJ, CAIN PA and ELLIS FR. Retrospective analysis of anaesthetics received by patients before susceptibility to malignant hyperpyrexia was recognised. *Br J Anaesth* 1979; **51**; 949–54.

17 HARRIMAN DGF, SUMNER DW, ELLIS FR. Malignant hyperpyrexia myopathy. *QJ Med* 1973; **42**: 639.

18 HARRISON GG. Althesin and malignant hyperpyrexia. *Br J Anaesth* 1973; **45**: 1019–21.

19 HARRISON GG. Control of the malignant hyperpyrexia syndrome in malignant hyperpyrexia susceptible swine by dantrolene sodium. *Br J Anaesth* 1975; **47**: 62–5.

20 HARRISON GG, SAUNDERS SJ, BIERUYCK JP, HICKMAN R, DENT DM, WEAVER V, TERBLANCHE J. Anaesthetic-induced malignant hyperpyrexia and a method for its prediction. *Br J Anaesth* 1969; **41**: 844–55.

21 ISAACS H, BARLOW MB. Malignant hyperpyrexia during anaesthesia: possible association with subclinical myopathy. *Br Med J* 1970a; **1**: 275–7.

22 ISAACS H, BARLOW MB. The genetic background to malignant hyperpyrexia revealed by serum creatine phosphokinase estimations in asymptomatic relatives. *Br J Anaesth* 1970b; **42**: 1077–84.

23 KALOW W, BRITT BA. Drug causing rigidity in malignant hyperthermia. *Lancet* 1973; **2**: 390–1.

24 KALOW W, BRITT BA, TERREAU ME, HAIST C. Metabolic error of muscle metabolism after recovery from malignant hyperpyrexia. *Lancet* 1970; **2**: 895–8.

25 LIERENSCHUTZ F, MAI C, PICKERODT VWA. Increased carbon dioxide production in two patients with malignant hyperpyrexia and its control by dantrolene. *Br J Anaesth* 1979; **51**: 899–903.

26 LISTER D. Correction of adverse response to suxamethonium of susceptible pigs. *Br Med J* 1973; **1**: 208–10.

27 LUCKE JN, HALL GM, LOVELL R, TAIT A, WHITE YS, LISTER D. The metabolic course of porcine malignant hyperthermia. *Br. J Anaesth* 1975; **47**: 905.

28 MOYES DG. Malignant hyperpyrexia caused by trimeprazine. *Br J Anaesth* 1973; **45**: 1163.

29 SATNICK JH. Hyperthermia under anesthesia with regional muscle flaccidity. *Anesthesiology* 1969; **30**: 472.

30 STEERS AJW, TALLACK JA, THOMPSON DEA. Fulminating hyperpyrexia during anaesthesia in a member of a myopathic family. *Br Med J* 1970; **1**: 341–3.

31 WILSON ME, ELLIS FR. Predicting malignant hyperpyrexia. *Br J Anaesth* 1979; **51**: 66.

32 WINGARD DW. A stressful situation. *Anesth Analg* 1980; **59**: 321–2.

Chapter 8
Neurological Disease

M. MARSHALL

In the majority of instances when an anaesthetist meets a patient with neurological disease the diagnosis has already been made and it only remains for the anaesthetist to understand the implications of that diagnosis for the patient and for his attendants. It is with these *implications* that this chapter is concerned and the descriptions of the diseases mentioned will be shorter than would be acceptable in a medical textbook. Surgical neurology is well covered in many texts concerned with anaesthesia for neurosurgery and will receive only limited mention in the following pages.

Patients in coma, however, may not have been diagnosed when first encountered by an anaesthetist. In the admission room, in the intensive care unit or following some catastrophe in the operating theatre, an examination and tentative diagnosis may therefore have to be made without expert neurological advice. For this reason and also because the production of reversible coma is one of the anaesthetist's skills, this chapter starts with a discussion of consciousness and its changes or aberrations.

CONSCIOUSNESS, SLEEP, STUPOR AND COMA

Being awake, conscious or aware, has two distinguishable components. One comprises the wakefulness itself and the other the activity associated with wakefulness—the content of consciousness. To be awake depends upon the normal functioning of certain parts of midbrain reticular formation. Both wakeful behaviour and the contents of consciousness depend upon the intactness and functioning of the cerebral hemispheres.

Hemispheral or cortical lesions produce recognizable alterations in function and in the contents of consciousness but do not in general produce alterations in consciousness that interfere with waking and sleeping patterns. Severe, diffuse cerebral damage may produce profound dementia or idiocy but sleeping and waking are still recognizable. Though the above is in general true, sudden massive cortical damage to both frontal and temporal lobes will result in unconsciousness and so will complete, or nearly complete, decortication. Such extensive lesions rarely occur without concomitant damage to other parts of the brain including the brain stem but cases of almost pure decortication have been reported. Plum and Posner [6] discuss the delayed results of acute hypoxia where occasionally the patient appears to make a complete recovery from the initial episode only to lapse later into deepening dementia and coma. This secondary deterioration is due to an almost complete demyelination of the hemispheral white matter without damage to the grey matter of the basal ganglia or brain stem. Some patients suffering deceleration head injuries have extensive shearing of the white fibres of the corona radiata which, in effect, permanently separates the cerebral cortices from all lower centres. At post-mortem such patients may show little brain stem damage though their cerebral hemispheres may be almost totally demyelinated. In life these patients though making some reflex movements and occasionally spontaneously opening their eyes do not convince their attendants that they are aware of their surroundings.

Conversely, patients with small limited lesions confined to the midbrain may remain permanently in coma although the remainder of the central nervous system appears to be intact.

Sleep and coma

In some circumstances, especially when patients are suffering from drug or metabolic intoxication, it is practically impossible to distinguish between coma and deep sleep. However, in spite of this difficulty it is useful, whenever possible, to distinguish between physiological and pathological alterations in consciousness.

As mentioned above, awareness depends upon the normal functioning of the midbrain reticular formation. The critical region would seem to be the tegmental grey matter on either side and below the aqueduct from the posterior hypothalamus rostrally to the level of the lower third of the pons caudally (see Fig. 8.1). Although

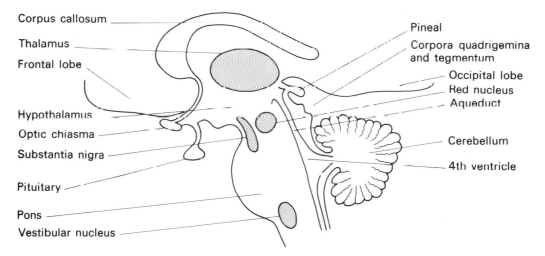

Fig. 8.1. Diagrammatic representation of a mid-line section of the brain stem and associated structures.

consciousness can be impaired when this area is intact, awareness is impossible when this area is destroyed. Stimulation of this area causes arousal and destruction causes coma. Other areas in the reticular formation in the posterior hypothalamus and also in the upper hind-brain seem to have an influence upon sleep. In animals stimulation of these regions produces apparently normal sleep while their destruction produces insomnia.

In normal sleep the depth of unconsciousness varies. The subject alters his position, his pattern of breathing and degree of muscle relaxation. He has periods when he has rapid eye movements (REM sleep) which are associated with profound muscle relaxation and dreaming. He sometimes twitches spontaneously. He is always rousable given a sufficiently strong and unfamiliar stimulus, and when roused is quickly alert and orientated.

Stupor

The distinction between sleep and stupor can be difficult. Drug-enhanced sleep following small doses of hypnotics can be identical with normal non-drugged sleep. With increasing doses of hypnotic drugs the signs typical of stupor develop. The subject becomes increasingly difficult to rouse and when woken is slow and confused. Left undisturbed he lies still, his breathing tends to be regular and sighing is diminished or absent. He fails to change position or to make spontaneous movements. Rapid eye movements do not occur. In all this he presents a picture very similar to that of the lightly anaesthetized patient except that he is rousable with a sufficiently painful stimulus.

The picture described above is most often seen following an overdose of sedative drugs where there is global depression of the central nervous system. Depression of the ascending reticular formation is presumed to be responsible for the lack of arousal and depression of the hemispheres for the slowness and confusion of thought. Lesions limited to the central grey matter of the posterior hypothalamus and rostral tegmentum can produce the same clinical picture but, when roused, the patient appears limp and apathetic rather than confused.

Coma

Just as sleep merges into stupor so stupor merges into coma. There is usually no difference in kind between the states but rather a difference in degree. A patient is described as 'comatose' when it is not possible to arouse him to the point where he gives the appearance of being 'conscious'. The terms are descriptive only and have little diagnostic significance except in so far as 'stupor' and 'coma' should only be used to describe conditions believed to be pathological. Later in this chapter a more objective method of describing unconscious or obtunded patients will be discussed.

EEG differences between sleep and coma

The standard EEG

In normal sleep the EEG shows slowing and an increase in amplitude of the wave form which reverts to the normal awake pattern on arousal.

In coma, such as that produced by light surgical anaesthesia, the EEG may be indistinguishable from the waking trace yet the patient is unrousable in spite of vigorous (surgical) stimulation. The EEG may also resemble a normal waking trace in some patients deeply unconscious with midbrain damage in whom the cerebral hemispheres have remained intact.

Evoked cortical potentials

In the intact animal, peripheral sensory stimulation will evoke an electrical potential in the appropriate part of the cerebral cortex; thus touch will evoke a potential in the contralateral post-central gyrus and visual and auditory stimuli will produce evoked potentials in the occipital lobes and in the superior temporal gyri, respectively.

Evoked cortical potentials have at least two major components: one fast and one slow. In the case of the potentials evoked by touch, the fast component is conveyed by the lemniscal pathways that subserve most forms of somatic sensation while the slow component travels along a parallel, polysynaptic pathway associated with the brain stem reticular formation. General anaesthetics selectively modify the slow component suggesting that, at least at first, they modify reticular formation activity while leaving the lemniscal pathway intact. They also leave relatively intact the cerebral cortex since the potentials that are recorded unmodified are from cortical cells. Also, at that level of anaesthesia at which the fast component of the evoked potential is intact and the slow component modified, stimulation of the precentral cortex will produce the appropriate motor response. Several anaesthetics would seem to interfere with reticular formation activity selectively and to do so before they modify cortical activity.

Narcolepsy

Narcolepsy is a clearly defined clinical entity in which at quite unpredictable times the subject has a sudden and irresistible desire to sleep. The attacks may continue for months or years with no other sign of intracranial disease being or becoming, apparent; are usually short-lived and are indistinguishable from normal sleep. During the attack the patient is easily aroused. Beforehand the subject feels suddenly drowsy but usually has time to ensure his safety before falling asleep. The EEG is normal.

This condition is mentioned here since it seems to be a disturbance of specific sleep centres which appear to be paroxysmally overactive. There is no apparent relationship to any form of epilepsy. The condition can be very disabling. Amphetamines have generally been used in treatment and protriptyline has also proved helpful.

Patients with chronically disturbed sleep are often unduly somnolent during the day and may be thought to suffer from narcolepsy. One group of such patients is discussed on page 289.

Sleep paralysis (night nurse's paralysis)

This is a frightening condition in which on waking the subject is momentarily quite unable to move. It has been reported by night nurses who have fallen asleep at their desks. The cause is unknown.

Cataplexy

In this disorder a sudden weakness occurs in response to emotional stimuli. The weakness may be partial, a temporary dropping of the head or limbs or a complete collapse with the subject falling to the ground. Consciousness however is never lost. The stimuli may be laughter, anger, fear or other emotional excitement. Imipramine has been used in its treatment. The condition is not a form of epilepsy.

THE NEUROLOGICAL EXAMINATION OF A PATIENT IN COMA

When examining a patient one should look first for those signs that indicate the possible need for urgent treatment or for urgent further investigation. Such signs have been summarized in Table 8.1.

Table 8.1 Neurological examination of a patient in coma.

Sign	Possible implications	Action indicated	Dangers
Inadequate or obstructed breathing		Intubation and (perhaps) mechanical ventilation	Possible masking of an expanding lesion by reducing brain bulk by over-ventilation
Neck stiffness	Meningitis, subarachnoid blood, posterior fossa mass lesion. Brain abscess	Lumbar puncture CT scan Angiography	'Coning' if there is a supratentorial mass lesion
Lateralizing signs	Mass lesion amenable to surgery	Surgical opinion CT scan, Angiography, Exploratory burr holes	Failure to treat an expanding lesion until irreparable damage has been done
Papilloedema	Raised intracranial pressure	Dehydration therapy: mechanical ventilation. CT scan	Masking an expanding lesion. Therefore the decision to investigate must precede the institution of dehydration therapy
Paraparesis/ paraplegia	Treatable mass lesion in spinal canal	Radiography of spinal column Myelography Decompression	Delay may result in permanent damage particularly to bladder function
Focal or generalized convulsions	Uncontrolled idiopathic epilepsy. Local lesion	Control of convulsive activity. CT scan/Angiography—for mass lesion EEG	The abnormal cortical discharge is damaging and should be suppressed by appropriate drugs. Control of the seizures should not preclude investigations for a treatable local lesion

Diagnosis takes second place to these considerations and the institution of life saving treatment may well precede accurate identification of the patient's condition. In the accident room and in the intensive care unit an anaesthetist may be one of the first people involved in the care and management of an unconscious patient and the following is written with this in mind.

Depth of coma

Anaesthetists are familiar with the signs of deepening or lightening general anaesthesia and these signs are applicable to many forms of 'metabolic' coma. 'Metabolic' in this context is used to describe global impairment of central nervous system (CNS) function whether this is due to drug intoxication or to metabolic disorders such as liver or renal failure or diabetes.

Depth of coma summarizes the degree of responsiveness to various stimuli. In very light coma the patient when stimulated appears almost to wake up. Painful stimulation will produce an appropriate response. Lash and corneal reflexes are present as are laryngeal and pharyngeal reflexes. The eyes tend to rove slowly and usually not conjugately. The rapid conjugate movements of REM sleep are not seen. The pupils react to light.

One frequently sees an examiner assessing a comatose patient's response to pain by rubbing his knuckles on the patient's sternum, twisting his ear lobe, pressing in the supra-orbital region or twisting the axillary folds between thumb and finger. These crude procedures result in a bruised patient and often little useful information for the examiner. In testing response to pain, a sharp, stinging stimulus should be presented to one side of the body at a time. An appropriate stimulus and one that does not leave bruising, consists in nipping the *epidermis only* of one anterior axillary fold between the *nails* of the thumb and middle finger. This provides a much sharper stimulus than blunt pinching. In testing responsiveness in the leg similar nipping of the skin in the popliteal fossa or scratching of the sole of the foot can be used.

In the lightest levels of coma the patient will groan, wince and try to brush away the examiner's hand. As coma deepens this response becomes diminished. The movements become less forceful and incomplete. Grimacing will be reduced to a slight twitch on one side of the face. Instead of brushing away the examiner's hand the arm flexes but makes no further movement. In the leg, stimulation will provoke at first vigorous withdrawal which becomes reduced, with increasing depth, to minimal flexion of the knee.

Some patients, when in metabolic coma deeper than the stages described above, become unresponsive to superficial stimulation though breathing may still be adequate and the cough reflex retained. Others may show responses which are typical of a decorticate or decerebrate state. The author has observed an occasional asymmetry of response during recovery from general anaesthesia which appears to be related to handedness. At a certain stage during awakening nipping the axillary folds produces purposive flexion of the dominant arm with flaccidity or extension on the non-dominant side. This stage lasts only a few minutes and is then replaced by a normal, symmetrical flexor reponse.

Pupillary signs

As metabolic coma deepens the pupils react less vigorously to light and dilate. In deep metabolic coma they are moderately enlarged and fixed showing only a minimal response to light. Unresponsive large pupils are a feature of severe widespread cerebral damage or of damage to the oculomotor nerves.

Oculocephalic and oculo-vestibular reflexes

Certain ocular reflexes are typical of coma that is due to global depression of the CNS without focal destruction.

The oculocephalic reflex is elicited by holding open the patient's eyes and turning his head sharply from side to side. As the head is turned there is a conjugate movement

9

of the eyes to the opposite side so that it appears as though the patient is maintaining a fixed gaze on an object directly ahead of him. Abrupt flexion of the head will produce a similar apparent fixity of gaze with the eyes moving upwards as the face is moved downwards. Sometimes the eyelids open spontaneously during this manoeuvre ('doll's-head eye phenomenon').

These two patterns of reflex eye movement depend upon an intact brain stem and are absent in conscious subjects. They do not depend upon an intact cortex nor upon ability to fix the gaze since they are retained in those with extensive cortical damage and in those who are blind.

The oculo-vestibular reflex (caloric response)

This is elicited by stimulating the lateral semicircular canal with warm or cold water. The patient's head is raised 30° above the horizontal to bring the lateral semicircular canal into a vertical position which maximizes the response. The ear is cleared of wax and ice-cold water trickled into the meatus. In the conscious patient cold water produces a nystagmus with the rapid phase directed towards the opposite side. The eye drifts towards the irrigated ear and then moves rapidly back to the central position. In the comatose patient with an intact brain stem there is a conjugate deviation of the eyes towards the irrigated ear. Warm water causes a conjugate deviation away from the irrigated ear.

In patients with metabolic coma these reflexes are retained when flexor responses to painful stimulation have been lost or replaced by extensor responses. In deepening metabolic coma the oculo-cephalic reflexes are lost before the oculo-vestibular.

Nursing observations on patients in coma.

Recently systems have been devised which rationalize and standardize the recording of nursing observations on comatose patients. Signs are recorded in graphic form or can be scaled giving a numerical value to each degree of deficit. The effect has been to improve the quality of the observations, to improve communication between

Table 8.2. The Glasgow coma scale.

Eye opening	Spontaneous	4
	To speech	3
	To pain	2
	None	1
Best verbal response	Orientated	5
	Confused	4
	Inappropriate	3
	Incomprehensible	2
	None	1
Best motor response	Obeying	5
	Localizing pain	4
	Flexing to pain	3
	Extending to pain	2
	None	1

From Teasdale and Jennett (1974) [8] by permission of the authors and the publishers of the *Lancet*.

attendant staff by simplifying and standardizing the descriptive vocabulary used and to facilitate the early recognition of changes in the patient's condition. Table 8.2 shows a coma scale described by Teasdale and Jennett [8] and Fig. 8.2 shows a record chart based on this scale.

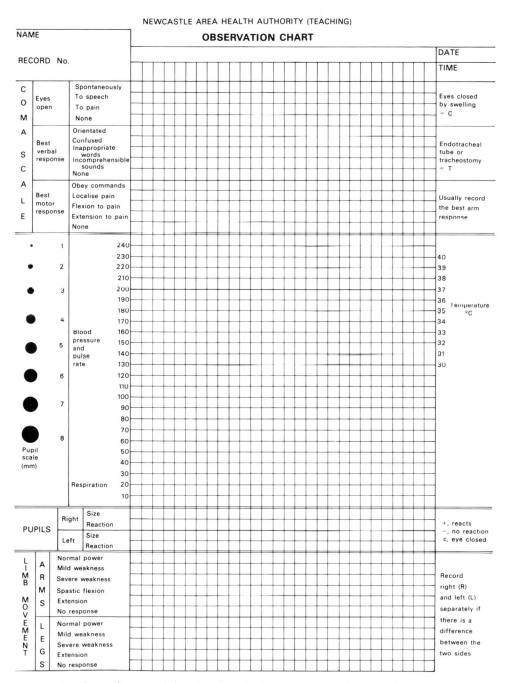

Fig. 8.2. An observation record chart based on the Glasgow coma scale (Teasdale, Galbraith and Clarke, 1975) [7]. Reproduced by permission of the authors and the editor of the *Nursing Times*.

Localizing signs

In the 'metabolic' model it is assumed that there is generalized and symmetrical impairment of CNS function and that this impairment is potentially reversible. In most patients in coma with neurological disease, signs due to areas of local damage are superimposed upon this relatively simple pattern.

Signs produced by corticospinal dysfunction

The signs of cortical dysfunction can be produced by interference with the cortical cells themselves or by interference with their axons in the long corticospinal tracts. Common causes of damage to the cells are contusion, compression or infarction and common causes of damage to the long tracts include shearing of the corona radiata from deceleration injuries, thrombosis or haemorrhage involving the internal capsule, compression of the cerebral peduncle and (rarely) demyelination.

In coma, damage to the frontal lobes produces disturbances of eye movements. Damage to one frontal cortex produces a conjugate deviation of the eyes towards the side of the lesion so that if the motor cortex is also involved the patient will appear to be looking towards the normal, nonparalysed side.

Irritation of one frontal cortex results in deviation of the eyes away from the side of the irritation. This is not a common finding but could occur in a patient in post-ictal coma whose seizure was provoked by a localized superficial lesion in one frontal area. In general, conjugate deviation away from the side of the lesion and look-towards the paralysed side is a sign of midbrain damage.

Frontal lobe damage is often associated with a grasp reflex on the side opposite to the lesion. Bilateral damage can produce bilateral grasp reflexes. Occasionally comatose patients will open their eyes in response to nonspecific stimulation and, if approached from the appropriate side, the combination of grasping the hand and the deviated gaze may give the impression of awareness. This impression can be corrected by approaching the patient in the same manner from the opposite side.

Damage to the motor cortex or to the corticospinal pathways produces different signs depending upon the severity and extent of the damage and upon the age of the lesion. Minor injury produces a weakened but essentially normal purposive response to painful stimulation. With increasing severity the weakness progresses to complete flaccidity. Later, tone and movement return and the arm is flexed in response to stimulation until it assumes the position typical of longstanding hemiplegia. The elbow is flexed until the wrist lies on the chest, the wrist and metacarpo-phalangeal joints are flexed and the phalangeal joints extended. In the leg, cortico-spinal damage results initially in either weakened normal responses or flaccid paralysis followed later by an increase in tone which results in the leg and foot being extended and internally rotated. Stimulation of the sole of the foot will produce a positive Babinski response: the big toe is extended while the other toes are flexed and fanned outwards.

For cortical lesions to produce coma in the absence of brain stem dysfunction, decortication has to be bilateral and virtually complete. Consequently signs of cortical damage, though commonly seen in conscious patients with circumscribed lesions, are usually modified or added to in patients in coma because of concomitant injury to the brain stem and other areas. In particular the flexor response typical of localized corticospinal damage is not commonly seen in comatose patients who almost invariably have other subcortical lesions which tend to extend the signs from those described as 'decorticate' to those described as 'decerebrate'.

Decerebration

When damage involves the subcortical hemispheral structures such as the basal ganglia as well as the cortex the patient is said to be decerebrate. The condition may involve one or both sides. Usually the lesion is not as anatomically precise as the term would suggest and the rostral brain stem is also involved and the patient is comatose. Very occasionally unilateral or bilateral decerebrate responses are seen in conscious patients with small, isolated brain stem lesions. The effect of decerebration is to disconnect one or both hemispheres from the middle and lower brain stem. In the intact animal the activity of the facilitatory parts of the brain stem is modified by suppressor influences from the cortex and basal ganglia, in particular by those from the caudate nucleus. Decerebration liberates facilitatory activity from this control resulting in increased muscle tone on one or both sides of the body. Since the extensor muscles are in general stronger than flexor muscles a generalized increase in muscle tone results in generalized extension. In the patient with unilateral corticospinal damage the side opposite to the lesion will show an extensor response to painful stimulation. In this the arm is extended and adducted, the forearm is pronated and the wrist flexed; the thumb and fingers are flexed at the metacarpo-phalangeal joints and extended at the interphalangeal joints.

The leg is also extended and adducted and the foot is plantar-flexed. The plantar reflex is extensor. The other side may at the same time make purposive or semi-purposive movements in response to stimulation.

In coma with bilateral decerebration both sides respond to stimulation as described above but the movements tend to be more violent. The trunk muscles are also involved and the patient tends towards opisthotonus with an arched back and extended neck. In the bilaterally decerebrate patient nonspecific stimulation often facilitates other activities apart from increasing muscle tone. As well as extending vigorously the patient may show vigorous overbreathing, dilatation of the pupils, raising of the upper eyelid and a rise in systemic blood pressure and pulse rate. Occasionally pilo-erection and sweating are also seen. The dilatation of the pupils can often be demonstrated in conscious subjects by stimulating the back of the neck (the ciliospinal reflex). It is much more readily elicited and recognized in the decerebrate.

In the decerebrate patient, middle and lower brain stem functions are retained or even exaggerated. Patients in coma with lesions below the level of the upper pons have usually stopped breathing and are quite unresponsive.

Particular patterns of coma and coma from particular causes

There are other patterns of coma not described above which are either of intrinsic interest because of their unusual nature or because they are particularly likely to be seen by anaesthetists. The following account is by no means exhaustive.

Prolonged decorticate or decerebrate coma

The patterns described above are those usually seen in the first few hours following the insult producing coma. When coma persists for several days, patients who are partially decorticate or decerebrate may start to show spontaneous movements which are related to some recovery in subcortical function. The decorticate cat can perform normally many everyday functions such as walking, eating, fighting and even avoiding objects obstructing its path. Decorticate primates and humans can only produce very limited motor activity of a nonpurposive kind. In patients, decortication or decerebration is often incomplete and may be demonstrable on only one side. In these circumstances the patient's response to stimulation may be a confusing mixture of apparently purposive and nonpurposive. Sometimes the response will vary during the course of the day. Spontaneous movements may include movements of the lips and jaws, eye opening and myoclonic twitching. In patients with lesions which include the region of the subthalamic nucleus, hemibalismus may appear. This consists in a one-sided thrashing movement most noticeable in the arm. Focal twitching and convulsions may also occur. Prolonged signs of decerebration suggest a very bad prognosis whatever the initial cause.

Although not showing signs of consciousness, decerebrate patients sometimes show variations in reactivity that seem to be the equivalent of sleeping and waking.

The energy expended by decerebrate patients showing vigorous extensor spasms and overbreathing can be of the order of 3,000 to 4,000 kcal a day. This high metabolic rate may be in part due to increased catecholamine release from midbrain sympathetic stimulation. The excessive activity should be controlled by sedation.

Raised intracranial pressure (ICP)

Pressure change inside the skull associated with a shift of intracranial contents is a frequent cause of coma with unilateral or bilateral motor impairment. The cause may be a discrete, expanding lesion such as an abscess or haematoma or may be generalized as in widespread cerebral oedema. For a rise in pressure to produce coma there must exist pressure gradients which result in parts of the brain being pushed into abnormal positions and distorted or compressed.

A typical pattern is shown in Fig. 8.3. Here a unilateral supratentorial lesion has produced a deviation to the side opposite the lesion with herniation below the falx cerebri and herniation of the uncal process of the temporal lobe through the tentorial hiatus. When the uncal processes of the temporal lobes are forced by high supratentorial pressure through the tentorial hiatus the moulded shape of the combined unci and brain stem as seen at autopsy is conical. The process producing a transtentorial pressure cone is colloquially known as 'coning'.

'Reverse coning' is sometimes seen when a lesion in the posterior fossa so raises the infratentorial pressure that the superior parts of the cerebellum are forced upwards through the hiatus.

Both 'coning' and 'reverse coning' can be produced by the inappropriate withdrawal of CSF. Lumbar dural puncture can lower the infratentorial pressure so rapidly that the gradient from above to below the tentorium increases abruptly and 'coning' is precipitated. Equally, though less commonly seen, the aspiration of CSF from the lateral ventricles in patients with high infratentorial pressure can precipitate 'reverse coning'.

In both types of 'coning', brain stem function is interfered with both directly by pressure and indirectly by disturbance of its blood supply. With the downward or upward shift of the brain stem its supplying vessels may be stretched or compressed. In both events a failure of brain stem function is observed.

Generalized cerebral oedema such as may follow an hypoxic episode or a gross water overload involves both cerebral and cerebellar hemispheres equally and there is therefore no pressure gradient across tentorium and no transtentorial pressure cone.

When the uncal processes of the temporal lobes are forced through the tentorial

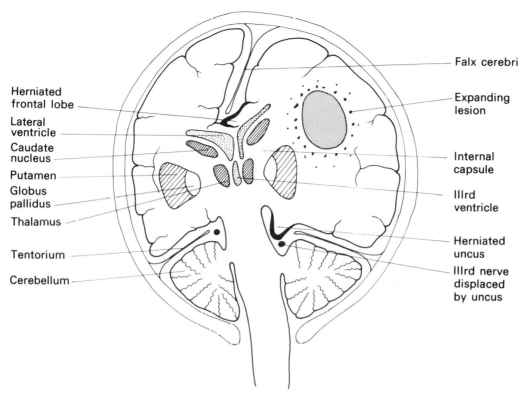

Falx cerebri

Herniated
frontal lobe

Expanding
lesion

Lateral
ventricle

Caudate
nucleus

Internal
capsule

Putamen

Globus
pallidus

IIIrd
ventricle

Thalamus

Herniated
uncus

Tentorium

IIIrd nerve
displaced
by uncus

Cerebellum

Fig. 8.3. A diagramatic representation of an oblique coronal section of the brain showing the distortion produced by an expanding cerebral lesion.

hiatus they impinge upon and stretch the oculomotor nerve. Patients with unilateral uncal herniation will show a partial or complete oculomotor (IIIrd nerve) palsy on the side of the lesion. This will be apparent before brain stem impairment is obvious. A patient who is in coma as a result of an expanding unilateral supratentorial lesion will already have considerable distortion of his intracranial contents and impaired brain stem function and a small further distortion or rise in pressure may cause irredeemable brain stem damage. Bilateral uncal herniation with bilateral third nerve signs produces greater brain stem compression and an earlier loss of consciousness. It is also a more urgent and precarious situation for the patient.

With acute rises in intracranial pressure papilloedema may or may not be present though it should always be looked for. Patients with unilateral expanding lesions sometimes show papilloedema only on the side of the lesion or show it more fully on that side. In the absence of direct measurement (which is increasingly used in neurosurgery) raised intracranial pressure usually has to be inferred from the patient's behaviour. Deepening coma with lateralizing signs is almost pathognomonic. Improvement with pressure lowering treatments such as head-up positioning, mechanical overventilation and dehydration therapy may show that a previous inference was correct.

Chronic subdural haematoma

One oddity which is worth mentioning in the context of raised intracranial pressure and brain shifts is the appearance of ipsilateral signs in patients with a chronic subdural haematoma. It seems that the diffuse gentle pressure over most of the surface of one hemisphere does not produce uncal herniation on that side but compresses the *opposite* cerebral peduncle against the free edge of the tentorium. The result is a weakness or paralysis on the same side of the body as the subdural haematoma. The paradigmatic presentation is of a patient with weakness or paralysis on one side in whom a skull X-ray shows a calcified pineal shifted towards the (opposite) normal side.

Basal ganglia disturbances

Some patients in coma may have disproportional damage to the basal ganglia on one or both sides. This may give rise to spontaneous athetoid or choreiform movements or give an athetoid component to the movements provoked by stimulation. For these disturbances to be apparent some cerebrospinal tracts must be intact: the patient cannot be decerebrate or at least not on the side responsible for the abnormal movements. There may, however, be considerable interruption of the specifically cortico-spinal pathways or again these may be relatively spared. In the latter case the movements can be seen to be purposive and the final goal is usually achieved though with much jerking and writhing during the performance.

Akinetic mutism

A curious type of coma is occasionally seen called 'akinetic mutism' in the English literature and 'coma vigile' in the French. The patient at times appears to be awake in that his eyes are open and they sometimes move in what appears to be a seeing way. Lash and corneal reflexes are present and he may sometimes blink in response to a threatening movement towards the eyes. He is mute and makes very few spontaneous movements. In response to pain his movements appear purposive but are feeble or incomplete. He is doubly incontinent. A wide variety of lesions has been described in association with this state but it is probable that the essential common factor is a disturbance of function in the reticular formation in the region of the posterior diencephalon and upper midbrain.

   The prognosis depends upon the cause and associated lesions but the condition is not necessarily irrecoverable. Transient akinetic mutism with recovery is sometimes seen after intracranial surgery.

Coma due to hypoxia

The CNS may be made hypoxic by profound hypotension or cardiac arrest or from breathing an atmosphere with a low or absent oxygen content. In hypotensive states cerebral damage may be patchy and areas between the arterial territories may be selectively damaged. This is not because the cells there are more vulnerable to hypoxia but because they are made more hypoxic because of their relatively precarious blood supply.

   In total hypoxia such as follows cardiac arrest, unevenness of damage is related to the different susceptibilities of different parts of the brain. Cells that are particularly liable to hypoxic damage are the Purkinje cells of the cerebellum and the cells of the basal ganglion especially those of the globus pallidus. Also susceptible are the myelin sheaths in the cerebral white matter. As a result of this differential susceptibility some patients who survive an hypoxic episode may have an apparently undamaged cerebral cortex but show various disorders of movement.

After an hypoxic episode a patient should regain his prehypoxic state within 45–120 minutes if he is to survive without some neurological diminishment. In patients who are under the influence of CNS depressant drugs at the time of the episode or immediately after it, recovery may be more prolonged but also more complete. This is due to the protective effect of agents that depress CNS metabolism and hence oxygen requirements. Occasionally recovery can apparently be complete even after several hours of coma and this seems to happen after carbon monoxide poisoning more often than after hypoxia from other causes.

Occasionally patients lapse again into coma some days after apparent recovery from the initial insult. This delayed response to hypoxia is due to demyelination of cerebral white matter. The process may result in complete decortication or may arrest spontaneously at a stage that still allows recovery. The phenomenon appears to be an immune response in which the patient produces antibodies to his own myelin. The formation of the antibodies is presumable triggered by the release of myelin or myelin breakdown products from white matter damaged during the initial episode.

The treatment of delayed recovery following an hypoxic episode is unsatisfactory. Hypothermia, dehydration therapy, sedation with barbiturates, overventilation and steroids have all been tried without apparent success. Dehydration therapy and over-ventilation with added oxygen are the measures most likely to be of use. Hypothermia and sedation offer considerable protection before the insult but are of little help after it. Steroids are often given but have little effect upon damage that is widespread. Steroids, and indeed the other treatments listed above, are effective in inverse proportion to the size of the cerebral lesion.

Cerebral fat embolism

This condition starts as a series of small cerebral infarcts and rapidly progresses to a generalized cerebral oedema. The patient is likely to have pulmonary fat embolism as well as cerebral embolization and is likely to suffer some respiratory embarrassment from this cause.

Treatment is with steroids and oxygen and with passive overventilation if the patient is unconscious or if he has difficulty in maintaining normal gas exchange because of pulmonary damage. The administration of CO_2 has been recommended for this condition in the hope that it would dilate the cerebral vasculature and allow the fat droplets to pass through. However, the suggestion is misconceived since the fat emboli normally pass through the precapillary arterioles (which are the vessels that dilate in response to a raised Pa,CO_2) but are too large to pass through the capillaries which they block. Dehydration therapy and the administration of barbiturates would both be reasonable treatments but are not commonly employed.

Recovery from fat embolism is extremely difficult to predict but it is probably true to say that the outlook is better than it would be for the same length and depth of coma if this were due to head injury.

Psychogenic coma

The term psychogenic coma is used to describe apparent coma which has no basis in organic disease and it includes frank malingering, hysteria, and extreme psychotic

9*

withdrawal and nonresponsiveness. All these conditions have some features in common which distinguish them from coma due to intoxications or structural damage.

Muscle tone. The limbs are rarely flaccid and often show increasing tone or resistance as the examiner moves them more vigorously. An arm lifted and allowed to fall will usually show a slowed or controlled return to rest. This is particularly noticeable if the arm is lifted and released so that it would be expected to fall on the patient's face. Tendon reflexes are normal and the plantor responses are flexor.

The response to painful stimuli. This is often minimal or absent and the patient shows an indifference to pain comparable to that shown by someone in an hypnotic trance. As with those in a trance, indignities or proposed indignities that threaten personal modesty or self esteem produce a more vigorous reaction than superficial pain.

Covering the nose and mouth to prevent breathing will usually unmask the hysteric or malingerer but may be accepted passively by the severely retarded psychotic.

Eye movement. The eyes usually fix straight ahead or roll upwards if the eyelids are lifted; they never rove as in light coma. Oculocephalic reflexes cannot be elicited and caloric stimulation of the middle ear produces nystagmus not deviation.

There is usually some resistance to lifting the eyelids and when released they close forcefully while the lids of a patient in coma tend to fall back into the closed position relatively slowly. A rapid movement towards the open eye will produce a blink.

Psychotic patients. These are usually easier to recognize than the malingerer or hysteric. They are often immobile but muscle tone is normal and they adopt and maintain a position that is typical of consciousness such as standing or sitting. On examination, their responses tend to be very slow and blunted but essentially normal. The most difficult imposter to detect is probably the informed person shamming psychosis.

HEMIPLEGIA AND DIPLEGIA

The recognition of corticospinal lesions in comatose patients was discussed in the previous section. Such lesions are not incompatible with consciousness and indeed the spastic gait of the hemiplegic or diplegic person is one of the most frequently seen and easily recognizable manifestations of serious neurological disease.

Stroke

A common cause of hemiplegia is a cerebrovascular accident in which the internal capsule is damaged by thrombosis or haemorrhage. The striate arteries deriving from the proximal part of the middle cerebral artery are peculiarly liable to rupture and, equally peculiar, when they do rupture the haemorrhage is often very limited so that the volume of nervous tissue destroyed is surprisingly small. It may be so small that on superficial examination the damage may seem to be confined to the cortico-spinal or pyramidal tract. Since the corticospinal fibres are intimately mixed with other descending fibres going from the cortex to the brain stem a pure corticospinal lesion is not possible and many of the signs shown by hemiplegic patients are due to destruction of these nonpyramidal, corticofugal pathways.

Immediately following a 'stroke' there is usually a flaccid paralysis of the side opposite to the site of the lesion. If the dominant hemisphere is involved the patient will also be aphasic or dysphasic. (Dominance for speech does not necessarily follow dominance for handedness. In some 40 per cent of left handed people speech is a function of the *left* cerebral hemisphere.) When the flaccidity passes off the patient becomes hyperreflexic. Some voluntary movement returns but is limited. The limitation is most noticeable in the hand and fingers which are often held immobile in the position described on page 248. Voluntary movements of the face are limited though wrinkling of the forehead is typically retained since this movement has bilateral cortical representation. Facial movements provoked by emotion are also retained and may even be exaggerated. Abdominal and cremasteric reflexes are lost on the affected side and the plantar response is extensor. The spasticity and hyperreflexia are partly due to interruption of the corticospinal fibres and partly due to interruption of the nonpyramidal fibres that accompany them. Projections from the cortex to brain stem normally exert an inhibitory influence on the facilitatory brain stem nuclei. Disinhibition of the red nucleus by disruption of corticorubral fibres results in spasticity especially of the proximal limb muscles and disinhibition of the vestibular nucleus by disruption of the corticovestibular fibres results in spastic extension of the leg.

The above description applies to hemiplegia produced by the most limited of lesions in the internal capsule. Frequently the damage is wider and involves the sensory limb of the capsule. Parts of the caudate nucleus, globus pallidus and thalamus may also be damaged.

Although a limited lesion in the internal capsule has been used as an example of the catastrophe referred to as 'stroke', other vascular lesions are covered by the term and hemiplegia may follow such accidents as carotid occlusion, embolization of the middle cerebral artery or its branches, cerebrovascular spasm and haemorrhage.

When hemiplegia or hemiparesis is caused by lesions above the internal capsule, that is in the corona radiata or the cortex itself or by pressure upon the cortex, the signs will vary depending upon the size, position and the rate of development of the lesion. It has been said that in hemiplegia the muscles of respiration are spared. This is certainly not true in the acute phase of hemiplegia due to a cortical lesion where there may be complete intercostal paralysis on the affected side. The diaphragm however seems to contract normally. The paralysis of the intercostal muscles reduces lung expansion on the affected side and the combined paralysis of intercostal and abdominal muscles reduces the effectiveness of coughing and serious consolidation/collapse can occur.

Apart from the possible interference with lung function, hemiplegia is also of interest to the anaesthetist since it is one of the conditions in which suxamethonium-induced hyperkalaemia is reported to occur [1]. As in chronic paraplegia this is puzzling since the muscles involved are not denervated. Dangerous rises in plasma potassium cannot be frequent since many patients with acute or long-standing hemiplegia have been given suxamethonium without ill effect.

The diagnostic use of a nerve stimulator in patients recovering from non-depolarizing neuromuscular blocking agents may be unreliable if the paralysed side is tested. There is an apparent resistance to block in the paralysed limbs suggesting that there is either a lowering of motor end-plate threshold or an increase in the number of acetylcholine receptor sites.

The spasticity following a stroke has recently been treated with dantrolene. This is a hydantoin derivative that acts directly upon muscle fibres, probably by interfering with calcium release. Phenothiazines will also reduce spasticity just as they reduce decerebrate rigidity and decerebrate spasms.

Diplegia

Congenital diplegia (Little's disease) was originally ascribed to birth trauma. It is now believed to result from intrauterine damage probably due to a viral infection. Similar symmetrical lesions sometimes follow viral infections in later life. The patient with diplegia could be described as having a bilateral hemiplegia in that the individual disabilities are of the same *kind* but affecting both sides. The *degree* of disability however is usually different. Hand movements are often better than in hemiplegia while control over the muscles innervated by the cranial nerves is less good. This latter disability may be so severe that coherent speech is difficult or virtually impossible. Chewing and swallowing may also be impeded. For the anaesthetist this means that such patients may have difficulty in maintaining an airway when they are not fully conscious and that they will have difficulty in coping with blood or vomit in the mouth or throat.

CONVULSIONS AND EPILEPSY

In epilepsy and other convulsive disorders, nerve cells become unusually excitable so that they may discharge spontaneously. The unusual excitability and spontaneous discharge may be limited to a small part of the brain, in which case the patient will show focal signs only, or they may become generalized in which case consciousness will be interrupted and the patient may have a typical convulsion. Overexcitability and spontaneous discharge can result from many different causes. Every person will convulse in response to a sufficient and appropriate stimulus, although in some the convulsive threshold would seem to be lower than in others. The term epilepsy, unqualified, is probably best reserved to describe the condition of those patients in whom no provocative focus can be identified but in whom the evidence suggests that an abnormal area in the diencephalon or upper brain stem is initiating the observed disturbance. Such patients could be described as suffering from 'idiopathic epilepsy'. In others the term epilepsy should be qualified depending upon the site of the provocative lesion and in general these patients could be described as suffering from 'symptomatic epilepsy'. Describing a patient as 'epileptic' implies a continuing liability to convulsions or some other manifestation of abnormal neuronal discharge and the term should not be applied to those who have one or more convulsions in response to an acute insult but who are thereafter free of convulsions.

TYPES OF EPILEPSY

Petit mal

This 'idiopathic' or 'centrencephalic' epilepsy typically presents with seizures consisting of brief periods of unconsciousness lasting only some seconds. The patient does not fall nor convulse and to the onlooker may appear transiently dazed or uncomprehending. The attacks have been described as 'absences'. The EEG during the attack shows a synchronous discharge over all areas of a repeated spike and wave pattern which is seen in no other condition.

Petit mal usually starts in childhood. Occasionally it precedes grand mal in which case the EEG pattern during the seizures changes to that typical of major epilepsy. Since the EEG patterns of grand mal and petit mal are different, it is assumed that the provocative lesion is differently sited in the two conditions. The change in seizure pattern from petit to grand mal presumably therefore represents a change in the site of the lesion.

Grand mal

This is another centrencephalic (idiopathic) epilepsy in which major seizures are preceded by a warning aura which is usually a nonspecific feeling of strangeness. When the initiating lesion is in one or other cerebral hemisphere, the aura has characteristics that depend upon the site of the lesion. The first phase of the convulsion is tonic; the subject loses consciousness and falls to the ground where he lies rigid, jaw clenched, breath held, arms adducted at the shoulder but flexed at the elbow and legs extended. After some 30 seconds the rigidity is replaced by spasmodic contraction and relaxation. At this stage he may thump his head or limbs rhythmically against the ground. Breathing will restart but spasms will interfere with it. The subject may also bite his tongue and frothy saliva may appear on the lips. He is often incontinent of urine and occasionally of faeces. The clonic phase lasts a minute or so and is followed by a period of unconsciousness lasting from a few minutes to half an hour. The subject then wakes but if undisturbed will probably sleep for perhaps several hours. Grand mal convulsions are sometimes followed by a period of automatism during which the patient behaves in an apparently ordered way but cannot explain his behaviour and has no memory of it.

The tonic and clonic phases of the convulsion are presumed to be due to abnormal discharges from the facilitator areas of the brain stem. The EEG shows repated high voltage spikes with no interspersed waves.

Seizures due to hemispheral lesions

An irritable focus in one or other cerebral hemisphere can act as the initiator of seizure activity. Sometimes the area of excitability spreads to include virtually the whole brain and a typical grand mal convulsion occurs. Sometimes it is limited, in which case consciousness may be retained in the presence of localized abnormal motor activity or involuntary and abnormal thoughts and sensations.

The temporal lobe is a common site for an irritable lesion and is often caused by birth trauma. Temporal lobe seizures can take many forms depending upon the function of that part of the lobe containing the lesion. Typically there is no grand mal convulsion but a period of altered consciousness during which the subject may experience tastes or smells, recall memories of past events, have perceptual disturbances (including the sensation of 'déjà vu'), have feelings of terror or extreme depression. Sometimes chewing and lip-smacking accompany sensations of taste and smell and this type of seizure has been called an 'uncinate fit'. Sometimes there is abnormal behaviour such as inappropriate rage, aggression or sexual activity. The provoking lesion can very occasionally be localized by electrocorticography and excised.

Lesions impinging upon the motor cortex can cause Jacksonian seizures (first described by Hughlings Jackson) in which the subject is liable to involuntary twitching. The twitching may be limited to one part, such as a hand or foot or the face, or may start in one part and spread until first the whole of one side of the body is jerking and then a generalized convulsion supervenes. After a Jacksonian seizure the patient may show a temporary paralysis of the limb in which the seizure started (Todd's paralysis).

Equivalent seizures may result from irritative lesions of the sensory cortex. In these the patient may be aware of abnormal sensations in some part but never of pain. The attack may be limited to localized paraesthesiae or may progress to a major convulsion.

Other parts of the hemisphere may contain an irritable focus which may be provoked by appropriate sensory input. Flicker can precipitate a seizure in some people and noise or music has also been known to do so.

Local and generalized disorders causing convulsions

Many local lesions can initiate convulsive activity; some of the more common include acute head injury, scarring from a previous injury, untreated depressed fracture of the skull, chronic subdural haematoma, abscess, subdural empyema, vascular malformation, tumour and parasitic cysts.

Generalized systemic disturbances causing convulsions include fever, hypoxia, carbon dioxide retention, uraemia, diabetic coma, hypoglycaemia, raised intracranial pressure, hypertension and water overload. Water overload or water retention with some degree of cerebral oedema probably accounts for attacks that occur in association with drinking bouts (though alcohol may also be a factor), in association with menstruation, pregnancy and the taking of an oestrogen containing contraceptive pill.

Seizures occurring for the first time during pregnancy are almost certainly provoked by water retention and the consequent slight cerebral oedema. In pregnant women already taking anticonvulsants an exacerbation of attacks may be due to altered pharmacokinetics in the pregnant state resulting in lower blood levels of the drugs. The convulsions of eclampsia are probably provoked by cerebral oedema secondary to both hypertension and water retention.

Overbreathing will produce convulsions in susceptible subjects. The exact mechanism is not clear. Probably it is the combination of cortical ischaemia, a raised pH and a lowered ionized calcium that is responsible. It has been suggested that the increased liability of pregnant women to convulsions might be due to their slight overbreathing. This seems improbable since the Pa,co_2 in pregnancy is rarely below 4 kPa (30 mmHg) while the Pa,co_2 associated with convulsions due to voluntary overbreathing is of the order of 2 kPa (15 mmHg) or less. Convulsive episodes were seen in the EEG during cooling for operations performed under profound hypothermia (core temperature 10–15°C). These were thought to be due to the very low levels of Pa,co_2 that occurred in those circumstances and the phenomenon was not seen when Pa,co_2 was kept near normal values by adding CO_2 to the anaesthetic gases.

Myoclonus

Some patients with grand or petit mal and some nonepileptic subjects make occasional jerking movements of the limbs. The movements, known as myoclonus, are associated with a brief cortical discharge. Both movements and discharge typically last less than a second. The twitching sometimes seen with the use of methohexitone and other induction agents has been described as myoclonic. This is however a misuse of the term since the methohexitone induced movements are not the symmetrical, vigorour jerks of true myoclonus and they are not associated with a cortical discharge.

THE PHARMACOLOGY OF EPILEPSY

The pharmacology of epilepsy is complicated and like the pharmacology of basal ganglia disturbances involves some unexplained paradoxical observations. Some drugs can produce different effects depending upon dosage. Lignocaine, a cell membrane stabilizer, can be used to control status epilepticus but in excessive dosage or directly applied to the cortex, it will induce convulsions. Thiopentone can be used to control convulsions. It has also been used to provoke discharges from epileptic foci (which show in the EEG as sharp spikes) though its use for this purpose has been abandoned in favour of the more effective methohexitone. Methohexitone and Althesin have been reported to cause convulsions yet both in larger dosage can control status epilepticus.

Drugs producing convulsions

Apart from analeptics many other drugs have been reported to cause convulsions both in known epileptics and in nonepileptic subjects. The anaesthetic drugs ether, halothane, methohexitone, Althesin, propanidid and ketamine have all been implicated. Enflurane in concentrations at twice MAC or more (i.e. more than 3 per cent) will regularly produce convulsive discharges in the EEG which are associated with frank convulsions if the patient is not paralysed. This convulsive activity is produced more readily if the Pa,CO_2 is below normal.

Drugs that are not commonly recognized as convulsants but which may either produce convulsions on their own or additively enhance the convulsive properties of other drugs, include penicillin (especially when given intravenously or intrathecally), oxacillin and carbenicillin, tricyclic antidepressants and the phenothiazines. The intrathecal contrast materials used in radiology, metrizamide and iophendylate can both, rarely, cause convulsions if allowed to enter the intracranial CSF. Metrizamide is much more likely than iophendylate to have this effect and it is recommended that it should not be used in known epileptics and that phenothiazines and butyrophenones should not be given before metrizamide radiography.

Drugs used in the treatment of convulsions

Some twenty or more different drugs are in regular use for the control of convulsive disorders and each has its particular indications and contraindications. Here it is only necessary to discuss in general the problems associated with anticonvulsant treatment.

Enzyme induction

Phenobarbitone and phenytoin are probably the most commonly prescribed anticonvulsants and both are active inducers of microsomal enzymes. The effects of this enzyme induction are often of importance to the patients receiving the drugs. The enzyme induction due to phenobarbitone increases not only the rate of destruction of phenobarbitone itself but also the rate of destruction of phenytoin. The induction produced by both drugs can increase the breakdown and inactivation of steroids with the result that osteomalacaia may occur from vitamin D deficiency, unwanted pregnancy from inactivation of the oestrogen component of the contraceptive pill and ineffective medication from dexamethazone and triamcinalone. The metabolism of other steroids is probably also interfered with but ill effects from this cause have not been reported. The metabolism of coumarin anticoagulants is also increased.

Direct adverse effects

These are numerous and phenytoin itself must have had attributed to it more unwanted actions than any other drug in common use. It has been held responsible for rashes of various sorts, fever, Stevens–Johnson syndrome, lupus erythematosus-like syndromes, hepatitis, renal failure, mononucleosis, eosinophilia, anaemia, thrombocytopaenia, leucopenia, lymphoid hyperplasia resembling lymphoma, pulmonary infiltrates, diffuse intravascular coagulation, thyroiditis, serum sickness, albuminuria and low circulating levels of the IgA globulin fraction. These reactions are not common; common unwanted effects are drowsiness and ataxia, gingival hyperplasia and megaloblastic anaemia due to a disturbance of folate metabolism (see page 343). Many of these side-effects are produced by other anticonvulsants. All patients on anticonvulsant treatment are liable to drowsiness and ataxia and alterations in mood and mental state. Congenital abnormalities have been reported following the use of trimethadione and paramethadione and phenytoin and carbamazepine have been shown to cause fetal abnormalities in mice.

Sodium valproate, a recent introduction in the management of epilepsy, can cause abnormal movements due to a disturbance of basal ganglia function. The anticonvulsant carbamazepine is of interest in that it is effective in the treatment of trigeminal neuralgia. It was first used for this purpose because it was thought that the spasmodic attacks of pain typical of the complaint might be some sort of 'epileptic equivalent' and that the attacks might therefore be modified by anticonvulsant therapy. Trigeminal neuralgia is no longer believed to be related to the epilepsies but carbamazepine remains a useful drug in its management.

Status epilepticus

In status epilepticus the patient convulses continuously or has a series of convulsions with only a very short interval between them without regaining consciousness. It may be precipitated by the sudden withdrawal or reduction of medication. It can occur after head injury or other direct cortical insult. It can follow the abrupt withdrawal of addictive drugs particularly of barbiturates, alcohol and diazepam. As in other convulsions, neuronal damage is caused by secondary hypoxia and also by the abnormal nervous activity itself. In treatment therefore it is not sufficient merely to control the motor manifestations by paralysis and ensure adequate ventilation and oxygenation, the abnormal electrical discharges must also be suppressed. Many drugs have been used to control status epilepticus. At present it seems usual practice to use intravenous diazepam or lorazepam in the first instance. If these fail or are only effective in very large doses it is the author's experience that chlormethiazole is an effective and convenient drug. The dose required to control the convulsions is often such that the patient needs to be artificially ventilated. Chlormethiazole has a shorter effective half-life in the body than diazepam or lorazepam so that recovery is quicker when the administration is stopped. The use of relaxants as well as sedation is recommended by some. If the patient is paralysed some form of monitoring of the EEG is needed to ensure that the abnormal neuronal activity is suppressed. A convenient machine for this purpose is the 'cerebral function monitor'. This is a modified and simplified EEG machine which records from two tempero-parietal electrodes and produces a record of the electrical output of the brain integrated with time. The vigorous electrical discharge associated with convulsive activity is readily recognizable in the write-out.

Paralysis is not usually necessary and in its absence the attendant staff can easily see the unsuppressed convulsions.

The anaesthetist and the epileptic patient

Epileptics are often ashamed of their condition and may suppress the fact that they are epileptic when they come into hospital. They may also leave their medication at home. The anaesthetist should ensure that medication is continued throughout the perioperative period and this may entail parenteral administration. Phenytoin is said to be poorly or erratically absorbed when given by intramuscular injection (though the author has seen no evidence of this in 20 years of practice in a neurosurgical unit) and more predictable blood levels are obtained when it is given by mouth or by nasogastric tube. Intravenous injection is effective but requires caution. Phenytoin has antidysrrhythmic effects upon the heart, depressing atrial and ventricular automaticity and has been recommended in the treatment of tachydysrrhythmias due to digitalis poisoning. Intravenous injection should therefore be in 50 mg increments given at 5-minute intervals; a total of some 200–300 mg may be required in an adult.

Treated epileptics are permanently a little sedated and smaller doses of anaesthetics are required than in normal patients. Phenothiazines and enflurane should be avoided.

Because of the possibility of folate deficiency and of bone marrow dyscrasia a full blood picture should be obtained before surgery.

Neurosurgical patients who have had a supratentorial craniotomy for aneurysm, head injury or for meningioma are particularly liable to convulsions and should be given prophylactic treatment for some 3 or 4 months postoperatively.

RAISED INTRACRANIAL PRESSURE AND CEREBRAL OEDEMA

Intracranial pressure can be raised by the presence of a mass lesion such as a tumour, abscess or haematoma or by an increase in CSF volume, intracranial blood volume, an increase in brain water or by a combination of these factors. Since the cranium is rigid and the intracranial contents are virtually incompressible the increase in volume of any one component has to be accommodated by a decrease in volume of some other component. The normal accommodation is for CSF to move from the intracranial compartment into the spinal dural sac.

When the brain becomes oedematous the excess water is found mainly in the glial cells in the grey matter and in the interstitial space in the white matter. The anatomical extracellular space in the brain is less than in other tissues occupying only some 10 per cent of the brain volume compared with 20–30 per cent in other tissues. The glial cytoplasm serves many of the functions performed by extracellular fluid elsewhere in the body. The exchange of water between the vascular compartment and the glial cytoplasm and extracellular space can be considered to follow Starling's hypothesis (see Fig. 8.4). The factors tending to increase brain water will therefore be systemic hypertension, arteriolar dilatation, increased capillary permeability, increased venous pressure and reduced plasma oncotic pressure. This latter is rarely important though the converse may be, in that the intentional raising of plasma oncotic pressure with intravenous, hypertonic, colloid solutions is an effective way of reducing raised intracranial pressure. Changes in plasma osmolality can be important and if the

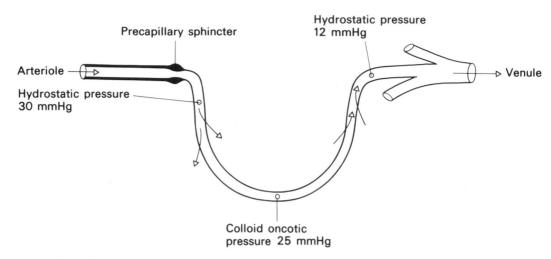

Fig. 8.4. This figure shows diagramatically *some* of the interconnections between the basal ganglia and functionally related nuclear masses.

plasma is hypotonic in relation to the brain cytoplasm, water will enter the cells causing cerebral oedema.

Systemic hypertension when mean arterial pressures exceed 150–160 mmHg cannot be accommodated by the autoregulatory mechanisms present in the cerebral vasculature and will result in a raised capillary filtration pressure. Arteriolar dilatation is caused by a rise in Pa,CO_2, a fall in Pa,O_2, a fall in pH and by many drugs and anaesthetic agents. Arteriolar dilatation not only encourages oedema formation by raising the filtration pressure in the capillaries but also raises the intracranial pressure by increasing intracranial blood volume.

Capillary permeability is increased by hypoxia, inflammation, accumulation of metabolites and by low blood cortisol levels. The sudden reduction of high blood glucocorticoid levels can also increase cerebral capillary permeability and the abrupt withdrawal of long term steroid therapy may precipitate cerebral oedema.

Signs and symptoms of raised intracranial pressure (ICP)

The signs and symptoms described below are common to all patients with raised ICP; however, patients with intracranial mass lesions may have superadded focal signs. The three classical hallmarks of raised ICP are headache, vomiting and papilloedema. There may also be complaints of drowsiness and giddiness and blurred vision or transient blindness. Double vision may occur from sixth nerve palsy which may be bilateral. Acute rises in intracranial pressure may result in coma and convulsions. A rise in blood pressure and slowing of the pulse typically accompanies acute rises in ICP. The signs and symptoms are worse on waking in the morning. This is probably due to a temporary exacerbation of the raised pressure due to raised CO_2 levels and recumbancy. There is mild CO_2 retention during normal sleep which is sufficient to cause some cerebral vasodilatation. Recumbancy results in a positive venous pressure in the head and neck in place of the negative pressure present when a person is upright. Bending the head downwards, coughing and straining, will all aggravate the symptoms. Due to the papilloedema there is an enlargement of the blind spot.

CAUSES OF CHRONIC RAISED ICP

Carbon dioxide retention

An arterial $P\text{CO}_2$ of 8 kPa (60 mmHg) or above can produce raised intracranial pressure and papilloedema. The patient often complains of headache. He may have a coarse, flapping tremor. He may have disturbed sleep with unpleasant dreams and he may show fluctuations in conscious level and have periods of confusion. The arterial CO_2 levels producing these signs and symptoms are not necessarily associated with obviously distressed breathing and the respiratory cause of the neurological signs may be overlooked. This is especially likely if the lungs are normal and the respiratory disability is due to reduced respiratory movements from such things as muscle weakness (myopathy), injury or gross obesity. The immediate cause of the cerebral oedema is again cerebral arteriolar dilatation.

Polycythaemia

In polycythaemia the blood viscosity is considerably increased and there is a compensating cerebral arteriolar dilatation which tends to maintain total cerebrovascular resistance within normal limits. There is however a concomitant increase in capillary pressure and cerebral oedema can result. The signs and symptoms of raised ICP which may be found in polycythaemia disappear when the haematocrit is returned to normal values.

Hypervitiminosis A

Hypervitaminosis is another cause of raised intracranial pressure with papilloedema. The patient complains of severe headache and sometimes also of nausea and vomiting. The condition is usually due to excessive self-medication and remits when this is stopped. The mechanism responsible is probably cerebral vasodilatation following lysosome breakdown and the release of lysosomal enzymes.

Benign intracranial hypertension

This, as yet, unexplained condition occurs most frequently in overweight young women, following pregnancy and/or in association with irregular menstruation. It is very rarely seen in men. Intracranial pressure is markedly raised, the ventricles are small and compressed and the brain is swollen. Papilloedema is extreme and the patient's vision is often at risk. Cerebral blood flow is increased. Diagnosis is by exclusion of other lesions. The condition is self-limiting, remitting spontaneously in three to six months. The danger to the patient is that during this time she may suffer permanent optic nerve damage and urgent surgical decompression is sometimes necessary to preserve vision. The increased cerebral blood flow suggests that the primary lesion is a cerebral arteriolar dilatation and that this results in increased capillary filtration pressure and increased passage of water into the brain tissues and an increase in intracranial blood volume. There is probably also an element of increased capillary permeability. The symptoms can be alleviated and the natural remission accelerated by measures that reduce ICP and cerebral oedema. Regular lumbar puncture and the removal of CSF; diuretics and osmotic dehydration regimes have been used singly or in combination. The steroids cortisone, hydrocortisone and prednisone have all been used effectively. Dexamethazone is now the steroid of choice. The puzzling element in this condition is that no precipitating factor has been identified though some disturbance of steroid metabolism seems probable.

CAUSES OF ACUTE RISES IN ICP

Disequilibrium

There are several acute 'non-surgical' causes of raised ICP. Most of these are due to an acute fall in plasma osmolality either in absolute terms or in relation to the cerebral intracellular osmolality.

Water 'intoxication'. Whenever a person drinks water at a faster rate than his kidneys can excrete it, generalized water overloading will eventually occur, the most serious effect of which is acute cerebral oedema. Water intoxication is not the most apt description of the condition since no toxins are involved but it is used here as a convenient and generally understood term. The classical circumstances for water intoxication occur when a patient with diabetes insipidus is treated with vasopressin but still allowed to consume his normal quantity of water. Similar circumstances can occur following the obstetric use of oxytocin.

In the absence of diuresis, water is retained and the more rapid the absorption, the more will the water be preferentially distributed to those organs with the richest blood supply. Since the brain at rest receives 20 per cent of the cardiac output, rapid water drinking is likely selectively to cause cerebral oedema.

The condition usually manifests itself by the patient lapsing, over a matter of minutes rather than hours, through stupor to coma with convulsions. Treatment is with sedation and diuretics, making sure that the airway and breathing are adequate. Frusemide will overcome the antidiuretic effect of both vasopressin and oxytocin.

Hypotonic fluid therapy can give rise to an exactly similar clinical pattern when solutions are used which are hypotonic in terms of those solutes that remain in the extracellular compartment. Solutions such as 5 per cent dextrose are 'isotonic' in the sense that red cells will not either become crenated or haemolysed when bathed in them but in terms of body distribution they enter the cells almost as readily as water. The important ion in this context is sodium since it is almost entirely retained in the extracellular compartment. Solutions low in sodium will mostly be distributed in the same way as water or 5 per cent dextrose, that is into total body water.

Beer drinking can result in water as well as alcohol intoxication. The anaesthetist is most likely to meet this combination in the drunken accident patient. He may also occasionally be asked to attend an EEG recording session where a defendant in legal proceedings is being investigated for temporal lobe epilepsy. Such a subject will be given sufficient beer to make him drunk while his EEG is examined for abnormal discharges. In these circumstances it is sometimes necessary to control violent anti-social behaviour or grand mal convulsions: both with some alacrity.

The replacement of sweat by hypotonic fluids is a not uncommon cause of acute cerebral oedema. Furnace beaters in steel works (who sweated profusely) were given 'small' beer with added salt. 'Small' here means low in alcohol content and the replacement solution they were drinking could be described as acceptably flavoured normal saline. Patients in respiratory failure are often grossly dehydrated both from sweating and from inadequate fluid intake. If their water deficit is made up with hypotonic solutions they are very liable to develop acute cerebral oedema.

Uraemic patients and those in hyperglycaemic, diabetic coma are liable to sudden reductions in plasma osmolality during the effective treatment of their condition. With dialysis or with insulin treatment, the blood urea, or glucose, level will fall very rapidly. Because of the impediment to the free movement of solutes between the brain and systemic circulation (known as the 'blood-brain barrier') the brain cells will be transiently hypertonic in relation to the plasma. The result of this will be a movement of water into the brain cells. Too rapid a reduction of blood urea or blood glucose levels can result in acute cerebral oedema with coma and convulsions.

An analogous disparity between brain cell and plasma osmolality is responsible for the 'rebound' cerebral swelling that occasionally follows dehydration therapy with agents such as hypertonic urea or hypertonic mannitol solutions. Gross overdose with hypertonic solutions, such as glucose, can also produce coma although the mechanism of this may be acute intracellular dehydration.

Intracranial disease such as chronic subdural haematoma, brain abscess or tumour can result in gross dehydration because the patient has been apathetic or stuporose and has not been given an adequate and appropriate fluid intake. To correct such dehydration with salt-poor solutions will almost certainly produce cerebral oedema. Isotonic saline should be given and if the serum sodium is below normal, a calculated volume of hypertonic saline should be added to the rehydration regime.

It may be thought that the preceding paragraphs have overelaborated a relatively simple problem but the author has seen the sequence: inappropriate fluid replacement, coma, convulsions and death more often than can be considered desirable in contemporary medical practice.

Steroids and intracranial pressure

The relationship between different endogenous and exogenous steroid compounds and intracranial pressure is not clear: different mechanisms seem to be present in different circumstances and sometimes the same compounds seem to be able both to cause and alleviate a rise in ICP.

As stated above, benign intracranial hypertension occurs almost exclusively in fat, young women with menstrual disturbances or a history of recent pregnancy and it is possible that steroid hormones play a part in its pathogenesis. A condition indistinguishable from benign intracranial hypertension has been seen in women taking an oestrogen/progestin contraceptive pill. These women have not been overweight and their condition improves as soon as the pill is stopped.

A previous generation of both general surgeons and neurosurgeons maintained that women bled more at operation if they were menstruating. Neurosurgeons also claimed that the brain was 'congested'. It is possible that salt and water retention results in some increase in cardiac output and peripheral vasodilatation and it is also possible that the general reduction in visceral smooth muscle tone at the end of the cycle (and during pregnancy) involves also the smooth muscle of the arterioles. If these changes applied to the cerebral vessels congestion and oedema would result. Some women have congested, watering eyes immediately preceding and during menstruation (so called 'menstrual red eye') and in some a premenstrual rise in intraocular pressure has been recorded. Since the eye and brain respond similarly to physiological changes it is easy to imagine that, at least in these women, the brain is also congested and contains excess water.

Patients treated with triamcinalone have developed a condition resembling benign intracranial hypertension which has improved when the drug has been withdrawn and returned when it was restarted. A similar pattern of response has probably also been seen in patients treated with prednisone. This type of adverse reaction is very unusual with either drug. A much commoner occurrence is the development of cerebral oedema when a patient on long term steroid therapy has his effective dose of steroid reduced. This may be due to a change in preparation, a misunderstanding regarding the equivalent effective doses of different steroids or a change in self-medication. Patients using steroid-containing ointments have also suffered from cerebral oedema when either they reduced the dose or were prescribed a preparation with a lower effective steroid content. An increase in effective dosage in these patients will reduce the raised intracranial pressure and allow the cerebral oedema to resolve.

Patients with Addison's disease are peculiarly liable to cerebral oedema which resolves when adequate steroid replacement therapy is given.

Steroids are not only effective in treating the cerebral oedema of benign intra-cranial hypertension; they are also effective in oedema from some other causes, the compound most commonly used being dexamethasone. The most dramatic results are obtained in patients with oedema associated with an intracranial tumour who may show an improvement in signs and symptoms within minutes of an intravenous injection. Dexamethasone is most effective when the oedema is limited to one part of the brain and it does little to improve the global oedema associated with head injury or that following an hypoxic episode.

Hydrocephalus

An abnormal accumulation of CSF may be due to a reduction in absorption or to a failure of normal CSF circulation because of a block in some part of the pathway. Occasionally the increase in CSF is due to increased production from a papilloma of the choroid plexus. The management is essentially surgical.

If the block is removable such as a tumour in the posterior fossa, it is removed; if the cause cannot be treated directly, CSF pressure is reduced by some form of shunting operation. Shunts containing a one-way valve can be placed between the lateral ventricles and the peritoneum, the lateral ventricles and the right atrium and between the spinal dural sac and peritoneum.

The anaesthetist not working in a neurosurgical unit is most likely to encounter patients with hydrocephalus after their condition has been relieved by a shunt when they come to operation for some unrelated condition. Shunts quite often become blocked and it is worth while asking the patient if he has any symptoms of raised intracranial pressure. If he has not, the presence of the shunt can be ignored and anaesthesia conducted as the operative requirements would normally dictate.

HEADACHE

Only a limited number of intracranial structures are pain sensitive. Pain is not normally felt in response to direct stimulation of the cerebral cortex and the parietal meninges are also insensitive. The basal meninges are sensitive particularly immediately around the sensory nerve foramina. Pain is produced when the larger arteries are stretched or dilated and it is probable that displacement or stretching of the falx cerebri and tentorium can also produce pain. Impulses arising in extracranial structures can be registered as 'headache' particularly disturbances of the external carotid circulation and abnormal contraction of the neck and jaw muscles. Contrary to popular belief, 'eye strain' does not produce headache.

The principle types of headache can be classified as tension, migrainous, other vascular, cluster headaches and those due to meningeal irritation.

Tension headache—psychogenic headache

This term is usually given to a generalized or principally frontal headache produced by prolonged, nonuseful contraction of the upper neck muscles and occasionally by contraction of the muscles of the jaw. It is also termed psychogenic headache because the presumed cause is an unconscious contraction of the muscles concerned in response to anxiety. The headache can sometimes be relieved by massage of the neck and occipital region though reassurance with the possible addition of anxiolytic drugs is more effective. It occurs much more commonly in women than in men.

A similar headache can follow the prolonged adoption of a relatively fixed position of the head and neck as in long distance driving. Headache may also be an early symptom of endogenous depression.

Occasionally disease of the upper cervical spine can cause pain in the head, particularly in the frontal region, rather than at the site of the lesion.

Migraine

The definition of 'migraine' is still argued. Here it will be assumed that it is a condition where a severe headache follows premonitory signs or symptoms that suggest spasm in some part of the cranial arterial tree. Typically the headache is one-sided and can be relieved by ergot preparations taken during the premonitory aura. Vomiting and nausea often accompany the headache. The attacks may come in bouts interspersed with attack-free periods. Each attack may last from a few hours to one or more days. There is a strong familial tendency and women are more commonly affected than men. Attacks in women may be related to the menstrual cycle or to the taking of a contraceptive pill containing oestrogen.

The premonitory signs are commonly visual and appear to be due to spasm in the posterior cerebral artery supplying one occipital lobe. The symptoms are consequently limited to one side of each visual field and may consist of scotomata, fortification spectra or shimmering and scintillating of objects seen. Visual disturbances may also be caused by constriction of retinal vessels. This is the pattern referred to as 'classical migraine'.

Premonitory symptoms are not always visual. There may be transitory dysphasia, or hemiparesis. If the basilar artery is involved there may be disturbance of lower brain stem and cerebellar function giving ataxia, diplopia, giddiness and sometimes loss of consciousness. The spasm may sometimes produce a neurological deficit lasting several hours or days and very occasionally the deficit may be permanent. These patterns are referred to as 'complicated migraine'.

Some women taking the pill experience a change in the nature of their attacks with more severe focal signs appearing during the prodrome such as severe weakness and/or severe dysphasia. In these women such a change is of serious import since it may herald a permanent arterial occlusion.

Pathogenesis of migraine

The prodrome is associated with cranial arterial spasm and the headache phase with arterial dilatation. The capillaries are dilated during the prodrome and the sufferer's face is flushed. During the headache the capillaries are constricted and the face is pale. Throbbing of the temporal arteries can be felt during the headache and compression of these vessels may ameliorate the pain. In a patient with a skull deficit and who also suffered from migraine, collapse of the scalp inwards over the deficit was observed during the prodromal phase and bulging during the headache [3]. Alterations in the circulating levels of serotonin (5 hydroxytryptamine) are probably responsible for the vascular changes observed. In the preheadache phase there is a slight rise in circulating serotonin and during the headache there is a pronounced fall. Serotonin produces arterial constriction and capillary dilatation. Reserpine lowers plasma serotonin and when given to migrainous subjects can precipitate a typical headache which coincides with the fall in serotonin level. Since a fall in serotonin has been observed in over 85 per cent of the patients investigated, migraine can be considered a 'low serotonin syndrome'. Various factors, both exogenous and endogenous, have been postulated as possibly being responsible for triggering the lowering of plasma serotonin. In those with 'dietary migraine' the tyramine contained in many foods and drinks has been held responsible. In those whose attacks are precipitated by chocolate, phenyl-ethylamine is probably the agent. Certain free fatty acids can cause a release of platelet serotonin and may be responsible both for some food precipitated attacks and also for attacks brought on by fasting.

Why only certain discrete parts of the cranial arterial tree respond to the circulating vasoactive substances remains a mystery.

Treatment and prevention of migraine

On the assumption that a migraine aura is initiated by selective vasoconstriction due to a small rise in plasma serotonin and that the headache is caused by a subsequent fall in plasma serotonin to below normal levels, it is reasonable to expect serotonin antagonists to prevent attacks beginning and a serotonin agonist to prevent or relieve the headache. Many lysergic acid derivatives have antiserotonin properties and of these methysergide has proved an effective prophylactic in migraine. Unfortunately its side effects, which include retroperitoneal fibroplasia, insomnia and hallucinations, have limited its use. Pizotifen is safer and almost equally effective. Many pheno-thiazines have antiserotonin properties which parallel their anti-α adrenergic activity. Chlorpromazine in particular has been recommended in migraine phrophylaxis. The α-blocker phenoxybenzamine has also been used. In children promethazine is said to be useful and the antidepressant amitriptyline is also often effective particularly in adolescents.

In the prevention or treatment of the headache ergotamine is the most widely used drug. Its vasoconstrictor activity appears to replace that of the diminished circulating serotonin. Prochlorperazine and metoclopramide have been used to

control the nausea and vomiting that may accompany the headache. Prochlorproma-
zine has also been used with benefit in migraine prophylaxis but the side-effects of
long term use make this inadvisable.

In the past, surgical treatment of migraine has been recommended in the belief
that the vascular phenomena were under sympathetic nervous control. Operations
such as stellate ganglionectomy, vascular stripping or ligation were performed but
were never effective and are no longer advocated. The vascular changes in migraine
are humorally mediated.

Periodic migrainous neuralgia or 'cluster headaches'

These are unilateral attacks of intense 'stabbing', 'burning' pain centred behind one
orbit and radiating to the temple, nose and cheek. The attacks last a half to two hours
and stop as abruptly as they start. They occur daily or several times a day for some
months when they remit for a year or more. During an attack the eye may be red and
watery and the ipsilateral nostril may be congested; there may also be flushing of the
cheek and prominent pulsation of the temporal artery. The attacks are sometimes
relieved by ergotamine.

The cause of the attacks is uncertain. They can be provoked by histamine and
small rises in circulating histamine have been discerned during attacks so it is possible
that the spontaneous release of endogenous histamine is responsible. No triggering
factors have been found and there is no explanation for the limitation of the vascular
disturbance to such a circumscribed area.

Other vascular headaches (common migraine)

Most headaches of intracranial origin are thought to be due either to the stretching
or dilatation of intracranial vessels. Intracranial masses can obviously distort and
stretch the vessels near them. Rises in systemic blood pressure and relaxation of
arterial tone can both cause an increase in the amplitude of pulsation. Conversely a
fall in intracranial pressure such as may follow lumbar puncture may increase the
arterial *transmural* pressure and again increase the amplitude of pulsation. In headaches associated with cerebral swelling two mechanisms may be present: the swelling
itself may stretch or distort vessels or the swelling and the headache may both be due
to arterial dilatation.

When morning headache is associated with hypertension, the slight rise in arterial
P_{CO_2} during sleep and recumbency may combine to both increase arterial dilatation
and produce some cerebral oedema. The headache associated with CO_2 retention has
also been discussed above and is presumably also caused by an increase in arterial
dilatation and some element of cerebral oedema. Vasoactive amines such as histamine
and tyramine present in common foods and drinks may cause headaches by their
direct action on cranial vessels. Sodium monoglutamate can also cause headache in
susceptible people and this has been termed the 'chinese restaurant syndrome'.
Typically the headache occurs some hours after the meal suggesting that a derivative
of the monoglutamate is responsible.

Headaches associated with menstruation or the taking of a contraceptive pill may
be due again to both arterial dilatation and/or cerebral swelling. Headache can
occur both at the time of peak oestrogen levels or following a fall in oestrogen. The
latter is frequently seen in pill takers, where headache occurs during the days when

they are not taking the pill. The mechanisms at work may therefore be due to excess steroids (probably oestrogen) or to abrupt steroid withdrawal.

Meningism

Irritation of the meninges by inflammation or extravasated blood produces a severe headache which is principally frontal but radiates to the neck and sometimes down the spine. The patient has neck stiffness and sometimes shows head retraction and strongly resists any attempt at head flexion.

Temporal arteritis (giant cell arteritis)

Temporal arteritis is a local manifestation of a generalized disease. Other vessels may be involved and there may be pain elsewhere apart from the head. The temporal vessels are enlarged and tender. The patient may complain of local or generalized headache. He or she is usually unwell with a low fever, malaise, loss of appetite and a raised sedimentation rate. The disease remits spontaneously but only after months or years of pain during which time the patient is liable to thrombosis of one or both ophthalmic arteries and the consequent irrecoverable blindness. The condition responds well to treatment with prednisone.

DISORDERS OF MOVEMENT

This section is concerned with those disorders of movement that have not been discussed in the sections on coma and epilepsy, paying particular attention to the pharmacological aspects of the various conditions.

Physiological tremor—essential tremor

Normal people show a fine tremor of their hands and fingers when asked to hold them in a steady unsupported position. The rate of movement is between 5 and 10 Hz. In some, the tremor is so fine that it is difficult to see; a sheet of paper placed on the outstretched fingers can be used to amplify the movement. The tremor is made worse by anxiety, fatigue, old age, thyrotoxicosis, β-adrenergic agonists, uraemia, pre-hepatic coma and by some intoxications including alcohol and lithium. It would seem to be due to the minimal cycling of the proprioceptive receptor-motor neurone servo-loop that is inherent in the system because of synaptic delay. The tremor can be reduced by β-adrenergic blockade. An exaggeration of this normal movement which is often familial is termed 'essential tremor'.

Disturbances of the basal ganglia—'extra-pyramidal' syndromes

Several different patterns of abnormal movement can be produced by dysfunction in different parts of the masses of subcortical grey matter known collectively as the 'basal ganglia'. The term 'basal ganglia' is used to include different structures by different authors. Generally, in anatomical writing, the term is used to embrace the caudate nucleus and its ultimate extension the amygdaloid nucleus, the globus pallidus, putamen and the claustrum. The globus pallidus and putamen are together known as the lentiform nucleus and the lentiform and caudate nuclei are together referred to as the striate body. Functionally the amygdala is separate from the other nuclei being part of the 'smell brain'. The ventrolateral and ventroanterior nuclei of the thalamus are concerned with the control of motor activity and so are the subthalamic nuclei, the substantia nigra and the red nucleus so that these structures should be included with the basal ganglia when thinking in functional rather than in anatomical terms.

The ventrolateral nucleus of the thalamus projects to the motor cortex and through this projection the basal ganglia can influence corticospinal activity. The final pathway mediating the abnormal movements of basal ganglion disease is the corticospinal tract. The term 'extra-pyramidal' to describe these conditions is therefore not strictly correct. Figure 8.5 is a diagram showing a *few* of the connections of the basal ganglia.

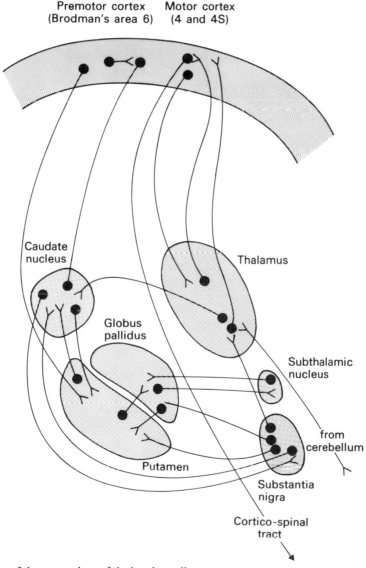

Fig. 8.5. A few of the connections of the basal ganglia.

In health, the different nuclei of the basal ganglia can be thought of as acting together in a balanced, coordinated way to modulate motor activity. In disease this balance is upset usually by damage to one or more parts which leaves the remainder relatively overactive.

There are several different patterns of abnormal movement associated with basal ganglia disease and almost all are associated with a generalized increase in muscle tone or rigidity. Peripherally, muscle tone is controlled by the muscle spindle. There are two γ-innervated muscle fibre components to each muscle spindle: the central 'nuclear bag' fibre and the peripheral 'nuclear chain' fibre. Each system has its own afferent innervation. The nuclear bag system is termed 'phasic' or 'dynamic' because it responds to movement of the parts concerned: the nuclear chain system is termed 'static' or 'tonic' because it is involved in the regulation or resting muscle tone. Releasing the nuclear bag γ-efferent system from the effects of descending inhibition results in hyperreflexia, an exaggerated response to movement of the part concerned. This is the condition seen when the inhibitory influence of corticospinal and rubrospinal tracts is removed. In basal ganglia disease there is typically a dis-inhibition of the *static*, nuclear chain γ-efferents which results in a permanent increase in tone but no hyperreflexia.

Several neurotransmitter substances are known to be involved in normal basal ganglion activity and these include serotonin, acetylcholine, GABA, dopamine, glutamine and enkephalins. More is known of the cholinergic and dopaminergic systems than of the others but even here knowledge is still very incomplete. In general the cholinergic and dopaminergic systems seem to counterbalance each other so that therapeutically, for instance, the lack of dopamine can be made good by either increasing local dopamine levels or by blocking cholinergic activity.

Many cholinergic drugs can cause basal ganglion disturbances but before discussing this and other unusual causes, a brief description of the classical syndromes will be given.

Parkinson's disease

Parkinsonism is a disturbance in which the patient suffers from a general increase in muscle tone or rigidity and a coarse regular tremor of 3–7 Hz. The tremor is most noticeable in the limbs particularly in the hands but may also involve the face and head. The akinesia or poverty of movement seen in Parkinsonism seems to be due to difficulty in overcoming the abnormal rigidity. The immobile, expressionless face is a well-recognized feature of the condition.

The Parkinsonian syndrome can follow encephalitis in which case the condition tends to appear in the third decade of life while arteriosclerotic Parkinsonism appears in the fifth decade or later. Postencephalitic Parkinsonism is associated with an increase in sweating and in the secretion of sebum, and with the occurrence of oculogyric crises. In these crises the eyes are deviated upwards and sideways and the head and neck rotated and extended. The spasms, which are very uncomfortable, may last a few minutes to a few hours. The attacks can be relieved or ameliorated by anticholinergic drugs.

In arteriosclerotic and postencephalitic Parkinsonism there are degenerative lesions in the substantia nigra and the condition seems to be due to the loss of dopaminergic input from this nucleus to the basal ganglia and thalamus. The imbalance produced by this can be redressed by giving anticholinergic drugs or by increasing brain dopamine levels. Surgical destruction of parts of the globus pallidus or of the ventro-posterolateral nucleus of the thalamus has also proved beneficial. The principal form of treatment for many years has been with anticholinergics of which benzhexol, benztropine and phenadrine have been the most widely used. Atropine is useful in the acute treatment of oculogyric crises.

Brain dopamine levels can be increased by giving the laevorotatory form of its precursor dihydroxyphenylanine (L-dopa) and this compound has proved very effective in the treatment of Parkinsonism. It is usually given with a dopa decarboxylase inhibitor which prevents its extracerebral destruction and lowers the dose required for effectiveness. Bromocriptine, a dopamine agonist, has been given with some benefit but its side effects limit its usefulness. (Recently sodium valproate has also been used without much success.)

Chorea (*St Vitus' dance*)

Sydenham's chorea is a disease affecting young people typically associated with rheumatic fever though it may occasionally follow other infections. It is three times more common in females than in males. It may occur without evidence of infection during pregnancy or while taking the contraceptive pill. The disease is self-limiting, usually remitting in a few months though recurrences can occur.

The involuntary movements of chorea are very quick and jerky. They may involve twitching and flinging movements of the arms and twitching and grimacing of the face. Voluntary movements are often impeded by the involuntary. When not impeded they are faster and brusquer and less accurate than normal. Unlike most other basal ganglion disturbances, chorea is associated with hypotonia.

In Sydenham's chorea there is generalized engorgement and swelling of the brain with the basal ganglia particularly affected and, of the basal ganglia, the caudate nucleus is said to be the most involved.

Treatment is with sedation. Phenobarbitone, chlorpromazine and diazepam have all proved useful. Improvement has also been reported following the use of dexamethasone.

Huntington's chorea is a degenerative disease of middle life. It is inherited as an autosomal dominant but some cases are thought to result from new mutations. Degenerative changes are widespread in the brain and progressive dementia is a regular feature of the disease, signs of which may appear before the abnormal movements. There is no effective treatment though sedation may help in the patient's management and the involuntary movements may be limited by tetrabenazine.

Athetosis

Athetosis is the term used to describe certain involuntary, writhing movements which are much slower and coarser than those seen in chorea. They involve the proximal muscles more than the distal. The condition can be bilateral or unilateral. Bilateral athetosis is usually the result of drug treatment but can occasionally be congenital due to brain damage or an inherited progressive disorder. It seems that the condition is caused by damage (or disproportionate damage) to the putamen.

Most cases are unilateral and the cause is usually some destructive lesion involving one cerebral hemisphere only. If the cortex or corticospinal tract is involved the abnormal movements may be combined with an associated hemiplegia.

The treatment of athetosis is unsatisfactory. Sedation with such drugs as diazepam may help a little and anticholinergics have also been tried.

Hemibalismus

Hemibalismus is a condition in which the patient has violent, repetitive, uncontrollable, flailing movements of one side of the body. The responsible lesion is in the opposite subthalamic nucleus, and is usually haemorrhage or infarction. The movements are so damaging and exhausting that radical treatment is justified and, since the involved side is useless for purposeful activity, section of the corticospinal tract has been employed to control them. The fact that corticospinal tract section is effective in stopping the abnormal movements is further evidence that 'extra-pyramidal' syndromes are mediated through the corticospinal (pyramidal) pathways.

Gilles de la Tourette syndrome

In this bizarre condition the sufferer makes spasmodic, jerking, tic-like movements which are often accompanied by grunting or other noises or by spoken obscenities. In between the spasms there is a restlessness and lack of attention and concentration. Treatment is usually with antidopaminergic drugs such as phenothiazines or butyrophenones. Though these produce some improvement it is at the expense of alertness and intellectual acuity. The reason for mentioning this condition here is that recently the antihypertensive agent clonidine has been found to be useful. There is evidence that the Tourette syndrome is due to a disturbance of catecholamine metabolism and it is aggravated by anxiety and stress. Clonidine is an noradrenergic agonist whose antihypertensive action appears to be centrally mediated. In low doses, however, it seems to reduce central noradrenergic activity.

Torticollis

This distressing condition usually occurs in middle age. It is a type of focal tortion dystonia in which clonic or tonic spasms involving the head and neck occur. The head is very forcibly rotated and flexed and often held in such a position that eating and drinking are impossible. Patients with this condition may become severely depressed and their depression is often worsened rather than relieved by being treated as though their problem were psychiatric. Treatment is very unsatisfactory. Anticholinergics such as benzhexol (Artane) may help as may sedatives such as diazepam. Surgical denervation of the abnormally contracting muscles is of little use, though still resorted to, and stereotactic lesions in the globus pallidus have also produced disappointing results.

Drug induced disturbances of movement

Most of the abnormalities of movement described above can be also caused by various drugs. In addition there are two patterns of behaviour that seem to be exclusively due to drugs: akathesia or pathological restlessness and tardive dyskinesia. Tardive dyskinesia, sometimes referred to as the buccolingual masticatory syndrome, consists in repetitive, chewing and sucking movements with grimacing and tongue protrusion.

It tends to occur in the elderly on long term treatment with phenothiazines or butyrophenones.

The pharmacology of basal ganglion disturbances is complicated and only very partially understood. A wide range of drugs can cause abnormal movements and often the same drug can both control abnormal movements and produce them. Sometimes the movements are made worse or first appear on withdrawal of the drug and sometimes increasing the dose may reduce the abnormal activity. Some drugs, particularly the phenothiazines and butyrophenones, produce different disturbances in different patients. There are several possible mechanisms involved and some drugs may act through more than one mechanism. Levodopa, methyldopa, bromocryptine and amantadine cause an increase in dopaminergic activity. Reserpine and tetrabenazine cause depletion of dopamine stores in the nerve endings.

Butyrophenones, phenothiazines and metaclopramide block dopamine receptors. They can also increase receptor sensitivity to dopamine and increase presynaptic dopamine release. It is commonly thought that a variation with time in the relative intensity in these different actions accounts for the different responses seen. Anticholinergic drugs such as benztropine and benzhexol can produce abnormal movements as well as relieve them.

Chorea has followed the use of phenytoin and dystonic movements have been seen following treatment with sodium valproate. In neither instance is the mechanism understood.

Contraceptive pills containing oestrogen can cause chorea. The mechanism in this case probably being a local vascular dilatation and oedema.

Drug-induced acute dystonias with head retraction and trismus have been mistaken for tetanus and abnormal drug responses should be suspected whenever a diagnosis of tetanus is not clear cut. The author has seen one patient with tetanus whose treatment included chlorpromazine and who developed dystonic spasms when the tetanus had nearly resolved.

The different movement disturbances produced by different drugs are summarized in Table 8.3.

Hypoxia

The nuclear masses forming the basal ganglia sometimes appear to be more susceptible to hypoxia or ischaemia than the cells of the cerebral cortex or cerebellum and it is not uncommon for patients who have suffered a hypoxic episode apparently to regain normal intellectual function but to be left with abnormal movements due to basal ganglia disturbance.

ATAXIAS

Hereditary ataxias

Several similar progressive degenerative diseases are included under this title, the best known of which is Friedreich's ataxia. This condition is familial and manifests itself in late childhood or early adult life. There is a diffuse progressive degeneration of the central nervous system which is particularly marked in the spinocerebellar and dorsal column tracts in the spinal cord. The main result of this degeneration is a severe reduction in the proprioceptive input which in turn results in an inability properly to

Table 8.3. Movement disturbances produced by different drugs.

Condition	Drugs Responsible	Probable Mechanism	Treatment
Parkinsonism	Tetrabenazine Reserpine	} Dopamine depletion	
	Phenothiazines Butyrophenones	} Dopaminergic blockade	Anticholinergics
	Methyldopa	? Dopaminergic blockade	(not levodopa)
	Tricyclic antidepressants	?	
Chorea	Levodopa	Dopaminergic enhancement	Tetrabenazine Haloperidol
	Phenytoin (very rare)	?	Drug withdrawal
	Oestrogen containing pill	? Local vascular	or reduced dosage
Acute dystonias (including oculogyric crises)	Sodium valproate	?	Drug withdrawal
	Phenothiazines Butyrophenones Metoclopramide	} Dopaminergic blockade and/or increased receptor sensitivity	Atropine
Akathisea	Phenothiazines Butyrophenones		Anticholinergics
Tardive dyskinesia	Phenothiazines Butyrophenones		None: may persist or worsen after drug withdrawal

control voluntary movements (an intention tremor) and generalized hypotonia. The fact that there are no involuntary movements at rest and that the limbs are hypotonic distinguishes intention tremor from the abnormal movements of basal ganglion disturbance. Although the predominant lesions are in the spinal cord there may also be signs of optic atrophy and nystagmus is usually present.

Of most interest to the anaesthetist is the concomitant occurrence of degenerative changes in the myocardium which may lead to frank heart failure.

In other similar ataxias, degeneration of the cerebellum is predominant.

Other causes of ataxia

Ataxia can occur as a result of raised intracranial pressure and ataxia associated with cerebellar signs can result from mass lesions in the posterior fossa. Vestibular disturbances due to drugs can present as ataxia, associated sometimes with cerebellar signs. Phenytoin has been suggested as a possible cause of cerebellar atrophy. Certainly it and other anticonvulsants such as phenobarbitone, carbamazepine and chlorazepam can all cause ataxia which is usually associated with nystagmus, giddiness and nausea.

Neurosyphilis: tabes dorsalis

Tertiary syphilis has become a rarity in recent years but a few people with arrested tabes dorsalis can be found and they often appear as patients at clinical examinations in medicine. The main point of interest for the anaesthetist is the probability of associated cardiovascular disease, particularly of aortitis.

The essential lesion in neurosyphilis is a vasculitis with perivascular inflammation and infiltration. In tabes this vasculitis results in ischaemia of the dorsal roots of the spinal cord and in their degeneration between the dorsal root ganglia and their entry into the cord. The larger fibres from the lower limbs are the first to be affected. Since these fibres are concerned with proprioception their destruction results in loss of position sense, ataxia and hypotonia. There is also loss of vibration sense and impairment of touch. Pain sometimes precedes overt ataxia. The pain is spasmodic and occurs first in the legs—so called 'lightning pains'. Pain may also occur in the abdomen and chest. These brief spontaneous spasms of pain are probably due to the loss of large fibre inhibitory input into the dorsal horn of the spinal grey matter. Large fibre stimulation produces inhibition of the second order neurones subserving pain. Removal of this inhibition may result in spontaneous discharge of these neurones and the consequent sensation of pain.

Although starting as degeneration of large fibre input in the lower part of the body the process progresses to include the whole length of the cord and to include the small as well as the large fibres. Small fibre destruction results in diminished appreciation of pain and temperature changes. Loss of pain sensation may result in tissue damage and trophic ulcers, particularly on the soles of the feet, and neuropathic arthropathy (Charcot's joints) are not uncommon.

Also typical of tabes is loss of bladder control, loss of anal sensation and an Argyll-Robertson pupil. In this latter condition the reflex constriction in response to light is lost while that in response to accommodation is retained.

Associated cardiovascular disease has been mentioned: also of interest to the anaesthetist is the general opinion that it is unwise to use spinal or epidural techniques for patients with spinal cord disease.

MOTOR NEURONE DISEASE (AMYOTROPHIC LATERAL SCLEROSIS)

This, one of the commonest purely neurological diseases, is a relentless degenerative process affecting both the upper and lower motor neurones. The patient consequently shows signs such as clumsiness and spasticity from corticospinal tract involvement and weakness, fasciculation, paralysis and atrophy from anterior horn cell destruction. The cause is unknown. There is a spontaneous and irreversible degeneration of the tracts and neurones involved. The onset is usually after the age of 50 and the progression from first symptoms to death rarely lasts longer than 2–3 years.

The first appearances of the disease are insidious and may follow one of three distinct patterns or any mixture of them.

Progressive bulbar paralysis. The lower motor neurones in the brain stem are sometimes affected early in the disease process causing weakness, wasting and loss of tone in the muscles of the palate, pharynx in particular the tongue, which also shows fasciculation. The patient becomes dysarthric and has difficulty in swallowing and coughing. Food is often inhaled into the lungs or regurgitated through the nose.

10

Progressive muscular atrophy. In this presentation the first signs and symptoms are predominantly in the hands and arms and are due to lower motor neurone degeneration. There is marked weakness, wasting and fasciculation.

Lateral tract degeneration. Sometimes degeneration of the corticospinal tracts to the lower parts of the body are affected early and the patient shows signs of a spastic paraparesis.

The patterns of onset described above may not be distinct but may merge into each other. Eventually the entire body musculature is involved and death is usually from respiratory failure or some associated condition such as chest infection.

The anaesthetist may be asked to advise on management of the airway when pharyngeal and laryngeal muscles are primarily involved or he may be asked to help when the respiratory muscles start to fail. The decision whether or not to interfere can be a difficult one since active treatment may only be prolonging temporarily an increasingly distressful existence. Respiratory weakness is sometimes disproportionate in that the patient may be able to walk or use his arms and hands, eat and talk and yet have respiratory distress. Such patients may benefit from periods of assisted ventilation during the day or complete mechanical ventilation at night. The rest given to the respiratory muscles in this way may allow freer and more comfortable activity during the remainder of the day.

The management of anaesthesia in such patients is considered on page 213.

Multiple sclerosis

In this condition, areas of spontaneous demyelination occur throughout the nervous system. The demyelination may be repaired with some functional recovery but is mostly followed by gliosis. The disease runs a protracted fluctuating course often over many years with alternating episodes of exacerbation and remission. Overall there is progressive loss of function leading to extensive paralysis, loss of sensation and often dementia. It has been said that the disease is accompanied by euphoria but this is unusual and the majority of sufferers become increasingly distressed by their condition.

The disease may present with the sudden appearance of one or more focal lesions, one of the commonest of which is optic neuritis, or it may present with an insidiously increasing weakness of one or both legs. When the onset is acute there is usually some improvement in the initial symptoms or even a complete remission. In established, moderately advanced cases there is evidence of multiple neurological deficits. There is a spastic paraparesis or paraplegia with painful flexor spasms of the legs and enhanced knee and ankle jerks. There is weakness, hypotonia and gross ataxia (intention tremor) in the arms and hands. There is patchy sensory loss. The optic discs are pale from optic atrophy and the eyes show nystagmus and often a divergent squint. Speech is slurred and may be staccato or scanning, this latter being as it were ataxic speaking. Sphincter control is lost eventually and occasionally early in the disease process.

The cause of the disease is unknown. A viral aetiology has long been suspected but not proven. Although the condition may be initiated by a viral infection the demyelination is probably at least in part due to an autoimmune process. Stress in the form of infection or injury may provoke an exacerbation. Many forms of treatment have been tried. Steroids or ACTH have been given especially during an acute exacerbation. Immunosuppressant drugs have been tried. Vitamin B_{12} has been given. Diets free from animal fats and diets free from gluten have also been advocated.

Because of the fluctuating cause of the disease the effects of treatment are difficult to assess but so far no treatment has been shown to be of very great benefit.

Anaesthetists are only likely to meet the disease professionally when patients with multiple sclerosis need surgery for some intercurrent condition. Because of involvement of the spinal cord it is usually considered best to avoid spinal or epidural techniques. It is conceivable that some suppression of the 'stress response' by heavy sedation with narcotics during and after operation might reduce the likelihood of an exacerbation of the disease but this is pure speculation.

ENCEPHALITIS, ENCEPHALOMYELITIS AND MYELITIS

These three conditions will be considered together because of the probable similarity in their aetiology and because they have similar implications for the anaesthetist. Distinct but uncommon disease entities such as encephalitis lethargica will not be discussed. Rabies is briefly considered on page 215.

Encephalitis

Encephalitis is usually taken to mean a non-suppurative inflammation of the brain. It can be caused by many different agents and the term covers many different disease entities, some acute, some chronic and many fatal. Two principal mechanisms are involved which may coexist. One is the direct invasion of nervous tissue by a virus with its resulting damage: the other is a type, or types, of hypersensitivity or auto-immune response. Experimentally, encephalitis, encephalomyelitis and peripheral neuropathies can all be induced by injections of suitably treated nervous tissue. The triggering antigen seems to be a breakdown product of myelin and the immunological response usually involves acute demyelination. In the central nervous system such an immune response can complicate direct viral invasion of the CNS or may follow some transient CNS damage. Much more common, however, is the delayed encephalomyelitic response that may follow any viral infection. The assumption in this case is that minimal involvement of the CNS by the original infection may be sufficient to release into the systemic circulation enough CNS antigen to produce an antibody response.

Signs and symptoms

The patient usually has a history of a mild febrile, influenza-like illness which may be a clearly recognizable disease entity such as measles, mumps, chickenpox or vaccination. This appears to resolve but is followed in a matter of days by headache and drowsiness which may proceed to stupor or coma. Meningism and photophobia may be present: occasionally, convulsions occur. On examination there may be slight papilloedema, and squints are common. Motor weaknesses are common and may proceed to complete paralysis: sensory disturbances, however, are relatively uncommon. Treatment is symptomatic: steroids and ACTH are often given but their usefulness is not proven.

Prognosis

This is extremely difficult. Some totally paralysed patients and some in deep coma can make a rapid and complete recovery. Others who were never so severely ill may be left with permanent deficits and some may die. In general, the longer coma and/or paralysis persist, the less probable is a complete return to normality. Of the two, coma carries a worse prognosis than paralysis.

These patients may require help from the anaesthetist either to control their convulsions (though this is unusual) or because of inadequate breathing which may be due to depth of coma or to paralysis. Occasionally, localized lesions such as cranial nerve palsies may put the airway at risk and temporary intubation or tracheostomy may be necssary. Patients with encephalitis or encephalomyelitis may be temporarily completely paralysed by their disease yet remain conscious and often with little or no disturbance of sensation. Once signs of motor weakness have appeared, the patient should be nursed in an area where complete respiratory failure can be immediately recognized and treated since it is not possible to predict which patients are liable to sudden deterioration. Mechanical ventilation is usually continued until recovery or death. At the time of instituting mechanical ventilation, the exact cause of the patient's condition is often in doubt but it may become clearer as the days go by. The attendants will then be faced with the problem of deciding on the management of a patient who cannot be labelled 'brain dead' but for whom there is no possibility of useful or even sentient activity.

Herpes simplex encephalitis differs from this picture in that localizing signs, usually a hemiparesis or hemiplegia, are superadded. The affected hemisphere becomes progressively swollen, haemorrhagic and necrotic. The hemiplegia may be accompanied or preceded by generalized convulsions and if the patient develops status epilepticus, the help of an anaesthetist may be sought. The disease is progressive and fatal in 80 per cent of cases. The diagnosis is made by excluding a discrete and possibly operable mass lesion, by brain biopsy and by finding a rising titre of antiherpes antibodies in the patient's blood.

Encephalomyelitis

The pathology, aetiology and symptomatology of encephalomyelitis are similar to that described above for encephalitis due to an autoimmune response, except that the encephalitic signs are less prominent and signs of brain stem and cord dysfunction predominate. Dysfunction in the pontine and lumbosacral regions is particularly noticeable. The anaesthetist is likely to be involved if breathing or the airway is threatened.

Myelitis

Sometimes the pathological processes described above are limited to the spinal cord or to the spinal cord and peripheral nerves. If the lesion appears to be limited to a few segments of the cord, the condition is called 'transverse myelitis' but if it progressively involves higher and higher segments, it is referred to as 'ascending' or Landry's paralysis. There may appear to be an element of peripheral nerve damage in these conditions and in some peripheral neuropathies there may appear to be some cord damage. If demyelination due to an autoimmune response is present, myelin may be lost from both central and peripheral nerve fibres. Thus there is probably a spectrum of disease processes all of similar aetiology extending from encephalitis, through encephalomyelitis, myelitis, polyradiculitis (Guillain–Barré syndrome) and some types of peripheral polyneuropathy. As stated above in relation to encephalitis, the more acute the development of the deficit and the quicker the resolution the better is the ultimate outlook for the patient. Patients with lingering or fluctuating signs and those with prolonged severe deficit are likely to have some permanent disabilities.

The role of the anaesthetist is again to help protect the airway and to maintain adequate ventilation.

One further point is worth making. Patients with spinal cord disease and/or with peripheral neuropathies, may have a loss of sympathetic function. This may be due to damage to the descending pathways in the spinal cord, to damage of the cells in the lateral horns of the thoracolumbar grey matter or to peripheral nerve damage. Patients with such damage have difficulty in accommodating to the change from spontaneous breathing to positive pressure ventilation. Their cardiac output may be improved by negative expiratory pressure, by raising the legs or by increasing the circulating blood volume.

For all those diseases where it is thought probable that there might be an allergic or autoimmune component, ACTH and steroids have been given. This treatment has not produced any obvious benefit and the consensus of opinion now is that because they reduce resistance to intercurrent infection such drugs are best avoided. In cases where there is a presumed active viral invasion of the CNS, antiviral agents such as amantadine and interferon have been used, again without obvious success.

ANTERIOR SPINAL ARTERY OCCLUSION

The major part of the spinal cord is supplied by the anterior spinal artery. Developmentally this artery is formed by fusion of the longitudinal anastomoses between each segmental artery. Segmental arteries enter each intervertebral foramen but in post-embryonic life only a few are of any significance. The artery is formed at the upper end by two symmetrical branches from the vertebral arteries. It receives major unilateral contributions in the lower thoracic or upper lumbar and the lower lumbar regions. Infarction following occlusion is usually limited to one of these territories so that three different clinical pictures can occur. The arrangement of the principal tracts in the spinal cord and the area supplied by the anterior spinal artery are shown in Fig. 8.6. It can be seen that occlusion of the artery will leave only the dorsal columns intact. Occlusions in the cervical region will result in a lower motor neurone paralysis of the arms and an upper motor neurone lesion below that level.

The infarct is usually between the spinal segments C4 and T5 and the diaphragm (supplied by C3, 4 & 5) is often spared. The patient may have difficulties due to the loss of forceful expiration as described on page 290. Pain and temperature sensation are lost below the level of the neck but proprioception, vibration sense and the perception of light touch are retained. This pattern is known as a dissociated sensory loss. It may also be seen in Syringomyelia (Chapter 7, page 211). A spastic paraplegia in flexion develops in the lower part of the body. Occlusion in the lower thoracic or upper lumbar region results in paraplegia below the mid-abdomen. Occlusion of the lowermost part of the artery may affect only the sacral segments resulting in partial paralysis of the lower limbs and loss of sphincter control.

There are several possible causes of occlusion. Systemic causes include hypotension, fat embolism, air embolism and decompression sickness (caisson disease). Apart from hypotension these causes are rare. Occlusion may be spontaneous without an apparent precipitating cause or there may be local lesions predisposing to occlusion. Local lesions include trauma, especially to the lower neck, compression against oestophytes

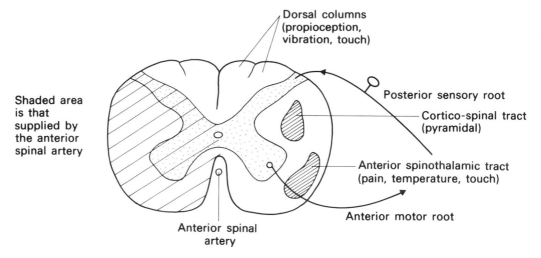

Fig. 8.6. The arrangement of the principal tracts in the spinal cord and the area supplied by the anterior spinal artery.

in cervical spondylosis, aortic aneurysm and disease of the aortic bifurcation. Aneurysms of the descending aorta may compromise the flow through the large feeding vessel that is usually present somewhere between T10 and L2. The conus medullaris and cauda equina receive their blood supply from a branch of one or other ascending lumbar artery. This artery arises from the iliolumbar branch of the internal iliac artery, and flow through it may be compromised by stenosis of the aortic bifurcation or a saddle embolus or by a temporary clamping of the aorta during operations for dissecting aneurysms. High occlusion may initially present an appearance very similar to transverse myelitis or polyradiculitis though the discovery of dissociated sensory loss will clarify the diagnosis.

The prognosis in anterior spinal artery occlusion is not good. There is usually some improvement upon the initial state but recovery is very unlikely to be complete. This is important since if the condition is mistaken for transverse myelitis or Guillain–Barré syndrome, an unjustifiably good prognosis may be given to the patient and relatives.

Because vasoconstrictors in the epidural space might reduce the blood supply to the cord it is generally advised that local anaesthetic solutions used for epidural anaesthesia should not contain adrenaline.

POLIOMYELITIS

Although poliomyelitis is now a rarity in the developed countries it is still endemic in some parts of the world and epidemics could again occur in Britain if the level of active immunization in the community were to fall significantly.

Signs and symptoms

The first indications of the disease are fever, headache and general malaise, often accompanied by sore throat and gastrointestinal symptoms. Insomnia may occur at this stage (and may also follow polio vaccination). In some patients recovery follows and no further symptoms develop. In others the disease progresses with pain in the back and limbs and neck stiffness. Paralysis may be preceded by fasciculation. Paralysis may be patchy, widespread or virtually total. In milder cases asymmetry in the pattern of muscles affected is typical. Occasionally paralysis starts in the legs and progresses upwards in a manner resembling ascending myelitis. Brain stem involvement can produce paralysis of the muscles of the head and neck, though the occular muscles are usually spared. In some patients paralysis is limited to muscles supplied by the lower cranial nerves—a condition referred to as 'bulbar polio'. Recovery from the paralysis is variable but there is usually a very considerable improvement upon the patient's condition at its worst.

The polio virus can be recovered from saliva, urine and faeces both during the disease and for some six weeks after the acute phase. Those in contact with the disease may also carry the virus for some weeks.

Other illness and injury were thought to predispose to the disease and it was usual to postpone nose and throat operations such as adenotonsillectomy during an epidemic. Exercise during the prodomal period tends to make the paralysis worse. There is a predisposition for the muscles most exercised to be those most severely affected.

Differential diagnosis

The allergic conditions described previously—encephalitis, encephalomyelitis, myelitis and polyradiculitis—can present in a way that is sometimes difficult to distinguish clinically from poliomyelitis. In poliomyelitis the CSF contains an excess of cells, both lymphocytes and granulocytes; in the other conditions the CSF cell count is normal. In both, the CSF protein is raised.

It is important to consider the possibility of poliomyelitis when treating any paralysed patient because of the possible risk to the attendants and because of the different prognosis. The treatment of the patient, which depends on his condition, will not necessarily be altered by a change in diagnosis. Complete recovery is less likely with poliomyelitis than with paralysis from autoimmune or allergic neurological disease. The risk to nonimmunized attendant staff looking after a patient with poliomyelitis is very real and all staff likely to be in contact with the disease—such as intensive care unit nurses—should be actively immunized. Further aspects of the management of such cases are discussed on page 214.

Pseudo-polio

In 1974, ten cases of a polio-like illness associated with asthma were reported from Australia [4]. Since then the same condition has been reported from Scandinavia, Britain and North America. All the patients have been children under the age of ten, and in all, paralysis has developed a few days after an acute attack of asthma. The paralysis is usually confined to one or more limbs and is severe with only little recovery. In the acute stage there is fibrillary twitching of the involved muscles. There is no sensory disturbance though there is pain and tenderness in the paralysed limb(s).

The lesion is presumed to be in the anterior horn cells but the cause is unknown. All the patients so far reported had been immunized against poliomyelitis. Viral and antibody studies have not been helpful.

The syndrome is not common but it may be met in anaesthetic practice since the asthmatic attack preceding the paralysis has sometimes been treated by mechanical ventilation.

The typical signs and symptoms of meningitis have been described above. Patients with meningitis may have respiratory inadequacy either because of some central derangement or because of concomitant pulmonary disease. Central depression of respiration does not necessarily carry a bad prognosis and these patients should receive whatever help they need.

In patients with a bacterial or purulent meningitis there is always the possibility of a mass lesion developing either in the form of a subdural empyema or intracranial abscess and the patient should be examined regularly for localizing signs.

An 'aseptic' form of meningitis can occur which is due to, or related to, a viral infection. The condition would seem to be essentially the same as the viral, or postviral encephalitis described above, with exaggeration of the meningitic component. Again, temporary mechanical ventilation may be required.

SUBACUTE COMBINED DEGENERATION OF THE CORD

This is a condition which occurs as a result of vitamin B_{12} deficiency. Vitamin B_{12} is necessary for neuronal nutrition and for forming and maintaining the myelin sheath. In its absence there is demyelination and axonal disruption. A similar pattern of damage may possibly be caused by folate deficiency. The anaemia associated with B_{12} deficiency neuropathy may not be severe in degree but blood and bone marrow studies show the typical megaloblastic picture. The term subacute combined degeneration of the cord is not wholly appropriate since the nervous damage is not confined to the cord but involves peripheral nerves and the brain. The word 'combined' was used to imply that degeneration occurred both in the dorsal sensory columns and also in the lateral corticospinal tracts and this distinguished the condition from tabes where lateral column degeneration does not occur. The signs and symptoms are predominantly those that would be expected from degeneration of those tracts to which may be added some due to cerebral and peripheral damage. The first symptoms tend to be sensory changes in the legs which spread upwards. These are followed by motor weakness and spasticity. Ataxia from loss of proprioceptive input is common. Reflexes may be absent or exaggerated depending upon the relative preponderance of dorsal or lateral column involvement. Occasionally there are mental changes and occasionally primary optic atrophy is present.

Treatment is with parenteral vitamin B_{12}. Folate may be given as well. Folate alone may worsen the patient's condition due to an increased uptake by the bone marrow of what little B_{12} is available to supply the needs of both bone marrow and the nervous system. With treatment there may be considerable improvement or there may be little more than an arrest of the destructive process.

The main interest to the anaesthetist in this disease lies in a recent report of an exactly comparable condition occurring after prolonged exposure to nitrous oxide [5]. The prolonged administration of nitrous oxide is known to interfere with bone marrow function and it is possible that it interferes in some way with B_{12} metabolism. The patients with nitrous oxide myeloneuropathy had normal blood B_{12} levels and had no signs of bone marrow dysfunction but they did show evidence of both spinal cord long tract damage and peripheral neuropathy. All improved or recovered when nitrous oxide was withdrawn.

The use of spinal, epidural or nerve block techniques in patients with such widespread neurological disease is best avoided.

CARDIOVASCULAR CAUSES OF NEUROLOGICAL DISEASE

Patients with neurological disease of cardiovascular origin form a large part of a neurologist's practice and a very wide variety of deficits can be produced by haemorrhage, thrombosis or embolism. To attempt to describe all these would not be of great benefit to the anaesthetist and consequently this section will be limited to some general observations and descriptions of a few selected syndromes.

General management of stroke

Following a cerebrovascular accident from whatever cause, the patient is liable to have an area of oedema and ischaemia round the lesion. Treatment of the oedema with steroids and/or dehydrating regimes has been shown to improve recovery following a stroke that is due to infarction, whether the cause is thrombosis or embolism. The same treatment has not proved effective after cerebral haemorrhage.

Improvement of oxygen delivery to ischaemic tissues has been shown to be improved by isovolaemic haemodilution, that is by a deliberate reduction of haematocrit without a reduction in blood volume. A haematocrit of 30 per cent (or haemoglobin of 10 g per cent) produces optimum oxygen delivery at rest. The reduction in viscosity (and hence improvement in flow) more than compensates for the reduction in oxygen carrying capacity. If, therefore, the patient's blood volume and haematocrit are being manipulated by his attendants, as it would be if the stroke had occurred in relation to some surgical operation, the benefits of isovolaemic haemodilution should be considered. Deliberate haemodilution has been recommended for stroke associated with polycythaemia.

Maintenance of systemic blood pressure and hence of cerebral perfusion pressure is important. Many patients with stroke already have a compromised cerebral circulation because of widespread arteriopathy. Autoregulation is often deficient or altered because of arteriolar rigidity. Sharp falls in systemic blood pressure should therefore be avoided and it is probably wise to maintain a systolic pressure of 120 mmHg or more.

Severe hypertension may precipitate a stroke or follow it. Systolic pressures above 180 mmHg should probably be treated and pressures above 200 mmHg should certainly be. Sedation may be sufficient; if not, for acute use, hydrallazine is safe and effective and can be given in 5–10 mg increments at 10 minute intervals until the desired reduction is achieved.

Embolism

The commonest source of a large cerebral embolus is the left atrium in a patient with atrial fibrillation. Clots can also form in the left ventricle following cardiac infarction and, occasionally, paradoxical embolization can occur when a clot from the venous

10*

side of the circulation passes through a patent foramen ovale from the right atrium to the left. The usual treatment is with anticoagulants.

Transient ischaemic attacks

In the instances mentioned above the emboli are pieces of blood clot. In arteriopathic subjects small pieces of debris from atheromatous ulcers in the arterial walls can separate and form emboli. These emboli consist of fibrin, platelets or cholesterol or a mixture of these. Common sources in the extracranial cerebral vessels are from atheroma at the bifurcation of the common carotid arteries or at the take off of the vertebral arteries from the subclavian. Typically the ischaemic attacks last a few minutes to some hours and each attack follows a stereotyped pattern. Embolism of the retinal vessels produces transient blindness or scotoma (amaurosis fugax). In middle cerebral artery embolism weakness, paralysis and/or parasthesiae can occur in the hand and face and there may be dysphasia. In the vertebral artery territory the signs may be due to embolism in the posterior cerebral artery distribution producing a hemianopia or there may be signs of brain stem disturbance such as giddiness, diplopia, faintness or drop attacks. The attacks may continue for months and remit spontaneously or they may herald a major stroke due to occlusion of the parent artery or one of its branches. Treatment with anticoagulants and endarterectomy of the atheromatous arterial segment when this is surgically practicable are often offered.

This syndrome has been mentioned partly because it is an interesting curiosity of cerebral blood flow that emboli from a source in the neck should repeatedly and accurately follow the same intracranial course and partly because of the serious implications of the condition. The fleeting and often trivial nature of the attacks may lead the patient or his medical advisers to dismiss them as unimportant. This is particularly likely to happen if the patient is hypertensive. The informed anaesthetist may be the first to recognize the pattern and its import.

Hypertensive encephalopathy

Severe hypertension can produce a pattern of neurological disturbance which has been termed hypertensive encephalopathy. The condition usually occurs when a patient who is already hypertensive has a further sharp increase in blood pressure. The signs are those of raised intracranial pressure with headache, nausea and vomiting. There may be transient focal signs such as dysphasia or paralyses: diplopia, blurring of vision and even complete blindness, may occur. Convulsions are almost invariable and lead to coma. Papilloedema and hypertensive retinopathy are almost always present. Diffuse cerebral oedema is not, however, always found at postmortem. Focal arterial spasm has been postulated as a cause of the symptoms but this has not been proven. Cerebral blood flow increases in severe hypertension when systemic blood pressure is above the upper limit of autoregulation, and the signs and symptoms can be satisfactorily explained as being due to raised intracranial pressure secondary to a sharp increase in intracranial blood volume, and an increase in brain water due to an increase in capillary filtration pressure (see page 262). Despite the dramatic nature of the condition the prognosis is good.

In eclampsia, a similar condition may appear at lower levels of blood pressure than in the established hypertensive probably because of the effect of water retention and cerebral oedema unrelated to blood pressure.

Acute nephritis may occasionally present as raised intracranial pressure because the hypertension and the renal signs are initially minimal and overlooked.

Treatment is with sedation and hypotensive agents. Chlormethiazole is useful to control convulsions: dehydration therapy with osmotic agents or diuretics is also useful. Hypertonic magnesium sulphate enemas used to be given to patients with eclampsia. They were probably effective for two reasons: first because of their dehydrating effect and secondly because of the sedative and anticonvulsive effect of magnesium ions.

Pontine haemorrhage

Spontaneous bleeding into the substance of the pons is not common but presents a recognizable clinical picture. The patient is usually elderly and hypertensive. He collapses without warning and quite soon becomes deeply comatose. Breathing is affected, becoming periodic or irregular before finally arresting. The patient is often totally unresponsive though sometimes the pupils react to light and sometimes there are flexor responses in the limbs to painful stimuli. The pupils are pinpoint and the eyes fixed in a central position. Oculovestibular and oculocephalic reflexes are absent. If the patient survives more than a few hours, body temperature rises. There may be a normal EEG if the patient has been protected from any hypoxic episode. This is because cortical function is undisturbed by the localized brain stem lesion although consciousness is lost as a result of destruction of essential parts of the midbrain reticular formation.

This particular pattern of coma can be produced by causes other than brain stem damage. The author was asked to see a patient who had stopped breathing whilst being anaesthetized for an aortogram. He had been returned to the ward and was being ventilated mechanically. His blood pressure was 190/90, he was flushed and felt hot. His pupils were pinpoint and not reacting to light. He was totally unresponsive to painful stimuli. A confident diagnosis of pontine haemorrhage was made but because of the fallibility of clinical opinion, treatment was continued. Two hours after the examination the patient woke up, pulled out the endotracheal tube and appeared to be unchanged from his preoperative state. Retrospectively a diagnosis of morphine overdosage and carbon dioxide retention was made. The patient had chronic bronchitis and had received 20 mg of papaveretum preoperatively.

DISORDERS OF BREATHING

In rapidly deepening coma whether due to an expanding intracranial lesion or to a metabolic disturbance, breathing tends to become slower and shallower until it finally stops. In more stable states of stupor or coma different patterns may occur.

Periodic (Cheyne–Stokes) breathing

This well known pattern where breathing waxes and wanes in regular cycles can be caused by at least three mechanisms. In those with a slow circulation time due to cardiovascular disease the delay between blood leaving the lungs and reaching the medulla is such that the fine control of breathing becomes coarsened and the system oscillates between overbreathing and underbreathing. In servo-system terms there is 'damping' in the feedback part of the loop.

Periodic breathing can follow voluntary overventilation. In this case damping of feedback is due to the slowness of the replenishment of the body's stores of carbon dioxide.

Periodic breathing due to primary neurological disease is usually associated with bilateral lesions in the cerebral hemispheres or diencephalon. The presumed mechanism is a reduction in the sensitivity or a slowed response of the respiratory centre to changes in CO_2 levels in both directions, i.e. less quick in response to both rises and falls in CO_2.

Although periodic breathing can occur due to the effect of expanding lesions in the posterior fossa, this is not common. It can also occur in patients in metabolic coma but probably only when the circulation time is simultaneously prolonged. The common change in breathing following metabolic disturbance or drug overdose or brain stem ischaemia is for it to become slower and shallower.

Decerebrate hyperventilation

In the decerebrate state the brain stem is freed from descending inhibitory control and is overactive. This overactivity is shown by extensor rigidity and often by sustained overbreathing. In response to stimulation the patient may have extensor spasms, sympathetic discharge (enlargement of the pupil and increase in pulse rate and blood pressure) and an even greater increase in rate and depth of breathing. This overbreathing serves no useful function and is wasteful of energy.

Gasping or apneustic breathing

Apneustic breathing consists of a series of, often irregular, inspiratory gasps. Inspiration is quicker and usually, but not always, deeper than normal, and peak inspiration is held for a second or two. Expiration is passive and the expiratory pause is prolonged.

This pattern of breathing is associated with destructive lesions at the level of the middle and lower pons that are usually irrecoverable. Agonal breathing is not normally apneustic. The last few breaths are often separated by long pauses but do not show the typical hold in peak inspiration.

Irregularly irregular (ataxic) breathing

Occasionally, particularly with lesions in the posterior fossa or lower brain stem, breathing becomes quite irregular both in depth and rate. Overall the rate tends to be slower than usual and ventilation is often inadequate. The volume of some breaths is greater than the normal resting tidal volume, and of others is smaller. There is no discernible pattern or sequence. This type of breathing occurring in patients with expanding lesions in the posterior fossa frequently heralds respiratory arrest.

Respiratory arrest

Patients dying from neurological disease usually die from some form of respiratory failure. While it is obviously necessary to ventilate patients mechanically when the cause of their respiratory arrest is in doubt, it is not desirable to do so when it is due to incurable disease.

Patients with expanding intracranial lesions will stop breathing when intracranial pressure becomes very high and the brain stem is compressed. If the cause of the raised pressure can be treated operatively, as for instance by draining an abscess or evacuating a haematoma, the patient may recover. If, however, the interval between the cessation of breathing and the surgical relief of pressure is more than some 15 minutes, recovery is doubtful. If more than an hour has passed since arrest, recovery is impossible.

Arrest from hypoxia is not usually recoverable if the patient remains apnoeic for more than a few minutes after re-establishment of adequate oxygenation.

Respiratory arrest from subarachnoid haemorrhage is irrecoverable unless a haematoma can be localized and evacuated within a matter of minutes—which is rarely possible. The same applies to arrest following a cerebrovascular accident.

Sleep apnoea

The term 'sleep apnoea' has been used to include at least three separate conditions.

Spontaneous failure of respiratory drive. Occasionally breathing stops when the subject falls asleep but restarts when he is woken and told to breathe. Rarely breathing also stops while the patient is awake and again restarts on command. The author has seen six instances of this condition all of which followed operations upon lesions in the posterior fossa. Breathing was precarious for five to ten days postoperatively and the patients were ventilated by machine for varying periods. Recovery was complete in all cases. The condition has also been seen following what appear to have been minor cerebrovascular accidents. It has not been satisfactorily explained.

Epileptic. True sleep apnoea can occur as a very rare manifestation of epilepsy. The attacks are usually sufficiently short for the patient to survive but they can be fatal. The diagnosis rests upon finding EEG abnormalities. Treatment is with anticonvulsants.

Obstructive apnoea. Respiratory obstruction can occur during deep sleep. This is not true apnoea since breathing efforts continue although there is no air flow into the lungs. The subject usually wakes after a few obstructed breaths. There are two components to this condition: one is a propensity to very deep sleep and the other is a configuration of the tongue and pharynx that makes the subject peculiarly liable to respiratory obstruction. Repeated episodes of obstructive apnoea can occur and up to 300 have been recorded in a single night. As a result, sleep is very disturbed and the patient is excessively somnolent during the day. This daytime somnolence has been mistaken for narcolepsy.

As well as daytime sleepiness the repeated periods of hypoxia associated with the obstructive episodes can result in pulmonary hypertension, right heart hypertrophy and right ventricular failure.

The obstruction of the upper airway can be fatal and even if not fatal the damage caused by repeated hypoxic episodes and the risk of death, can make a permanent tracheostomy the safest form of treatment. Antidepressive drugs and amphetamines have been used to lighten sleep but without much benefit. Acromegalics are liable to this syndrome because of the disproportionate overgrowth of the tongue and the soft tissue of the pharynx and larynx.

Children with enlarged tonsils and adenoids have also occasionally been found to suffer from the combination of obstruction, daytime drowsiness, pulmonary hypertension and right heart strain. All their symptoms and signs have resolved after adenotonsillectomy.

The obesity hypoventilation (or Pickwickian) syndrome

This is an association of obesity, episodic somnolence and hypoventilation. Neuro-logically, they seem to be in the same predicament as patients with muscular dystrophy or motor neurone disease. Though obviously no conscious decision is made, it is as though the effort of breathing were so great that they opt for an insensitivity to CO_2 rather than to attempt to maintain normal gaseous exchange. There are secondary circulatory abnormalities as well as changes in lung function. These aspects are discussed more fully in Chapter 12 (page 402).

The effects on breathing of spinal cord transection

High transection of the spinal cord can result in respiratory embarrassment. The diaphragm is supplied by the 3rd, 4th and 5th cervical segments so that transections below this level will leave diaphragmatic activity intact. If there is transection imme-diately below this level all intercostal and abdominal muscle activity will be lost. The principal effect of this upon breathing is the removal of all active or forced expiration. Expiration becomes purely passive. This can sometimes be helped a little by com-pression of the chest and belly by an attendant but not usually enough to produce an effective cough. The effect on the respiratory pattern as seen on spirometry is shown in Fig. 8.7. The major part of the inspiratory reserve volume is due to diaphragmatic contraction and there is no severe reduction in vital capacity. The expiratory reserve

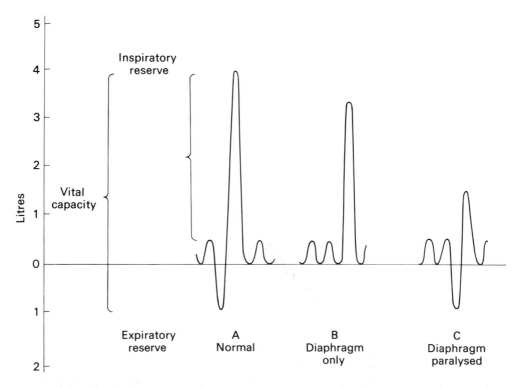

Fig. 8.7. The diagram shows the sort of spirometry trace that might be obtained from: (A) a healthy young man, (B) the same after cord transection at C6–C7 and (C) the same following bilateral phrenic nerve palsy.

however is lost because this depends upon the forced expulsion of air after the lungs and chest wall have recoiled to their resting position. The paralysis of the expiratory muscles makes an explosive cough impossible and patients with such high cord lesions may need a permanent tracheostomy if their lungs are to be kept free from accumulating secretions.

For contrast the effect of bilateral phrenic palsy is also shown in Fig. 8.7. The paralysed diaphragm acts in the same way as a flail segment in thoracic trauma, moving paradoxically with each breath, and there is considerable reduction in vital capacity. Looking at patients with the two conditions, high cord transection produces a pattern of breathing where the belly moves outwards noticeably on inspiration and the chest is less noticeably drawn inwards while bilateral phrenic palsy produces a pattern where there is a very vigorous expansion of the chest during inspiration and an indrawing of the belly; at no time during inspiration is there any outward movement of the abdominal wall.

Unilateral phrenic palsy is of little moment but bilateral palsy can produce serious limitation of maximum breathing capacity. Bilateral palsies can occur as part of a peripheral neuropathy or (rarely) can follow operations on the neck such as bilateral stellate ganglionectomy.

Sympathetic outflow is from $T1–L1$ or 2. High cord transection therefore separates the sympathetic efferent neurones in the lateral horns of the spinal grey matter from higher control. This will result in a loss of sympathetic function below the level of the transection with consequent vasomotor instability.

BRAIN DEATH

The concept of 'brain death' implies irrecoverable damage to the central nervous system in the presence of adequate cardiovascular and pulmonary function. The term is most often used when a patient shows no evidence of any cerebral or brain stem function. It is also sometimes used when some evidence of brain function persists but the patient remains are flexic and apnoeic.

Various investigations have been advocated to establish the diagnosis of brain death, such as blood flow studies and EEG recordings. These investigations do not improve upon the information obtainable from a clinical examination combined with a CO_2 challenge repeated at an interval of several hours. Indeed, an EEG recording in these circumstances can be positively misleading. Fast cortical activity with runs of clearly defined α-rhythm, can occasionally be recorded from patients who are apnoeic from fatal intracranial disease. Usually such records are obtained from patients who have suffered a brain stem haemorrhage or infarct but who have not been subjected to any prolonged hypoxia because of the prompt institution of mechanical ventilation.

To establish brain death includes testing for response to painful stimuli, testing for the presence of various cranial nerve reflexes and observing the lack of response to a CO_2 challenge.

The cranial nerve reflexes tested are the pupillary, corneal and gag reflexes and the oculovestibular reflex or caloric response as described on page 246.

The CO_2 challenge consists in observing the patient's respiratory response, or lack of it, to an arterial CO_2 tension slightly above normal (6–7·3 kPa; 45–55 mmHg). The raised CO_2 can be achieved by administering 5 per cent CO_2 in O_2 through the ventilator or by incorporating a dead space in the ventilator tubing. The actual level of CO_2 should be checked by arterial blood gas analysis and there should be no element of hypoxia while the test is being conducted. It is important that the patient's core temperature should be normal or above normal when this test is performed and if his core temperature has fallen below 36°C he should be warmed.

Some spinal reflexes may be retained in the presence of irrecoverable intracranial disease and these should not be allowed to mislead the clinician nor to give false hope to the relatives.

It should be emphasized that the decision to resuscitate or not and the decision to continue or discontinue life support systems depend upon the interrelationship between the certainty of the diagnosis and the length of time that the patient has been observed. When the diagnosis is certain and the prognosis hopeless, a decision can be reached very quickly. When the diagnosis is in doubt, support must be maintained for at least 12 hours and perhaps for up to 48 or 72 hours.

Even when the diagnosis is known and the prognosis is hopeless, there may be indications for maintaining a vegetative 'life' for at least some hours. One of these is to help the patient's relatives to accommodate to the situation and another is the possibility of using organs for transplant.

A joint statement from the Royal Colleges contains a full discussion of the problems associated with removing life support systems from brain-dead patients [2].

REFERENCES

1 COOPERMAN, LH. Succinylcholine-induced hyperkalaemia in neuromuscular disease. *J Am Med Assoc* 1970; **213**: 1867–71.
2 CONFERENCE OF MEDICAL ROYAL COLLEGES AND THEIR FACULTIES IN THE UNITED KINGDOM. The diagnosis of brain death. *Lancet* 1976; **2**: 1069–70.
3 GOLTMAN AM. The mechanism of migraine. *J Allergy* 1936; **7**: 351–5. Quoted in: Pearce J. Migraine: *Clinical features, mechanisms and management*. Springfield: Charles C Thomas, 1969 (original not consulted).
4 HOPKINS IJ, SHIELD LK. Poliomyelitis-like illness associated with asthma in childhood. *Lancet* 1974; **1**: 760.
5 LAYZER RB. Myeloneuropathy after prolonged exposure to nitrous oxide. *Lancet* 1978; **2**: 1227–30.
6 PLUM F, POSNER JB, eds. *The diagnosis of stupor and coma*. 2nd ed. Philadelphia: Davis Co, 1972.
7 TEASDALE G, GALRRAITH S, CLARKE K. Acute impairment of brain function—2 observation record chart. *Nurs Times* 1975; **71** (25): 972–3.
8 TEASDALE G, JENNETT B. Assessment of coma and impaired consciousness: a practical scale. *Lancet* 1974; **2**: 81–4.

RECOMMENDED FURTHER READING

BOWSHER D. *Mechanisms of nervous disorder: an introduction*. Oxford: Blackwell Scientific, 1978.
MATTHEWS WB, MILLER H. *Diseases of the nervous system*. 3rd ed. Oxford: Blackwell Scientific, 1979.
PLUM F, POSNER JB, eds. *The diagnosis of stupor and coma*. 2nd ed. Philadelphia: Davis Co, 1972.

ACKNOWLEDGEMENT

I would like to thank Dr. J. B. Foster for his very helpful criticism and advice in the preparation of this chapter.

Chapter 9
Medical Genetics Relevant to Anaesthesia

M. D. VICKERS

There are many abnormal conditions which are inherited, and many more which are present at birth. It is important, however, to distinguish between these two groups. A disorder present at birth is congenital, but it may not necessarily have been inherited. Conversely, some inherited disorders may not be manifest at birth, or indeed may never be manifest at all.

All human variability is a result of the interaction of hereditary and environmental factors. If a condition occurs only in persons of a certain genetic constitution and when this is present, it *always* occurs, one has complete hereditary determination. Usually, however, some effect of environment or some combination of inherited factors is necessary to produce the condition so that the inherited disorder is not always fully expressed.

Some common conditions occur in persons of *any* genetic constitution, but have different frequencies in persons of different genetic constitution. Such an example is provided by the different blood groups in which there is a different susceptibility to various apparently unrelated diseases.

When, however, the condition occurs in persons of any genetic constitution, and in the same frequency whatever the genetic make-up, it is assumed to be entirely determined by environment.

It is, to a certain extent, a matter of definition as to what is, or is not, an inherited disorder. Many conditions, such as diabetes or hallux valgus, are more common in related individuals than in the general population. To attempt to encompass them all would be counterproductive and only conditions in which patterns of inheritance can usually be clearly traced, and which override environmental influences, are considered here.

This chapter attempts a short résumé of human genetics and the terminology employed, illustrated by examples of interest to anaesthetists. Many haematological, neurological, and musculoskeletal disorders in particular have an inherited basis and the clinical aspects of the more important are discussed in Chapters 7, 8 and 11.

GENES AND CHROMOSOMES

GENES

All inherited features are determined by the nature of an individual's genes. The basic structure of the genes is simple although its elucidation was one of the finest pieces of scientific detective work of recent times [8].

Each gene consists of about 1,500 linked molecules of desoxyribonucleic acid (DNA). Each molecule of DNA consists of two out of four possible bases linking molecules of a pentose sugar and phosphate. Fig. 9.1 shows the arrangement. The four possible bases are adenine (A), thymine (T), cytosine (C) and guanine (G). Adenine etc.   etc.

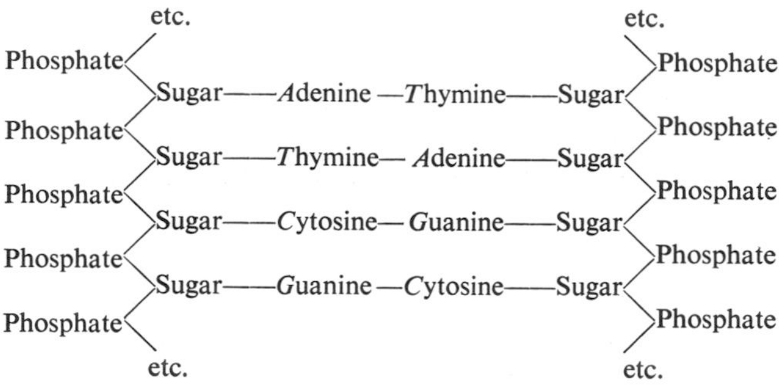

Phosphate⟨   ⟩Phosphate
        ⟩Sugar——*A*denine —*T*hymine——Sugar⟨
Phosphate⟨   ⟩Phosphate
        ⟩Sugar——*T*hymine— *A*denine——Sugar⟨
Phosphate⟨   ⟩Phosphate
        ⟩Sugar——*C*ytosine— Guanine——Sugar⟨
Phosphate⟨   ⟩Phosphate
        ⟩Sugar——*G*uanine —*C*ytosine——Sugar⟨
Phosphate⟨   ⟩Phosphate

etc.   etc.

Fig. 9.1. The four possible base pairs which link the strands of the double helix of DNA.

is always paired with thymine and cytosine with guanine, but as the order of the pairs down the complete structure is significant, adenine-thymine has a different significance to thymine-adenine. There are thus four possible base pairs. A sequence of three such base pairs (called a *codon*) is necessary to encode for the structure of each amino acid and each gene therefore consists of about 500 such codons which is the order of magnitude of the number of amino acids in a polypeptide chain.

The genes are aggregated into structures called chromosomes. These appear to be somewhat squat and fat but this is deceptive and in fact each is a tightly coiled, fine spiral filament of considerable length. This spiral is composed of a large number of genes in a linear order. The number of genes which go to make up a chromosome is not known but it has been estimated that there are between 20,000 and 40,000 different pairs of genes in total.

The information which is encoded in the genes is replicated at the time of normal cell division because each DNA molecule divides between the two bases, and each temporarily freed base attracts its complementary partner base from the substrate and this results in the reconstitution of two identical DNA molecules.

The chromosomes, with one exception, are aggregated into similar pairs. For most characteristics, therefore, a pair of genes are present and determine the genetic constitution. Such a gene pair is called a *locus*. The exceptions are the sex chromosomes (see below) on which a single unpaired gene occupies a locus.

There are at least three kinds of genes, structural, operator and regulator.

Structural genes act as the basic template which determines the structure of each person's characteristic enzymes and proteins. They do not do this directly: the code is first transferred to a strand of ribonucleic acid (messenger RNA) which migrates to the cytoplasm where transfer RNA provides the appropriate amino acids to construct the polypeptides and proteins which were originally specified by the DNA of the chromosome. If the specification produces a structurally abnormal enzyme this will result in a complete or partial inhibition of the metabolic pathway in which that enzyme functions. So will failure to elaborate any enzyme at all. This can be called a *silent* gene. Several examples are now well documented. The absence of genes to encode for phenyl-alanine hydroxylase means that tyrosine (an essential amino acid) cannot be formed from phenylalanine, resulting in the condition called phenylketonuria. The absence of galactose-l-phosphate uridyl transferase likewise results in galactosaemia.

The absence of glucose-6-phosphate dehydrogenase (G6PD) is an example of a silent gene which is sex-linked (see below). It is also an example of a condition which requires both a particular constitution as well as environmental influences, since it only gives rise to serious disease (haemolytic anaemia) when fava beans are ingested (favism) or after the administration of certain drugs such as primaquine and sulphon-amides.

There are both silent genes and abnormal structural genes for plasma cholinesterase as described more fully later.

Each cell contains the complete genetic information to enable replication of the appropriate substances to take place. Cellular differentiation, however, means that all the cells of the body do not actually undertake replication of all substances of which they are theoretically capable, and *operator genes* are assumed to exist to provide the necessary mechanism to determine which potentialities shall be expressed. *Regulator genes* determine when the operator genes shall be switched on and off.

Abnormalities in operator genes exert influences such as rate-limiting or a failure to rate-limit a particular metabolic pathway, and such an abnormality is probably a factor in porphyria.

CHROMOSOMES

In the somatic cells of human females there are 23 identical pairs of chromosomes and 22 identical pairs and 1 nonidentical pair in the human male. The 22 pairs of chromosomes which are the same in both male and female are called *autosomal* chromosomes; the 23rd pair are the X and Y chromosomes and are the *sex* chromosomes. Females have two X chromosomes, and males, one X and one Y.

During maturation of ova and spermatozoa there is a reduction in the number of chromosomes by half, with one of each pair normally going into each of a pair of cells. Cells containing the half number of chromosomes are called *gametes*. An important histologically identifiable structure in each chromosome is the *centromere*; at one stage during the reduction division the pairs of chromosomes appear to be joined only at centromere and at this stage visual identification of the various chromosomes is possible.

An agreed, internationally standardized, format for the identification and display of chromosome abnormalities is the Denver-London system. This chromosome picture is called a *karyotype* (Fig. 9.2). The chromosomes are grouped according to size and according to whether the centromere is median or near median (metacentric), midway to one end, or terminal (acrocentric).

A nonpictorial international system to categorize chromosome abnormalities is the Chicago system. A normal female is designated 46,XX and a normal male 46,XY. 47,XY,G+ indicates an extra chromosome in the G group in a male. Because the centromere is rarely median most chromosomes have short and long arms, and these are designated p and q respectively. Thus 46,XX,4p− indicates that the short arm only of chromosome 4 is missing in a female.

A number of abnormal conditions are associated with an additional chromosome or the absence of part or all of one chromosome. An additional chromosome is a *trisomy* disorder. Down's syndrome (mongolism) is a well-known example and is due to an additional chromosome 21 (47,XX,21 + or 47,XY,21 +, depending on sex). This abnormality arises because both the 21 chromosomes migrate into one gamete during cell division. This implies an equal number of gametes without a 21 chromosome and a clinical abnormality (antimongolism) does exist corresponding to the genetic pattern 45,XX,21 − but is rare. These children have many serious malformations and generally do not survive long. This is an example of a general truism that the absence of a chromosome is more of a catastrophe for the organism than an extra chromosome, and

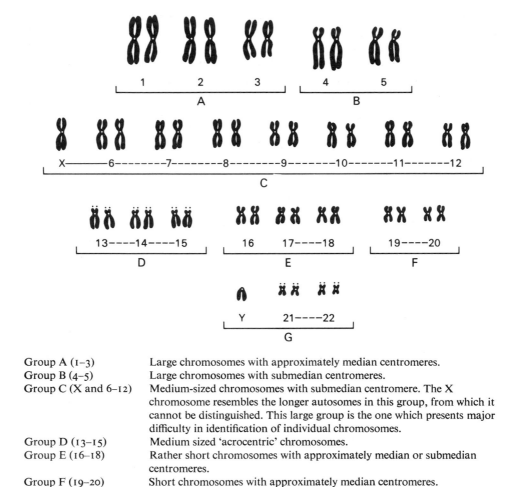

Group A (1–3)	Large chromosomes with approximately median centromeres.
Group B (4–5)	Large chromosomes with submedian centromeres.
Group C (X and 6–12)	Medium-sized chromosomes with submedian centromere. The X chromosome resembles the longer autosomes in this group, from which it cannot be distinguished. This large group is the one which presents major difficulty in identification of individual chromosomes.
Group D (13–15)	Medium sized 'acrocentric' chromosomes.
Group E (16–18)	Rather short chromosomes with approximately median or submedian centromeres.
Group F (19–20)	Short chromosomes with approximately median centromeres.
Group G (Y and 21–22)	Very short, acrocentric chromosomes. The Y chromosome is usually distinguishable from the autosomes of this group.

Fig. 9.2 A normal male karyotype, 46, XY. Agreed description of the human chromosomes (Denver-London System). The dotted lines indicate uncertainty, and the solid lines very great uncertainty, of individual chromosome identification by this technique.

often results in a nonviable fetus or early death. Two other trisomy disorders have now been identified, Edward's syndrome (trisomy of chromosome 17 or 18) and Patau's syndrome (trisomy 13). Both have skeletal and facial disorders and, usually, congenital heart disease.

   Additional sex chromosomes have much less effect than extra autosomal chromosomes. This is not unexpected since all individuals have to be able to function effectively, whether they have one or two X chromosomes. Consequently those chromosome abnormalities which are found in nearly normal individuals mostly turn out to be abnormalities of the sex chromosomes. The disorder arises whenever both sex chromosomes go to one pole during cell division, so that there are ova which are either XX or O or spermatozoa which are XY or O. Any of these combinations can unite at conception with a normal ovum or spermatozoan, to give an individual with either an extra

X or an absent X or Y. (The uniting of an abnormal ovum with an abnormal spermatozoan is very improbable.)

A 47,XXY, chromosome structure gives rise to Kleinfelter's syndrome, which manifests as a male with feminine traits (small genitalia, testicular atrophy, gynaecomastia). This is a common abnormality, affecting about 1 in 400 males. A 45,XO pattern gives rise to Turner's syndrome and these may come to anaesthetic attention because of aortic stenosis, which is a common finding in this syndrome. Typically they have a web neck and no gonads. A 47,XXX pattern is fairly common (1 in 1,250) and these appear to be almost normal looking females although with a tendency to mental subnormality.

It may be noted that the Y contributes a lot of 'maleness' and 47,XXY, 48,XXXY and even 49,XXXXY are all obviously males. However, if the Y is absent, the individual is always female.

One plausible explanation for the innocuous behaviour of additional X chromosomes is that all but one become inactivated in somatic cells. Dark staining spots of chromatin 1μ in diameter are found on the inner surface of the nuclear membrane in the cells of those individuals, and are called Barr bodies after their discoverer; these are always one less in number than the number of X chromosomes.

Other congenital abnormalities arise from loss of a segment of a chromosome—called a *deletion*. There can also be reciprocal translocation when a broken off part of one of a pair of chromosomes is exchanged for a broken off part of one of another pair. (This is not a cross-over as discussed below, a normal event which involves the exchange of parts of chromosomes between a pair of chromosomes.)

It has been estimated that as many as 4 per cent of conceptions have chromosome abnormalities, 90 per cent of which are eliminated by the abortion of a nonviable fetus.

PATTERNS OF INHERITANCE

In many inherited conditions, no chromosome abnormality can be detected microscopically. Sometimes, however, the pattern of inheritance is such that it can be confidently ascribed to the X chromosome, and such a condition is said to be sex-linked. Haemophilia, colour-blindness, a common type of muscular dystrophy, are all controlled by genes in the X chromosome. Only one condition linked to the Y chromosome has been described and even this is uncertain. Most of the important abnormal sex-linked genes rarely produce an abnormality in females, for reasons which will emerge.

Abnormalities which are due to genes on autosomal chromosomes are usually not ascribable to any specific chromosome pair although with the technique of genetic linkage (see below) chromosome mapping is advancing, and already a few conditions, principally biochemical abnormalities, can be ascribed to particular chromosomes.

When both genes appear to be acting identically, the individual is said to be *homozygous* for that characteristic. If either the inheritance pattern or other evidence shows that the genes are having different effects, that individual is said to be heterozygous. (A male, because he possesses only one X, is strictly speaking *hemizygous* for characteristics carried on the X chromosome. If the gene is abnormal he is affected—if it is normal he is not affected.)

It is important to realize that the apparent physical condition of the individual (the phenotype) is not a reliable guide to the underlying genetic situation (the *genotype*). If the 'abnormal' gene produces something which is ineffective but harmless, the 'normal' gene may have enough activity to make the individual indistinguishable from a normal homozygote. Increasingly, however, the differences between a normal homozygote and, say, a normal/silent heterozygote are being uncovered by various sophisticated techniques. In their absence, adequate family studies which often need to span two or more generations can elucidate the genetic make-up and it is for this reason that patterns of inheritance are studied.

Mendel, in his original work, identified certain characteristics which were *dominant* and others which were *recessive*. A recessive characteristic was one which was overt only when the appropriate (recessive) gene was present on both chromosomes; dominant homozygotes and dominant/recessive heterozygotes both exhibited the dominant characteristic. In a mating between two heterozygous individuals, one quarter of the next generation exhibited the recessive characteristic and three quarters exhibited the dominant one (Fig. 9.3).

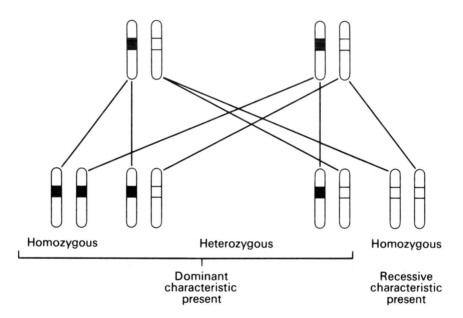

Fig. 9.3. A mating between two heterozygous individuals, one quarter exhibit the recessive characteristic whilst three quarters exhibit the dominant characteristic. = dominant gene, = recessive gene.

Similarly, in human genetics, a dominant characteristic is one which is present whenever the abnormal gene is present and a recessive characteristic is one which produces an effect only when the appropriate gene is present in both chromosomes. These are facts of observation. There are, however, an increasing number of intermediate situations, when the heterozygous condition can be identified and found to be intermediate between the homozygous conditions so that the homozygous abnormal is just *more* abnormal than the heterozygous abnormal. If the heterozygotes can be detected, the gene must be regarded as an incomplete recessive. In some conditions not all the heterozygotes can be detected. Thus while there *may* be such a phenomenon as complete dominance there may not be such a phenomenon as complete recessiveness.

It is as well to realize also that with some rare conditions, dominance has been assumed because of the inheritance pattern, although because of the rarity of the gene, the homozygous condition may never have been observed. Whether or not it would be more severely abnormal than the heterozygotes which have been observed may not therefore have ever been ascertained. For example, multiple telangiectasis (Osler's disease) is regularly inherited as a simple dominant and usually manifests itself in early adult life with epistaxis and telangiectatic spots. These tend to increase with age and occasionally there may be a severe haemorrhage. In one case, however, a child whose parents were both affected, had a large haemangioma at birth, developed telangiectasia fairly rapidly during the first four weeks of life, then suffered haemorrhages from various sites and died of the consequences of multiple organ haemorrhages before the age of three months.

DOMINANT INHERITANCE

An abnormality which is inherited as a dominant must either have arisen as a new mutation or it can be clearly traced through the family since, whenever this gene is present its effect is produced. When an individual possesses a gene giving rise to a dominant abnormality, half the gametes will receive the abnormal gene and half the normal gene during the reduction division. In a mating with a normal individual, half of the resulting offspring can be expected to receive a normal gene from both parents whilst half will receive the abnormal gene (a 1 : 1 ratio obviously cannot be expected exactly in small numbers.)

The genetic constitution of the affected children is, of course, the same as that of their affected parent, and when they themselves mate with a normal individual the same consequences will follow (see Fig. 9.4).

Thus, unless we are observing a mutation,
1 affected individuals have an affected parent;
2 when affected individuals mate with a normal, they have affected and normal children in approximately equal numbers;

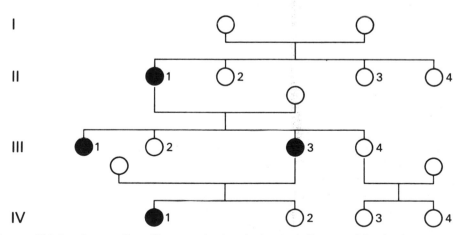

Fig. 9.4. This imaginary pedigree illustrates the three basic criteria for recognizing dominant inheritance. The mutant gene (●) arises in II 1 (i). All affected individuals thereafter have an affected parent. (ii) Normal offspring (III4) married to another normal produce only normal offspring (IV 3 and 4) (iii). The mutant gene occurs in half the children (III 1 and 3, IV 1) of affected individuals.

3 when the *normal* offspring mate with normals, there are *no* affected offspring.

Variegate porphyria presents an almost classic example of a condition inherited as an autosomal dominant and is discussed later.

Relative importance of inheritance and mutation in dominant conditions

Whilst the above is true of relatively minor conditions, when one examines dominant defects which affect survival or fertility it becomes clear that most of the affected individuals in the population must have arisen as new mutations, and the frequency of the defect in the population represents the balance between new mutation and elimination.

A good illustration of this has been provided by a study of achondroplasia. This condition gives rise to dwarfs with normal sized heads. The characteristic mutation rate producing this abnormality was found to be 1 in 20,000 genes, or 1 in 10,000 individuals. It was also found that 80 per cent of achondroplasic dwarfs die in the first year of life. On such figures a stable population of ten million people would contain 1,000 new mutations, augmented by only 200 children of the surviving dwarfs of the previous generation, 40 grandchildren from the generation before that, eight great grandchildren, etc., i.e. approximately 1,250 cases in all, nearly 80 per cent of whom are new mutations.

Mutation

Mutations are not rare events. They are caused by high energy ionizing radiation, by ultraviolet rays, by certain chemicals such as mustard gas, and as an inevitable consequence of increasing age of the germ cells. Most mutations affect only a single gene and most are harmful presumably because a random change in a well-ordered system is likely to do more harm than good. They are single events, so that only one child in the family is affected. There is, however, a condition of *gonadal mosaicism*, in which only part of the ovary or testis carries the mutant gene. If this occurs the 1 : 1 ratio of affected offspring discussed above, no longer applies.

RECESSIVE INHERITANCE

With conditions caused by recessive genes, quite other conclusions emerge. Firstly, the condition only occurs, typically, when two individuals who are heterozygous for the same gene produce a child. Since they are heterozygous, the parents will be normal with regard to the relevant characteristic. A well-known example is albinism. Albinos are usually born to 'normal' parents. Because the parents are both 'carriers' it is quite possible that they will produce more than one abnormal child, and indeed such conditions were regarded at one time as 'familial' rather than as 'hereditary'. In a mating between heterozygous individuals one in four of the children can be expected to be abnormal. Because the majority of cases arise from the mating of heterozygous individuals, in whom the gene can be present undetected through several generations, an undue proportion of consanguineous marriages is found amongst the *parents* of affected individuals.

Simple arithmetic shows that the gene frequency must be quite high even for quite rare recessive disorders. For example, if the gene is present in 2 per cent (1 in 50) of individuals (gene frequency—1 in 100), random mating will give a homozygous incidence of only 1 in (100 × 100) or 1 in 10,000 affected individuals. Quite rare recessive characteristics are thus common in the gene pool, and it is estimated that most normal individuals are heterozygous for between 3 and 5 recessive genes which would give rise to known abnormalities if present in the homozygous form.

INTERMEDIATE INHERITANCE

Increasingly, with sensitive biochemical methods, conditions are being identified in which the heterozygous state can be detected and shown to be abnormal, although less so than the homozygous state. Such is the case with sickle-cell disease and with the cholinesterase variants discussed below. Frequency considerations such as those used in the preceding paragraph show that unless the heterozygotes are very common the homozygote abnormal must be extremely rare. For example:

Frequency of gene	*Frequency of heterozygote* (Double the frequency of the gene)	*Frequency of homozygote* (Random mating) (Frequency of gene^2)
1 in 100	1 in 50	1 in 10,000
1 in 1,000	1 in 500	1 in 1,000,000
1 in 10,000	1 in 5,000	1 in 100,000,000.

In the case of the commonest of the cholinesterase variants (the dibucaine-resistant gene) the relevant frequencies are approximately:

Gene	*Heterozygote*	*Homozygote*
1 in 60	1 in 30	1 in 3,600.

PENETRANCE AND EXPRESSIVITY

In human genetics the situation is rarely as straightforward as the foregoing might suggest. For example, a hereditary disorder may have many features which are commonly found: yet in any one individual, not all may be present. Likewise, the degree of abnormality may vary. In the syndrome of congenital anonychia, for example, there may be an abnormality of the nails only, or quite severe deformities of the hands and feet. Such a variation in severity, or in the number of associated abnormalities, is called variable expressivity.

An alternative form of variation can be visualized. All genes must produce their effect in the presence of other genes and against different environmental circumstances; in some of these the gene produces its effect, and in others it fails to do so. The term penetrance is used to categorize the expression or nonexpression of the effects of a gene. The consequence of incomplete penetrance is to destroy the ratios which would be found if straightforward dominant, intermediate, or recessive inheritance patterns were operating.

GENETIC LINKAGE AND GENE MAPS

During the process of chromosome division, a part of a chromosome is often exchanged with the other one of the pair. This must be so, or large blocks of characteristics represented by all the genes on the chromosome would always be inherited together. Even so, family resemblances which cannot depend on a single gene are so common that groups of linked genes obviously must often stay associated. The process of crossing-over is shown diagrammatically in Fig 9.5 where both a single and double cross-over are illustrated.

Clearly, if there were a relatively common genetic marker, the frequency of its

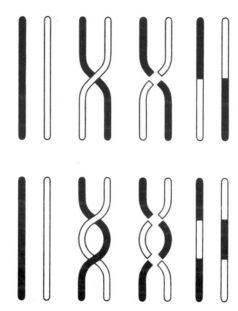

Fig. 9.5. Diagram to illustrate the interchange of segments in crossing-over between the members of a chromosome pair. Above, a single cross-over; below, a double cross-over.

occurrence in association with another feature determined by a single gene would give valuable information concerning the location of the respective genes. Suppose, for example, the two characteristics are determined by pairs of genes on *separate* pairs of chromosomes. Since cross-over exchanges take place between the two chromosomes of a single pair, the frequency with which the two characteristics are associated will be unaffected by cross-over and determined by chance alone. They would be found together as often as they would be found separate.

Suppose, however, the two marker genes are on the same chromosome pair. On the left in Fig. 9.6 is shown diagrammatically two pairs of genes Aa and Bb which are on the same chromosome pair. In the absence of crossing-over, one gamete will receive AB and the other ab. Suppose this individual mated with a person without either dominant gene, as shown on the right. If no cross-over occurs, only two kinds of offspring occur, those with two dominant characteristics and those with none.

Suppose the gene pairs are reversed, so that the double heterozygote has gene pattern A with b and a with B (Fig. 9.7) and again mates with a double recessive individual. Again, there are only two kinds of offspring, but this time half the offspring have *one* dominant characteristic and the other half have the other. None has both of the dominant features and none is without one of them.

If a number of such matings were observed and no crossing-over existed, the same four types of offspring would be found and there would be no obvious evidence that they were not an independent assortment of unlinked genes. However, unlike genes on different pairs in which any mating might result in *any* of the four outcomes, attention to the matings would show that some mating would yield *only* two kinds and the remaining matings would yield *only* the other two.

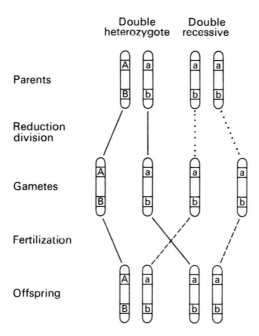

Fig. 9.6. Chromosome diagram showing the transmission of the genes (in the absence of crossing-over) in a mating between a double heterozygote and a double recessive, the two gene pairs being situated upon the same chromosome pair. The double heterozygote carries the two dominant genes upon one chromosome and the two recessive alleles upon the other.

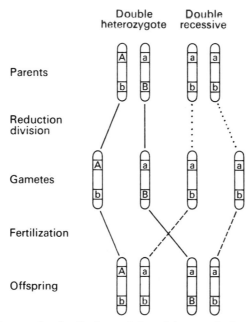

Fig. 9.7. Chromosome diagram showing the transmission of the genes in the same mating as that of Fig. 9.6, except that in the double heterozygote each chromosome bears one dominant and one recessive gene.

When a cross-over occurs, however, a different situation arises. Instead of the uncrossed gametes in Fig. 9.6 being AB and ab, crossing-over gives rise to gametes

Ab and aB. If a cross-over occurs only 5 per cent of the time, then 95 per cent of the offspring will have either both dominants or neither as before, but 5 per cent will have one or other dominant. If, however, the two dominants were originally on opposite chromosomes (as in Fig. 9.7) the same percentage of cross-over would yield the opposite result—95 per cent would have only one or other dominant (as before) but 5 per cent would have both or neither. Looking at a whole range of such matings we see that some have an excess of two kinds of offspring whereas the other matings give rise to an excess of the other two kinds of offspring. The deviation from 100 per cent is the percentage of cross-overs. Where the figure is 100 per cent, the genes are so closely associated that they are never switched by a cross-over.

The likelihood of a cross-over occurring between two genes is obviously higher the further the distance between them. The percentage of cross-overs calculated in this way is the unit of map-distance. Once the cross-over percentage reaches 50 per cent the situation cannot be distinguished from a free assortment of independent genes.

The blood group genes provide such a system of markers, since there are a number of blood group systems, each with well-defined genetics. Any association between one of these groups and any other abnormality can easily be detected.

There are now about 30 useful autosomal marker genes of which 10 are blood group genes, three or four are serum genes detected by antigen/antibody reactions and the remainder detected by electrophoresis.

Another technique which has recently been found to be of value involves creating hybrid cells in cell cultures between human and animal cells. During cell division, these artificial cells tend to lose chromosomes from one of the species. If that species is the only one to have a chromosome with the gene encoding for a particular enzyme, it may be possible to correlate its loss with the loss of a certain enzyme activity. By such means the location of several genes has been established.

EXAMPLES OF INHERITED CONDITIONS

Nearly 2,000 different genetically determined disorders have been reported [5], in less than 10 per cent of which reasonably precise information is known concerning the specific biochemical abnormality. Fortunately inherited conditions which give rise to serious disease tend to be rare although some inherited conditions of importance to anaesthetists are common in some populations (e.g. sickle-cell disease). Others are so innocuous that they are not normally regarded as diseases. Those which give rise to diseases of importance have generally been considered in the relevant chapter. Rarities that may have some practical significance to anaesthetists have been well covered by Katz and Kadis [4] and useful summaries of the more frequently met rarities are given in chapters 12 and 19 of Stevens [7]. It only remains to consider in this chapter a few conditions which deserve a fuller discussion and which have not been fully dealt with elsewhere in the book.

SICKLE-CELL DISEASE

The haematology of this condition is considered in Chapter 11.

The sickle-cell trait corresponds with the heterozygous state and its frequency in some African Negro populations may be greater than 40 per cent. The anaemia is the homozygous form of the abnormality. In the heterozygous state about 40 per cent of the haemoglobin is haemoglobin S but in the homozygous state *all* the haemoglobin is haemoglobin S. This form of haemoglobin has a tendency to aggregate as liquid crystals or tactoids in the reduced form and the polymerized haemoglobin causes deformity and rupture of red cells when oxygen tension falls. It is due to the replacement of glutamic acid by valine as the sixth amino acid in the β-chain of the globin part of the molecule.

About 4 per cent of African Negro children are homozygous and fail to survive to reproduce. The elimination rate is thus enormous and it is inconceivable that the observed stable incidence in the population is being maintained by new mutations at a similar rate. The heterozygous individuals must therefore have some advantage over normal homozygotes and have a higher replication rate. Such an advantage has been ascribed to a greater degree of resistance to malignant tertian malaria.

One would expect that if this advantage were to be lost, elimination would bring the population incidence steadily down. Such an instance is provided by the Negroes transported from West Africa to the U.S.A. where the present incidence in American Negroes is lower than in West African Negroes and corresponds remarkably well with calculations based on the assumption that heterozygous advantage ceased some 200–300 years ago.

Haemoglobin S is present *instead* of haemoglobin A because of an abnormal structural gene which is occupying the same *locus* as that normally occupied by the usual gene.

These genes are said to be *allelomorphic* or *alleles*. Haemoglobin C, which is also found in West African/American Negroes is also allelomorphic, and is due to yet another substitution, lysine, for glutamic acid at the same position in the β-chain. Allelomorphism implies that only one kind of haemoglobin can be elaborated from each gene, and even in heterozygotes a maximum of two types of haemoglobin can be present. In this situation individuals can, of course, be heterozygous for *two* abnormal genes rather than for a normal and abnormal one. There are several other much rarer haemoglobinopathies due to various abnormal substitutions in either the α- or β-chain. Whether or not they are also allelomorphic is not certain; the evidence so far is that they are.

THALASSEMIAS

The thalassemias are a group of disorders in which there is a defective rate of synthesis of one or more of the globin chains of haemoglobin. There are two main groups of thalassaemias, the α- and the β-thalassaemias characterized by a deficiency of α- or β-chain synthesis respectively. In both of these groups there are several genetically distinct disorders.

The clinical picture in these syndromes is due to the nonproduction of normal haemoglobin and to the unbalanced globin chain synthesis which results in aggregates which precipitate and damage the red cell. There is persistence of fetal haemoglobin (Hb F). The genetic presentation bears many resemblances to that of the sickle-cell disorders in that the homozygous abnormals (and those heterozygous for two different abnormal genes) are associated with life-shortening anaemia, whilst those heterozygous for one abnormal gene may be symptomless or have only mild anaemia. Again, like the sickle-cell disorders, there must be factors which confer advantages on the heterozygotes. The gene tends to be present in highest frequencies in areas where malaria is endemic but not in all such areas.

The basic molecular defects in the various thalassaemias is unknown but there is evidence of a deficiency of messenger RNA in some of them [9].

PORPHYRIA

The porphyrias are a group of diseases which are related to defects in the metabolism of porphyrins. These compounds are essential to the elaboration of respiratory pigments. They form coordination complexes with various metals—magnesium to form chlorophyll and with iron to form the haem of haemoglobin and to form cytochromes.

GENETICS

One type of porphyria, the South African variegate porphyria (VP), is a classical example of autosomal dominant inheritance. This disease arose as a mutation in either Gerrit Janz van Deventer or Ariaantje Adriansse, one of the original forty couples who colonized the Cape. Nine thousand cases have been traced to one or other of their four children and the incidence is now 1 in 500 in South Africa generally and 1 in 250 in Eastern Cape province. One would naturally wonder how an obviously unfavourable mutation has been able to increase in this way. The answer is that the general growth of population from the initial settlers to the present population has in fact been at a *greater* rate than this. Identical cases have now been described in Europe and North America, arising presumably, by new mutation. Acute intermittent porphyria (AIP) erythrohepatic protoporphyria (EHP) and hereditary coproporphyria also show autosomal dominant inheritance. Congenital erythropoietic porphyria (CEP) however is a recessive trait: porphyria can also be acquired (when there is strong association with alcoholic liver disease) and has also been described in association with hexachlorabenzene poisoning.

BIOCHEMISTRY

The synthetic pathway of porphyrin production starts with the elaboration of δ amino laevulinic acid (δALA). This is the rate-limiting step in the pathway and the activity of the enzyme δALA synthetase which catalyses this process is normally subject to negative feed-back by the end product, haem, which not only inhibits the enzyme, but is also able to control its synthesis. This regulating mechanism must be very efficient judging by the small quantities of free porphyrins and other precursors which are normally excreted. The synthetic pathway is found in both liver and bone marrow and a failure of regulation at one or other site is responsible, respectively, for the hepatic and erythropoietic porphyrias.

The rest of the synthetic pathway is shown diagramatically in Fig. 9.8. The nomenclature of the porphyrins is determined by the side chains on the pyrrole group (marked X in Fig. 9.8) and the I series and III series are optical isomers. Only the III series is the precursor of haem synthesis.

Whilst increased δALA synthetase activity is found in all the porphyrias, it is usually secondary to a block elsewhere in the pathway of haem synthesis. Fig. 9.8 shows four points at which enzyme defects occur in four of the hereditary porphyrias. In the

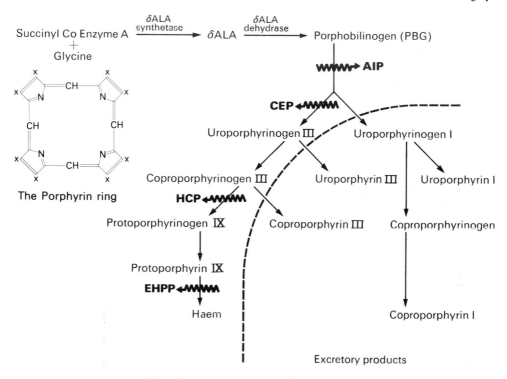

Fig. 9.8. Pathways of porphyrin metabolism.

case of VP there are at least two defects involving both the conversion of protoporphyrin to haem and coproporphyrinogen III to protoporphyrin IX (see Fig. 9.8). Depending on the site of blockage there is a particular pattern of abnormally increased excretory products, which are produced in excess because of the lack of negative feedback from haem.

CLINICAL SYNDROMES

The usual classification of porphyrias is as follows:

Erythropoietic	*Erythrohepatic*	*Hepatic*
Congenital erythropoietic porphyria (CEP)	Erythrohepatic protoporphyria (EHPP)	Acute intermittent porphyria (AIP)
		Hereditary coproporphyria (HCP)
		Variegate porphyria (VP)
		Symptomatic porphyria (SP).

The *erythrohepatic* and *erythropoietic* porphyrias are extremely rare and are mainly associated with photosensitivity. They are of no special significance in anaesthesia.

Of the *hepatic porphyrias*, AIP and VP are of chief importance to anaesthetists because they commonly present with lesions in the central and peripheral nervous systems and because acute attacks can be precipitated by a variety of drugs. Furthermore, the acute symptoms may mimic an abdominal emergency.

There has been much interest in the relationship between the biochemical lesions and the symptoms (see Fig. 9.9). If only the precursors, δALA and PBG, are produced

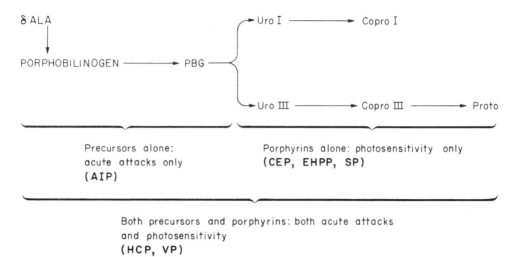

Fig. 9.9. Relationship between the biochemical lesions in the porphyrins and the pattern of symptons.

the patient suffers acute attacks of demyelination and presents as AIP. If only porphyrins are produced in excess, the patient only exhibits photosensitivity (CEP, EHPP). When both precursors and porphyrins are produced, the patient suffers both acute attacks and photosensitivity (HCP and VP). Photosensitivity is due to the accumulation of porphyrins in the skin where they absorb light of wavelengths 360–400 nm and undergo reduction with the production of singlet oxygen (O_2^-). This in turn damages lysosomes which then release chemical mediators, causing itching and erythema. The acute illnesses of AIP and VP may be associated with axonal damage and demyelination in various parts of the central, peripheral and autonomic nervous systems, although symptoms do not depend on this and may be biochemical in origin. δALA has been shown to have several neuropharmacological effects in animal preparations: it can inhibit synaptic transmission, Na^+/K^+-dependent ATP-ase and interfere with the metabolism of γ-amino butyric acid. It does not seem, however, to be neurotoxic.

Acute relapses alternate with latent phases: the predominant symptom is abdominal pain with tenderness, diarrhoea, and vomiting or ileus. These may all be part of an autonomic neuropathy. The other neurological abnormalities are very varied. Psychological disturbances may lead to a diagnosis of hysteria. A variety of motor and sensory neuropathies occur, and weakness of respiratory and bulbar muscles may need prolonged supportive treatment. Autonomic neuropathy is also associated with tachycardia and hypertension and indeed the pulse rate is a good guide to the progress of an acute attack.

Electrolyte disturbances are common, giving rise to hyponatraemia. Partly this is due to vomiting, but there may also be inappropriate secretion of antidiuretic hormone, indicating hypothalamic involvement. There is also fever and leucocytosis.

Table 9.1. Porphyrinogenic drugs.

All barbiturates	Sulphonamides
Althesin	
Meprobamate	Adrenal hormones
Chlordiazepoxide	Aminopyrine
Flunitrazepam	
Ergometrine	
Glutethimide	Griseofulvin
Methyprylone	
Ethyl alcohol	
Phenytoin	
Steroids	
Nikethimide	

Precipitating factors

There are a number of known precipitating factors, including infection and pregnancy; however, by far the most important is the intake of a porphyrinogenic drug. They may precipitate an attack, or intensify a chronic condition. Once an acute attack has started there is no known way of modifying it. Opinion on whether a drug is porphyrinogenic has, in the past, been acquired by reportage of clinical experiences. In recent years animal models have been developed in which a sensitizing chemical is used in conjunction with the drug under investigation [1]. If the model can reliably classify agents whose porphyrinogenity is already established, it can then be used to make predictions about new agents.

The drugs listed in Tables 9.1 and 9.2 are included either because of good clinical information or on the basis of animal model predictions. Amongst the precipitating drugs, the most important are the barbiturates, all of which are absolutely contraindicated. Other well-authenticated and currently used precipitating drugs are listed in Table 9.1.

ANAESTHETIC MANAGEMENT

If the diagnosis is known, there is little danger of precipitating an attack and a wide range of agents are available, as listed in Table 9.2.

Local analgesics are not specifically incriminated and extradural, caudal and

Table 9.2. Drugs which can be given to patients with porphyria.

1 *Preoperative drugs*
   (i) Sedatives—Chlorpromazine, promazine, promethazine
   (ii) Analgesics—Morphine, pethidine
   (iii) Hypnotics—Chloral hydrate
2 *Induction agent*
   Propanidid, etomidate, minaxolone
3 *General anaesthetics*
   Nitrous oxide, diethyl ether, cyclopropane. (Halothane probably safe also)
4 *Relaxants*
   Suxamethonium, *d*–tubocurarine, gallamine
5 *Adjuvants*
   Atropine, neostigmine, pentolinium, syntocinon

pudendal blocks have been employed safely. However, they are liable to be blamed for any unpredictable neurological deterioration which may occur and it would be wise to discuss the matter fully with the patient before use.

PLASMA CHOLINESTERASE VARIANTS

These provide examples of many of the terms and principles already introduced. An intermediate inheritance pattern has been delineated purely on the basis of biochemical investigation, and without any overt way of detecting heterozygotes. Several alleles have been identified, and there is now an allele for a second locus.

The Enzyme Commission has given the enzyme the systematic name acylcholine acylhydrolase with the code number EC 3.1.1.8. It is elaborated in the liver and is found in the plasma. It serves no obvious essential function and no pathological condition has been noted in the few individuals who appear to be without it. It may be that it is predominantly a liver enzyme which prevents pharmacologically active esterases in the diet from progressing beyond the liver.

GENETICS

Investigation of suxamethonium-sensitive individuals and their families has revealed the existence of several genotypes. These have been identified with the aid of inhibitors. Activity of the enzyme is normally determined, for the sake of biochemical convenience, using benzoylcholine as substrate. Numerous substances have been shown to inhibit the activity of the enzyme against this substrate in low concentrations. In practice, two inhibitors have been found most useful, cinchocaine (Nupercaine, Dibucaine) and sodium fluoride, both in 10^{-5}M concentration. The percentage inhibition produced by these inhibitors under carefully defined conditions of temperature and concentration have been called the dibucaine and fluoride numbers respectively.

The 'usual' enzyme, which is highly effective in metabolizing suxamethonium, is sensitive to the effects of both these inhibitors and would typically have a dibucaine number (DN) of about 80 (80 per cent inhibition), and fluoride number (FN) of about 60–65 (see Table 9.3).

Table 9.3. Dibucaine and fluoride numbers, frequency, and suxamethonium sensitivity of genotypes at the E_1 locus.

	DN	FN	Frequency	Sensitivity
Homozygotes $E_1{}^uE_1{}^u$	80	62	97%	Not sensitive
$E_1{}^aE_1{}^a$	20	22	1:3,000	Very sensitive
$E_1{}^fE_1{}^f$	65	35	Very rare	Moderately sensitive
$E_1{}^sE_1{}^s$	..	..	Very rare	Very sensitive
Heterozygotes $E_1{}^uE_1{}^a$	60	50	3%	Slightly sensitive
$E_1{}^uE_1{}^f$	75	52		depending on total
$E_1{}^uE_1{}^s$	80	62		activity
$E_1{}^aE_1{}^f$	50	35	Uncertain	Very sensitive
$E_1{}^aE_1{}^s$	20	22		Very sensitive
$E_1{}^fE_1{}^s$	65	35		Moderately sensitive

The Motulsky nomenclature [6] is usually employed in the anaesthetic literature, and uses E (for Esterase). A superscript symbol is used to designate the type of gene found at that locus. The 'usual' enzyme has been designated E_1^u and homozygotes, $E_1^u E_1^u$, constitute about 97 per cent of the population. The E_1 locus has been provisionally assigned to chromosome 1, sandwiched between transferrin (TF) and phosphogluconate dehydrogenase (PGD) [2]. A second locus (E_2) has been described but has not been assigned to any chromosome.

The commonest variant, at the E_1 locus and the first to be identified, is the dibucaine-resistant gene, designated E_1^a (for atypical). This variant is allelomorphic with the usual gene. Homozygotes $E_1^a E_1^a$ occur with a frequency of about 1 in 3,000. These individuals have a DN and FN of about 20–24. The atypical enzyme is unable to catalyse the hydrolysis of suxamethonium to any measurable extent at the concentrations found with clinical doses of suxamethonium.

The heterozygotes, $E_1^u E_1^a$ constitute about 3 per cent of the population and have a DN of about 60 and an FN of about 50. It is clear that the quantity of usual enzyme is sufficient to catalyse the breakdown of suxamethonium since the majority are clinically indistinguishable from normal homozygotes. In fact, if one has a high index of suspicion and investigates minor degrees of apnoea, quite a significantly higher percentage of heterozygotes can be detected than would occur with random sampling.

Another atypical gene, also allelomorphic has been identified because of atypical fluoride numbers. A few presumed normal and presumed heterozygous individuals, as identified by the dibucaine number, were noted to have a much lower fluoride number than expected, and family studies have now also identified homozygous individuals. The $E_1^f E_1^f$ homozygote is very much rarer than the $E_1^a E_1^a$ homozygous atypical. These variants are presumed to be due to the inheritance of an abnormal structural gene.

Another variant which has now been clearly identified is the so-called 'silent' gene, E_1^s and this is also allelomorphic with the usual, atypical and fluoride-resistant genes. Heterozygotes have normal DN and FN, of course, but about half the normal level of activity. In fact there are two, or even three silent variants which may be differentiated immunologically, electrophoretically or by inhibition studies: some homozygotes are truly anenzymic whilst others have very low activity [10]. It would not be surprising if many other variants exist: the molecule consists of four polypeptide chains, each of molecular weight about 80,000 daltons. Each chain contains about 400 aminoacids, thus giving enormous scope for structural variants.

The variant at the E_2 locus is present in about 10 per cent of the population. This variant has also been called the C_5 variant because it was originally identified as a slower moving band on electrophoresis [3]. Possessors of this variant exhibit up to 30 per cent more cholinesterase activity than normal but this is not normally detectable clinically as 'resistance' to suxamethonium although one case has been reported in which it was.

REFERENCES

1 BLEKKENHORST GH, HARRISON GG, COOK ES, EALES L. Screening of certain anaesthetic agents for their ability to elicit acute porphyric phases in susceptible patients. *Br J Anaesth* 1980; **52**: 759–62.

2 CHAUTARD-FREIRE-MAIA EA. Probable assignment of the serum cholinesterase (E) and transferrin (TF) loci to chromosome 1 in man. *Hum Hered* 1977; **27**: 134–42.

3 HARRIS H, HOPKINSON DA, ROBSON EB, WHITTAKER M. Genetical studies on a new variant of serum cholinesterase detected by electrophoresis. *Ann Hum Gen* 1963; **26**: 359–82.

4 KATZ J, KADIS LB. *Anesthesia and uncommon diseases: Pathophysiologic and clinical correlations.* Philadelphia: WB Saunders, 1973.

5 MsKUSICK VA. *Mendelian inheritance in man: Catologs of autosomal dominant, recessive and X-linked phenotypes.* 2nd ed. Baltimore: John Hopkins, 1968.

6 MOTULSKY AG. Pharmacogenetics, In: Steinburg AG, Bearn AG, eds. *Progress in Medical Genetics.* Vol III. New York: Grune and Stratton, 1964.

7 STEVENS AJ. *Preparation for anaesthesia.* Tunbridge Wells: Pitman Medical Ltd, 1980.

8 WATSON JD. *The double helix.* New York: Atheneum, 1968.

9 WEATHERALL JD. The Thalassaemias, In: Stanbury JB, Wyngaaden JB, Fredrickson DS, eds. *The metabolic basis of inherited disease.* 3rd ed. New York: McGraw-Hill, 1970.

10 WHITTAKER M. Plasma cholinesterase variants and the anaesthetist. *Anaesthesia*, 1980; **35**: 174–97.

ACKNOWLEDGMENTS

I am indebted to J. A. E. Roberts for permission to reproduce Figs. 9.2, 9.3, 9.4, 9.5, 9.6 and 9.7 from *Introduction to Medical Genetics*, 6th ed. (1973) Oxford University Press, Oxford.

Chapter 10
Acute Biochemical Disorders

D. R. BEVAN

'A genuine understanding of the functions of sodium, potassium, calcium, magnesium and their salts in the organism would necessitate a comprehension of the nature of protoplasm and its behaviour in living cells, something we have not begun to attain.' (J. J. Peters and D. D. Van Slyke, 1931 [14])

The half-century since this statement was made has seen considerable progress in the understanding of acute biochemical disturbances. In part, this stems from a greater ability to measure, quickly and accurately, the biochemical variables concerned but also from the rapid increase in knowledge of the controlling factors involved. In particular, greater understanding of renal function and the hormonal environment in which it operates have allowed therapy to be directed in a logical sequence. Acute biochemical disturbances affect, mainly, the excitable tissues of the central nervous, cardiovascular and musculoskeletal systems and such perturbations may seriously jeopardize the safety of the patient under general anaesthesia. The major manifestations of the disturbances were well known 50 years ago and it is important to appreciate that all the changes are potentially reversible with appropriate therapy.

In this chapter, the causes, effects and therapies of major disturbances of water metabolism, electrolyte and acid–base balance will be reviewed briefly, with particular emphasis on those disorders which affect the surgical patient.

WATER METABOLISM

Approximately 60 per cent of adult body weight is made up of water, of which two-thirds is intracellular and one-third extracellular. An average 70 kg man consumes in his diet about 1,500 ml fluid and a further 500 ml from solid food. In addition, 200 ml are generated by metabolic activity. Thus, the daily requirement for a sedentary man is approximately 30 ml $kg^{-1}day^{-1}$. All this fluid must be excreted if intake and output are to be balanced. The water is lost in the urine, 1,200 ml, faeces, 200 ml, and from the lungs, 600 ml, and skin, 200 ml.

Control mechanisms

Maintenance of the volume status of the individual is essential for cardiovascular stability. Equally important, is the maintenance of constant concentration of solute throughout the body water because with a few exceptions, the body does not tolerate osmotic gradients. Consequently, it is not surprising that both volume and osmotic factors are concerned in the control of the volume and composition of body fluid.

In conscious man, water intake is governed by the sensation of thirst which is stimulated by several factors (Table 10.1) which also increase the synthesis and release of antidiuretic hormone (ADH) to reduce renal water losses (Fig. 10.1). Thus, the control of water balance is dependent on the integration of thirst mechanisms, ADH secretion and the ability of the kidney to modify the concentration of the urine [3].

Disorders of volume homeostasis

These conditions are characterized by an increase or decrease in body water and its distribution although the concentration of solute, osmolality, is unchanged. Such pure disturbances are rare and even when they occur are brief because the compensatory changes that they evoke result in secondary changes in electrolyte concentrations. For instance, loss of blood by acute haemorrhage or of extracellular fluid from a burn result in redistribution of fluid from intracellular to extracellular sites and renal water conservation by ADH secretion, both of which lead to hyponatraemia. These mixed disturbances will be discussed below.

Disorders of osmolar homeostasis

The development of a sensitive radioimmunoassay for ADH (arginine vasopressin, AVP) has demonstrated the close correlations between serum osmolality and AVP

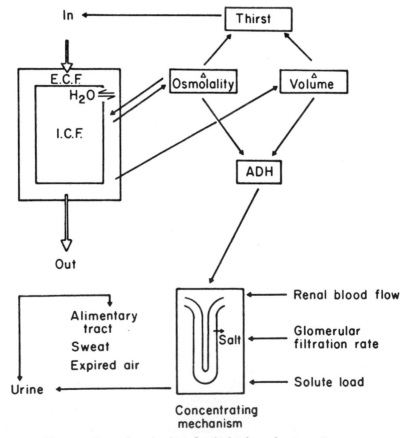

Fig. 10.1. Control mechanisms for the intake and output of water.

Table 10.1. Stimulants of thirst and ADH secretion

Osmotic	ECF hyperosmolality	
Non osmotic	Hypotension	Aortic, atrial and renal Baroreceptors
	Pain	
	Emotional stress	
	Hyperthermia	
	Drugs	Opiates
		Anaesthetics
		β agonists
		Cholinergic agents
		Chlorpropamide
	Renin–angiotensin stimulation	

concentration and the consequent changes in urine osmolality (Fig. 10.2) to preserve constant body osmolality [21]—serum osmolality 285 ± 5 mosmol kg^{-1}. Hypoosmolar syndromes are more common than hyperosmolar because, in the latter, the preservation of thirst allows osmolar homeostasis even if this necessitates the drinking of several gallons of water per day, e.g. diabetes insipidus.

The clinical manifestations of both hyper- and hypo-osmolar states affect mainly central nervous system function as a result of the passive swelling or shrinking of the cells of the brain which acts as an osmometer. The severity of the symptoms depends upon the rate of change of osmolality as well as the absolute values achieved. In chronic hyperosmolar states the brain volume is gradually restored by the generation of new, nonelectrolyte intracellular solute in the brain—'ideogenic osmoles' [15].

Hyperosmolar syndromes

Hyperosmolality (> 300 mosmol kg^{-1}) is usually the result of body fluid depletion when water is lost in excess of sodium. Less commonly, it accompanies accumulation

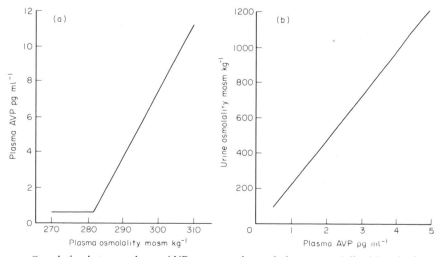

Fig. 10.2. Correlation between plasma AVP concentration and plasma osmolality (a) and urine osmolality (b) (modified from Robertson *et al.*, 1976, with permission).

Table 10.2. Hyperosmolar syndromes and aetiology.

Water depletion

(a) Normal renal function	Reduced fluid intake
	Excessive sweating
	Vomiting and diarrhoea
	Burns
	Comatose patients
(b) ADH failure	Diabetes insipidus
	Essential hypernatraemia
	Head injury or tumour
(c) Renal concentrating failure	Chronic renal disease
	Osmotic diuresis
	Flouride toxicity
	Hypokalaemia
	Hypertonic parenteral dialysis

Solute accumulation

(a) Glucose	Diabetes mellitus
	Glucose infusion
(b) Sodium	8·4% Sodium bicarbonate
	Saline enemata
	Infant feeding
	Primary aldosteronism
	Cushing's syndrome
(c) Alcohol	
(d) Urea	Renal failure
(e) Solute loading	Mannitol
	Urea

of endogenous or exogenous solute and rarely is associated with failure of ADH secretion or of the renal concentrating mechanism (Table 10.2).

Water depletion. This is common in the very young and very old who may be incapable of responding to thirst. In infants, this may be exacerbated by high solute feeding with modified cows milk and, in the elderly, by high protein diets. Similarly, large water losses may occur from the respiratory tract in pneumonia or from the skin in pyrexial patients.

Solute accumulation. The commonest cause of hyperosmolality in Western cultures is from alcohol ingestion. The increased osmolality is a combination of the alcohol as solute and the inhibition of ADH secretion. Hyperglycaemia in the absence of ketosis has been described in adult-onset diabetes—nonketotic hyperosmolar coma [20] in whom the endogenous insulin secretion, although limited, prevents the development of ketosis. Half these patients die. Hyperosmolality in the surgical patient may also result from the administration of hyperoncotic fluids—hypertonic saline, hypertonic sodium bicarbonate, mannitol, sorbitol and fructose.

Clinical features. Hyperosmolality is always associated with thirst unless the patient is comatose or unconscious. Indeed, hypernatraemia from water deficits does not develop unless thirst is not permitted to operate.

When the serum osmolality exceeds 300 mosmol kg^{-1} there are usually neurological and cardiovascular signs although the rate of its development is also important. Sudden increase of osmolality leads to brain shrinkage and subsequent tearing of dural vessels. Neurological features include hyperpnoea, hallucinations and disordered sensorium, stupor, coma, and occasionally, focal signs. Mild pyrexia is common. Cerebrospinal fluid contains increased protein and is xanthochromic from the small haemorrhages. Children are irritable, crying and may develop myoclonus, muscular rigidity and tremor. Transient chorea or convulsions may follow focal haemorrhage.

Hyperosmolality from fluid deficits leads to tachycardia, hypotension, oliguria and poor tissue perfusion from hypovolaemia. The blood shows an increased concentration of all constituents, haemoglobin, electrolytes, protein and urea.

Treatment. Body water deficits should be managed by the administration of hypotonic fluids by oral, rectal or intravenous routes. Correction should be achieved slowly, if time permits over 48–72 hours, to prevent violent swings of brain cell volume. Rapid rehydration may cause convulsions. The volumes required for total correction can be calculated from measurement of serum osmolality or plasma sodium concentrations and assuming that the deficit exists throughout the total body water.

Hypo-osmolar syndromes

Hypo-osmolality is seldom the result of simple water excess because, unless the volume ingested exceeds 15–20 l day^{-1}, urinary diluting mechanisms maintain serum osmolality within normal limits. All hypo-osmolar patients are also hyponatraemic although the converse may not be true: hyperosmolality from hyperglycaemia or mannitol infusion induces the movement of water from cells to ECF with a subsequent reduction in serum sodium concentration. Rarely, hyponatraemia without hypo-osmolality is seen when the nonaqueous fraction of plasma is increased in hyperlipidaemia, myeloma or hyperproteinaemia. In this 'factitious hyponatraemia' the sodium concentration in the aqueous portion of plasma is unaffected.

The major causes of hypo-osmolality can be divided into three categories depending upon the status of the body sodium and water compartments (Table 10.3) [17]. In the

Table 10.3. Hypoosmolar syndromes and aetiology (Adapted from Schrier & Berl [17])

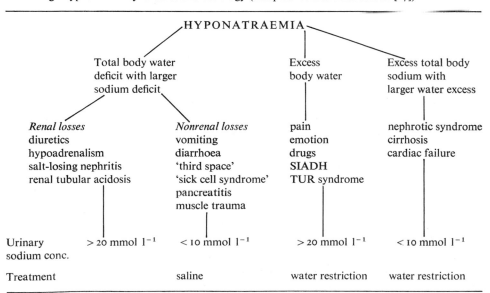

	HYPONATRAEMIA		
Total body water deficit with larger sodium deficit		Excess body water	Excess total body sodium with larger water excess
Renal losses diuretics hypoadrenalism salt-losing nephritis renal tubular acidosis	*Nonrenal losses* vomiting diarrhoea 'third space' 'sick cell syndrome' pancreatitis muscle trauma	pain emotion drugs SIADH TUR syndrome	nephrotic syndrome cirrhosis cardiac failure
Urinary sodium conc. > 20 mmol l^{-1}	< 10 mmol l^{-1}	> 20 mmol l^{-1}	< 10 mmol l^{-1}
Treatment	saline	water restriction	water restriction

first group, reduction of ECF volume leads to stimulation of the renin–angiotensin system, thirst and ADH secretion. The postoperative hyponatraemia common after major surgery can be included, in part, in this group where salt losses may occur into a 'third space' of traumatized tissue or remain intracellularly by failure of the sodium pump in the 'sick cell syndrome'. Urinary sodium concentration in this group is low, < 10 mosmol l^{-1}. Hypovolaemic hypo-osmolality can also occur when electrolyte-rich fluid losses (gastro-intestinal fluid) are replaced with water.

The second group accounts for the majority of hyponatraemic patients in the hospital population. It results from a moderate expansion of all fluid compartments together with a small decrease in total body sodium. These patients exhibit a failure of excretion of free water. This may accompany inadequate urinary dilution, i.e. solute diuresis, diuretics, reduction of nephron mass or the many factors which impair renal medullary osmotic stratification. More commonly it is associated with circulating concentrations of ADH greater than that required for osmolar homeostasis, e.g. Table 1 and the syndrome of inappropriate secretion of ADH (SIADH) [12] Table 10.4.

Table 10.4. Inappropriate ADH secretion.

From neurohypophysis
    CNS disorders: infection (meningitis, encephalitis,
                        abscess, Guillain–Barré)
                        intracranial tumours
                        trauma (head injury, subarachnoid
                        haemorrhage)
                        acute intermittent porphyria
    Pulmonary disorders (tuberculosis, pneumonia,
    chronic infection, aspergillus)
    Endocrine disorders (Addison's disease, myxoedema,
    hypopituitarism)
From tumours
    Ca lung, duodenum and pancreas
    Thymoma

These factors are also concerned in the hyponatraemia of the early postoperative period which are compounded by the injudicious i.v. administration of sodium-free fluids.

Acute hypo-osmolar volume expansion following irrigation of the bladder with hypotonic solutions during transurethral resection of the prostrate has been described [19]. Serum sodium concentration may decrease to 100 mmol l^{-1} with an acute brain syndrome and pulmonary oedema. However, spontaneous recovery usually occurs with a diuresis of 6–7 l day^{-1}.

The third group includes oedematous states in which excess total body sodium exists with a greater excess of water. Separation of the groups can usually be determined from clinical history and measurement of urine sodium concentration.

Clinical features. Cerebral symptoms of headache, anorexia, nausea, lethargy, confusion and psychosis usually occur when serum sodium concentration is less than 120 mmol l^{-1}. Muscle twitching, tremors and cramps (miner's cramps) are frequent but focal or generalized convulsions are rare. Similar cerebral symptoms occur if the blood urea is suddenly reduced by dialysis and are a result of brain osmolar disequilibrium. Permanent brain damage may follow if treatment is delayed. Cardiovascular signs of hypovolaemia are only present in the water deficient group.

Treatment. This is based upon the correction of the underlying condition (Table 10.3). When serum sodium concentration is less than 120 mmol l^{-1} hypertonic saline (2N or 5N) should be provided. As in hyperosmolar syndromes correction should be made assuming deficits throughout the body water, proceeding slowly, 48–72 hours.

In the seriously ill patient in whom 'sick cell syndrome' is suspected, restoration of the sodium pump and correction of the hyponatraemia is helped by a glucose-potassium-insulin regimen. Initially, a 50 per cent glucose solution with potassium, 40 mmol l^{-1}, and insulin, 120 u l^{-1}, is infused rapidly as a bolus of 50 ml at the start of each hour. Insulin and potassium additions are adjusted according to blood glucose and serum potassium measurements. These must be performed 2–3 hourly because rapid changes in glucose tolerance are common.

Colloid osmotic pressure

Starling's formula related the transcapillary movement of water to the balance of hydrostatic and osmotic forces:

$$V = K_f[(P_C - P_{IF}) - (\pi p - \pi_{IF})],$$

where V is the rate of liquid movement, K_f the capillary filtration coefficient, P_C and P_{IF} the hydrostatic pressures in the capillary and interstitial fluids, and πp and π_{IF} the plasma and interstitial fluid oncotic pressures.

The use of pulmonary artery catheters and the simple measurement of plasma colloid osmotic pressure (COP) tempted several investigators to measure Pc (Pulmonary wedge pressure—P_{AW}) and πp (COP) and to derive the COP-P_{AW} gradient as an estimate of the forces encouraging pulmonary oedema. It was suggested that oncotic therapy, with salt-free albumen, be administered to reduce pulmonary oedema if the

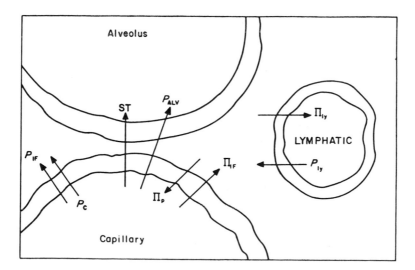

Fig. 10.3. Physical forces affecting fluid exchange in the lung where Pc, P_{IF}, P_{ly} are the hydrostatic pressures and πp, π_{IF}, π_{ly} the oncotic pressures in the pulmonary capillaries, interstitial fluid and lymphatics; ST is the alveolar surface tension and P_{AW} the alveolar pressure (after Robin *et al.* [22]).

gradient was less than about 5 mmHg. Unfortunately, such measures have not been universally successful, probably because several other factors, particularly pulmonary lymphatic flow and alveolar forces, are concerned in the maintenance of an increase in lung water (Fig. 10.3). At the present time the place of oncotic therapy in noncardiac oedematous states is uncertain. In cardiogenic pulmonary oedema, digitalis, diuretics, oxygen and narcotics remain first-line therapy. Oncotic therapy should only be considered when these have failed and when COP is known to be low [4].

SODIUM

Sodium is the principal cation of the extracellular fluid which accounts for most of the total exchangeable sodium in man (40 mmol kg^{-1}). Yet salt is a rare and precious commodity which is still recognized in the language of fiscal reward—'salary'. On land, it is only found where the oceans have receded leaving their evaporated solutes behind. The average European diet contains 100–300 mmol sodium per day and almost all of this is lost by the kidneys which are able to compensate for large variations in the diet.

Sodium excretion

More than 99 per cent of the filtered sodium is reabsorbed by the kidney at four sites:

    (i)   proximal tubule: 50–70 per cent, active iso-osmotic reabsorption;
    (ii) ascending loop of Henle: 10–20 per cent, secondary to active reabsorption of chloride;
    (iii) distal tubule: 10 per cent ⎫ active reabsorption under
    (iv) collecting duct: 1 per cent ⎬ influence of aldosterone.

Bulk reabsorption occurs at the proximal tubule but the eventual sodium concentration of the urine is dependent upon distal tubular control.

Several factors have been implicated in the control of sodium excretion but the renin–angiotensin–aldosterone system (RAAS) seems to play the key role. Renin is relased from storage granules of the juxta-glomerular apparatus in response to decreased renal perfusion pressure, sympathetic stimulation, decreased sodium load at the macula densa and hyperkalaemia. The RAAS is also activated during and after major surgery as part of the hormonal response to stress. Renin cleaves its substrate, an α_2 globulin synthesized in the liver to produce the decapeptide (angiotensin I (AI)) which is hydrolysed by converting enzyme, found in the lung, plasma and kidney, to the octapeptide (angiotensin II (AII)). Angiotensin II is a potent vasoconstrictor but is also the most important stimulant to aldosterone secretion. In addition, AII leads to the release of ADH.

Clinical disorders

Sodium and water metabolism are intimately related although controlled by separate mechanisms. The movement of sodium is always accompanied by water to maintain osmotic equilibrium. Thus, in conditions of sodium depletion or accumulation there is always an associated shift of water and these together with the aetiology, clinical features and therapy of hypo- and hypernatraemia have been discussed already.

Anaesthesia and surgery

Major surgery is almost always accompanied by sodium conservation. As for water retention, its intensity and duration depend upon the magnitude of the surgical trauma. Paradoxically, the retention is often accompanied by a mild hyponatraemia, serum sodium concentration 130–135 mmol l^{-1}. Several factors have been implicated but the relative importance of each remains controversial.

Activation of the RAAS again plays a key role. The stimulation, as part of generalized stress hormone activation, is reinforced by third space losses producing hypovolaemia. Although such losses may have been overemphasized in the past there is little doubt that ECF accumulates in traumatized tissue, peritonitis, burns, inflammatory lesions, crush injuries and ascites. The only question that remains is the size of this 'functional' reduction of ECF in the uncomplicated patient.

Postoperative sodium conservation appears to be unaltered in adrenalectomized patients and in those treated with aldosterone antagonists. Thus aldosterone does not appear to be essential for the response. It has been suggested that AII alone may be sufficient, acting by diverting renal blood flow to the sodium-conserving juxtamedullary nephrons.

Hyponatraemia is mainly the result of nonosmotic release of ADH, in part as a component of the stress response but also from stimulation by AII. In addition, the failure of the sodium pump in damaged tissue and particularly with sepsis, encourages the intracellular accumulation of sodium. The hyponatraemia appears to be unimportant and requires no treatment as long as sodium containing fluids are prescribed to replace all known losses. In particular, allowance should be made for third space losses which should be replaced with fluid similar in electrolyte content to ECF, e.g. Ringer's lactate. Probably the commonest fluid and electrolyte disorders in the uncomplicated surgical patient are iatrogenic: fluids administered in ignorance of the volume and electrolyte requirements of the patient.

Perioperative fluid therapy

Fluid administered over the operative period must provide daily maintenance of water and electrolytes, fluid to replace losses of ECF, blood or other abnormal losses, e.g. fistulae, gastric suction, diarrhoea.

Maintenance

The minimal daily water requirement is the sum of the amount of water required to excrete the solute load and the amount required to replace insensible loss, less the water available from endogenous metabolism.

A 70 kg man after operation produces for excretion a daily solute load of approximately 600 mosmol and the maximum urine concentration in the postoperative period is 1000 mosmol kg^{-1}. Therefore at this concentration 600 ml water will be needed to cover the solute load. If the urine is less concentrated (300 mosmol kg^{-1}), then 2 l fluid will be necessary.

Insensible losses in the postoperative period are relatively constant over the customary ranges of environmental temperature and humidity. The rate of loss in afebrile patients is about 40 ml m^{-2}h^{-1} over the environmental temperature range of 20–25°C and relative humidity of 20–60 per cent. This amounts to about 1400 ml day^{-1}

in a 70 kg patient. Endogenous water production is of the order of 300 ml (70 kg)$^{-1}$. Therefore, the total daily water requirement to replace insensible loss is about 1100 ml day^{-1}. In febrile patients insensible losses increase by about 12 per cent for each degree Celsius that the temperature is above 38°C. Respiratory water losses are, of course, reduced in patients receiving humidification during controlled ventilation.

The total daily water requirements can be met by the infusion of 30–40 ml kg^{-1} day^{-1}. The requirements for sodium and potassium are about 1 mmol kg^{-1}day^{-1}, although potassium is not usually added until the second or third postoperative day when normal renal function has been established.

ECF replacement

Transudation into traumatized areas should be replaced with fluid of a composition similar to ECF and administered in addition to the replacement of blood loss. During major abdominal surgery, Ringer's lactate can be infused to replace these losses at a rate of 5 ml kg^{-1}h^{-1} without risk of overload.

Blood replacement

In patients with normal cardiopulmonary function, the tissue demands for oxygen can be met without difficulty down to a haemoglobin concentration of 8 g (100 ml)$^{-1}$. Thus the avoidance of hypovolaemia takes precedence over the infusion of haemoglobin. The three choices of fluid for blood replacement are crystalloid solutions (saline or Ringer's lactate), colloid solutions (plasma or plasma substitutes) and blood. One must remember that crystalloids are distributed throughout the ECF and the blood volume will be maintained only if three times the blood loss is administered. Such large volumes of fluid limit their usefulness if the syndrome of overinfusion is to be avoided.

POTASSIUM

Potassium is an ubiquitous element so that a diet sufficient for energy requirements will also contain ample potassium. The normal daily requirement for potassium is 1–2 mmol kg^{-1}, mostly excreted in the urine to maintain potassium balance. Potassium is also secreted into the bowel lumen and its concentration increases along the gut

Table 10.5. Potassium content of gastro-intestinal fluid.

	Max. volume per day (ml)	Concentration (mmol l^{-1})	Daily total (mmol)
Gastric juice	500	5–10	2·5–5
Mixed secretions (e.g. intestinal obstruction)	3000	10–15	30–45
Diarrhoea (e.g. ulcerative colitis)	4000	20	80

so that considerable quantities may be lost in diarrhoeal fluid (Table 10.5). The total body potassium is about 40–50 mmol kg^{-1}, distributed mainly intracellularly, with the result that the serum potassium concentration is a poor guide to total body potassium and also that cellular damage, e.g. trauma, crush injury, haemolysis and succinylcholine, encourages an exodus from the cells to produce hyperkalaemia.

Renal potassium handling

The glomerulus filters 600–900 mmol potassium each day. Most of this is reabsorbed and the potassium in the urine originates mainly as the result of potassium secretion in the distal tubule and collecting duct. An active pump in the pericapillary membrane transfers K$^+$ into the cell against a large concentration gradient. Once within the cell the electronegativity of the luminal membrane encourages secretion of K$^+$ into the tubular lumen. The transport of K$^+$ into the cell is loosely coupled with the outward transport of Na$^+$. The activity of the pump is stimulated by small increases in plasma K$^+$, by aldosterone and by alkalosis but is inhibited by acidosis. Potassium secretion is also stimulated by increased delivery of volume and Na$^+$ to the distal nephron.

Clinical disorders of K$^+$ metabolism accompany alterations in renal function, acid–base balance and diet.

Hyperkalaemia

Aetiology

Of the many causes of hyperkalaemia (Table 10.6) the most important to the anaesthe-

Table 10.6. Actiology of hyperkalaemia.

1 Increased input	(a) exogenous; diet
	(b) endogenous; haemolysis, alimentary haemorrhage, crush injury, catabolism, malignant hyperpyrexia
	(c) release after succinylcholine; burns, trauma, paraplegia, motor neurone disease, tetanus
	(d) transfusion of stored blood
2 Acidaemia—respiratory and metabolic	
3 Renal failure	(a) acute
	(b) chronic, GFR < 15 ml min^{-1}
4 Impaired K$^+$ secretion	(a) decreased distal delivery of Na$^+$ and volume
	(b) impaired renin, angiotensin aldosterone axis
	(c) renal disease; sickle cell disease, amyloid, post renal transplant, SLE
	(d) drugs: spiranolactone, triamterene amiloride, digitalis
5 Abnormal K$^+$ distribution	(a) insulin deficiency
	(b) aldosterone deficiency
6 Factitious	(a) laboratory error
	(b) haemolysis, thrombocytosis, leucocytosis

tist are renal failure, acidosis and those occurring following the release of K^+ from damaged tissues or by succinylcholine.

Clinical features

Symptoms of hyperkalaemia are seen mainly in the gastrointestinal tract leading to nausea, vomiting, abdominal colic and diarrhoea. The important effects of hyperkalaemia are upon the heart. At plasma concentrations exceeding 7 mmol l^{-1} arrythmias appear and above this, ventricular fibrillation can occur. The ECG is characterized by high, tent-shaped T waves, wide QRS complexes and absent P waves.

Renal failure. In acute renal failure the rate of increase of serum K^+ depends upon K^+ input; when chronic, hyperkalaemia is rare until GFR decreases below 15 ml min^{-1} because K^+ secretion is increased by the remaining tubules. Gastro-intestinal K^+ secretion is enhanced and there is increased movement of potassium into the tissues.

Acidosis. Hyperkalaemia is common in acidosis in part as a result of inhibition of the K^+ pump but also because as the acidosis develops hydrogen ions move into the cells and this is associated with an efflux of K^+.

Succinylcholine. In normokalaemic patients succinylcholine, 1 mg/kg, results in a small, 10 per cent, increase in serum K^+ and this increase is not greater in the normokalaemic patient in renal failure. However, increases of more than 80 per cent have been reported when administered to patients with cell membrane instability. particularly those with severe burns or multiple trauma but also in subjects with paraplegia, motor neurone disease, tetanus and muscular dystrophy [23].

Treatment

Hyperkalaemia is a life-threatening condition and must be treated promptly to reduce serum K^+ below 6 mmol l^{-1}. This is best achieved with an infusion of 100 ml 5 per cent dextrose containing 24 units soluble insulin and 10 ml 10 per cent calcium gluconate. In addition, sodium bicarbonate, 50–100 mmol, encourages cellular potassium uptake.

Hypokalaemia

Aetiology (Table 10.7)

The commonest causes of hypokalaemia in the surgical patient are inadequate dietary intake, renal losses associated with diuretic therapy, gastro-intestinal losses (Table 10.5) and the hormonal response to stress.

Clinical features

Symptoms from hypokalaemia seldom occur until plasma potassium concentration is less than 2·5 mmol l^{-1} and then are predominantly of muscle weakness. All muscles, including the diaphragm and intestinal smooth muscle are affected. Cardiovascular changes include bradycardia, postural hypotension, dysrrhythmias, ventricular fibrillation and sensitivity to digitalis. The ECG shows QT prolongation, sagging of the ST segments and, occasionally a U wave. Postural hypotension with reduced respon-

Table 10.7. Aetiology of hypokalaemia.

---

1 Decreased input: diet, inadequate parenteral nutrition
2 Alkalosis
3 Gastrointestinal losses—diarrhoea, fistulae
4 Renal losses   (a) increased fluid+salt delivery;
                    saline loading, proximal renal tubular
                    acidosis
                    diuretics
                    diabetes mellitus
        (b) increased aldosterone secretion,
                    primary, secondary, 'stress response'
                    carbenoxolone
        (c) alkalosis
5 Abnormal distribution—insulinoma
6 Factitious—laboratory error

---

siveness of the peripheral vasculature to catecholamines may produce postoperative hypotension. Severe hypokalaemia is associated with metabolic alkalosis, decreased renal concentrating ability, and increased sensitivity to the competitive neuromuscular blocking drugs [7].

Diuretics. Potassium secretion is stimulated by increased distal delivery of salt and fluid by diuretics acting at the proximal tubule (e.g. thiazides), or loop of Henle (e.g. frusemide) and by those which produce a solute diuresis (e.g. mannitol). However, the mild hypokalaemia, plasma K^+ 3–3·5 mmol l^{-1} seen during long-term diuretic therapy reflects only a small decrease in total exchangeable potassium unless it is further complicated by severe heart failure or renal or liver disease [11].

Stress response. Increased renal potassium excretion is a constant accompaniment of severe injury, trauma, burns and major surgery. In part, this reflects the release of intracellular K^+ following cellular trauma, but the increased mineralocorticoid activity is also important so that the average loss after major surgery is about 100 mmol day^{-1}.

Treatment

Pre-existing K^+ deficiency should be treated, whenever possible, before surgery. Orally, the most reliable absorption is obtained with potassium chloride as a liquid with the taste disguised by fruit juices. Up to 15 g daily (195 mmol) can be administered by this route.

When oral therapy is not possible KCl may be added to intravenous infusion fluids but particular care should be taken to avoid a high concentration of K^+ reaching the myocardium and producing ventricular fibrillation. Potassium chloride additions to intravenous fluid should not exceed 40 mmol l^{-1} for a flow rate not exceeding 1 l in 2 hours. This allows the addition of 120–160 mmol day^{-1} and, as deficits rarely exceed 400 mmol, they can be corrected rapidly.

If urgent operation is necessary in a patient known to be hypokalaemic the ECG should be monitored and K^+ administered only if there is a clear indication to do so.

After operation, it is traditional to avoid K^+ therapy until the urine output is adequate. This is not necessary as long as the prescriber understands the control of therapy. Indeed, in the face of known K^+ deficits such practice is foolhardy.

CALCIUM

Almost all of the body's stores of calcium (99·5 per cent) is found in bone bound to phosphate and carbonate. The daily intake is 1–2 g; most of which is excreted via the gut and only 200 mg via the kidney. Half the serum calcium (2·1–2·6 mmol l^{-1}) is unionized and bound to protein. The remainder, free ionized calcium, is responsible for its many actions which include cardiac and neuromuscular excitability, cell division and growth, blood coagulation and the coupling of a variety of electrical, chemical and hormonal stimuli. The free ionized calcium concentration is increased in acidosis and hypoproteinaemia.

Control of serum calcium concentration

The normal serum calcium concentration, 2·1–2·6 mmol l^{-1} (9–11 mg 100 ml^{-1}) is controlled by the interaction of parathyroid hormone, vitamin D and perhaps calcitonin. *Parathyroid hormone* (*PTH*) formation and release are stimulated in response to hypocalcaemia and result in an increase in serum calcium by its action on bone (increased resorption), kidney and gut (increased reabsorption). The actions on bone and gut also require 1,25 dihydroxycholecalciferol (1,25 DHCC) the active metabolite of *vitamin D* (cholecalciferol) which is converted to 25 hydroxycholecalciferol in the liver and then to 1,25 DHCC in the kidney. In animals, hypercalcaemia stimulates the release of *calcitonin* which decreases serum calcium by reducing osteoclast activity and increasing renal calcium excretion. However, it is uncertain whether it has a physiological role in man.

Hypercalcaemia

The commonest causes of hypercalcaemia in surgical practice are excess PTH secretion, bone metastases, lymphoma, hyperabsorption (milk–alkali syndrome), immobilization after trauma and the use of thiazide diuretics.

The symptoms are usually vague and include tiredness, decreased memory and concentration, hallucinations, delirium and eventually coma. Abdominal pain and itching are common. The ECG shows a typical shortening of the Q–T interval. Hypercalcaemia increases the inotropic but also the toxic effects of digitalis. Infusion of calcium results in increased BP with peripheral vasoconstriction and catecholamine release. Prolonged hypercalcaemia leads to dehydration from polyuria and renal acidification is impaired.

Nevertheless, calcium induced cardiac dysrhythmias during anaesthesia are rare unless serum calcium concentration exceeds about 3·5 mmol l^{-1} [9]. If serum calcium exceeds 5 mmol l^{-1} death is common and calcium reduction is urgent. This is best achieved by a combination of ECF volume expansion with saline and correction of hypokalaemia with the possible addition of chelating agents (EDTA), steroids, sodium sulphate or haemodialysis.

Hypocalcaemia

Hypocalcaemia is seen in association with acute pancreatitis, soft tissue infection, and pancreatic and small bowel fistulae. It always occurs after parathyroidectomy unless calcium supplements are given and in severe renal failure as a result of decreased

1,25 DHCC synthesis. Rapid, massive blood transfusion may cause transient hypocalcaemia.

The commonest symptom is tetany because of increased irritability of the motor nervous system. Initial symptoms include numbness, tingling and burning of the extremities, hyperactive reflexes, carpopedal spasm, muscle and abdominal cramps, and stridor as a result of laryngeal muscle spasm. Mental function is depressed and emotional lability and psychosis are common in adults. Eventually convulsions may occur. Tetany may first appear during hyperventilation and anaesthesia; alkalosis reduces the ionized Ca^{++} [6]. Chronic hypocalcaemia causes thinning and loss of hair, dry skin and lenticular cataracts. The ECG is characterized by a prolonged Q–T interval.

Treatment with calcium chloride or gluconate produces rapid relief of the motor symptoms.

Renal osteodystrophy

Severe, chronic renal disease is usually associated with serious bone disease. In children this presents as growth retardation and in adults as osteomalacia, osteosclerosis and osteoporosis. Secondary hyperparathyroidism results from hypocalcaemia which has a multifactorial aetiology. The most important factors include decreased 1,25 DHCC synthesis, phosphate retention, skeletal resistance to PTH and an altered feedback between serum calcium and PTH release. Even after successful renal transplantation 15–35 per cent of patients develop secondary hyperparathyroidism.

Bone pain and pathological fractures are common, myopathies and muscle weakness occur despite normal serum creatine phosphokinase and electromyography.

MAGNESIUM [13]

About half of the total body content of magnesium, 1000 mmol, is found in bone and the remainder is distributed, like potassium, mainly intracellularly. The normal serum magnesium concentration is 0·75–1·0 mmol l^{-1}. The normal daily intake is about 4 mmol and it is excreted mainly in the faeces with fine control by urinary excretion although the details of its control are poorly understood.

Magnesium is a chelating agent with many biological functions. In particular, it is an activator of many enzymes concerned with intermediary metabolism, protein synthesis and genetic transfer.

Hypermagnesaemia

Hypermagnesaemia usually occurs either associated with advanced renal disease or as an iatrogenic complication of magnesium therapy. The major signs and symptoms affect the central nervous and cardiovascular systems and neuromuscular conduction. Drowsiness and light coma are common. The cardiovascular system is affected by impaired conduction in the myocardium and depression of sympathetic ganglia. These result in hypotension, bradycardia and an abnormal ECG which shows increase in the QT interval and conduction defects. Cardiac arrest occurs when serum magnesium concentration exceeds 7–8 mmol l^{-1}. Neuromuscular conduction is decreased as a result of impaired release of acetylcholine and complete paralysis, excluding the diaphragm, occurs at serum levels exceeding 7 mmol l^{-1}. Hypermagnesaemia is associated with potentiation of both competitive and depolarizing muscle relaxants [8].

Treatment is by removal of the source, and positive pressure ventilation. Rapid symptomatic relief may follow administration of calcium, 2–5 mmol, or a glucose–potassium–insulin regimen to encourage intracellular shift of magnesium.

Hypomagnesaemia

Symptomatic hypomagnesaemia is associated with inadequate magnesium intake, from starvation or long term magnesium-free parenteral nutrition, gastrointestinal losses, from malabsorption or diarrhoea, and renal losses, in renal tubular disorders. It is also seen in pancreatitis, primary aldosteronism, diabetic acidosis, diuretic therapy and after renal transplantation. The commonest cause in Western society is chronic alcoholism.

Clinical symptoms are extremely variable. Episodic confusion, irritability, surliness and anorexia are common. The neuromuscular and central nervous hyperactivity resemble hypocalcaemia: increased tendon reflexes and tetany with positive Chovstek's and Trusseau's signs. Cardiovascular effects include supraventricular tachycardia, flat T waves, paroxysmal ventricular fibrillation and tachycardia, and increased sensitivity to digitalis—the last a result of a decrease in intracellular K^+ concentration.

Treatment is by the intravenous administration of 20 ml, 50 per cent magnesium sulphate over 2–4 hours although care must be taken to avoid hypermagnesaemia particularly in the patient with hypovolaemia or impaired renal function.

HYDROGEN ION

Clinicians are confused by disorders of acid–base balance and, too often, make therapeutic decisions using ill-understood and erroneous mathematical formulas. Their confusion arises from three causes. First, acid–base terminology is based upon complicated physico-chemical concepts which are seldom comprehended. Second, a multiplicity of 'simple' diagrams and associated jargon has evolved attempting to separate the metabolic and respiratory components from any set of acid–base data. Third, it has been erroneously assumed that the change in pH which occurs in blood tonometered with gases of differing CO_2 tensions is similar to the change in whole body pH which occurs when the P_{CO_2} of the patient is altered.

Assessment of acidity

The range of hydrogen ion (H^+) concentrations found in aqueous bodily solutions is large, 10^{-1}–10^{-15} mol l^{-1}. For convenience, these concentrations are expresssed by exponential arithmetic (Table 10.8).

One basic difficulty is that it is not possible to measure either the actual H^+ concentration or its activity in biological systems. The pH numbers, produced by electrometric measurement, are defined by an operational scale based upon standard buffer solutions at fixed temperatures of measurement [2]. They do not relate precisely to H^+ concentration or activity.

The normal value for arterial pH in man, at a P_{a,CO_2} of 5·3 kPa (40 mmHg) is 7·4 with a range of 7·35–7·45. For venous blood the range is 7·32–7·42.

Table 10.8. Conversion of H^+ concentration ($mol\,l^{-1}$ and $nmol\,l^{-1}$) to pH units.

$[H^+]$ ($mol\,l^{-1}$)	pH	$[H^+]$ ($nmol\,l^{-1}$)
$0\cdot001 = 10^{-3}$	3	1 000 000
$0\cdot00001 = 10^{-5}$	5	10 000
$0\cdot0000001 = 10^{-7}$	7	100
$0\cdot000000001 = 10^{-9}$	9	1

Assessment of acid–base state

In vivo CO_2 titration

Consideration of the Hendersen–Hasselbalch equation is the core to the understanding of acid–base balance:

$$pH = pK' + \log\frac{[HCO_3^-]}{\alpha PCO_2} \qquad (\alpha = \text{sol. coeff. for } CO_2).$$

Both metabolic and respiratory factors are represented. Unfortunately some established methods of assessing acid-base balance have linked pH to the molar concentrations of bicarbonate and carbonic acid in plasma or blood *in vitro* and assumed that similar changes would be found *in vivo*. In addition, it is now appreciated that the constants in the equation cannot be predicted accurately.

Nevertheless, the equation allows us to expect that an *in vivo* alteration of PCO_2

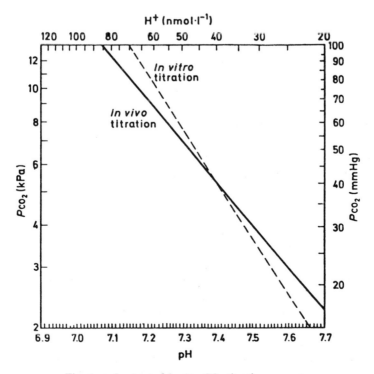

Fig. 10.4. *In vivo* and *in vitro* CO_2 titration curves.

will be associated with a predictable change in pH. Such an association has been confirmed in animals and in man [10, 16]. If the Pa,co_2 is either increased or decreased, and time allowed for a steady state to be reached, an *in vivo* CO_2 titration curve (straight line using a pH/log Pco_2 plot) is obtained (Fig. 10.4). When such a titration is performed in animals made deliberately acid, with varying amounts of hydrochloride acid, a family of curves, approximately parallel to, and to the left of the normal curve is found. The more acid that is added the further is the curve shifted to the left. Similarly, in man, a nonrespiratory acidosis produces curves shifted to the left and a nonrespiratory alkalosis to the right. Buffering capability increases with increasing nonrespiratory acidosis so that left shifted curves are more vertical than the normal (Fig. 10.5).

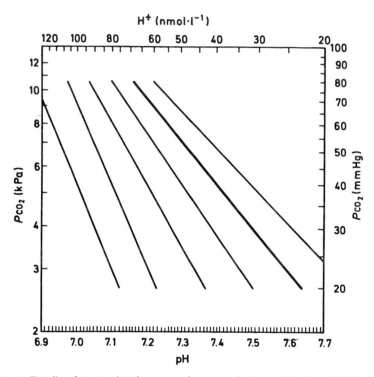

Fig. 10.5. Family of *in vivo* titration curves in nonrespiratory acidosis and alkalosis.

Acidosis, alkalosis and acidaemia, alkalaemia

The terms acidosis, acidaemia and alkalosis, alkalaemia are often used interchangeably, but this is not correct.

Acidaemia should be defined as existing if the arterial pH is less than 7·35. Similarly, an alkalaemia is present if the pH is above 7·45. If a primary nonrespiratory (metabolic) tendency towards acidaemia is accompanied by a tendency towards respiratory alkalaemia so that the resulting pH still lies within the normal range, the acid–base state should be known as nonrespiratory acidosis accompanied by a respiratory alkalosis. By definition, if the Pco_2 is above 6·0 kPa (45 mmHg) or less than 4·7 kPa (35 mmHg) a respiratory acidosis or alkalosis, respectively, is present. If the set of pH-Pco_2 values produces a point on the *in vivo* CO_2 titration curve to the left or right of the normal curve, then a metabolic acidosis or alkalosis, respectively is present.

NONRESPIRATORY (METABOLIC) ACID–BASE CHANGES (Table 10.9)

Nonrespiratory acidosis

Nonrespiratory acidosis may be caused by an increasei n the production of non-volatile acids during anaerobic metabolism in starvation, diabetes mellitus, hypoxia,

Table 10.9. Nonrespiratory disturbances of acid–base status.

Acidosis	Acid load	Anaerobic metabolism
		Starvation
		Diabetes mellitus
		Sodium nitroprusside
		Lactic acidosis
	Loss of base	Diarrhoea
		Pancreatic/biliary fistula
	↓ Acid excretion	Renal acidosis
	Dilutional	Saline excess
Alkalosis	Alkaline load	$NaHCO_3$ infusion
		Oral alkali
	Acid loss	Vomiting
		Gastric fistula
	K^+ loss	Hypokalaemia
		1° aldosteronism
		Diuretics

after cardiac arrest and following administration of large amounts of sodium nitro-prusside. A nonrespiratory acidosis also accompanies excessive loss of base from diarrhoea or pancreatic and biliary fistulae. Severe renal disease or isolated distal tubular defects cause an acidosis by a net reduction in renal acid excretion. An uncommon, but probably overemphasized, cause of nonrespiratory acidosis occurs if extracellular bicarbonate is diluted by overenthusiastic replacement with saline. Such administration only occurs during the resuscitation of the severely hypovolaemic patient in whom the restoration of circulatory volume by an isotonic fluid is an urgent requirement to restore tissue perfusion and aerobic metabolism.

Biochemically, the *in vivo* CO_2 titration curve is shifted to the left in non-respiratory acidosis. Ventilation is stimulated by peripheral chemoreceptor drive so that arterial and CSF P_{CO_2} and $[HCO_3^-]$ are lowered until pH returns almost to normal. If the pH is corrected rapidly by the administration of bicarbonate, CSF P_{CO_2} will rise and pH fall stimulating central chemoreceptors and replacing the arterial non-respiratory acidosis with a respiratory alkalosis.

The correction of a nonrespiratory acidosis is probably the commonest thera-peutic manipulation of acid–base status. Exact, single-dose, correction could only be achieved if it were possible to know whether the patient was improving or deteri-orating and if the volume of distribution of H^+ were known precisely. Only empirical general guidelines can be given. Correction should be by the slow administration of sodium bicarbonate, over ten minutes, and monitored by repeated blood gas analysis to prevent overcorrection. A simple guide is to calculate the change in pH which would have occurred if no respiratory compensation had taken place. This is achieved by drawing a line parallel to the normal *in vivo* CO_2 titration curve to pass through the point at which the patient lies (Fig. 10.4). For a 70 kg patient, 100 mmol $NaHCO_3$ should then be given for each 0·1 decrease in pH from 7·4. A further set of P_{CO_2}-pH values should be obtained in 30 minutes and the process repeated.

Lactic acidosis

Lactic acidosis is best defined as the combination of a pH of less than 7·25 and a blood lactate concentration of more than 5 mmol l^{-1} [1]. Care must be taken to exclude other conditions, e.g. renal failure and ketoacidosis, where the elevation of lactic acid is not alone responsible for the acidosis.

Aetiology

Cohen and Woods [5] have simplified the classification of lactic acidosis by defining two types: type A due to tissue hypoxia and anaerobic metabolism; type B due to other causes.

Type A lactic acidosis. The association of metabolic acidosis with circulatory collapse and hypoxia is well recognized. Impaired tissue perfusion may be the result of any form of shock and tissue oxygenation is further compromised by severe anaemia and hypoxaemia. Blood lactate concentration, although seldom measured, is closely correlated with mortality. There is a mortality of 73 per cent in patients with blood lactate from 4·4 to 8·9 mmol l^{-1}, but only 18 per cent mortality with lactates of 1·3–4·4 mmol l^{-1}.

Treatment entails removal of the cause and alkali therapy.

Type B lactic acidosis. There are many causes of type B lactic acidosis (Table 10.10) although biguanide therapy and agents used for parenteral nutrition have received recent attention.

Table 10.10. Aetiology of type B lactic acidosis.

β1	β2	β3
Common disorders	Drugs and toxins	Inherited
Diabetes mellitus	Biguanides: phenformin	Glycogen storage disease
Renal failure	metformin buformin	Fructose 1,6-diphosphate deficiency
Hepatic disease	Parenteral nutrition:	Leigh's syndrome
Infection	fructose sorbitol	Methylmalonic acidaemia
Leukaemia	xylitol ethanol Salicylates Methanol	

The treatment of type B lactic acidosis is difficult. If possible the cause should be removed. Large amounts of alkali are necessary due to the continuing lactate production. Attempts have been made to remove the lactate by dialysis or by stimulating pyruvate dehydrogenase to encourage conversion of lactate to pyruvate by the removal of the latter via the tricarboxylic acid cycle.

Non-respiratory alkalosis

Most of the causes of nonrespiratory alkalosis are iatrogenic either by the administration of excessive alkali, sodium bicarbonate, or oral antacids, or by failing to recognize hypokalaemia due to diuretic therapy. Acid may be lost from the body either from the stomach by prolonged vomiting, or from the kidney by hypokalaemia with its paradoxical combination of acid urine and alkaline ECF. Severe non-respiratory alkalosis (pH > 7·55) has a high mortality [24].

Biochemically, the *in vivo* CO_2 titration curve is shifted to the right. There is usually some respiratory compensation, although less than in a metabolic acidosis, so that the P_{CO_2} is elevated, which reduces CSF pH and leads to an increase in CSF $[HCO_3^-]$.

Correction of a nonrespiratory alkalosis is achieved, predominantly, by treating the cause. In particular, potassium loss should be replaced using potassium chloride. One-sixth molar NH_4Cl has been used as a source of acid as two molecules NH_4Cl condense to form one molecule urea and two molecules HCl. It is contraindicated in hypokalaemic patients as further K^+ loss is induced. The place of intravenous acid, as 0·3 molar HCl given by a central venous catheter, is not widely accepted. If correction is contemplated, the same criteria as those suggested for the treatment of a nonrespiratory acidosis should be used. Correction should be slow and with frequent acid–base monitoring. Acid dosage should be based upon the degree of shift of the *in vivo* CO_2 titration curve.

Pyloric stenosis

Prolonged vomiting by patients with pyloric stenosis presents a characteristic biochemical picture. In addition to the nonrespiratory alkalosis with elevated serum bicarbonate concentration (35–50 mmol l^{-1}) they demonstrate severe hypokalaemia (1·8–3 mmol l^{-1}) and hypochloraemia (40–80 mmol l^{-1}) and they excrete acid urine. The hypokalaemia and acidaemia occur in response to gastric loss of chloride. In the absence of chloride, sodium can be conserved by the kidney only if it takes part in cation exchange initially with potassium, producing hypokalaemia, and then with hydrogen ion, which potentiates the alkalosis. The alkalosis can be corrected with saline infusion and even in the alkalosis associated with severe potassium deficiency the provision of chloride is essential [18].

REFERENCES

1 ALBERTI KGM, NATTRASS M. Lactic acidosis. *Lancet* 1977; ii: 25–9.

2 BATES RG. *Determination of pH. Theory and practice.* New York: Wiley, 1964.

3 BEVAN DR. Osmometry. 2. Osmoregulation. *Anaesthesia* 1978; **33**: 801–8.

4 BEVAN DR. Colloid osmotic pressure. *Anaesthesia* 1980; **35**: 263–70.

5 Cohen RD, Woods HF. *Clinical and biochemical aspects of lactic acidosis.* Oxford: Blackwell Scientific Publications, 1976.

6 Drop LJ, Miller EV. Biochemical alterations during tetany. *Anesthesiology* 1980; **52**: 82–3.

7 Feldman SA. Effect of changes in electrolytes, hydration and pH upon the reactions to muscle relaxants. *Br J Anaesth* 1963; **35**: 546–51.

8 Ghonheim MM, Long JP. The interaction between magnesium and other neuromuscular blocking agents. *Anesthesiology* 1970; **32**: 23–7.

9 Gunst MA, Drop LJ. Chronic hypercalcaemia secondary to hyperparathyroidism: a risk factor during anaesthesia. *Br J Anaesth* 1980; **52**: 507–11.

10 Kappagoda CT, Linden RJ, Snow, HK. An approach to the problems of acid–base balance. *Clin Sci* 1970; **39**: 169–82.

11 Morgan DB, Davidson C. Hypokalaemia and diuretics: an analysis of publications. *Br Med J* 1980; **i**: 905–8.

12 Newsome HH. Vasopressin: deficiency, excess and syndrome of inappropriate antidiuretic hormone secretion. *Nephron* 1979; **23**: 125–9.

13 Paymaster NJ. Magnesium metabolism: a brief review. *Ann R Coll Surg Engl.* **58**: 309–14.

14 Peters JJ, Van Slyke DD. *Quantitative clinical chemistry* Vol. 1. 1st ed. Baltimore: Williams & Wilkins, 1931: 764.

15 Pollock AS, Arieff AI. Abnormalities of cell volume regulation and their functional consequences. *Am J Physiol* 1980; **239**: F195–F205.

16 Prys-Rorerts C, Kelman GR, Nunn JF. Determination of the *in vivo* carbon dioxide titration curve of anaesthetized man. *Br J Anaesth* 1966; **38**: 500–9.

17 Schrier RW, Berl T. Disorders of water metabolism. In: Shrier RW, ed. *Renal and electrolyte disorders.* Boston: Little Brown and Company, 1976: 36.

18 Schwartz WB, Cohen JJ. The nature of the renal response to chronic disorders of acid–base equilibrium. *Am J Med* 1978; **64**: 417–27.

19 Still JA, Modell JH. Acute water intoxication during transurethral resection of the prostate using glycine solution for irrigation. *Anesthesiology* 1973; **38**: 98–9.

20 Tyler FH. Hyperosmolar coma. *Am J Med* 1968; **45**: 485–7.

21 Robertson GL, Shelton RL, Athar S. The osmoregulation of vasopressin. *Kidney Int* 1976; **10**: 25–37.

22 Robin ED, Cross CE, Zelis R. Pulmonary odema. Parts I and II. *N Engl J Med* 1973; **288**: 239–46 and 292–304.

23 Vaughan RS, Lunn JN. Potassium and the anaesthetist. *Anaesthesia* 1973; **28**: 118–31.

24 Wilson RF, Gibson D, Percinel AK, *et al.* Severe alkalosis in critically ill surgical patients. *Arch Surg* 1972; **105**: 197–203.

ADDITIONAL READING

Maxwell MH, Kleeman CR. *Clinical disorders of fluid and electrolyte metabolism.* 3rd ed. New York: McGraw-Hill, 1980.

Orloff J, Berliner RW. *Handbook of physiology.* Section 8. Renal physiology. Washington: American Physiological Society, 1973.

Schrier RW. *Renal and electrolyte disorders.* Boston: Little, Brown & Co, 1976.

Bevan DR. *Renal function in anaesthesia and surgery.* London: Academic Press, 1979.

Kinney JM, Egdahl RH, Zuidema GD. *Manual of preoperative and postoperative care.* New York: WB. Saunders, 1971.

Chapter 11
Haematological Disorders

T. HILARY HOWELLS AND JOHN E. PETTIT

Haematology is a subject principally concerned with the cellular structure and function of the blood and blood forming tissues. The disorders encountered are numerous and reflect either primary blood anomalies or derangements secondary to disease processes elsewhere. It is hardly surprising then, that haematological tests are prominent during the early investigation of so many conditions and subsequently become a necessary part of monitoring disease progress and its therapy.

The starting point of all haematological study comprises a haemoglobin measurement, blood cell counting and the microscopic examination of blood film characteristics. Few surgical patients are denied this basic screening because a knowledge of the oxygen capacity and the leucocyte responses, for example, are essential for the correct anaesthetic and surgical management. Frequently, the anaesthetist will need to be aware of the coagulation status of his patient and, as indicated, the platelet count or the haemoglobin genotype. Less frequently he may require an assessment of the red cell enzymes or assays of specific coagulation factors and fibrin degradation products.

Normal values (in S.I. units) are given in Table 11.1. Appendices I and II to this chapter list the principle abnormalities during blood film examination and their clinical associations.

Table 11.1. Normal haematological values.

Haemoglobin	11·5–18·0 g/dl
PCV	0·35–0·54
Red cell count	$3·9–6·5 \times 10^{12}/l$
Mean cell haemoglobin	27–32 pg
Mean cell volume	76–96 fl
Mean cell haemoglobin concentration	30–35 g/dl
Reticulocytes	0·2–2·0%
	$10–100 \times 10^9/l$
White cell count	$4·0–11·0 \times 10^9/l$
Platelets	$150–400 \times 10^9/l$
Serum iron	14–29 μmol/l
Total iron binding capacity	45–75 μmol/l
Serum B_{12}	160–925 ng/l
Serum folate	3–20 μg/l
Fibrinogen	1·5–4·0 g/l

ANAEMIA

The first step in the diagnosis of anaemia is its detection. This requires the accurate measurement of haemoglobin or haematocrit and a comparison of these values with suitable reference values for a healthy population (see Table 11.2). It must be remem-

Table 11.2. Normal haemoglobin and haematocrit
(PCV or VPRC) values.

	Haemoglobin g/dl	Haematocrit
Men	13·5–18·0	0·40–0·54
Women	11·5–16·5	0·35–0·47
Full-term infants	13·6–19·6	0·44–0·62
Children: 3 months	9·5–12·5	0·32–0·44
Children: 1 year	11·0–13·0	0·36–0·44
Children: 10–12 years	11·5–14·8	0·37–0·44

bered that the mean normal value and the lower limit of the 'normal' range (defined by the mean value minus twice the standard deviation) depend on the age and sex of the subject and the altitude of residence. After puberty the values for males are higher than for females. Although statistical interpretation of normal distribution curves would suggest that 2·5 per cent of a healthy population might have haemoglobin or haematocrit values lower than 2 standard deviations below the mean, it is essential to show that disease is absent in every patient in whom the values fall below the limits given.

The accurate definition of anaemia requires thorough clinical evaluation of the patient and haematological investigation. As well as eliciting the patient's symptoms enquiry should be made about occupation, diet, chemical exposure and family history of blood disorders. Apart from pallor, physical signs particularly relevant to the diagnosis of anaemia include jaundice, glossitis, splenomegaly, liver and lymph node enlargement. With modern automated electronic counters, accurate computed red cell indices (MCV, MCH and MCHC) readily indicate the morphological class of anaemia, e.g. hypochromic microcytic, macrocytic or normocytic, from which the patient is likely to be suffering. Examination of the blood film provides an essential check on these indices and the rest of the blood count and in many patients identifies the type of anaemia present, e.g. macrocytic anaemia with oval macrocytes and hypersegmented neutrophils suggests a megaloblastic anaemia; spherocytosis and polychromasia would point to a haemolytic anaemia. The reticulocyte count, a valuable index of the erythropoietic response to anaemia, is also of great value in the initial definition of anaemia. Often the exact diagnosis can only be made after detailed laboratory studies. These definitive tests are discussed in following sections.

Anaemia develops as a result of an abnormality of red cell production or because there is an excessive loss of these components. It may be congenital or acquired, primary or secondary to other disease. In many patients anaemia is not a diagnosis in itself but merely reflects the presence of an underlying systemic disorder and a final diagnosis must include the pathogenesis of the anaemia, e.g. iron deficiency due to chronic haemorrhage from carcinoma of the stomach. Correct treatment of anaemia depends on knowledge of the pathogenesis.

When dealing with anaemic patients it is important to know when and how to correct the condition and also when not to—of particular importance with patients in stable chronic anaemia. Although anaemia results in a depletion in the oxygen-carrying capacity of the blood due to a reduction in red cell numbers, their haemoglobin concentration or both, the level of tissue oxygenation is not dependent on haemoglobin concentration alone. The oxygen dissociation curve of the patient's haemoglobin is also important and a compensatory increase in cardiac output also improves oxygen delivery in anaemic patients. In many patients with chronic anaemia an increase in the level of the glycolytic intermediate 2, 3 diphosphoglycerate in red cells results in a shift of the oxygen dissociation curve to the right, i.e. oxygen is given up more readily than normal to the tissues. In those patients in whom this right shift is greatest, e.g. in sickle-cell disease, pyruvate kinase deficiency, and as recently recognized, in renal failure, it may be unnecessary to transfuse or treat in any other way. Experience with severely anaemic haemodialysis subjects has led to an acceptance of far lower haemoglobin levels than formerly so that an oxygen capacity deficit of up to 50 per cent need not cause undue anxiety provided the haemodynamic compensation is optimal and the patient is evidently coping with the compensatory demand. Features which indicate compensatory failure are fatigue, dyspnoea on exertion, angina, palpitation, sustained tachycardia or signs of heart failure. Conversely, if the oxygen dissociation curve is shifted to the left and oxygen is given up to the tissues less readily than normal, as in rare patients with abnormal haemoglobins, the patient may need to maintain a haemoglobin level above the normal range to ensure adequate oxygen supplies to the tissues.

IRON DEFICIENCY

Iron deficiency is the commonest single cause of anaemia. It has been estimated that 10 20 per cent of the world population is deficient in iron; in Western countries it is the commonest nutritional deficiency, affecting mainly women, children and the poor.

IRON BALANCE

The healthy male body contains about 4 g of iron, some 65–70 per cent present as haemoglobin, about 25–30 per cent as ferritin and haemosiderin in stores, with the remainder present as cellular enzymes containing iron and circulating iron bound to transferrin. Circulating haemoglobin iron and iron stores are a third less in females. Daily loss of iron means that iron requirements amount to about 1 mg in adult males and children, 1·5–2·0 mg in menstruating females and up to 3 mg or more in a normal pregnancy. An average Western diet contains 10–20 mg iron daily and iron balance is controlled by absorption which occurs maximally through the duodenum and jejunum. It is restricted to about 5–10 per cent of intake and just matches daily loss. Although absorption can be increased in the presence of increased requirements, e.g. during growth, pregnancy or iron deficiency, the amount absorbed seldom exceeds 20–30 per cent of food iron, the exact figure depending on the type of food taken, iron from animal sources usually being better absorbed than iron in vegetables.

CAUSES OF IRON DEFICIENCY

Physiological. Iron deficiency is common in infancy and adolescence—the expanding red cell volume during periods of growth creates increased demands for the vital metal—and in women of child-bearing age because dietary intake may not be sufficient to meet the increased demands created by menstruation, pregnancy, parturition and lactation.

Blood loss. Gastrointestinal haemorrhage from oesophageal varices, hiatus hernia, peptic ulceration, aspirin ingestion, gastric or colonic carcinoma, hookworm infestation, ulcerative colitis or haemorrhoids, is an important cause of iron deficiency. Less commonly the bleeding is from the renal tract as haematuria or is due to chronic intra-vascular haemolysis with haemoglobinuria and haemosiderinuria. In women, apart from the physiological causes of blood loss already mentioned, excessive uterine bleeding, e.g. from fibroids or menorrhagia, is an additional cause.

Poor diet. Iron deficiency due solely to inadequate iron intake is unusual. However, where a poor diet is taken continually, particularly from childhood as in undeveloped countries, inadequate intake may be the most important factor. Dietary iron deficiency also occurs frequently in infants taking unsupplemented milk diets. Cow's milk intolerance has also been implicated in occasional infants with gastrointestinal haemorrhage as an additional factor [3, 26].

Malabsorption of iron. Malabsorption of iron is a less common cause of iron deficiency. In untreated coeliac disease, whether in adults or children, iron deficiency is usual and there is associated folate deficiency. With other gastrointestinal lesions, e.g. atrophic gastritis, partial gastrectomy or Crohn's disease it is likely that excess iron loss due to exfoliating cells or haemorrhage aggravates deficiency.

CLINICAL FEATURES

Symptoms include those due to the anaemia, e.g. lassitude, weakness, dyspnoea on exertion and, in many patients, those due to the disorder responsible for the iron deficiency, e.g. peptic ulcer. Repeated mild infections may be a problem in iron deficient infants and children. Pallor is usually present and, in long-standing cases, epithelial changes such as angular stomatitis, glossitis and koilonychia occur. There is associated atrophic gastritis and achlorhydria in a small proportion of patients and rarely a post-cricoid oesophageal web may result in dysphagia (Plummer–Vinson syndrome). Splenomegaly when present is mild and only seen in severe cases.

DIAGNOSIS

Iron deficiency anaemia is hypochromic and microcytic with a mean cell volume (MCV) of less than 80 fl (femtolitres) mean cell haemoglobin concentration (MCHC) less than 30 g/dl and mean cell haemoglobin (MCH) less than 27 pg.

Blood film examination usually confirms the absolute red cell values with prominent red cell hypochromia, microcytosis, anisocytosis, poikilocytosis and variable numbers of 'pencil' and 'target' red cell forms. When the anaemia is mild, however, the film may be normochromic and normocytic. The platelet count may be raised (above 350×10^9/l), particularly if haemorrhage is occurring. The serum iron is low, e.g. morning samples less than 14 μmol/l and the iron binding capacity raised, e.g. morning samples above 70 μmol/l. The serum ferritin is low—less than 14 μg/l. When iron deficiency develops, the stores become completely depleted before anaemia occurs. Bone marrow examination reveals micronormoblastic erythropoiesis and iron cannot be demonstrated in tissue stores or as siderotic granules in developing erythroblasts. The most frequent diagnostic mistakes occur when other hypochromic anaemias, e.g. the anaemia of chronic disorders or, less frequently, sideroblastic anaemia or thalassaemia, are diagnosed as iron deficiency. The combination of serum ferritin, serum iron, iron binding capacity and bone marrow examination should help to distinguish iron deficiency from these other hypochromic anaemias.

TREATMENT

The treatment of iron deficiency includes measures to replace the iron deficit of circulating haemoglobin and stores and those directed towards correcting the underlying cause. Chronic anaemia is usually corrected at leisure by iron therapy and should be completed if possible before nonurgent elective surgery.

Oral Iron. Iron is usually given orally for about six months. Ferrous sulphate, gluconate, succinate or fumarate are equally effective; ferrous sulphate the cheapest, should be used in the first place. Doses of 200 mg (60 mg elemental iron) t.d.s. are used; larger doses cause frequent toxicity with nausea and epigastric pain. Liquid preparations may be used in children and are sometimes preferred in adults with gastrointestinal lesions which make tablets unsuitable.

With oral iron therapy the speed of response depends on the bone marrow's capacity to form haemoglobin and not on the amount of iron given. Haemoglobin levels should rise 1–1·5 g/dl per week with a reticulocyte response beginning on the 4th or 5th day peaking at about 5–15 per cent between the 7th and 10th days of therapy. Inadequate responses to oral iron are not infrequent. The patient may not be taking the tablets or may have an intolerance or malabsorption of oral iron. The cause of the deficiency, especially haemorrhage, may be continuing or there may be an underlying condition such as malignancy, chronic inflammation or renal failure which inhibits marrow response. Occasionally the lack of response is the result of an additional cause for anaemia, e.g. folate or vitamin B_{12} deficiency.

Parenteral iron. Intramuscular iron (iron dextran or iron sorbitol) is given when the patient is intolerant to oral iron, when bleeding continues or when the patient has a gastrointestinal disorder that may be aggravated by iron. Although the response during the first week is marginally greater than that observed with oral iron, after this time the response rates are similar.

A total dose intravenous infusion of iron dextran in saline over a period of several hours may be used to correct the total body iron deficit. The incidence of toxic effects is low but, particularly in subjects with an allergic history, vasomotor or allergic reactions may occur and deaths from anaphylactic shock have been reported. Total dose infusion is used only when correction of iron deficiency by other methods is not possible. Calculation of dose is made from the deficit in circulating haemoglobin: a 1 g/dl fall equals approximately 170 mg or iron in a 70 kg male; in addition, 1–1·5 g are needed to replenish body stores.

Blood transfusion. Occasionally the patient's clinical state is severe or urgent surgery is required. In these rare situations a carefully monitored delivery of plasma reduced red cells is indicated. Bearing in mind the circulatory hyperdynamic state in such patients the anaesthetist must be aware of undue myocardial depression when using intravenous narcotic agents and slowed induction time using inhalational agents.

In the event of acute haemorrhagic anaemia, rapid replacement of the 'acutely' lost blood by whole blood is safe even in the presence of pre-existing anaemia. Following acute haemorrhage, haemodilution is not complete for some two days so that early haemoglobin estimations are misleading. Blood volume estimations are neither readily available nor particularly accurate and replacement therapy is best controlled by clinical observation and measurement of blood losses and patient responses. Central venous pressure measurements are useful during blood volume restoration but should not be relied upon as the overriding guide to replacement therapy.

MEGALOBLASTIC ANAEMIA

Megaloblastic anaemia is usually caused by vitamin B_{12} or folate deficiency [19]. Apart from the anaemia, one should remember the association of pernicious anaemia with myxoedema, folate deficiency with alcoholism and anticonvulsant therapy. The megaloblastic anaemias may be associated with nutritional states and hepatic disease. Patients with vitamin B_{12} deficiency may have difficulty in walking, parasthesiae, muscle weakness or mental disturbances, associated with bilateral peripheral neuropathy or degeneration of lateral and posterior columns of the spinal cord (subacute combined degeneration) (see page 284). Disturbed vision may be caused by retrobulbar neuritis with optic atrophy. The neurological complications seen in vitamin B_{12} deficiency, may lead the anaesthetist to be wary of epidural or subarachnoid analgesia.

Diagnosis

Although often suspected on clinical grounds because of pallor, jaundice, glossitis or neurological signs, the diagnosis of megaloblastic anaemia depends on the association of red cell macrocytosis with bone marrow 'megaloblastic change'. The MCV is greater than 100 fl and figures in excess of 120 fl are frequent; MCH and MCHC are usually normal; oval macrocytes, red cell anisocytosis and hypersegmented neutrophils are characteristically found during blood film examination.

In severe cases leucopenia and thrombocytopenia are also present and the bone marrow is hypercellular. Megaloblastic features include a dissociation of nuclear and cytoplasmic maturation in erythroblasts and granulopoietic cells with a fine, open, stippled appearance of nuclear chromatin, generalized enlargement of cells and an increased proportion of primitive cells. Raised levels of serum bilirubin, iron, lactic dehydrogenase and lysozyme are usually found. The severity of all these changes correlates well with the degree of anaemia. Coincident iron deficiency occasionally masks the changes found in erythropoiesis but not those seen in developing granulocytes.

The estimation of serum vitamin B_{12}, serum and red cell folate levels is required to establish which deficiency is responsible for the megaloblastic change. When these tests are not available or when the results are all low a therapeutic trial may be used. In this, after a period of baseline observation, the response of the anaemia to parenteral physiological doses of vitamin B_{12} (1–2 μg) or folic acid (100–200 μg) daily is followed.

VITAMIN B_{12}

Vitamin B_{12} exists in several forms all of which have the same cobalamin nucleus. The daily requirement is 1–2 μg and the stores in adult man amount to 2–3 mg, i.e. enough for 3 to 4 years if supplies are completely cut off. Gastric and intestinal juices release vitamin B_{12} from protein complexes in food. The absorption of adequate quantities of vitamin B_{12} requires intrinsic factor. This glycoprotein, normally produced by the stomach, binds the vitamin and transports it to specific receptor sites on the brush border surface of the distal ileum where absorption takes place.

The causes of vitamin B_{12} deficiency are listed in Table 11.3. Malabsorption of the vitamin is the usual cause and pernicious anaemia is the most important vitamin B_{12} deficiency disorder in Great Britain. Inadequate dietary intake, rare in Western

Table 11.3. Causes of vitamin B_{12} deficiency.

1. *Nutritional*—Vegans
2. *Malabsorption*
   - Pernicious anaemia
   - Gastrectomy
   - Intestinal stagnant-loop syndrome
     - jejunal diverticulosis
     - ileo-colic fistula
     - intestinal stricture
     - anatomical blind loop
   - Fish tapeworm
   - Tropical sprue
   - Ileal resection
   - Selective malabsorption and proteinuria
     - (Imerslund's syndrome)

countries, is seen in Vegans (religious Hindus of India) who omit both animal meat and animal products such as milk, eggs and cheese from their diet.

Pernicious anaemia

In adult pernicious anaemia the megaloblastic change is the result of a severe lack of intrinsic factor due to gastric atrophy. The incidence of pernicious anaemia in Great Britain is 120 per 100,000 population. The disease occurs more commonly than by chance in close relatives and usually presents over the age of 40. There is an equal sex incidence and patients with this disorder have an increased incidence of gastric carcinoma. It appears likely that the underlying gastric atrophy is 'autoimmune' in origin since: (1) plasma cells and lymphocytes invade the stomach; (2) steroid therapy has temporarily improved the gastric lesion in some cases; (3) parietal cell antibodies are found in 90 per cent and intrinsic factor antibodies are present in 60 per cent of patients; (4) there is an association with hypogammaglobulinaemia and possible autoimmune diseases such as 'autoimmune' thyroiditis and myxoedema, Addison's disease and hypoparathyroidism.

Two rare types of childhood pernicious anaemia occur. In the first there is congenital intrinsic factor deficiency, morphologically normal stomach, normal acid secretion and no parietal cell or intrinsic factor antibodies in the serum. The second type resembles adult pernicious anaemia with gastric atrophy and gastric antibodies. This latter type may be associated with an endocrinopathy.

Gastrectomy

The usual body stores of vitamin B_{12} are exhausted 3 to 4 years following total gastrectomy. A proportion of patients with extensive partial gastric resections also develop megaloblastic anaemia after this period of time. More frequently than not the vitamin B_{12} deficiency is associated with coincident iron deficiency. In most post-gastrectomy patients the vitamin B_{12} deficiency results from resection of intrinsic factor secreting tissue and atrophy of the remaining stomach. In occasional patients the creation of an intestinal blind loop or the development of abnormal jejunal flora may aggravate the malabsorption.

Intestinal causes of vitamin B_{12} deficiency

In the 'stagnant loop syndrome' colonization of the small intestine by colonic bacteria is thought to be responsible for the deficiency. Removal of more than four feet of terminal ileum causes malabsorption of vitamin B_{12}. Deficiency in advanced Crohn's disease may result from heavy involvement of the terminal ileum; fistulae and blind loops may also contribute. The vitamin B_{12} malabsorption in patients with tropical sprue usually improves after folic acid and antibiotic therapy.

FOLATE

Pteroylglutamic acid (folic acid) is the parent compound of a group of compounds collectively called folates. Adult daily requirements for folate are about 100 μg and the normal Western diet contains about 600 μg folate mostly in the polyglutamate form. Folates are easily destroyed by cooking at high temperatures. The pteroyl polyglutamates are deconjugated following ingestion to monoglutamates and maximum absorption occurs through the duodenum and jejunum.

The main causes of folate deficiency are listed in Table 11.4.

Table 11.4. Causes of folate deficiency.

1 *Nutritional*
2 *Malabsorption*
    Tropical sprue
    Coeliac disease+dermatitis herpetiformis
    ? Anticonvulsant therapy
3 *Excess requirement or loss*
    Pregnancy
    Hyperactive haemopoiesis
    Homocystinuria
    Excessive urinary loss:
      Congestive heart failure
      Active liver disease
    Haemodialysis, peritoneal dialysis
4 *Antifolate drugs*
    Aminopterin, methotrexate
    Alcohol
    ? Anticonvulsants

Nutritional folate deficiency

The intake of folate is not greatly in excess of daily requirements and because body reserves are slender, folate deficiency develops rapidly when the diet is inadequate. An inadequate diet is the dominant cause of folate deficiency and, indeed, in most patients with folate deficiency, a nutritional element is present. Folate deficiency is particularly common in countries with 'subsistence agriculture', e.g. India, where there is a marked seasonal variation in folate intake. Folate deficiency may occur in scurvy and kwashiorkor and in infants with repeated infections or fed solely on goats' milk which has a very low folate content. Dietary deficiency occurs also with old age, poverty, chronic invalids, psychiatric patients, and in some post-gastrectomy patients. The clinical features are discussed in Chapter 12.

Other causes of folate deficiency

Malabsorption of folate occurs in coeliac disease, dermatitis herpetiformis and tropical sprue. Low serum folate levels in patients receiving anticonvulsant therapy have been attributed to a reversible drug-induced malabsorption of folate but the mechanism of deficiency with these drugs remains to be established—inhibition of the action or synthesis of folate dependent enzymes and displacement of folate from its plasma transport proteins are alternative theories. Malabsorption may also contribute to folate deficiency in some patients following partial gastrectomy or jejunal resection.

Although anaemia in pregnancy is often due to multiple nutritional deficiencies, e.g. iron, folate and occasionally vitamin B_{12}, two thirds of anaemic pregnant women are folate deficient. Pregnancy increases severalfold the daily requirements for folate and most obstetricians give routine folic acid supplements. Clinical evidence has suggested that severe folate deficiency in pregnancy may be associated with complications other than anaemia, e.g. abortion and premature separation of the placenta.

The folate deficiency seen in liver disease is due to poor diet, impaired hepatic storage and increased urinary loss. Alcohol may have a direct inhibitory effect on folate metabolism.

Differential diagnosis and treatment

Once it is known that an anaemia is megaloblastic and whether vitamin B_{12} or folate deficiency is responsible, the cause of the deficiency must be found. The clinical history may offer an immediate answer, e.g. past gastrointestinal surgery or an inadequate diet.

Vitamin B_{12}. Vitamin B_{12} deficiency from whatever cause, is corrected and body stores of vitamin B_{12} replenished with six intramuscular injections of 1000 μg hydroxocobalamin given at intervals over two to three weeks. In pernicious anaemia and most other causes of vitamin B_{12} deficiency, therapy is needed for life; 500 μg or 1000 μg hydroxocobalamin is given once every three months.

Folic acid. Once vitamin B_{12} deficiency has been excluded as the cause of the megaloblastic anaemia 5 to 15 mg folic acid daily by mouth for a few days is sufficient to saturate body stores of folate (about 10 mg) in all patients, even those with malabsorption of the vitamin. The dose is continued for four months to ensure that the red cells are replete with folate. The decision about maintenance therapy depends on whether the cause of the deficiency can be corrected; such measures as improved diet, a gluten-free diet for coeliac disease, or the end of a pregnancy, may mean that the deficiency is unlikely to recur.

The severely ill case. When a patient is admitted to hospital with megaloblastic anaemia and heart failure or a severe infection it is often mandatory to give both vitamin B_{12} and folic acid in large doses immediately after the initial blood count, bone marrow aspiration and blood withdrawal for vitamin B_{12} and folate assays. Heart failure should be managed in the usual way with digoxin and diuretics and antibiotic therapy instituted after cultures have been taken if infection is present. Whenever possible, transfusion should be avoided, particularly in the elderly, since death from circulatory overload is possible in patients who have adjusted to the slowly progressive anaemia. However, if urgent surgery is required, or the patient is in late pregnancy or if severe anaemia is causing dangerous cardiac problems, transfusion may be necessary; one or two units of plasma reduced cells should be administered slowly, possibly with the simultaneous removal of an equivalent amount of blood from the other arm and with careful monitoring for signs of heart failure.

Because fatal hypokalaemia has occurred during the initial response of megaloblastic anaemia to therapy it may be prudent to give oral potassium during the first week of therapy to patients with heart failure or with initial hypokalaemia.

OTHER NUTRITIONAL ANAEMIAS

Other nutritional anaemias may occur, the most important being those found in conjunction with scurvy, severe protein deficiency and riboflavin deficiency. They are considered in Chapter 12.

SIDEROBLASTIC ANAEMIA

Sideroblastic anaemia presents as a hypochromic or dimorphic anaemia which is refractory to iron therapy. Bone marrow examination reveals increased iron stores and characteristic 'ring sideroblasts'. In the primary form, sideroblastic anaemia may be inherited as a sex-linked condition which occurs in males only or it may be acquired. Approximately one-third of patients respond to pyridoxine with or without the addition of folic acid. Secondary forms of sideroblastic anaemia may be associated with drugs (including isoniazid and cycloserine), alcohol, other haematological disorders, particularly the myeloproliferative disorders, and occasionally with carcinoma and other conditions. In some of these conditions the anaemia is reversible if the underlying cause, e.g. alcohol or antituberculous chemotherapy, is removed. In some secondary cases the sideroblastic changes may disappear with pyridoxine and/or folic acid therapy. General tissue iron overload complicates this disorder, especially in patients who need regular blood transfusion or have received large quantities of iron tablets before the correct diagnosis was made.

SECONDARY ANAEMIAS

The secondary anaemias form the largest group of anaemias seen in clinical practice. Causative disorders include infections, connective tissue disorders, malignancy, endocrine and liver disorders and renal failure. These anaemias respond to the alleviation of the causative disease; standard haematinics such as iron, folic acid and vitamin B_{12} usually have little effect.

Anaemia of chronic disorders

Three components appear to contribute to the pathogenesis of the normochromic or hypochromic normocytic anaemia which occurs in patients with chronic inflammation or malignant disease: (i) reduced iron release from reticuloendothelial stores; (ii) an inadequate erythropoietin response to the anaemia; and (iii) a reduced red cell survival. Both serum iron and total iron binding capacity are low, serum ferritin is usually normal; bone marrow iron stores are adequate but siderotic granulation of erythroblasts is reduced. The severity of anaemia is proportional to the activity of the underlying disease and if the haemoglobin is less than 9·0 g/dl there is likely to be an additional cause for the observed anaemia such as associated haemorrhage, iron or folate deficiency, marrow infiltration or haemolysis.

Anaemia in endocrine disease

Anaemia is found in most patients with hypothyroidism. In some this is due to associated pernicious anaemia or iron deficiency. In hypopituitarism the mild anaemia is probably principally due to reduced erythropoiesis and responds to replacement therapy with thyroxine, corticosteroids and androgens which raise the basal metabolic rate and may also act as direct marrow stimulants. The mild anaemia found in Addison's disease responds to corticosteroids.

Anaemia in hepatic cirrhosis

Many factors may contribute to the anaemia seen in patients with hepatic cirrhosis. Blood loss may result from bleeding oesophageal varices or from the haemostatic defects of reduced coagulation factors and thrombocytopenia. Hypersplenism, folate deficiency and a reduction in red cell survival may occur. Alcohol has a direct toxic action on bone marrow and megaloblastic change associated with folate deficiency or sideroblastic anaemia is also seen in heavy drinkers. The blood film in cirrhosis is usually macrocytic and variable numbers of 'target' cells or acanthocytic red cells are frequently present. In Zieve's syndrome a self-limiting acute haemolytic episode associated with hyperlipidaemia is observed following a period of sustained alcoholic intake.

Anaemia of renal disease

Both acute and chronic renal failure are accompanied by an anaemia which is due to a reduced erythropoietic response and to shortened red cell survival. In many patients blood loss, infection, iron and folate deficiency and microangiopathic haemolytic anaemia may complicate the issue. Patients undergoing regular haemodialysis require prophylactic iron therapy and those with folate deficiency require folic acid as well.

HAEMOLYTIC ANAEMIAS

Haemolytic anaemias are defined as those anaemias which result from an increase in the rate of red cell destruction. Jaundice, splenomegaly, characteristic red cell changes, e.g. spherocytes, and fragmented red cells, and an increase in absolute reticulocyte levels above $200 \times 10^9/l$, are findings that suggest active haemolysis. Because of the erythropoietic hyperplasia which accompanies chronic haemolytic anaemia the rate of red cell destruction may need to be increased severalfold before the patient becomes anaemic. Definitive diagnosis of the type of haemolytic anaemia often requires detailed laboratory tests and in patients who present acutely with severe anaemia it is important to initiate these tests before transfusing since dilution of the patient's red cells with donor red cells may delay an accurate diagnosis. The life span of the normal red cell is 120 days; in haemolytic anaemia a variable shortening occurs and in severe haemolysis the cells survive only a few days. If serious doubt about haemolysis exists, a [^{51}Cr] chromium labelled red cell survival study may be needed.

Anaesthetists meet patients with haemolytic anaemia when splenectomy is recommended. There is a likelihood of continuing high platelet counts and consequent risk of thromboembolism in those cases whose haemolysis is not cured by the operation and in infancy and early childhood splenectomy carries with it an increased risk of serious infection. As well as the management of anaemia anaesthetists need to remember that some patients, e.g. those with autoimmune haemolytic anaemia may be receiving steroid therapy. Gallstones are frequently a problem in chronic haemolysis and cholecystectomy is sometimes necessary. The hazards of anaesthesia in the presence of sickle-cell disease are now well-known and many hospitals insist on screening patients of Negro origins or from the Eastern Mediterranean, Middle East and Indian subcontinent for this possibility before an anaesthetic is given. Glucose-6-phosphate dehydrogenase (G6PD) deficiency is also widespread in populations where the sickle-cell gene is prevalent and haemolysis in this condition may be triggered by many drugs. A classification of the more important haemolytic anaemias is given in Table 11.5.

Table 11.5. Haemolytic anaemias.

Hereditary red cell defects—1 *Membrane*, e.g. hereditary spherocytosis
                                          hereditary elliptocytosis
                      2 *Metabolism*, e.g. G6PD deficiency
                                          pyruvate kinase deficiency
                      3 *Haemoglobin*, e.g. sickle cell disorders
                                          unstable haemoglobins
                                          thalassaemic disorders
Acquired membrane defects—Paroxysmal nocturnal haemoglobinuria
Extracorpuscular abnormality—Immune haemolytic anaemias, e.g. autoimmune
                                          drug induced
                                          haemolytic disease of the newborn
                                          isoimmune transfusion reaction
                      Red cell fragmentation syndromes
                      Hypersplenism
                      Miscellaneous—Drugs, chemicals, toxins and infections

---

DISORDERS OF RED CELL MEMBRANE

Hereditary spherocytosis

Hereditary spherocytosis is inherited as an autosomal dominant but the degree of expression is remarkably variable. Although most patients present in childhood or early adult life with anaemia and jaundice, occasionally the condition remains undetected until later years. The diagnosis is suspected when spherocytes are detected during blood film examination and confirmed by finding a negative direct antiglobulin (Coombs') test, an increase in red cell osmotic fragility and increased autohaemolysis which shows partial correction with glucose. Infections, particularly viral, may precipitate haemolytic or aplastic crises and the increased bilirubin load of chronic haemolysis may be associated with pigment gallstones, cholelithiasis and biliary obstruction. Mild degrees of haemolysis may cause marked jaundice in patients who are congenitally unable to deal with the bilirubin load, e.g. with Gilbert's disease.

Splenectomy invariably relieves the anaemia though spherocytes remain, albeit with less marked forms. Even if the disease is mild, the operation can be recommended in patients with clinical jaundice, continuous anaemia or a history of aplastic crises both to reduce the risk of gallstone formation and to improve general health. As splenectomy in infancy is associated with an increase in morbidity and mortality from bacterial infections, particularly pneumococcal, the operation should be delayed until the child is at least six and preferably until the later years of childhood.

Hereditary elliptocytosis

Hereditary elliptocytosis or familial ovalocytosis is also inherited as an autosomal dominant with variable expression. No treatment is necessary for most patients as haemolysis is either absent or mild. In occasional patients with overt haemolytic anaemia, splenectomy should be performed; the consequent reduction in haemolysis, although considerable, is somewhat less than in hereditary spherocytosis.

HAEMOLYTIC ANAEMIAS DUE TO DEFECTIVE RED CELL METABOLISM

Glucose-6-phosphate dehydrogenase deficiency

Numerous variants of the enzyme glucose-6-phosphate dehydrogenase (G6PD) have been characterized and many are associated with less activity than the 'normal' Western or type B G6PD. The principal racial groups affected are West African, Mediterranean and South East Asian but sporadic G6PD deficiency occurs in all populations. The inheritance is sex-linked, affecting mainly males in the hemizygous state. The dominant problem is acute *drug-induced haemolytic anaemia*. *Favism* (haemolytic sensitivity to the broad bean *vicia fava*), *hereditary nonspherocytic haemolytic anaemia* and *neonatal jaundice* are other manifestations of particular types of G6PD deficiency.

Bacterial and viral infections, diabetic acidosis and other acute illnesses, may also trigger haemolysis in G6PD deficient subjects. A large number of drugs have been associated with acute haemolytic anaemia in G6PD deficiency (Table 11.6). These drugs or their metabolites are usually oxidant compounds related to the 8-amino-quinolines or derived from an aniline base. Because the normal reduction of methaemo-globin is impaired in this condition, prilocaine is contraindicated. The clinical picture is of rapidly occurring intravascular haemolysis but the severity is partly determined by the nature of the enzyme variant: Negroes with the A-type of deficiency often suffer from less severe anaemia than that observed in the rarer variants found in Northern Europeans. The anaemia improves rapidly following cessation of the offending drug but in Negroes with the A- deficiency, even with continuation of the offending drug, the haemolytic anaemia is self-limiting because the young red cells produced in response to haemolysis have near normal G6PD activity and resist haemolysis. Patients presenting with symptoms from severe anaemia must be treated with red cell trans-fusions. Adequate fluid intake is important as high urine volumes should be maintained during crises of intravascular haemolysis.

Haemolytic anaemias caused by other metabolic defects

Patients with rare deficiencies of other enzymes associated with the pentose phosphate pathway, e.g. *glutathione reductase deficiency*, *glutathione peroxidase deficiency* and

Table 11.6. Agents which may cause haemolytic anaemia in G6PD-deficient patients.

Analgesics	*Sulphonamides and Sulphones*
Phenacetin	Sulphanilamide
Paracetamol	Sulphapyridine
Aminopyrine	Sulphadimidine
Acetanilide	Sulphafurazole
	Sulphacetamide
Antibacterial Agents	Salazosulphapyridine (salazopyrine)
	Sulphamethoxazole*
Nitrofurans—Nitrofurantoin	Dapsone
—Nitrofurazone	Aldesulphone
—Furaxolidone	Thiazosulphone
Penicillin	Glucosulphone
Chloramphenicol	
p-Aminosalicylic acid	*Miscellaneous*
Streptomycin	
Isoniazid	Prilocaine
Nalidixic acid	Stibophen
	Probenicid
Antimalarials	Dimercaprol (BAL)
	Naphthalene (moth balls)
Primaquine	Vitamin K (water soluble analogues)
Pamaquine	Quinidine
Quinacrine	Methylene blue
Quinine	Arsine
Chloroquine	Phenylhydrazine
Pyrimethamine	Acetylphenylhydrazine
	Trinitrotoluene
	Fava beans and other vegetables

* Combined with trimethoprim as 'Septrin' or 'Bactrin'.
N.B. Aminoquinolines and aniline-base derived drugs are always a risk.

glutathione deficiency may also present with an acute haemolytic anaemia following exposure to oxidant drugs.

Inherited defects of enzymes in the glycolytic pathway usually result in hereditary (nonspherocytic) haemolytic anaemia. *Pyruvate kinase* (PK) deficiency which is inherited as an autosomal recessive is the most frequently encountered disorder of this type. PK deficient patients tolerate moderate anaemia particularly well as there is an increased delivery of oxygen to the tissues due to the build up of the glycolytic intermediate 2, 3 diphosphoglycerate in PK deficient red cells which causes a shift to the right of the haemoglobin oxygen dissociation curve. However, in severe disease, symptoms of anaemia occur, and regular red cell transfusions may be required. Splenectomy results in only a partial improvement in the degree of anaemia.

Other enzyme deficiencies causing a congenital nonspherocytic haemolytic anaemia include those of *triose phosphate isomerase, phosphoglycerate kinase, hexokinase and diphosphoglycerate mutase*, and in the first two of these a serious neurological disorder may be present due to lack of the enzyme in tissues other than red cells.

ABNORMALITIES OF HAEMOGLOBIN STRUCTURE OR SYNTHESIS

Anaemia may result either from the synthesis of an abnormal haemoglobin (the haemoglobin variants or haemoglobinopathies) or from the defective synthesis of normal haemoglobin (the thalassaemia disorders). A very large number of haemoglobin disorders have now been discovered and characterized [27]. If the haemoglobin variant becomes insoluble under conditions of hypoxia an increase in red cell rigidity may produce haemolytic anaemia, e.g. Hb S and Hb C diseases.

Instability of the haemoglobin molecule may result in congenital Heinz body anaemia (unstable haemoglobin disease), e.g. Hb Koln, Hb Hammersmith, Hb Bristol; or a proneness to oxidant drug induced haemolysis, e.g. Hb Zurich, Hb Gun Hill. The haemoglobin variant may also produce clinical effects by altered function of the haemoglobin molecule: oxidation of the haem ferrous atom to ferric may be associated with congenital cyanosis and methaemoglobinaemia, e.g. the haemoglobin M's of Boston, Iwate, Hyde Park, Saskatoon; alteration of the oxygen affinity of the molecule produces congenital polycythaemia, e.g. haemoglobins Chesapeake, Kempsey, Yakima and Ranier.

Successful management depends on establishing a specific diagnosis by measurement of haemoglobin A_2 and F, heat stability, O_2 dissociation, electrophoretic, sickling and other studies of the patient's haemoglobin and, if possible, of the haemoglobins of the parents and siblings.

Homozygous haemoglobin C, D and E states produce mild haemolytic states with target cells. No treatment is needed. The unstable haemoglobin disorders are rare, and splenectomy in some of these patients is of benefit [46].

Sickle-cell disorders

The abnormal haemoglobin (Hb S) in the sickle-cell disorders may be found in association with more or less equal amounts of normal adult haemoglobin (Hb A) in the heterozygous state designated sickle-cell trait or Hb AS. The homozygous state or sickle-cell anaemia (Hb SS) is generally the most hazardous of the disorders. Combinations of the sickle-cell gene with Hb C, sickle-cell C disease (Hb SC) or with thalassaemia, sickle-cell thalassaemia (Hb S-thal) may also give rise to severe disease.

The special characteristic of Hb S is its tendency to form tactoid 'crystals' when exposed to low oxygen tensions, which result in altering the red cell into a sickle shape (sickling) in which form the cells increase blood viscosity and may 'clump' causing an infarctive crisis. They also possess a shortened life span and are liable to rupture. The degree of sickling is roughly proportional to the concentration of Hb S in the cell for any given (lowered) oxygen tension and pH. Thus in sickle-cell anaemia (HbSS) when the Hb S fraction may be 90 per cent, the cells will sickle at a Po_2 of approximately 5·6 kPa (40 mmHg) while in sickle-cell trait (Hb AS) with a Hb S concentration of, say, 40 per cent, sickling may not occur significantly until an oxygen tension of 2·8 kPa (20 mmHg) is reached. When it is remembered that the normal mixed venous Po_2 is about 5·6 kPa (40 mmHg) and that some organ venous tensions are considerably lower it is not surprising that the cells of patient with sickle-cell anaemia are sickling chronically during his lifetime and conferring on him his chronic haemolytic anaemia.

Which patients should be sickle tested as a routine precaution before anaesthesia? It is generally agreed that all those of negro descent should be screened for the presence of HbS. It is understandable that in many developing regions, especially those where HbS is prevalent and clinically well-recognized, routine sickle testing is not performed. Subjects from the Balkans, North Africa, Middle East, Eastern Mediterrania and the Indian subcontinent may possess a sickle-cell haemoglobino-

12*

pathy. While Hb S is often detected in Arabian patients it is <u>rare in Indians</u> and because of the low yield of Hb S detection in the latter race many units have abandoned routine screening tests in these peoples. The answer to the question must therefore be that it must be left to the informed anaesthetist who will consider the probability of race incidence and the resources and experience of the environment in which he practices. If the patient proves to be 'sickle positive' electrophoretic genotyping must be performed in elective cases or when surgery is not urgent. When Hb S is found in a patient presenting with acute abdominal pain, the possibility of splenic or mesenteric infarct must be included in the differential diagnosis. If rapid screening facilities cannot be easily obtained from the laboratory, the anaesthetist must obtain a quick test such as the 'Sickledex' for his own use in theatre when emergencies present.

If the patient proves to be sickle positive and time does not permit genotyping the clinicians must, in addition to knowing the haemoglobin content of the blood, ask for a blood film examination. Should the haemoglobin content be near the normal and the film shows no cellular abnormalities, then the anaesthetist may proceed under the assumption of Hb AS. However, even when anaemia is absent, if cellular abnormalities are present in the blood film and surgery is required immediately, anaesthesia should proceed under the assumption of high hazard sickle haemoglobinopathy. This is because the anaemia of HbSS may be masked by dehydration and because Hb SC disease and Hb S thal. may not show significant anaemia. Tourniquets should be avoided in all sickle-cell disorders. When a tourniquet is considered essential for surgery, the limb must be maximally exsanguinated.

Sickle-cell trait

Although during normal life most patients with sickle-cell trait (Hb AS) usually require no treatment, infarctive and sequestration crises may occur at low oxygen tensions: <u>should not fly in unpressurized aircraft.</u>

It has been reported that these patients experience <u>sickling under general anaes-thesia for even simple surgery</u> [22, 25, 30] but when major thoracic operations are performed the risks are considerable [31]. Even so, with attention to detail it is possible to minimize these to acceptable proportions [23].

The sickle-cell trait (carrier) should be well <u>hydrated, warm</u> and free from inter-current <u>infection</u> when presenting for general anaesthesia. Premedication should not significantly disturb respiration or pre- and postoperative ambulation. Preoxygenation for several minutes should precede induction and the maintenance of anaesthesia should include a technique that gives the best assurance of oxygenation, clear airway and avoidance of circulatory stasis. Postanaesthetic oxygen therapy is essential until full clinical recovery, at least, has occurred. While many doctors might say that these recommendations comprise the recipe for any good anaesthetic, the anaesthetist will know that many patients dislike being faced with a mask and that to 'guarantee' an uncompromised airway may require endotracheal intubation.

Sickle-cell anaemia

The homozygous form of Hb S disease is characterized by a 'steady state' of chronic haemolysis which is interrupted by periodic crises. In the 'steady state' haemoglobin levels of <u>6 to 9 g/dl</u> are usual but patients tolerate this degree of anaemia well because Hb S has a <u>lower oxygen affinity</u> than Hb A.

General management is directed toward preventing and treating the periodic crises which tend to be more frequent in childhood. The aplastic, haemolytic, sequestration and infarctive crises which dominate the clinical course of sickle-cell disease require intensive treatment in hospital. Precipitating factors include infections, dehydration, exposure to cold, intense muscular activity, hypoxia and acidosis. Complications of the crises include pulmonary fibrosis, cardiac enlargement, hepatic necrosis, renal papillary necrosis and the nephrotic syndrome, aseptic bone necrosis and leg ulcers. The maintenance of high standards of nutrition, personal hygiene and housing are most important. Regular folate, 5 mg daily, reduces the frequency and severity of crises. Early identification and treatment of infections (often pneumococcal or salmonella) is essential. Because of their inability to concentrate urine, the patients are vulnerable to dehydration and early fluid replacement may avert an impending crisis.

Rest, analgesics, hydration and use of viscosity-reducing plasma volume expanders are mainstays of management of a crisis. Plasma-reduced red cell transfusions are only necessary if severe anaemia is causing symptoms. In very severe cases exchange transfusions may be more effective but these must be carried out with careful neutralization of citrate by calcium and control of blood pH, in an intensive care unit. The aim of transfusion should be to restore the patient's haemoglobin to the 'steady state' level of between 6 and 9 g/dl. Greater transfusion incurs the risk of crisis due to increased blood viscosity. Some workers, however, hold a more liberal attitude towards pre-operative blood transfusions [5]. In dehydrated patients an intravenous infusion of 5 per cent glucose is used; the increase of plasma volume helps prevent stagnation of sickled cells and isotonic glucose has its own antisickling effect. Administration of sodium bicarbonate to prevent and treat acidosis is of established value in the management of infarctive crises.

Anaesthesia. Surgery must be undertaken with reluctance and seldom as an urgent event because emergency operations are very risky. The patient should be in a 'steady phase', warm, hydrated and infection-free as a general preparation for elective surgery. The haemoglobin level should be corrected for major surgery if it is found to be below 7–8 g/dl. Plasma-reduced blood transfusion is desirable by slow delivery in the days leading up to operation, while during surgery fresh blood should be available to replace significant haemorrhage. For major abdominal or thoracic operations an exchange transfusion must be considered. Prophylactic broad spectrum antibiotic cover is necessary to minimize postoperative chest infections which may be disastrous. The position concerning pre- and pre-operative alkalinization is yet to be resolved. While it confers an antisickling environment, it results in a shift of the oxygen dissociation curve to the left so that the tissue cell may lose oxygen availability. However, experience of excellent functional recovery of exsanguinated animals following transfusion with 2,3 diphosphoglycerate (2,3DPG) depleted blood (with extremely low P50s) strongly suggests that the antisickling value of alkalinization (which also lowers the P50) greatly outweighs the somewhat theoretical disadvantage of impeding tissue oxygen delivery. Furthermore, the anaemic sickler has red cells enriched with 2,3DPG which already places his oxygen–haemoglobin dissociation curve well to the right. Therefore, it may be wise to infuse isotonic bicarbonate at about 3 m mol per kg/hour during surgery as a compromise.

Premedication should avoid respiratory depression. Preoxygenation should always precede induction followed by endotracheal intubation and controlled moderate hyperventilation with nitrous oxide–oxygen mixtures (30 per cent oxygen is optimal) and a judicious dose of halothane to promote vasodilation without causing significant hypotension. Body warmth, hydration and circulation must be well maintained and renal output kept up. Accordingly heat-retaining blankets, dextran, mannitol and fruse-mide are usefully employed.

Controlled oxygen therapy must be continued well into the postoperative period, especially following abdominal or thoracic surgery. Early ambulation, chest physio-therapy and control of chest infection are essential. It is noteworthy that morbidity and mortality have a much greater incidence in the postoperative period than during the course of anaesthesia [20]. Regional nerve blocks and local infiltrations should be used where applicable instead of general anaesthesia but tourniquets and blood stasis should be avoided.

Pregnancy is a major risk. In the past the associated maternal death rate has been approximately 10 per cent and the fetal and neonatal mortality has approached 50 per cent. Regular folate therapy is essential and early treatment should be instituted for such complications as toxaemia and pyelonephritis. The possible advantage of partial exchange transfusions during the later months of pregnancy is currently being evaluated. Difficult and prolonged labour must be avoided at all costs.

Sickle-cell C disease and sickle-cell thalassaemia

In general terms, the recommendations laid out for Hb SS pertain to these conditions if they are associated with high Hb S concentrations, abnormalities in the blood film and anaemia. These patients may possess no normal Hb A and may have a similar tendency to sickle as Hb SS in the presence of hypoxia. However, the sickle cell thalassaemic red cell contains a significant percentage of Hb F. This protects against sickling because its greater affinity for oxygen effectively maintains a store of oxygen within each red cell. This may be transferred to the Hb S molecules if they become deoxygenated during exposure to low oxygen tensions. On the other hand, the existence of Hb C with Hb S within the erythrocyte promotes sickling because Hb C is relatively insoluble and readily precipitates to disturb the intracellular environment.

Management of the out-patient 'sickler'

The ambulant day case or out-patient who presents for anaesthesia and is found to be 'sickle positive' on a screening test deserves special consideration. Full genotyping and general haematological survey is essential, because hospital admission is indicated in the high risk case requiring general anaesthesia. When sickle trait is confirmed and local analgesia for the proposed surgery is not relevant, a full appraisal of the patient's general condition and the type of surgery intended is necessary before deciding to embark on a general anaesthetic. The sickle trait patient requiring treatment for a dental abscess is a typical example of the dilemma facing the anaesthetist. Interim antibiotic therapy which controls the infection may allow subsequent extraction under local analgesia. Where a general anaesthetic appears the only answer, management should be undertaken within a hospital department where suitable resources are readily available [21].

The thalassaemia disorders

While of widespread distribution, they are found mainly in the Mediterranean, Middle and Far East and comprise some of the more complicated genetic haematological conditions [45]. Normal adult haemoglobin (Hb A) contains two α and two β polypeptide globin chains while fetal haemoglobin (Hb F) contains two α and two γ chains. The thalassaemic disorder is a failure to produce normal quantities of either the α chains (α-thalassaemia), or the β chains (β-thalassaemia). In each type, the failure of the one chain production leads to excess of the other chain, resulting in imbalance, the excess fraction precipitating.

α-Thalassaemia

The most severe homozygous form of α-thalassaemia, which is seen predominantly in South East Asia, is incompatible with life beyond the late fetal stage and the condition results in stillborn hydropic fetuses. Excess γ chain is generated resulting in γ_4 haemoglobin molecules (Hb Barts). There is no effective treatment. Patients with haemoglobin H disease, a less severe form of homozygous α-thalassaemia in which β chain excess is generated resulting in β_4 molecules (Hb H), commonly present with moderate anaemia. They may also experience severe haemolysis when taking drugs similar to those which cause haemolysis in G6PD deficient patients. α-Thalassaemic subjects may be managed in the same way as those suffering from the β variety.

Homozygous β-thalassaemia

This condition is also known as Thalassaemia major, Cooley's anaemia or Mediterranean anaemia. Most patients with homozygous β-thalassaemia have severe disease and survival beyond the first few decades is uncommon. The very severe anaemia often requires regular transfusions to sustain life. Growth retardation, iron overload and hypersplenism are dominant clinical problems.

Excess free α chain precipitates to form insoluble inclusions and Heinz bodies in red cells and erythroblasts leading to severe haemolysis, and a compensatory marrow hyperplasia often produces bone erosion and overgrowth. Hepatosplenomegaly may be gross. The peripheral blood film shows prominent erythroblastosis and reticulocytosis with marked red cell polychromasia, hypochromia, targetting, anisocytosis poikilocytosis and stippling. Much of the functional haemoglobin in adult life persists as Hb F. Indeed up to 90 per cent may be of the fetal variety. In severe disease regular blood transfusions are given to maintain Hb over 8 g/dl. Recently iron chelation therapy has been introduced to prevent or reduce iron overload. Desferrioxamine is given by daily subcutaneous infusions (1–4 g over 8–12 hours) and added to each unit of blood transfused (2 g). Daily vitamin C increases the excretion of iron. Splenectomy is recommended in older children to reduce blood transfusions.

Both liver and renal failure occur and heart muscle is often damaged by haemosiderin deposits. Although severely anaemic, patients retain a high blood volume and compensate for their oxygen capacity deficit by maintaining a hyperdynamic circulation. Patients are very prone to infection, especially if neutropenic, and to bleeding, if there is appreciable thrombocytopenia.

Before splenectomy or surgery for some coincidental disease the patient should be transfused to achieve a Hb level of about 10 g/dl.

Some cases of homozygous B thalassaemia are mild (Hb 7–10 g/dl) and do not require repeated transfusions.

β-Thalassaemia trait

Patients with the heterozygous form of β-thalassaemia are usually symptomless. They may present with a mild hypochromic anaemia, or they may be detected during studies of relatives of patients suffering from thalassaemia. Occasionally during pregnancy or infection the severity of the anaemia may increase. β-Thalassaemia trait may be differentiated from iron deficiency by finding, in nearly all cases, raised haemoglobin F or haemoglobin A_2 and normal serum iron and transferrin levels. Iron therapy is contraindicated.

Hb C-thalassaemia is a relatively mild condition while Hb S-thalassaemia may give rise to serious problems and is discussed under the sickle haemoglobinopathies above.

Paroxysmal nocturnal haemoglobinuria

Paroxysmal nocturnal haemoglobinuria (PNH) is due to an acquired defect of the red cell membrane which renders it abnormally sensitive to lysis by complement [17, 36]. Platelets and granulocytes are also sensitive to complement. The diagnosis is confirmed by finding a positive acidified serum lysis test. This condition may occur alone, in patients who have aplastic anaemia or a previous history of marrow hypoplasia and in association with myelosclerosis [10]. The chronic intravascular haemolysis is classically maximal during sleep and episodes of enhanced haemolysis occur during infections.

There is no specific treatment available. *Red cell transfusions* are reserved for those patients with severe anaemia. To reduce the risk of increasing haemolysis during transfusion, donor red cells must be washed three times in saline to remove the complement in the donor's plasma. Iron deficiency commonly develops as a result of the constant haemosiderinuria and iron therapy may produce a partial improvement in the anaemia. Splenectomy has no influence on the degree of haemolysis. All operations are dangerous and should be avoided if possible; there is an unacceptable post-operative mortality from massive venous thrombosis and pulmonary emboli.

IMMUNE HAEMOLYTIC ANAEMIAS

Immune haemolytic anaemias are caused by antibodies reacting against antigens present on the red cell surface or by the absorption of antigen-antibody complexes to the red cell surface. A positive direct antiglobulin (Coombs') test is the hallmark of these conditions (see p. 568).

Autoimmune haemolytic anaemia (AIHA)

In autoimmune haemolytic anaemia, the body reacts against its own red cell surface antigens. In many instances this event occurs during another illness such as infections, lymphoproliferative or connective tissue disorders. More frequently no other disease is found and these acquired haemolytic anaemias are referred to as 'idiopathic' [11].

'Warm' AIHA

When the free antibodies in serum and on the surface of the red cells are best detected at 37°C the condition is referred to as the 'warm type' AIHA. When only the IgG subclass of immunoglobin coats the red cells, destruction occurs mainly in the spleen.

However, when complement fixation occurs, the whole reticuloendothelial system takes part in red cell destruction and, rarely, in severe cases there may be intravascular lysis.

High dose steroid therapy is the initial treatment. Splenectomy is considered in all patients who fail to respond to steroids and in those patients who require maintenance therapy of more than 15 mg prednisolone daily. Best results are obtained in those patients with an IgG only coating of the red cells and patients in whom ^{51}Cr surface counting studies have identified dominant splenic red cell destruction. The value of immunosuppressive therapy is not well established.

'Cold' AIHA

Patients are described as having 'cold type' AIHA when serological investigations indicate that their antibodies combine optimally with the red cell antigens at 4°C with progressively less affinity at higher temperatures. These cold agglutinins are usually IgM and the antiglobulin test is positive due to complement on the red cell surface.

The acute haemolytic anaemias seen rarely in *Mycoplasma pneumoniae* infections and infectious mononucleosis are of this cold antibody type. Although occasionally associated with a malignant lymphoma, chronic cold agglutinin disease in the majority of patients is 'idiopathic'. Exposure to the cold produces recurrent episodes of intravascular haemolysis, haemoglobinuria and Raynaud's phenomenon. Red cells for transfusion should be washed since, as in PNH, it is essential to avoid giving donor complement components. Splenectomy and corticosteroids are of little or no value. Alkylating agents, e.g. chlorambucil or cyclophosphamide, have improved some patients with severe disease.

Drug-induced immune haemolytic anaemia

Enquiry into recent drug therapy should be made in all patients who present with an immune haemolytic anaemia. Although the documented list of drugs causing immune haemolysis is small it is expected that many further drugs will be incriminated in the future. In the haemolytic anaemia associated with high dose *penicillin* therapy a haptenic mechanism is operative. Haemolysis is mediated by an IgG antibody directed against penicillin attached to the red cell membrane. *Phenacetin, quinidine, quinine, stibophen, para-aminosalicylic acid, izoniazid* and *chlorpromazine* have also been associated with haemolysis which is drug-dependent and ceases rapidly when the drugs are discontinued. With these drugs an attachment of an IgM or IgG antibody-drug complex to the red cell membrane triggers haemolysis through complement fixation. Blood transfusions may be required for symptomatic relief.

In the autoimmune haemolytic anaemia associated with *methyldopa* the autoantibodies which have an anti-Rh specificity may be detected with normal cells without the addition of the drug. Although 20 per cent of patients taking this drug develop a positive direct antiglobulin test only 0·5 per cent show evidence of overt haemolytic anaemia. The drug should be discontinued only in the exceptional patients with haemolytic anaemia. Severely affected patients may require blood transfusion and corticosteroid therapy. The haemolysis usually ceases a few weeks after discontinuing the methyldopa, though the direct antiglobin test may remain positive for 12–18 months. The development of similar autoantibodies with positive antiglobulin tests have also been described in patients taking *mefenamic acid, indomethacin, hydantoins, methysergide* and *L-dopa* [47].

Haemolytic disease of the newborn

Feto-maternal Rhesus D (Rh D) incompatibility is by far the most important cause of isoimmune haemolytic disease of the newborn. Maternal antibodies directed against other antigens of the Rhesus, Kell, Duffy or Kidd blood group systems are rare causes and occasionally IgG anti-A or anti-B may cross the placenta to haemolyse fetal red cells.

Prevention of Rh D sensitization. Passive immunization of previously unsensitized Rh negative mothers by injecting Rh immune globulin within 72 hours of their giving birth to a Rh positive infant has been responsible for a dramatic fall in incidence of Rhesus haemolytic disease of the newborn. Delivery is the time of greatest risk of sensitization from the feto-maternal leakage of red cells and the protection offered by passive immunization is greater than 90 per cent.

Treatment of Rhesus Disease. In sensitized Rh D negative women antenatal antibody screening, tests on the husband for Rh D homozygosity and measurement of bilirubin peaks in fluid obtained by amniocentesis, have all contributed to more accurate predictions of prognosis and better management. A maternal antibody titre of 1 in 16 or more is usually taken as the need to examine amniotic fluid.

Intrauterine transfusions. Have been associated with a salvage of 50 per cent of severely affected fetuses. Depending upon the anticipated severity, delivery is planned two to four weeks before term. *Exchange transfusions* are given at birth for severe anaemia and repeated, if necessary, to prevent kernicterus. In affected infants, small top-up transfusions are occasionally required two to six weeks after delivery.

Haemolytic transfusion reactions

Most severe immediate haemolytic transfusion reactions are the result of ABO incompatibility. More rarely, IgM antibodies directed against other blood group antigens may be the cause. Severe haemolytic reactions are accompanied by pain along the vein into which the blood is being transfused, flushing of the face, feelings of head throbbing and chest constriction and lumbar pain. Tachycardia, hypotension, urticaria, peripheral circulatory collapse, rigors and pyrexia accompany these symptoms. Many of these reactions are abolished by anaesthesia. Either a fall in blood pressure or an increase in pulse rate may warn the anaesthetist but often the first sign of a haemolytic transfusion reaction in an anaesthetized patient is bleeding at a previously dry operation site. The clinical presentation of transfusion reactions due to Rhesus incompatibility or other IgG mediated reactions is less severe. The diagnosis is confirmed by finding a positive direct antiglobulin test on samples taken from the patient at the time of the reaction and in severe reactions there will be marked haemoglobinaemia.

Apart from stopping the offending transfusion, treatment must be directed towards maintaining the circulating blood volume; plasma volume expanders are given until further compatible blood becomes available and an intravenous injection of a corticosteroid and an appropriate antihistamine may prove beneficial. An infusion of 500 ml of 10 per cent mannitol and the administration of sodium bicarbonate are believed to reduce the risk of anuria following severe haemolytic reactions. If *in vitro* haemostasis testing indicates the presence of disseminated intravascular coagulation, heparin therapy and platelet transfusions should be considered.

With less severe and delayed haemolytic transfusion reactions urgent treatment is not required. However, many patients will require further transfusion with compatible blood.

Other immediate transfusion reactions

The infusion of *infected blood* results in symptoms similar to those described for ABO incompatibility with profound shock, hypotension, vomiting and frequently widespread bleeding from disseminated intravascular coagulation. The fatality rate is 50–80 per cent. Immediate diagnosis is essential and Gram stains should be performed on smears made from the plasma of the infected blood. The causative organisms are usually endotoxin-producing pseudomonads, coliform or achromobacteria which are capable of growing at low temperatures. Treatment includes restoration of the blood volume with compatible fresh blood transfusion, intravenous methyl prednisolone, inotropic agents, e.g. dopamine, high doses of appropriate antibiotics, e.g. gentamycin and metronidazole, and intravenous heparin if disseminated intravascular coagulation is present. If the patient survives the initial few hours it is likely that further management will include the treatment of acute renal failure.

The febrile reactions which were caused by the transfusion of bacterial pyrogens are now rare because of the widespread use of disposable sterile plastic transfusion sets. Rises of temperature to 40°C accompanied by headache may be the result of white cell or platelet incompatibility. White cell and platelet isoantibodies are generally not found until the patient has had many transfusions or pregnancies. Although these reactions may be unpleasant they are rarely serious; aspirin therapy and slowing the drip-rate may allow completion of the transfusion. The use of washed red cells, or leucocyte filters may diminish or prevent such reactions.

Very rarely anaphylactic reactions occur in patients lacking IgA who have a potent anti-IgA in their plasma which reacts with donor IgA. Immediate treatment with subcutaneous adrenaline 1 mg (1 ml of 1:1000), intravenous hydrocortisone (100 mg or more) and an intravenous antihistamine is indicated. In such patients, repeatedly washed red cells have still invoked reactions and full protection may be provided only by transfusing blood from rare donors lacking IgA.

Red cell fragmentation syndromes

Red cell fragmentation haemolytic anaemias are caused by physical injury to circulating red cells by abnormal surfaces or fibrin deposition in large or small blood vessels. The haemolytic anaemias associated with malfunctioning heart valves or patch grafts may continue until surgical correction of the 'bare' surface is carried out. Microangiopathic haemolytic anaemia occurs in association with such diverse conditions as bacterial septicaemias (particularly Gram-negative or meningococcal), abruptio placenta, mucin-secreting adenocarcinomas, malignant hypertension, the haemolytic uraemic syndrome, and in thrombotic thrombocytopenic purpura. The haemolytic anaemia is often of secondary importance in these conditions and treatment must be first directed against the primary disorder. When the red cell fragmentation is associated with disseminated intravascular coagulation it remains controversial whether or not heparin therapy is beneficial [33].

Hypersplenism

Anaemia is common in patients with massive splenomegaly from any cause. Contributing factors include splenic red cell pooling, the dilutional element of the associated increase in plasma volume and a moderate haemolytic component.

The hyperplastic enlargement of the spleen in many primary haemolytic disorders may itself contribute to the pathogenesis of the observed anaemia. In patients receiving regular transfusions for aplastic or refractory anaemias, progressive splenic enlargement may be responsible for increased transfusion requirements. Neutropenia and thrombocytopenia are usually present and the relative severity of the cytopenias depends to some extent on the nature of the underlying disease.

A reduction in splenic size by appropriate therapy, e.g. cytotoxic drugs or radiation for myeloproliferative or lymphoproliferative disorders; treatment directed towards malaria, Leishmaniasis, brucellosis or tuberculosis; and portosystemic anastomosis for portal hypertension, may all produce considerable relief of anaemia. The place of splenectomy in the management of some of the primary haemolytic anaemias has already been mentioned. Splenectomy may also alleviate anaemia, neutropenia and thrombocytopenia in nonhaematological disorders associated with splenomegaly, e.g. lipid-storage diseases, sarcoidosis and Felty's syndrome, and reduce the need for transfusion in patients with refractory or hypoplastic anaemia and associated splenomegaly.

Miscellaneous haemolytic anaemias

Haemolytic anaemias may be caused by extensive burns, chemical poisoning e.g. chlorates, drug overdoses, clostridial and bartonella infections, malaria and following snake and spider bites. The treatment in these conditions is directed primarily towards elimination of the causal agent and the prevention of shock and renal failure by well-judged blood transfusion and fluid replacement. Carefully controlled exchange transfusions should be considered in moribund patients with haemolytic anaemias associated with circulating toxic agents.

MISCELLANEOUS HAEMOGLOBIN VARIANTS

Whenever haemoglobin is in a form other than its oxygenated or unoxygenated state, the molecule is unavailable for oxygen transport. Although such haemoglobin states rarely produce a functional anaemia of significant proportions they may be considered conveniently under this section.

Methaemoglobin (Met Hb)

This is continuously formed and reduced in the normal subject during the process of haemoglobin deoxygenation. An abnormal state of methaemoglobinaemia exists when circulating concentrations exceed 2 per cent of the total haemoglobin. Such occasions arise when congenital aminoacid substitutions occur in the polypeptide chains of the molecule and render haemoglobin stable in the ferric form—as already noted in the Hb M discussion earlier. Alternatively, abnormal methaemoglobinaemia may occur if either of the Met Hb reduction enzyme systems is either congenitally deficient or overloaded. The direct reduction system is NADH diaphorase and the shunt system relies on G6PD. The latter route is blocked by prilocaine metabolites, phenacetin, etc., while either system may be overloaded by oxidizing drugs (e.g. higher oxides of nitrogen). Central cyanosis is apparent at about $1\cdot5$ g/dl (10 per cent Met Hb).

The condition may be reversed with weak acids such as ascorbic acid or methylene blue.

Sulphaemoglobin

This variant is not normally present but is also created by oxidizing agents such as sulphonamide and phenacetin. Unlike Met Hb it cannot be reversed to normal haemoglobin and requires red cell destruction and subsequent excretion.

Carboxyhaemoglobin (HbCO)

HbCO is formed when haemoglobin is metabolized to biliverdin during transformation to bilirubin. Thus, in the normal subject who is neither a smoker nor within a polluted environment, levels of up to 2 per cent of circulating haemoglobin may be in the carboxy form. Levels above this can be considered abnormal and may reach 15 per cent in the cigarette chain-smoker.

Because of the high affinity of Hb for carbon monoxide and because of the long half-life of the association, heavy smokers may enter general anaesthesia with a significant reduction of their functional oxygen capacity. In this context, cessation of smoking for 24 hours before general anaesthesia is advocated.

Acute carbon monoxide poisoning becomes life-threatening over 50 per cent HbCO and requires treatment by life support measures and displacement of carbon monoxide by oxygen on the haemoglobin molecule.

APLASTIC ANAEMIA

In aplastic anaemia there is pancytopenia which results from a reduction in the amount of haemopoietic bone marrow. The haemoglobin, granulocyte and platelet levels vary from patient to patient but sustained neutrophil counts of less than $0.5 \times 10^9/l$ and platelet counts of less than $20 \times 10^9/l$ are associated with a poor prognosis. The normochromic red cells usually show moderate anisocytosis and poikilocytosis and the reduced number of white cells and platelets seen in the peripheral blood do not include primitive or abnormal forms. The reticulocyte count is usually, but not invariably, low. Hepatomegaly, splenomegaly or lymphadenopathy are unusual.

Bone marrow examination is essential to differentiate aplastic anaemia from other causes of pancytopenia, e.g. aleukaemic leukaemia, megaloblastic anaemia, hypersplenism, infiltration of the marrow with carcinoma or myeloma. The replacement of myeloid tissue by fat is not usually complete and, in most patients, small foci of haemopoietic tissue are evident in marrow aspirates or trephine biopsies. If doubt exists about the diagnosis, ferrokinetic studies with ^{59}Fe show a slow clearance and a predominantly hepatic uptake of the label; plasma iron turnover and red cell iron incorporation are low.

In about half the patients aplastic anaemia follows exposure to a toxic agent such as a drug, chemical or virus (see Table 11.7). *Chloramphenicol* and *phenylbutazone* are the two most frequently associated drugs in Europe and North America. In other cases, aplasia is due to a chemotherapeutic agent used for therapy of other conditions, e.g. busulphan for chronic granulocytic leukaemia. Aplastic anaemia may also occur during infections, especially viral hepatitis and disseminated tuberculosis. A group of

Table 11.7. Toxic factors associated with bone marrow depression.

Agents whose effect is dose dependent
  1 Ionizing radiation
  2 Benzene and its derivatives
  3 Arsenic
  4 Cytotoxic drugs

Agents whose effect depends on idiosyncrasy

Antibiotics:	Chloramphenicol, streptomycin, penicillin, sulphonamides, tetracyclines, isoniazid, amphotericin B
Anti-inflammatory drugs:	Phenylbutazone,* indomethacin, acetylsalicylic acid, colchicine, Gold salts†
Anticonvulsants:	Mephenytoin,* trimethadione,* paramethadione,* phenytoin, primidone
Antithyroid drugs:	Carbimazole,* Thiamazole,* thiourea, thiocyanate, $KClO_4$
Hypoglycaemic drugs:	Tolbutamide, chlorpropamide
Psychotrophic drugs:	Chlorpromazine,* promazine,* meprobamate,* pecazine,* amitriptyline,* imipramine,* chlordiazepoxide
Miscellaneous:	Chlorothiazides,† organic arsenicals,† hair dyes, acetazolamine, quinidine, CCl_4, trinitrotoluene, mepacrine, hydralazine
Insecticides:	DDT, Lindane, Parathion
Viruses:	Congenital rubella, hepatitis, infectious mononucleosis

---

* Selective neutropenia usual toxic effect.
† Selective thrombocytopenia usual toxic effect.

congenital aplastic anaemias occurs in children. *Faconi's anaemia* presents during the first decade of life with pancytopenia and there may be abnormalities of skin, bones, genital development, spleen and kidneys. The inheritance is autosomal recessive.

Treatment

Supportive therapy

Red cell transfusions are given to raise the patient's haemoglobin to a symptom free level, e.g. 9–11 g/dl; three units every month is usually adequate. Fresh red cells are preferred and these should be washed to avoid isoimmunization to transfused leucocytes and platelets. Patients with massive haemorrhage should receive *fresh whole blood* supplemented by *platelet concentrates*. Platelets are also indicated with less severe degrees of continuing haemorrhage. The place of prophylactic platelet transfusion is more controversial. Many patients with aplastic anaemia are continuously at risk from severe thrombocytopenia for months or years. As sudden catastrophic haemorrhage is a principal cause of death soon after presentation, there is a place for regular platelet transfusions in the early management of patients with repeated minor haemorrhage. If possible HLA matched platelets should be used because frequent platelet concentrates lead to isoimmunization with subsequent reduced survival of donor platelets.

Infections are a principal cause of death in patients with aplastic anaemia. Because of the paucity of neutrophils recognition of early infection is difficult; febrile responses are often atypical, exudates are scanty and rises in blood white cell levels minimal. In febrile patients blood cultures should be taken and vigorous attempts made to identify the responsible organism by direct examination of possibly infected material as well as by culture methods. Many lethal infections originate from the patient's own microbial flora, e.g. pseudomonas, *E.coli*, proteus, anaerobes, *staphylococcus aureus*. Persistent unexplained pyrexia should be treated with empirical *broad spectrum bactericidal antibiotics*, e.g. gentamycin and carbenicillin or cephalothin. As soon as the infective agent and its sensitivities are known appropriate changes in the antibiotic regimen may be made. If cell separator facilities are available *leucocytes* from normal donors or patients with chronic granulocytic leukaemia (CGL) should be given to patients with life-threatening infections due to neutropenia. To reduce the risk of graft-versus-host reaction the leucocytes should be irradiated with 15Gy to destroy the lymphocyte population prior to their transfusion. HLA matched leucocytes are preferable but it is usually not possible to obtain them.

Androgens, particularly the 17-alkalated anabolic variety, e.g. oxymethalone, have been successful in stimulating erythropoiesis and, less frequently, granulopoiesis and thrombopoiesis in some patients with aplastic anaemia. A haemopoietic response is seldom observed before three months' therapy.

It is controversial whether *splenectomy* influences haemopoietic regeneration in aplastic anaemia but it may reduce transfusion requirements in patients with red cell isoantibodies and improve the response to platelet transfusions. However, even with readily available platelet concentrates, in severe aplasia, the operative risks are great.

Bone marrow transplantation [9] (see Table 11.10) is considered in severe cases when the patient is under the age of 40 and has a compatible HLA matching sibling. Successful results with long-term survival may now be expected in 60–70 per cent of these patients. Death during or after transplantation is usually the result of overwhelming infection particularly if there is graft rejection or acute or chronic graft–versus–host disease (manifest by skin rashes, liver and gastrointestinal problems).

Red cell aplasia

In this disorder the marrow hypoplasia is confined to the erythroblastic series and the patient presents with a normochromic anaemia and reticulocytopenia. A rare constitutional form (the Blackfan–Diamond Syndrome) presents in early infancy. Acquired forms have a number of aetiologies. Regular blood transfusions and corticosteroids are the mainstays of therapy.

THE NONLEUKAEMIC MYELOPROLIFERATIVE DISORDERS

The 'myeloproliferative disorders' are a group of diseases in which a proliferative process involves one or more of the haemopoietic components in the bone marrow and, in many cases, the liver and spleen. They are closely related, transitional forms occur and in many patients an evolution from one entity into another occurs during the course of the disease (see Fig. 11.1). Polycythaemia vera, essential thrombocythaemia and myelosclerosis comprise the 'nonleukaemic myeloproliferative disorders'. Many consider essential thrombocythaemia simply as a variant of polycythaemia vera.

Polycythaemia vera

The term 'polycythaemia' or its synonym 'erythrocytosis' refers to a pattern of blood cell change that usually includes an increase in haemoglobin above 18 g/dl, a red cell

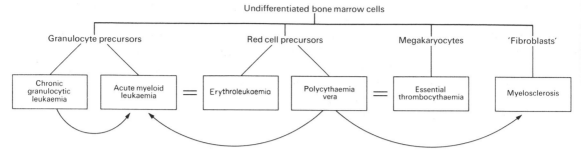

Fig. 11.1. Relationships of the myeloproliferative disorder.

count above 6.0×10^{12}/l and a haematocrit above 0.55. The causes of polycythaemia are listed in Table 11.8. Initial blood volume studies are required to establish whether the polycythaemia is 'real' where there is an increase in red cell volume or 'relative' where there is no increase in red cell volume. The red cell volume may be determined

Table 11.8. Classification of polycythaemia

Primary
  Polycythaemia vera

Secondary
  1 *Due to compensatory erythropoietin increase in:*
  High altitudes
  Cardiovascular disease
  Pulmonary disease and alveolar hypoventilation
  Heavy smoking
  Increased affinity haemoglobins (familial polycythaemia)
  Methaemoglobinaemia (rarely)
  2 *Due to inappropriate erythropoietin increase in:*
  Renal diseases, e.g. hydronephrosis, vascular impairment, cysts, carcinoma
  Massive uterine fibromyomata
  Hepatocellular carcinoma
  Adrenal tumours
  Cerebellar haemangioblastoma

Relative
  'Stress' or 'spurious' polycythaemia
  Dehydration: water deprivation, vomiting
  Plasma loss: burns, enteropathy

by ^{51}Cr or ^{99m}Tc labelled red cell methods and the plasma volume should be measured separately using the ^{125}I-albumin dilution method.

The normal results using these methods are:

> Red cell volume, men: 26–33 ml/kg
> women: 22–29 ml/kg
> Plasma volume: 40–50 ml/kg

Polycythaemia is considered real if the red cell volume is greater than 36 ml/kg in men and 32 ml/kg in women.

In polycythaemia vera the increase in red cell volume is caused by endogenous myeloproliferation. The underlying defect is probably of the marrow stem cell for in most patients there is also an overproduction of leucocytes and platelets. Clinical symptoms are due to hypervolaemia and hyperviscosity; headaches, plethora, pruritis, dyspnoea, blurred vision, parasthesias, thrombosis and haemorrhage; and to hyper-metabolism: night sweats and weight loss. Occasional patients suffer from gout and one third of patients have associated hypertension. Supportive findings that suggest polycythaemia vera rather than a secondary polycythaemia include: leucocytosis and thrombocytosis, marrow hyperplasia involving granulopoiesis and thrombopoiesis as well as erythropoiesis, splenomegaly, raised levels of serum uric acid, leucocyte alkaline phosphatase and serum vitamin B_{12} and vitamin B_{12} binding capacity. Radiological studies, measurement of arterial oxygen concentration and haemoglobin studies may be required to exclude a cause of secondary polycythaemia.

Thrombosis and haemorrhage are common and vascular accidents are a frequent cause of death in patients with polycythaemia vera. The increased viscosity, vascular stasis and high platelet levels may predispose towards thrombosis. Haemorrhage is promoted by vascular distension, defective platelet function and interference with clot formation by the increased red cells in the fibrin meshwork.

Therapy

Treatment is directed at reducing the red cell volume and consequently the blood viscosity. This is achieved by repeated venesection, the administration of radioactive [^{32}P] phosphorus or by myelosuppressive drugs, e.g. busulphan or chlorambucil. Venesection is particularly useful when a rapid reduction of red cell volume is required, e.g. at the start of therapy. Viscosity is decreased after the restoration of plasma volume from extravascular sources. In elderly patients with cardiovascular disease venesection should be carefully monitored; it must not be done too rapidly since the expanded blood volume sustains the increased cardiac output essential for tissue oxygenation with the viscous polycythaemic blood. Repeated venesections as a means of long-term therapy are associated with a high mortality and morbidity from thrombosis and haemorrhage for which the sustained high platelet levels may be partly responsible. The mean survival of patients treated by venesection alone is 3·5 years from the time of diagnosis. Most patients achieve a complete haematological remission with ^{32}P and this therapy is preferred in most clinics in Great Britain. Sustained myelosuppression may also be achieved with cytotoxic drugs; the main disadvantage of this form of therapy is that prolonged close supervision and regular blood counts are mandatory. The median survival of patients treated by ^{32}P or chemotherapy is 13 to 16 years from the time of diagnosis.

Transition from polycythaemia to myelosclerosis occurs in 20 to 30 per cent of patients. Some 10 to 15 per cent of patients develop a blast cell leukaemia, with or without an intervening period of myelosclerosis.

Therapy in secondary polycythaemia

In patients in whom polycythaemia represents a homeostatic adjustment to hypoxia, the polycythaemia has been shown to improve tissue oxygenation; the beneficial effect of increased blood volume more than offsets the potentially hypoxic effects of the sluggish blood flow. Although treatment should be directed towards causative cardio-vascular or pulmonary disorders, in most patients no reduction in red cell volume is desirable. However, if heart failure develops in patients with haematocrits of greater than 65 per cent carefully monitored venesection may lead to clinical improvement.

Surgery and polycythaemia

Surgery in patients with uncontrolled polycythaemia vera carries with it a 75 per cent incidence of major haemorrhage or thrombosis with an associated mortality approaching 30 per cent. Patients effectively controlled at the time of surgery have a low incidence of complications [13, 44]. When major elective surgery is indicated patients should be treated with ^{32}P or myelosuppressive drugs until a near normal blood count has been achieved and maintained. In the case of an emergency procedure a rapid haemodilution should be attempted by venesection. This should be accompanied by an infusion of equivalent amounts of an electrolytic solution or low molecular weight dextran. Heat loss and circulatory stasis should be avoided. The circulation time may be considerably slowed in polycythaemic patients, a factor which must be remembered when inducing anaesthesia. If surgical bleeding occurs, the use of fresh blood is recommended.

Essential thrombocythaemia

In this myeloproliferative syndrome megakaryocyte proliferation and overproduction of platelets is the dominant feature; there is a sustained platelet count of more than $1000 \times 10^9/l$. In the blood film the platelets often appear to be abnormally large and megakaryocyte fragments are frequently seen. Platelet function tests are consistently abnormal. Recurrent haemorrhage and thromboses dominate the clinical course. There may be anaemia (often due to iron deficiency from chronic gastrointestinal bleeding) or the thrombocythaemia may be accompanied by polycythaemia. Although splenic enlargement is frequently observed early in the disease, splenic atrophy occurs in the later stages in about half the patients. Radioactive phosphorus, busulphan or chlorambucil may be employed to reduce platelet levels; the doses required are usually less than those needed in classical polycythaemia vera. In some patients a fall in platelet level results in control of haemorrhage and an increase in red cell volume to polycythaemic levels occurs.

MYELOSCLEROSIS

In myelosclerosis, or agnogenic myeloid metaplasia, haemopoietic cell proliferation is more generalized with splenic and hepatic involvement in addition to that of the bone marrow. There is an associated increase in fibre production with the consequence that bone marrow is usually unobtainable by aspiration. Trephine biopsies in the early phases of the disease show hypercellular marrow with an increase in reticulin fibres; in the later stages an increase in intercellular substance with variable collagen deposition may occur.

Myelosclerosis usually has an insidious onset in older people and anaemia is the most frequent presenting feature. Weight loss and night sweats occur in some patients. While leucocyte and platelet counts are often elevated at the time of presentation, later in the disease pancytopenia is common. Splenomegaly is frequently massive and carries with it the problems of 'hypersplenism' with prominent splenic red cell 'pooling' and destruction. A third or more patients with myelosclerosis have a history of previous polycythaemia vera and some patients present with clinical and laboratory features of both disorders.

Therapy in myelosclerosis is palliative and unsatisfactory. Periodic blood transfusion may be required, folic acid supplementation is necessary in many patients and occasionally the anaemia responds to androgen therapy. Splenic irradiation and therapy with alkylating agents, e.g. busulphan, may diminish the enlarged spleen and the hypermetabolism. Anaesthetists are occasionally confronted with the myelosclerotic patient when splenectomy has been recommended. Opinion remains divided about the value and timing of splenectomy in myelosclerosis. In the later stages of the disease the operative risk is great; the patients are in poor general condition and there is an unacceptable postoperative mortality from infection and haemorrhage. Routine early splenectomy is unjustified since not all patients develop massive splenomegaly and this aggressive approach probably involves a number of unnecessary dangerous operations and may be contraindicated because of a high risk of postoperative thromboembolism. A moderate approach to splenectomy is indicated: it should be considered for patients with unacceptable transfusion requirements who show erythrokinetic evidence of increased splenic red cell destruction and red cell pooling, in patients with massive splenomegaly causing distressing symptoms uncontrollable by radiotherapy or chemotherapy, and when severe thrombocytopenia is associated with recurrent haemorrhage.

NEUTROPENIA

Some of the causes of selective neutropenia are given in Table 11.9. A variety of congenital neutropenic syndromes have been described and a mild asymptomatic reduction in neutrophil levels are found in many people of West African ancestry. Frequently, neutropenia is part of a general bone marrow failure or due to hypersplenism with accompanying anaemia and thrombocytopenia. Bone marrow examination is essential to determine whether the neutropenia is a result of depressed granulopoiesis or of accelerated removal of neutrophils from the blood; this procedure may

Table 11.9. Causes of neutropenia.

1 *Selective neutropenia*
Drug induced
Idiopathic
Familial syndromes
Cyclical

2 *Bone marrow failure*
Aplastic anaemia
Leukaemia
Malignant infiltration
Multiple myeloma

3 *Splenomegaly*

4 *Megaloblastic anaemia*

5 *Miscellaneous*
Viral infections, e.g. hepatitis, influenza
Fulminant bacterial infection, e.g. typhoid, miliary tuberculosis
Hypersensitivity and anaphylaxis
Paroxysmal nocturnal haemoglobinuria
Felty's syndrome
Systemic lupus erythematosus

also reveal such important causes as leukaemia, megaloblastic change or marrow infiltrations. Neutropenia may be the earliest sign of drug-induced marrow damage and if the drug is stopped at this stage further toxicity may be prevented. Drugs which may cause selective neutropenia include the phenothiazines, antithyroids, anticonvulsants, sulphonamides, phenindione and phenylbutazone (see Table 11.7). Although a drug-hapten antibody mechanism was responsible for the agranulocytosis which occurred with aminopyrine and dipyrone therapy, drug-dependent antibodies have rarely been identified in neutropenias associated with other drugs which probably have a more direct myelotoxic action [32].

Patients with acute severe neutropenia (absolute neutrophil counts $<0.2 \times 10^9$/l) usually present because of fever and infection. They should be admitted to hospital and nursed in separate rooms with 'reverse barrier' isolation techniques or placed in 'laminar flow rooms' or plastic isolators if these intensive care facilities are available. The infective organism should be isolated and treated vigorously as already described. The use of corticosteroids in neutropenia is dangerous and contraindicated; the anti-inflammatory action of these drugs may mask infection and the raised neutrophil levels that may be observed result from retardation of neutrophil migration and do not indicate increased granulopoiesis. If cell separator facilities are available, leucocyte transfusions prepared from chronic granulocytic leukaemic donors, or from normal donors, have given encouraging results in neutropenic patients with life threatening septicaemias not responding to antibiotics.

Although many drug-induced neutropenias are reversible and recovery occurs one to two weeks after stopping the drug in other patients, the bone marrow damage is permanent. Before the introduction of antibiotics the early mortality of patients presenting with acute severe neutropenia was 80 per cent. With modern treatment the prognosis is still poor: 20 per cent of patients are dead within a month of their presentation.

Infection remains the dominant problem in patients with chronic neutropenia. Early recognition of infection is essential and antibiotic and supportive therapy must be initiated without delay. Even trivial infections should be treated vigorously. Once infection is established appropriate therapy may be required for extended periods.

Occasional patients with acquired chronic neutropenia have large spleens and bone marrow examination reveals normal or hyperplastic granulopoiesis. This group includes patients with Felty's syndrome, occasional patients with systemic lupus erythematosus and rare patients with no apparent associated disease in whom the syndrome is labelled 'Primary splenic neutropenia'. Splenectomy should be considered in these patients; favourable results are obtained in about half the cases [43]. The results of splenectomy in neutropenic patients with reduced granulopoiesis however (and this includes the majority), have been disappointing.

THE LEUKAEMIAS

The leukaemias comprise a group of disorders of unknown aetiology characterized by the accumulation of abnormal white cells in the bone marrow. Common but not essential features include abnormal white cells in the peripheral blood, a raised white cell count, evidence of bone marrow failure, anaemia, neutropenia, thrombocytopenia; involvement of organs other than marrow, e.g. liver, spleen, lymph nodes, brain, skin, and gums. Approximately 2,500 deaths occur from leukaemia in England and

Wales each year [15]. The classification of leukaemia is somewhat confused partly because of a mixture of terms based on morphology, or clinical course or supposed cell of origin has been used.

THE ACUTE LEUKAEMIAS

The acute leukaemias are generally associated with a predominance of undifferentiated cells. 'Lymphoblastic leukaemia' is thought to derive from cells of the lymphoid series and the acute myeloid leukaemias are classified into various subclasses depending upon the dominant cell type present, e.g. myeloblastic, promyelocytic, myelomonocytic, monocytic and erythroleukaemia.

The common presenting manifestations of the acute leukaemias are anaemia, fever, infections and haemorrhage. Blood counting reveals progressive anaemia, neutropenia and thrombocytopenia; white cell levels are frequently elevated up to 100×10^9/l.

Chemotherapy with cytotoxic drugs, e.g. vincristine, cytosine arabinoside, rubidomycin, thioguanine, mercaptopurine, methotrexate, cyclophosphamide and prednisolone has been associated with improved prognosis particularly in lymphoblastic leukaemia in childhood. Using vincristine and prednisolone the clinical and haematological remission rate in childhood lymphoblastic leukaemia is 90 per cent. A less satisfactory remission rate of less than 70 per cent is obtained in acute myeloid types. In an attempt to continually reduce the 'hidden' leukaemic cell population most modern regimens employ rotating cycles of different cytotoxic drugs for up to two years after an initial remission has been induced. The benefit of prophylactic central nervous system irradiation, intrathecal methotrexate and cytosine arabinoside, have significantly improved prognosis in childhood acute leukaemia. Supportive measures such as intensive antibiotics, leucocyte transfusions, isolation procedures for infections and pyrexia, platelet transfusions for thrombocytopenia and haemorrhage and red cell transfusion for anaemia are of great importance in management. (See under aplastic anaemia.)

Trials employing bone marrow transplantation (Table 11.10) are currently under way [40, 41]. Allogeneic (HLA and mixed lymphocyte culture compatible sibling) bone marrow transplantation is considered in patients under 40 with acute myeloid leukaemia in first remission and in lymphoblastic leukaemia patients who relapse and achieve a second successful remission after reinduction therapy. Transplantation is performed to repopulate the patient's haemopoietic system after total body irradiation and intensive chemotherapy is given to eradicate all remaining leukaemic cells. If an identical twin is available transplantation is recommended in all acute leukaemias at the time of first remission.

Should the anaesthetist be concerned with acute leukaemia in relapse, particular care is required with regard to manipulative endotracheal trauma and if there is a severe bleeding tendency, intramuscular premedication should be avoided. The anaesthetist may be required for bone marrow harvesting, marrow biopsy and Hickman central venous cannulation to provide a long term cytotoxic route. Reverse isolation barrier conditions often prevail and in remote ward areas oral lorazepam followed by ketamine usually provides satisfactory anaesthetic management.

In untreated patients with acute leukaemia the median survival is less than three months. Recent trials have indicated that the median survival of children with lymphoblastic leukaemia treated with intensive chemotherapy and prophylactic central nervous system irradiation is greater than five years. In acute myeloid leukaemia,

Table 11.10. Bone marrow transplantation.

Indications	Severe aplastic anaemia [9] Acute myeloid leukaemia in first remission [40] Acute lymphoblastic leukaemia in second remission [41] Chronic granulocytic leukaemia—acute phase Combined immunodeficiency disease
Donor	SYNGENEIC—identical twin ALLOGENEIC—HLA lymphocyte culture (MLC) matched sibling or unrelated donor AUTOLOGOUS—self after marrow storage e.g. chronic phase of CGL for acute phase CGL
Preparation of recipient	Large doses of cyclophosphamide in days 5, 4, 3, 2 before the transplant. This is modified and total body irradiation added in cases of acute leukaemia
Technique	500–1000 ml of bone marrow ($> 10^9$ nucleated marrow cells) is harvested from donor by multiple aspirations, filtered and infused intravenously into recipient.
Post transplant management	Supportive measures include preventing infection with antibiotics, leucocyte concentrates, platelet concentrates. Intermittent methotrexate is given to help prevent graft–versus–host disease
Main complications	Graft rejection Graft–versus–host disease Severe infections

remissions are shorter, the value of maintenance therapy less obvious and the median survival of treated patients is less than about one year.

CHRONIC GRANULOCYTIC LEUKAEMIA

Chronic granulocytic leukaemia (CGL) comprises 20 per cent of all the leukaemias, and is seen most frequently in middle age. In most patients there is a replacement of normal bone marrow by cells with an abnormal G group chromosome (the Philadelphia or Ph^1 chromosome). A great increase in total body granulocytes occurs with high blood leucocyte counts, e.g. $50–600 \times 10^9$/l, massive splenomegaly and symptoms of hypermetabolism such as weight loss, lassitude, night sweats, anorexia and fever. There is often failure of red cell and platelet production with anaemia and thrombocytopenia but the platelet count is sometimes elevated. The differential leucocyte count reveals a predominance of neutrophils and myelocytes and occasionally a basophilia. The neutrophil alkaline phosphatase score is invariably low and serum levels of vitamin B_{12} and its binding protein are elevated.

CGL has a surprisingly constant clinical course with a very predictable response to palliative therapy in the chronic phase of the disease. Busulphan is the treatment of choice. This drug is one of the alkylating agents—chemicals which disrupt nucleoprotein by covalent linkage. Other forms of therapy include the drugs dibromomannitol and hydroxyurea, splenic irradiation and splenectomy. There is a high rate of 'conversion' or 'metamorphosis' to an inconstant but more acute disorder sometimes referred to as 'the blastic crisis'. Associated features of this 'metamorphosis' include the patient becoming refractory to therapy, anaemia, thrombocytopenia or thrombocytosis, leucocytosis or leucopenia, an increase of blast cells in the peripheral blood and bone marrow, blasts cell infiltrations of lymph nodes, other organs and soft tissues, new chromosome abnormalities, splenomegaly and a high neutrophil alkaline phosphatase score.

The median survival is 3–4 years. Death usually occurs from 'metamorphosis', or from intercurrent haemorrhage or infection; 20 per cent of patients survive ten years.

Cryopreserved peripheral blood white cells from patients with chronic granulocytic leukaemia in the chronic phase can function as an autograft. Autotransplantation of cryopreserved stem cells holds promise of significant prolongation of remission in selected patients undergoing blast cell transformation. Trials are proceeding but in the few patients who have had the chronic phase of chronic granulocytic leukaemia recycled, the prolongation of life has only been modest [16].

CHRONIC LYMPHOCYTIC LEUKAEMIA

Chronic lymphocytic leukaemia comprises 25 per cent of the leukaemias seen in clinical practice and occurs chiefly in the elderly. Although classified as a lymphoproliferative disorder in most patients there is little evidence to support an aggressive proliferation of the abnormal lymphocytes. The accumulation of large numbers of apparently 'mature' lymphocytes (up to 50–100 × normal) in the blood, bone marrow, spleen and liver may be related to immunological nonreactivity and excessive life span. With advanced disease, in addition to hepatosplenomegaly, there is often generalized discrete lymphadenopathy and bone marrow failure with anaemia, neutropenia and thrombocytopenia. Associated hypogammaglobulinaemia frequently results in an increased susceptibility to infections. However, many patients with early CLL are asymptomatic without abnormal physical findings. Skin manifestations are more frequent than in other leukaemias and include local and generalized infiltrations, herpes zoster and excessive reaction to insect bites and smallpox vaccination.

Although most patients with CLL have a leucocytosis of $30–300 \times 10^9$/l (70–99 per cent lymphocytes) the diagnosis should be suspected if there is a persistent lymphocytosis of more than $5 \cdot 0 \times 10^9$/l. Lymphocytes comprise more than 30 per cent of the nucleated cells seen in marrow aspirates. 15–20 per cent of CLL patients develop a secondary autoimmune haemolytic anaemia (see page 354).

The lymphocytes of CLL are sensitive to alkylating agents, steroids and irradiation. There is no good case for treating patients with early disease. Patients in bone marrow failure should be treated initially with prednisolone. When platelet, neutrophil and haemoglobin levels recover, continuous treatment with chlorambucil or cyclophosphamide successfully reduces total lymphocyte mass and may prevent bone marrow failure for periods of up to several years until the lymphocytes become refractory to these agents. No improvement of immunological capacity occurs with this therapy and special attention must be directed towards the prophylaxis and treatment of infections. Splenectomy is occasionally indicated for autoimmune haemolytic anaemia which does not respond to steroids and for those patients with massive splenomegaly refractory to therapy which is causing symptoms of 'hypersplenism'. A reduction in spleen size may be achieved with irradiation which is also useful for treating lymph nodes or local deposits causing pressure symptoms.

MULTIPLE MYELOMA

In multiple myeloma a neoplastic proliferation of plasma cells in the bone marrow causes lytic bone lesions, bone marrow failure and homogenous serum and/or urinary globulin elevations. 80 per cent of patients present after the age of 40 and in Britain this disorder is responsible for an annual death rate of 9 per million population [14].

Common presenting features include back pain, pathological fractures, normo-chromic normocytic anaemia, neutropenia and thrombocytopenia. Deposition of Bence-Jones protein, hypercalcaemia and pyelonephritis, may all contribute to renal failure. Repeated infections are related to deficient antibody production. Associated amyloid disease in some patients may also lead to renal failure, cause macroglossia or a 'carpel tunnel' syndrome. Interference of coagulation factor activity by the myeloma proteins and thrombocytopenia may produce a haemorrhagic diathesis. Rarely poly-merization of myeloma IgG or IgA causes a 'hyperviscosity syndrome' with heart failure, disturbed vision, nervous system manifestations or purpura. This syndrome is more frequently seen in the related monoclonal IgM gammopathy, Waldenstrom's macroglobulinaemia. The median survival in patients with multiple myeloma is two years.

Diagnosis

A monoclonal protein in the serum, urine or both is found in 98 per cent of patients. The serum protein is more frequently IgG than IgA and 50 per cent of patients with serum protein elevations excrete the low molecular weight Bence-Jones protein. In 15 per cent of patients urinary Bence-Jones protein is the sole abnormality [18].

In the majority of patients bone marrow aspiration reveals an infiltration by large numbers of plasma cells often with abnormal or 'myeloma' forms.

Skeletal radiology shows osteolytic lesions in 60 per cent of patients and generalized bone rarefaction in a further 20 per cent of patients.

Other laboratory findings include uraemia and hypercalcaemia which is not associated with a raised serum alkaline phosphatase unless there has been a recent pathological fracture. There is a high ESR. The blood film occasionally shows leuco-erythroblastic change and plasma cells are present in 15 per cent of cases.

Therapy

The alkylating agents melphalan and cyclophosphamide as well as prednisolone effectively relieve pain, reduce plasma cell proliferation in the marrow permitting improved normal marrow function and reduce the serum levels of paraprotein. Unfortunately, many patients become resistant to this palliative therapy.

Other supportive measures include blood transfusions for anaemia; hydration, prednisolone and neutral phosphate for acute hypercalcaemia; irradiation for single painful skeletal lesions and plasmapheresis for the hyperviscosity syndrome or bleeding due to paraprotein interference of coagulation.

Compression paraplegia occasionally necessitates an emergency laminectomy and prevalent vertebral compression fractures also require protection from displacement during incidental surgery. The presence of rib pain or fracture renders myeloma patients susceptible to postoperative chest infection. Deep vein thrombosis is common and requires prophylactic attention to reduce the incidence of pulmonary embolism.

The abnormal serum proteins may lead to unpredictable action by many drugs whose plasma binding normally influences distribution and activity.

MALIGNANT LYMPHOMA

The malignant lymphomas are divided into Hodgkin's disease and non-Hodgkin's lymphoma. In both disorders there is replacement of normal lymph node architecture by collections of abnormal cells, Hodgkin's disease being characterized by the presence of Reed-Sternberg giant cells and the non-Hodgkin's lymphomas by diffuse or nodular collections of abnormal lymphocytes, immunoblasts or, rarely, histiocytes.

HODGKIN'S DISEASE

Hodgkin's disease, in many patients, is localized initially to a single lymph node region and its subsequent progression is by direct contiguity within the lymphatic system. After a variable period of containment within the lymph nodes, the natural progression of the disease is to disseminate to involve nonlymphatic tissue.

Selection of appropriate treatment depends on accurate staging of the extent of disease. Lymphangiography is used to detect clinically silent pelvic and paraortic nodal involvement. In order to cannulate lymphatics in the dorsum of the feet (which then provide injection routes for radio-opaque media) their pathways are demonstrated by the absorption of dye injected into the toe skin-webs. Because this procedure is lengthy and disturbing, children are usually given general anaesthesia. Anaesthetists should be prepared for the development of a significant and persistent central cyanosis derived from the systemic absorption of the dye (currently Bleu Patent V). Because of the unreliability of other methods of clinical staging many clinicians advocate the performance of laparotomy with abdominal lymph node and liver biopsies and splenectomy in all cases who do not have overt evidence of disease dissemination.

It is now clear that many patients with localized Hodgkin's disease may be cured by high-dose radiotherapy to involved nodes and contiguous lymph node areas. Cylical chemotherapy with combinations of 3 or 4 cytotoxic drugs such as mustine, vincristine, procarbazine, prednisone, cyclophosphamide, bleomycin and adriamycin, is the treatment of choice for patients with advanced disease.

NON-HODGKIN'S LYMPHOMA

The clinical presentation and natural history of non-Hodgkin's lymphomas are more variable than in Hodgkin's disease, the pattern of spread is not as regular and a greater proportion of patients present with extranodal disease. Some of these lymphomas are closely related to chronic lymphocytic leukaemia or Waldenstrom's disease and others may terminate with leukaemic manifestations. Staging procedures, including lymphangiography and diagnostic laparotomy, are sometimes performed but the extent of the disease is less clearly related than histological type to prognosis.

The approach to treatment is similar to that for Hodgkin's disease. Localized disease is treated with high-dose radiotherapy and advanced disease with combination chemotherapy. Non-Hodgkin's lymphomas with cells resembling small lymphocytes, and those with nodular histology, have a more favourable prognosis than those with immunoblastic and histiocytic cytology or diffuse architectural patterns.

HAEMORRHAGIC DISORDERS

Normal haemostasis depends on an interaction between circulating platelets, blood vessel wall and the clotting factors. Platelet and coagulation factor deficiency and, more rarely, defects of the microcirculation, result in prolonged bleeding.

In considering surgical and anaesthetic management of any haemorrhagic disorder medication should generally be given orally or intravenously. When endotracheal intubation is specially indicated, manipulations must be extremely gentle and assisted by good conditions of muscular relaxation choosing the oral and not the nasal route. Otherwise it is better to avoid intubation whenever possible. However, general anaesthesia is preferable to regional analgesia for fear of haematoma formation at deep injection sites.

The diagnostic approach to a bleeding disorder requires thorough clinical and laboratory assessment. It must be established whether the bleeding tendency has been lifelong and whether there is a family history of bleeding. While purpura, excessive bleeding from superficial cuts or abrasions, and mucosal haemorrhage suggest a platelet disorder, deep haematomas, haemarthroses, haematuria and delayed wound healing are more characteristic of coagulation factor deficiency. Bruising occurs with both types of defect although large, spreading bruises are more suggestive of a coagulation disorder. Table 11.11 lists the commonly employed tests used to characterize bleeding disorders. The bleeding time and platelet count are used to detect quantitative and qualitative platelet defects. The prothrombin time is sensitive to deficiencies of coagulation factors II, V, VII and X and is typically prolonged in liver disease, vitamin K deficiency and during oral anticoagulation. The activated partial thromboplastin time is sensitive to deficiencies of factor V, VIII, IX and X and thus is able to

Table 11.11. Tests used in the diagnosis of bleeding disorders.

USUAL SCREENING TESTS	Bleeding time (B.T.)
	Coagulation time (C.T.); Clot retraction (C.R.)
	Prothrombin time (P.T.)
	Activated partial thromboplastin time (A.P.T.T.)
	Thrombin time (T.T.)
	Platelet count
	Blood film examination
	Test for fibrin degradation products (FDP)
SOMETIMES USED	Capillary resistance test (C.R.T.)
	Test for fibrin stabilizing factor (f.XIII)

Platelet defects		*Coagulation defects*		*Defibrination (D.I.C.)*
(Abnormal B.T., C.R.T., C.R.)		(Abnormal P.T.)	(Abnormal C.T., A.P.T.T.)	(Small clot, low platelet count, abnormal T.T., P.T., A.P.T.T. and presence of FDPs in serum)
Low platelet count	Normal platelet count	Assays for factors II	Assays for factors VIII	
|	|	V	IX	Fibrinogen titre
Bone marrow examination	Platelet aggregation studies	VII	and { XI	Fibrinogen assay
		X	rarely { XII	Euglobulin clot lysis time
|				Fibrin plate lysis
Platelet survival studies				Plasminogen assay
				Factor V and VIII assays

detect the most important hereditary coagulation disorders, haemophilia (deficiency of factor VIII) and Christmas disease (deficiency of factor IX). This latter test is also sensitive to the presence of heparin. In disseminated intravascular coagulation low fibrinogen levels and raised fibrin degradation products can be detected by the fibrinogen titre, the thrombin time and one of the screening tests for fibrin degradation products; thrombocytopenia should be confirmed by platelet counting and prolongation of prothrombin time and activated thromboplastin time indicates reduced levels of coagulation factors. The whole blood coagulation time is prolonged in severe haemophilia and during heparin therapy. The observation of clot retraction after one hour's incubation provides a guide to platelet function and smaller than normal clots indicate fibrinogen deficiency. More definitive tests listed in Table 11.11 are discussed in the following accounts of the different bleeding disorders. The results of haemostasis screening tests in patients with the rather ill-defined vascular purpuras are usually normal.

THE VASCULAR PURPURAS

Scurvy. Perifollicular haemorrhages on the flexor surfaces of the legs and buttocks are a characteristic sign in vitamin C deficiency. With severe scurvy there is more widespread bruising and painful periosteal haemorrhage occurs in children.

Henoch-Schönlein purpura. This hypersensitivity reaction is usually seen in childhood. A purpuric rash which typically involves the buttocks and limbs may be accompanied by localized subcutaneous oedema, painful joint swelling, haematuria and abdominal pain with or without melaena. Although in most cases this disorder is self-limiting, occasional patients develop renal failure.

Hereditary telangiectasia. The dilated microvascular lesions of this condition appear during childhood and become more numerous with age. In addition to extensive involvement of the skin and mucous membranes, A-V fistulae may be found in the liver, spleen and lungs. Chronic gastrointestinal bleeding, epistaxis and haemoptysis produce a state of severe iron deficiency which requires intensive iron replacement therapy (see page 339). Ethinyloestradiol has diminished the bleeding in some patients.

Ehlers–Danlos syndrome. In this rare hereditary condition defective perivascular connective tissue results in recurrent ecchymoses, muscle haematomata, gastrointestinal bleeding and haematuria. There is no effective treatment.

THROMBOCYTOPENIA

The main causes of thrombocytopenia are listed in Table 11.12.

CHRONIC IDIOPATHIC THROMBOCYTOPENIC PURPURA (ITP)

This relatively common disorder has an immune origin; sensitive tests are now able to demonstrate an antiplatelet IgG in the serum of most patients [12, 24]. Chronic ITP occurs predominantly in adults, particularly in women between 20 and 50 years. The onset is insidious with petechial haemorrhage, easy bruising and menorrhagia. Mucous

13

Table 11.12. Causes of thrombocytopenia.

Failure of platelet production
i. *Selective megakaryocyte depression*
Drugs, chemicals, viral infections
ii. *Part of general bone marrow failure*
  Aplastic anaemia
  Leukaemia
  Myelosclerosis
  Marrow infiltration: Carcinoma
  Lymphoma
  Multiple myeloma
  Paroxysmal nocturnal haemoglobinuria

Abnormal distribution of platelets
  Splenomegaly

Abnormal destruction of platelets
  Idiopathic thrombocytopenic purpura
  Secondary immune thrombocytopenia
    (rarely in SLE, CLL and lymphomas)
  Drug-induced immune thrombocytopenia
  Neonatal isoimmune thrombocytopenia
  Post-transfusion purpura
  Disseminated intravasular coagulation
  Thrombotic thrombocytopenia

Dilutional loss
  Massive transfusion of old blood to bleeding patients

---

membrane bleeding occurs in severe cases but intracranial haemorrhage is fortunately unusual. Most patients have platelet counts between 10 and 50×10^9/l on presentation and the platelets in the blood film appear large. Patients with ITP often show less haemorrhage than patients with similar degrees of thrombocytopenia resulting from marrow production failure. This has been attributed to a predominantly young, functionally superior, platelet population in ITP, due to the short platelet life-span. Increased numbers of megakaryocytes are seen in marrow aspirates. The bleeding time is prolonged, the capillary fragility test is positive and there is impaired clot retraction. Other tests of coagulation are normal.

It is important to exclude a drug as the cause of the thrombocytopenia and the direct antiglobulin test, tests for antinuclear factor (ANF), LE cells and for disseminated intravascular coagulation, should be done to exclude other causes. Secondary immune thrombocytopenia occurs sporadically with systemic lupus erythematosus, sarcoidosis, tuberculosis, carcinoma, lymphoma and with autoimmune haemolytic anaemia.

Treatment

Less than 10 per cent of adult patients with chronic ITP recover spontaneously. It is usual to treat with prednisolone in a dose of 1 mg/kg and to reduce the dose after 2 or 3 weeks. Phagocytic activity, particularly in the spleen, is reduced so that the antibody coated platelets survive longer.

Splenectomy is recommended in patients who do not recover within three months of starting steroid therapy or who require more than 5–10 mg prednisolone daily to maintain a platelet count above 50×10^9/l. About 75 per cent of patients are improved by splenectomy; in some, platelet counts rise to normal and remain so; in others, the dose of prednisolone which is needed is reduced. Platelet transfusions are necessary for patients with major haemorrhagic episodes although the transfused platelets seldom survive longer than the patient's own. Platelet transfusions may also be indicated to cover the operative period during splenectomy in those patients with severe thrombocytopenia. Immunosuppressive drugs, e.g. azathioprine, cyclophosphamide, vincristine or vinblastine are given with some success to those patients resistant to both corticosteroids and splenectomy.

ACUTE IDIOPATHIC THROMBOCYTOPENIC PURPURA

Acute ITP has an equal sex incidence but is more common in children. It usually follows vaccination or an infection such as chicken pox, measles, rubella or glandular fever. An allergic reaction is presumed but has not yet been proven. Typically, petechiae or ecchymoses develop rapidly and bleeding may occur from the gums, nose, vagina, gastrointestinal and urinary tracts. Rarely, death from intracranial haemorrhage occurs but more commonly the disease remits or passes into the chronic form. Treatment consists of blood and platelet transfusions and corticosteroid therapy, for example 1 mg/kg prednisolone daily for a week with subsequent gradual reduction.

DRUG-INDUCED THROMBOCYTOPENIA

Although thrombocytopenia may occur as a result of generalized toxic marrow depression, or with some drugs such as chlorothiazides and tolbutamide due to selective megakaryocyte depression, it is now believed that most drug-induced thrombocytopenias are caused by an allergic mechanism. The list of drugs causing immune thrombocytopenia is very large. The most frequently reported drugs have been quinidine, quinine, apronal, paraminosalicylate, sulphonamides, chloroquine, digitoxin, stibophen, rifampicin and the gold salts. Initially with Sedormid [2] it was postulated that the drug, acting as a hapten, attached to the platelet membrane and the antibody was directed against the drug-platelet antigen. However, it is now considered that most drug-induced immune thrombocytopenias are caused by an immune complex mechanism where antibody is directed against an antigen consisting of drug and a plasma protein binder and the platelet is damaged as an 'innocent bystander' [28]. Whether drugs can stimulate autoantibody formation to platelets, as methyldopa does to red cells, remains undetermined, though a few patients receiving methyldopa have developed thrombocytopenia [4].

Drug-induced thrombocytopenia may have a gradual onset or present with an acute bleeding syndrome. The latter presentation may be heralded by a chill, headache and flushing with severe bleeding from mucous membranes, skin, and the gastrointestinal, urinary or female genital tract. Recovery occurs after a few hours or days with rapidly metabolized drugs but may take months in gold sensitivity. The platelet count is frequently below $10 \times 10^9/l$, normal or increased megakaryocytes are found in marrow aspirates and drug dependent antibodies against platelets may be detected by *in vitro* techniques. Negative *in vitro* results may arise because an active metabolite is involved in the allergic reaction rather than the drug itself.

All suspect drugs should be stopped, or if these are essential the drugs should be replaced by others with similar actions. Corticosteroids are given in the hope that they improve capillary fragility, and platelet concentrates are administered for severe haemorrhage. Dimercaprol (BAL) is given in cases due to gold sensitivity.

The patient must avoid the offending drug and any structurally related drugs.

NEONATAL THROMBOCYTOPENIA

Destruction of fetal platelets by maternal IgG antibodies which pass across the placenta, directed against paternally inherited antigens, causes thrombocytopenia in about 1 in 5,000 births. Generalized petechiae develop within hours of birth and severe, life-threatening internal or external haemorrhage may occur. The platelet count falls to its lowest levels within hours of birth and rises spontaneously after about two weeks. Infants born to mothers with chronic ITP frequently have a similar syndrome.

POST-TRANSFUSION PURPURA

This rare syndrome occurs 5 to 8 days after a blood transfusion. It has similar clinical features to acute drug-induced thrombocytopenia, lasts up to 3 weeks, is self-limiting, and has only been reported in women who have previously been pregnant, and who are among the 1 per cent of the population lacking the platelet antigen, PL^{A1}. Anti-PL^{A1} antibody can be detected in the affected patient's serum and it is thought that PL^{A1} antigen-antibody complexes are deposited on the recipient's own platelets [1, 38].

HEREDITARY THROMBASTHENIA

In this rare condition there is recurrent epistaxis, bruising, gastrointestinal bleeding and menorrhagia. The inheritance is autosomal recessive. Although the platelet count is normal, the bleeding time is prolonged, there is capillary fragility, clot retraction is abnormal and the platelets do not aggregate with ADP and thrombin [8]. Severe bleeding episodes should be treated with platelet concentrates.

ACQUIRED QUALITATIVE PLATELET DEFECTS

Functionally defective platelets are largely responsible for the bleeding tendency in uraemia. There is defective platelet factor 3 release and the dysfunction is reversed by dialysis. Abnormal platelet function has also been demonstrated in the myeloproliferative disorders, in patients with macroglobulinaemia and in liver disease.

Aspirin therapy is associated with an irreversible inhibitory effect on the platelet release reaction and this may contribute to the associated gastrointestinal bleeding seen in some patients. Occasionally there is mild purpura, abnormal surgical bleeding occurs, the bleeding time is prolonged, and *in vitro* platelet aggregation tests with collagen and adrenaline are abnormal. Aspirin ingestion may accentuate bleeding in patients with other haemorrhagic disorders.

COAGULATION FACTOR DEFICIENCY

Ten factors are necessary for normal clotting. Deficiencies may be congenital, usually of a single factor, or acquired, when several factors may be reduced. Haemophilia.

Christmas disease and Von Willebrand's disease are the most frequently encountered hereditary conditions. Liver disease, anticoagulant overdosage and disseminated intravascular coagulation dominate the scene concerning the acquired coagulopathies. Table 11.11 outlines the tests which are used in diagnosis.

HAEMOPHILIA

It has been estimated that there are 3,000–4,000 severely affected haemophiliacs in Great Britain [35] and there may be an equal number of mildly affected patients. Although the sex-linked inheritance pattern is well established as many as 25–30 per cent of haemophiliacs have no family history of the disease. The defect in haemophilia is an absence or low plasma level of functional coagulation factor VIII activity (VIII:C). Immunological studies show normal quantities of factor VIII-related protein (VIIIR:AG) in the plasma [7].

The clinical problems associated with haemophilia correlate well with the plasma factor VIII activity; patients with severe disease usually have less than 1 per cent factor VIII activity. In many boys the condition has been revealed by post-circumcision haemorrhage. Joint haemorrhages which are painful and may lead to deformity and subsequent crippling dominate the clinical problems. Muscle haematomas cause nerve and blood vessel compression and occasionally result in serious contractures and haematuria is a frequent problem. Operative and post-traumatic haemorrhage are life threatening in both severely and mildly affected cases. Fortunately intracranial haemorrhage is rare.

The whole blood coagulation time and the activated partial thromboplastin time are usually prolonged. However, these are relatively insensitive tests and factor VIII assays should be performed in all suspected haemophiliacs.

Because of the lability of factor VIII at 4°C, stored blood is of little value in replacement therapy; bleeding episodes should be treated with fresh plasma, fresh frozen plasma, cryoprecipitate (which is selectively rich in factor VIII and fibrinogen) or freeze dried factor VIII concentrates. The circulating level required to initiate and maintain haemostasis varies with the type of bleeding, remembering that the half life of factor VIII in the circulation is only 12 hours.

Spontaneous minor bleeding and early haemarthroses usually respond well to fresh plasma or cryoprecipitate and the factor VIII level should be elevated to 5–20 per cent of normal. Gentle splinting and rest are required for 24–48 hours. In recent years prophylactic cryoprecipitate or concentrate injections have successfully reduced the incidence of bleeding episodes.

To treat dangerous muscle haematomas effectively or to cover multiple dental extractions, the level of factor VIII should be elevated above 20 per cent. A typical regime for dental extractions in the haemophiliac is the following [35]. The patient is given factor VIII or cryoprecipitate transfusion on the morning of operation sufficient to achieve (by calculation) a factor level of 50 per cent normal. This is followed by tranexamic acid intravenously 30 mg/kg/body weight prior to surgery. After operation, it is given orally in the same dose six hourly for 7–10 days. No further factor VIII is given unless the tooth sockets start to bleed. Tranexamic acid is less toxic than its predecessor ε-amino-caproic acid (EACA) and is an inhibitor of plasminogen and therefore impedes the normal clot lysing process. Nonirritant oral analgesics may be given postoperatively but aspirin derivatives should be avoided because of erosive action on gastric mucosa and interference with blood coagulation.

For major surgery and serious accidents it is essential to maintain a level of factor VIII above 40 per cent for a period of 6–10 days during and after the operation or following trauma. Before haemorrhagic surgery begins factor VIII levels of 100–150 per cent may be required and other clotting factors may become essential during the procedure. Such levels may be achieved only by using large quantities of cryoprecipitate or factor VIII concentrates.

Antibodies to factor VIII develop in 5–10 per cent of haemophiliacs. With many patients this resistance to injected factor VIII may be overcome by massive replacement therapy. Plasmapheresis may also have a place in treating bleeding episodes in patients with factor VIII antibodies. Nowadays, cryoprecipitate and fresh frozen plasma have been largely superseded by factor VIII concentrates.

CHRISTMAS DISEASE

The inheritance pattern and clinical features of patients with Christmas disease are identical to those of haemophilia [6]. Although in severe cases there is prolongation of whole blood clotting and activated partial thromboplastin times the factor VIII activity is normal. The diagnosis is made by demonstrating low or absent plasma factor IX activity.

The principles of management are similar to those in haemophilia. Bleeding episodes are treated with fresh plasma, fresh frozen plasma or factor IX concentrates. The plasma half life of factor IX is 20 hours and the activity levels required to maintain haemostasis under variable stresses are similar to those described for haemophilia.

VON WILLEBRAND'S SYNDROME

This bleeding disorder has an autosomal dominant inheritance and affects both sexes [29]. Operative and traumatic haemorrhage are frequently a problem and excessive bleeding occurs from superficial cuts and scratches and from mucous membranes. Haemarthroses and muscle haematomas are rare.

In severely affected patients the bleeding time is prolonged, the capillary fragility test is positive and there is a variable deficiency of factor VIII coagulant activity (VIII:C) and comparable reduction in factor VIII-related protein (VIII:AG) by immunoelectrophoretic techniques [48]. Most patients show an absence of Ristocetin-induced platelet aggregation and poor retention of platelets in glass bead columns [37]. These findings indicate that the deficient factor VIII protein has relevance both to factor VIII clotting activity and to platelet function. The laboratory results in mildly affected patients are somewhat variable.

Treatment consists of fresh-frozen plasma, cryoprecipitate or factor VIII concentrates. Single infusions are associated with sustained and often delayed increases of factor VIII activity.

LIVER DISEASE

Biliary obstruction results in impaired absorption of vitamin K with a consequent decreased synthesis of factors II, VII, IX and X by the liver parenchymal cells. With severe hepatocellular disease, as well as a deficiency of these factors there is often reduced levels of factor V and fibrinogen and increased levels of plasminogen activator. The hypersplenism which occurs with portal hypertension is frequently associated with thrombocytopenia. These multiple abnormalities contribute to increased surgical bleeding and bruising in patients with liver disease and may exacerbate haemorrhage from oesophageal varices. The degree of haemostatic defect is best judged by prolongation of prothrombin and bleeding times.

Patients with liver disease should receive 20–50 mg vitamin K_1 daily 3–4 days prior to liver biopsy or imminent surgery. Fresh-frozen plasma will replace the deficient clotting factors and surgical blood loss should preferably be replaced by fresh whole blood which provides platelets in addition to coagulation factors. In the most severely affected patients, concentrates of coagulation factors II, VII, IX and X are most effective and if severe thrombocytopenia exists, platelet concentrates may be required.

ANTICOAGULANT OVERDOSAGE

The coumarin and indancdionc anticoagulants arc vitamin K antagonists and produce anticoagulation by decreasing the liver synthesis of factors II, VII, IX and X. Serious haemorrhage is the principal side-effect of this therapy. An increased responsiveness to these drugs occurs in patients with obstructive jaundice or liver disease. Alcohol may increase their action by inhibiting the oxidative process concerned with their elimination, and certain drugs, e.g. phenylbutazone, chloral hydrate and clofibrate, may potentiate their action by displacing them from their plasma protein binding sites. Haemorrhage due to anticoagulants may be worsened by salicylates because of their antiplatelet actions and their irritant effect on the gastric mucosa. With overdosage there is usually an excessive prolongation of prothrombin time or a very low thrombotest result.

Treatment consists of vitamin K_1 20–50 mg intravenously and, with severe bleeding, fresh-frozen plasma, fresh blood, or factor II, VII, IX, and X concentrate.

DISSEMINATED INTRAVASCULAR COAGULATION (DIC)

Widespread intravascular deposition of fibrin with consumption of coagulation factors and platelets occurs as a consequence of many disorders and may be associated with a fulminant haemorrhagic syndrome. This process may be triggered by the entry of procoagulant materials into the circulation, e.g. in patients with premature separation of the placenta, amniotic fluid embolism, haemolytic transfusion reaction, disseminated mucin-secreting adenocarcinoma, promyelocytic leukaemia, or it may result from widespread endothelial cell damage with collagen exposure, e.g. during shock, viraemia, acidosis or hypothermia. The trigger mechanisms appear to centre around the vascular endothelium. Intact vascular endothelial cells synthesize a prostaglandin known as prostacyclin which inhibits platelet adhesion. Endothelial damage results in a loss of this inhibitory prostaglandin and exposure of endothelial collagen promotes platelet adhesion and aggregation. Once platelets are aggregated they release serotonin and adenosine diphosphate which promote the formation of thrombin [34]. Septicaemia with Gram-negative organisms is a frequent cause. In acute syndromes the blood may fail to clot because of gross fibrinogen depletion and high concentrations of fibrin degradation products may result in grossly abnormal fibrinogen titre and thrombin times. Thrombocytopenia is usual and fragmented red cells may or may not be seen on blood film examination. Although screening tests for coagulation factor deficiency, e.g. prothrombin time, activated partial thromboplastin time, are prolonged in the acute syndrome, with more chronic disease an increased synthesis may result in normal levels of coagulation factors and normal screening test times. Fibrinogen assays are required to document the severity of fibrinogen depletion. Reduced concentrations of a number of other coagulation factors are present but the pattern is not consistent except that factor V and factor VIII are nearly always low [33]. Although plasminogen levels are reduced in acute syndromes, tests for systemic fibrinolysis (euglobulin clot lysis time, fibrin plate lysis) usually show no increase in circulating plasminogen activator.

The haemolytic–uraemic syndrome in children and postpartum nephritis are associated with local renal fibrin deposition and platelet consumption may produce laboratory results similar to those found in DIC. Thrombotic thrombocytopenic purpura is a disorder in which there is widespread platelet aggregation in small blood vessels but in many patients there is no major consumption of clotting factors.

The main therapeutic efforts in patients with DIC are directed towards urgently correcting or treating the causative disorder. In acute syndromes supportive therapy with fresh blood, fibrinogen and platelet concentrates are often required. The place of heparin therapy remains controversial [33]. Although it is unlikely that heparin could influence the basic disease present its powerful anticoagulant action should prevent the continuing fibrin deposition associated with this syndrome. In many transitory forms of DIC heparin is definitely not indicated. For example, in premature separation of the placenta, fibrin deposition rapidly ceases when the uterus is evacuated and heparin may increase the risk of major haemorrhage and shock. Benefit has been claimed for heparin therapy in acute but continuing DIC associated with septicaemia in septic abortion, purpura fulminans, meningococcal septicaemia, haemolytic transfusion reaction, promyelocytic leukaemia and drug-resistant *Plasmodium falciparum* malaria. However, the role of heparin has often been difficult to evaluate because it has been combined with other specific and supportive therapy. It remains doubtful whether or not this anticoagulant has improved prognosis in the haemolytic–uraemic syndrome. Long-term heparin therapy is unsatisfactory and there is no evidence that oral anticoagulants are effective in the management of chronic forms of DIC. Fibrinolytic agents, e.g. streptokinase, urokinase, have been used in isolated patients with DIC to accelerate the recanalization of thrombosed areas of the microcirculation. The potentially harmful effects of these agents, including fibrinogenolysis and further coagulation factor depletion, probably outweigh any potential advantage. Local activation of plasminogen within the thrombi in DIC is beneficial and there is usually no increase in circulating plasminogen activator; the use of antifibrinolytic agents, such as tranexamic acid, EACA and aprotinin, should be firmly discouraged.

MASSIVE TRANSFUSION BLEEDING SYNDROME

During massive haemorrhage treated by stored blood and nonsanguine blood volume replacement there is a dilution of clotting factors. Unless these are replaced, uncontrollable bleeding will result. If factor assays are not immediately available it may be essential to transfuse one unit of rewarmed fresh frozen plasma (FFP) and one unit (from 5 donations) of platelet concentrate for every 5–7 units of stored blood or plasma substitutes rapidly administered. Calcium gluconate therapy is generally recommended for rapid blood transfusions of large proportion although evidence of benefit is sparse. Calcium chloride may cause ventricular hyperexcitability. Microfiltration of stored blood is widely recommended. Although debris and microaggregates are undoubtedly removed it is not certain that these are causal agents of 'shock lung' or DIC [39].

2,3 DPG DEPLETION

It is well established that during storage blood loses the substrate 2,3 diphospho-glycerate (2,3 DPG) from its red cells. The amount of this substrate in the red cells is normally similar to haemoglobin and determines the degree of association of oxygen with haemoglobin. When cells are stripped of 2,3 DPG, the p50 for haemoglobin/oxygen is very low so that while haemoglobin's oxygen uptake is great, oxygen release to tissues is apparently inhibited. The loss with citrate phosphate dextrose (CPD) is less than when acid citrate dextrose (ACD) is used as an anticoagulant preservative and the former has generally replaced the latter. In CPD blood stored at 4°C, the 2,3 DPG level is, in fact, well retained up to 10 days storage after which time depletion soon occurs. Because stored blood is issued such that most patients receive the oldest product it is inevitable that most transfused blood is severely 2,3 DPG depleted. When large demands for transfusion are being met, however, it is likely that blood banks are forced to issue increasingly fresh products. Although the half-life recovery time for 2,3 DPG within the donated red cells appears to be some 5 hr or so [42], clinical experience of rapid, massive transfusion of old stored blood with successful resuscitation suggests that 2,3 DPG is not such a vital factor in oxygen delivery.

REFERENCES

1 ABRAMSON N, EISENBERG PD, ASTER RH. Post-transfusion purpura; immunological aspects and therapy. *N Engl J Med* 1974; **291**: 1163–6.
2 ACKROYD JF. The pathogenesis of thrombocytopenic purpura due to hypersensitivity to sedormid. *Clin Sci* 1949; **7**: 249–85.
3 ANYON CP, CLARKSON KG. Cow's milk: a cause of iron deficiency anaemia in infancy. *NZ Med J* 1971; **74**: 24–5.
4 BENRAAD AH, SCHOENAKER AH. Thrombocytopenia after use of methyldopa. *Lancet* 1965; **2**: 292.
5 BENTLEY PG, HOWARD ER. Surgery in children with homozygous sickle cell anaemia. *Ann R Coll Surg Engl* 1979; **61**: 55–8.
6 BIGGS R, DOUGLAS AS, MacFARLANE RG, et al. Christmas disease: a condition previously mistaken for haemophilia. *Br Med J* 1952; **2**: 1378–82.
7 BLOOM AL. The biosynthesis of factor VIII. *Clin Haematol* 1979; **8**: 53–77.
8 CAEN JP, CASTALDI PA, LECLERC JC, et al. Congenital bleeding disorders with long bleeding time and normal platelet count I. Glanzmann's thrombasthenia. *Am J Med* 1966; **41**: 4–26.
9 CAMITTA BM, THOMAS ED, NATHAN DG, et al. A prospective study of androgens and bone marrow transplantation for treatment of severe aplastic anaemia. *Blood* 1979; **53**: 504–14.
10 DACIE JV, LEWIS SM. Paroxysmal nocturnal haemoglobinuria. Clinical manifestations, haematology, and nature of the disease. *Ser Haematol* 1972; **5**: 3–23.
11 DACIE JV, WORLLEDGE SM. Auto-immune hemolytic anemias. *Prog Hematol* 1969; **6**: 82–120.
12 DIXON R, ROSSE W, ERBERT L. Quantitative determination of antibody in idiopathic thrombocytopenic purpura. *N Engl J Med* 1975; **292**: 230–6.
13 FITTS WT Jr, ERDE A, PESKIN GW, FROST JW. Surgical implications of polycythaemia vera. *Ann Surg* 1960; **152**: 548–58.
14 GALTON DAG. Myelomatosis. In: Hoffbrand AV, Lewis SM, eds. *Postgraduate haematology*. London: Heinemann, 1981: 513–42.
15 GALTON DAG. Leukaemia. In: Hoffbrand AV, Lewis SM, eds. *Haematology*. London: Heinemann, 1972: 451–83.
16 GOLDMAN JM, CATOVSKY D, HOWS J, SPIERS ASD, GALTON DAG. Cryopreserved peripheral blood cells functioning as autografts in patients with chronic granulocytic leukaemia in transformation. *Br Med J* 1979; **I**: 1310–13.

17 GOTZE O, MULLER-EBERHARD HJ. Paroxysmal hemoglobinuria; hemolysis initiated by the C_3 activator system. *N Engl J Med* 1972; 286: 180–4.

18 HOBBS JR. Immunochemical classes of myelomatosis. *Br J Haematol* 1969; 16: 599–606.

19 HOFFBRAND AV. Megaloblastic anaemia. In: Hoffbrand AV, Lewis SM, eds. *Postgraduate haematology*. London: Heinemann, 1981: 72–111.

20 HOMI J, REYNOLDS J, SKINNER A, HANNA W, SERJEANT G. General anaesthesia in sickle-cell disease. *Br Med J* 1979; 1: 1599–601.

21 HOWELLS TH. Anaesthesia and blood diseases. In: Hewer CL, Atkinson RS, eds. *Recent advances in anaesthesia and analgesia, 12*. London: Churchill Livingstone, 1976 120–30.

22 HOWELLS TH, HUNTSMAN RG, BOYS JE, MAHMOOD A. Anaesthesia and sickle-cell haemoglobin. *Br J Anaesth* 1972; 44: 975–87.

23 HUEHNS ER. Diseases of haemoglobin synthesis. In: Baron DN, Compston N, Dawson AM, eds. *Recent advances in medicine*. 16th ed. Edinburgh: Longman, 1973: 365–411.

24 KARPATKIN S, STRICK N, KARPATKIN MB, SISKIN GW. Cumulative experience in detection of antibody in 234 patients with idiopathic thrombocytopenic purpura, systemic lupus erythematosus and other clinical disorders. *Am J Med* 1972; 52: 776–85.

25 KONOTEY-AHULU FI. Anaesthetic deaths and the sickle cell trait. *Lancet* 1969; I: 267–8.

26 KRAVIS LP, DONSKY G, LECKS HI. Upper and lower gastrointestinal tract bleeding induced by whole cow's milk in an atopic infant. *Pediatrics* 1967; 40: 661–5.

27 LEHMANN H, HUNTSMAN RG. *Man's haemoglobins*. Amsterdam: North-Holland, 1974.

28 MIESCHER PA. Drug induced thrombocytopenia. *Semin Hematol* 1973; 10: 311–25.

29 NILLSON IM, HOLMBERG L. Von Willebrand's disease today. *Clin Haematol* 1979; 8: 147–68.

30 ODURO KA. Anaesthesia in Ghana. *Anaesthesia* 1969; 24: 307–16.

31 ODURO KA, SEARLE JF. Anaesthesia in sickle cell states—a plea for simplicity. *Br Med J* 1972; 4: 596–8.

32 PISCIOTTA AV. Immune and toxic mechanisms in drug-induced agranulocytosis. *Semin Hematol* 1973; 10: 279–310.

33 PITNEY WR. Disseminated intravascular coagulation. *Semin Hematol* 1971; 8: 65–83.

34 PRESTON FE. Haematological problems associated with shock. *Br Journal of Hospital Medicine* 1979; 21: 232–47.

35 RIZZA CR. Haemorrhagic disorders. *Medicine* (London) 1974; 24: 1449–56.

36 ROSSE WF, DACIE JV. Immune lysis of normal red cells and paroxysmal nocturnal hemoglobinuria (PNH) red cells. I. The sensitivity of PNH red blood cells to lysis by complement and specific antibody *J Clin Invest* 1966; 45: 736–45.

37 SALZMAN EW. Measurement of platelet adhesiveness. A simple *in vitro* technique demonstrating an abnormality in von Willebrand's disease. *J Lab Clin Med* 1963; 62: 724–35.

38 SHULMAN NR, ASTER RH, LEITNER A. Immunoreactions involving platelets. V. Post-transfusion purpura. *J Clin Invest* 1961; 40: 1597–620.

39 SOLIS RT, WALKER BD. Does a relationship exist between massive blood transfusion and adult respiratory distress syndrome? *Vox Sang* 1977; 32: 319–20.

40 THOMAS ED, BUCKNER CD, CLIFT RA, *et al.* Marrow transplantation for acute nonlymphoblastic leukaemia in first remission. *N Engl J Med* 1979; 301: 597–9.

41 THOMAS ED, SANDERS JE, FLOURNOY N, *et al.* Marrow transplantation for patients with acute lymphoblastic leukaemia in remission. *Blood* 1979; 54: 468–76.

42 VALERI CR, HIRSCH NM. Restoration *in vivo* of erythrocyte adenosine triphosphate, 2,3-diphosphoglycerate, potassium ion, and sodium ion concentrations following the transfusion of acid-citrate-dextrose-stored human red blood cells. *J Lab Clin Med* 1969; 73: 722–33.

43 VINCENT PC, LEVI JA, MACQUEEN A. The mechanism of neutropenia in Felty's syndrome. *Br J Haematol* 1974; 27: 463–75.

44 WASSERMAN LR, GILRERT HS. Surgical bleeding in polycythaemia vera. *Ann NY Acad Sci* 1964; 115: 122–38.

45 WETHERALL DJ, CLEGG JB. *Thalassaemia and related disorders*. 3rd ed. Oxford: Blackwell Scientific Publications, 1979.

46 WHITE JM, DACIE JV. The unstable hemoglobins—molecular and clinical features. *Prog Hematol* 1971; 7: 69–109.

47 WORLLEDGE SM. Immune drug-induced hemolytic anemias. *Semin Hematol* 1973; 10: 327–44.

48 ZIMMERMAN TS, RATNOFF OD, POWELL AE. Immunologic differentiation of classic hemophilia (factor VIII deficiency) and von Willebrand's disease. *J Clin Invest* 1971; 50: 244–54.

APPENDIX I

Common Red Cell Abnormalities and Associated Conditions

RED CELL ABNORMALITY	ASSOCIATED CONDITIONS
Anisocytosis	Nonspecific finding in many blood disorders
Macrocytosis	Vitamin B_{12} or folate deficiency, liver disease, with reticulocytosis of haemolytic states or haemorrhage
Microcytosis	Iron deficiency, thalassaemia
Poikilocytosis	Nonspecific finding of many blood disorders, myelosclerosis, malignant infiltration of marrow, iron deficiency, vitamin B_{12} or folate deficiency
Hypochromia	Iron deficiency, thalassaemia, haemoglobinopathy, sideroblastic anaemia
Polychromasia	During reticulocytosis of haemolytic disorders or haemorrhage, myelosclerosis, malignant infiltration of marrow, thalassaemia
Spherocytosis	Hereditary spherocytosis, other haemolytic anaemias
Elliptocytosis	Hereditary elliptocytosis, iron deficiency, myelosclerosis
Target cells	Iron deficiency, liver disease, thalassaemia, haemoglobinopathy postsplenectomy
Acanthocytes	Liver disease, postsplenectomy, hereditary abetalipoproteinaemia
Red cell fragments and irregularly contracted cells	Drug-induced haemolytic anaemia, disseminated intravascular coagulation or microangiopathic haemolytic anaemia, uraemia
Howell-Jolly bodies (nuclear remnants)	Postsplenectomy, hyposplenism, during severe marrow hyperplasia, acute haemolysis or severe megaloblastic anaemia
Basophilic stippling	Dyshaemopoietic anaemias, thalassaemia, lead poisoning
Siderotic granules (Pappenheimer bodies)	Postsplenectomy, sideroblastic anaemia, thalassaemia
Erythroblasts	Myelosclerosis, malignant infiltration of marrow, leukaemia, in rapidly developing or severe anaemia

APPENDIX II

Leucocytes: Normal Values, Common Abnormalities and Their Associated Conditions

NEUTROPHILS	Normal Values: $2 \cdot 5$–$7 \cdot 5 \times 10^9$/l
Neutrophilia	Bacterial infection, haemorrhage, trauma, polycythaemia vera, malignant tumours, connective tissue disease, chronic granulocytic leukaemia
Neutropenia	Marrow hypoplasia, agranulocytosis, splenomegaly, vitamin B_{12} or folate deficiency, malignant infiltration of marrow, leukaemia
Reduced nuclear segmentation with metamyelocytes and myelocytes	With above causes of neutrophilia, myeloid leukaemia
Pelger forms	As benign hereditary anomaly, 'pseudo' forms in myeloid leukaemia, severe infection
Increased nuclear segmentation	Vitamin B_{12} or folate deficiency, renal failure
Increased granulation	Infection, some aplastic anaemias, Alder–Reilly anomaly
Decreased granulation	Myeloid leukaemia
Dohle bodies	Severe infection, May–Hegglin anomaly
EOSINOPHILS	Normal Values: $0 \cdot 04$–$0 \cdot 44 \times 10^9$/l
Eosinophilia	Allergy, parasitic infection, skin disorders, drug administration, Hodgkin's disease, chronic granulocytic leukaemia
BASOPHILS	Normal Values: $0 \cdot 00$–$0 \cdot 10 \times 10^9$/l
Basophilia	Myeloproliferative disorders, chronic granulocytic leukaemia, mast cell disease.
MONOCYTES	Normal Values: $0 \cdot 2$–$0 \cdot 8 \times 10^9$/l
Monocytosis	Chronic infections, protozoal and rickettsial infections, Hodgkin's disease, monocytic or myelomonocytic leukaemia
Myelomonocytic forms	Myeloid leukaemia
LYMPHOCYTES	Normal Values: $1 \cdot 5$–$3 \cdot 5 \times 10^9$/l
Lymphocytosis	Pertussis, exanthemata, infectious mononucleosis, hepatitis, lymphocytic leukaemia, lymphocytic lymphoma. Normal infants and children have higher values than adults
Lymphopenia	During irradiation, steroid or immunosuppressive therapy
Atypical reactive forms	Infectious mononucleosis, hepatitis, many viral infections
Plasmacytoid 'Turk' cells	Viral infections, especially rubella

Chapter 12
Nutritional Disorders

A. P. ADAMS

NUTRITION

Nutrition is the study of all processes by which microorganisms, plants and animals absorb and utilize food substances. Good nutrition cannot be achieved without a satisfactory diet. Nutritional diseases and disorders result from adverse effects of a deficiency or an excess of certain nutrients in the body tissues. These effects are most often caused by a faulty diet that is either lacking or excessive in one or more essential nutrients or food groups. Less commonly they result from constitutional metabolic defects that prevent optimum digestion, absorption or utilization of ingested food. These defects include disease processes, structural defects or chemical disorders. Deficiencies may also result from increased requirements or the defective incorporation of a vitamin or trace element into an enzyme or cofactor, and more than one mechanism may be operative in any situation.

The body of a young male adult weighing 65 kg consists of 11 kg protein, 9 kg fat, 1 kg carbohydrate, 4 kg minerals and 40 kg water [15]. Most of the protein is an essential component of the cells but about 2 kg can be lost without serious results. About 400 g of tissue protein are turned over each day but about 40 g a day of protein is the minimum safe level required in the diet [39]. The essential amino acid composition of the diet, related to the body's requirements determine its protein quality. The body's requirements for both protein and essential amino acids vary with age and are determined by the rate of turnover. Of the 9 kg of fat, not more than about 1 kg is essential, the remainder represents a store which can be drawn on in times of need. In contrast the body can be depleted at most by 200 g of carbohydrate [28]. During starvation the carbohydrate store is continuously replenished by synthesis from the reserves of protein and fat. The body can lose about 10 per cent of its total water and at least a third of the mineral content of the skeleton without serious consequences.

The average adult male in economically developed countries consumes over 3,000 kilocalories (12·54 MJ) a day, but in less developed areas the underprivileged may consume less than 1,000 kilocalories (4·18 MJ) a day. Not only is the quantity of food inadequate but its quality is poor. In these deprived parts of the world, malnutrition has its greatest impact on the young. Recommended intakes of nutrients vary for different countries and populations.

The commonest nutritional disorder that anaesthetists encounter in economically advanced countries is obesity whereas hunger and starvation are common in underprivileged parts of the world. Little is known about the interaction between specific effects of malnutrition and anaesthesia, and in the underdeveloped countries the anaesthetist usually has to make the best of the situation and probably is not often in a position to have much choice regarding drugs and techniques. Local anaesthetic techniques may be recommended in preference to general anaesthesia even when neurological complications of disease processes are known to exist.

Advances in medicine have led to the recognition of the importance of the balanced provision both in quantity and quality of energy requirements, proteins, carbohydrates, fats, vitamins, elements and water. The anaesthetist should be able to prevent, recognize and treat both general and specific nutritional disorders. Patients who have undergone extensive gut resections and anastomoses may develop complications such as fistulae, adhesions, peritonitis and obstruction. The presence of a pre-existing poor state of nutrition is a serious handicap in such patients. Blind loops, diverticulosis of the jejunum or any 'cul-de-sac' present in the gut after operation are classical causes

Table 12.1. Mechanisms of malabsorptive disorders.

Loss of absorptive surface and digestive enzymes	Artificial openings, stomas, fistulae; short-circuiting of absorptive areas; e.g. duodenum (important site for iron absorption) pancreatic malfunction
Fast transit through gut lumen	Motility disorders; anomalous secretion of hormones acting on gastrointestinal motility; short intestine after resection
Destruction of mucosal surface	Inflammatory reactions, ischaemia, radiotherapy, toxic effects of drugs
Disruption of absorptive pathways	Tumour infiltration, inflammation, etc.
Inhibition of absorption or competitive utilization of nutrient by bacterial flora of gut	Blind-loop and cul-de-sac syndromes

of malabsorption (Table 12.1). The malabsorption syndrome is characterized by a deficiency of essential nutrients and vitamins with changes in the water, acid–base and electrolyte balance of the body. Steatorrhoea is a common finding and can result in diminished absorption of the fat-soluble vitamins (vitamin K and vitamin D, with consequences as described later). Deficiency of specific water-soluble vitamins leads to anaemias and neuropathies with changes in epithelial tissues affecting the mouth, tongue and cornea. Acid–base disturbances and electrolyte losses result from protracted vomiting, diarrhoea or loss of fluids through fistulae.

Alcoholism is associated with vitamin B complex deficiencies because the requirements for the vitamin are increased whilst the intake of vitamin is decreased. This is due to gastritis, loss of appetite and reduced food intake and because alcoholics eat less food during their drinking sessions. In economically advanced countries beriberi cardiac disease is seen in chronic alcoholism and pellagra occurs as a complication of alcoholism or the malabsorption syndrome. Alcoholics appear to require slightly increased amounts of anaesthetic agents and attention should be paid to this during anaesthesia with muscle relaxant drugs lest awareness occurs. On the other hand, an alcoholic peripheral neuropathy may predispose the patient to hypotension because vasoconstrictor responses are impaired.

Anorexia nervosa is a voluntary starvation in young women; the intake of food is highly selective, and there is rarely evidence of protein deficiency. However, the tendency is to follow the energy-protein-malnutrition condition (see below) with hypotension, bradycardia, hypothermia, hypokalaemia, anaemia, decreased endocrine function and dehydration with changes in the electrocardiogram and cardiomyopathy.

MALNUTRITION

Nutrition becomes disordered as a result of any deviation from the normal. Malnutrition means simply disordered nutrition and may be due to deficiency (undernutrition) or to excess (overnutrition) of nutriment. Primary nutritional disorders are those directly due to dietary disorder; secondary nutritional disorders result from disease processes in the body. Many diseases interfere with a number of essential functions and treatment of disease may, as a side-effect, interfere with the body's nutrition, for example resection of the gastrointestinal tract.

Malnutrition may also develop in a patient consuming a satisfactory diet if he has certain diseases or disorders that interfere with the proper usage of food. This is sometimes called conditional malnutrition. Undernutrition characterized by thinness is due to imbalance between the calories available and those expended.

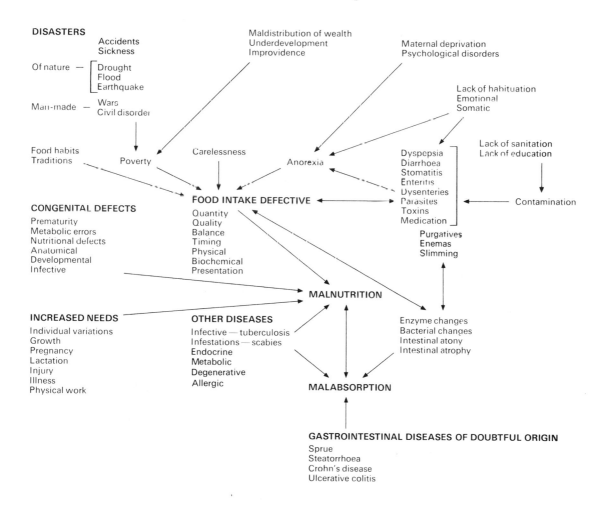

Fig. 12.1. Some causes of malnutrition. (Modified from Williams, C.D. [38].)

STARVATION

Starvation implies absolute or relative lack of all foodstuffs including vitamins and mineral elements, which are necessary for life. The individual adapts by drawing on body stores but later tissue protein is catabolized to provide basic calorie needs .There is bradycardia, lowered systolic and diastolic arterial pressures, low venous pressure, reduced cardiac output and heart size. Vital capacity, respiratory rate, minute volume and respiratory efficiency are all reduced. Secretion of thyrotrophic and adrenotrophic hormones are not affected but growth hormone is decreased. Hypothermia is frequent and contributes to death. Anaemia is usually mild, of a normochromic, normocytic type with a hypoplastic marrow. There is a considerable expansion of the plasma volume and a depression of erythropoiesis. Neurological changes are rare in general starvation. The nature of famine oedema, which is of a dependent type, is ill-understood although plasma proteins are usually slightly reduced.

ENERGY-PROTEIN-MALNUTRITION
(EPM)

Energy-protein-malnutrition was formerly termed Protein-Calorie-Malnutrition (PCM), the change in terminology being due to the adoption of the Joule as the basic unit of energy instead of the Calorie while 'Energy' takes precedence over 'Protein' because of accumulating evidence for the paramount importance of energy deficit. Energy-Protein-Malnutrition is one of the most serious and widespread health problems in underdeveloped countries in the world today. It has recently been estimated that at any one time there are 400 million preschool children throughout the world suffering in some degree from EPM which is largely responsible for the fact that half the children born do not survive to the age of 5 years. EPM characteristically occurs in children under the age of 5 years whenever the diet is poor in energy and protein.

Severe EPM can be regarded as a clinical spectrum of malnutrition with the condition of marasmus at one extreme and that of kwashiorkor at the other. Between these two extremes are forms in which the clinical features vary according to the combinations of deficiency of protein and energy, together with deficiencies of vitamins and minerals and associated infections; these forms are sometimes called marasmic-kwashiorkor. Intensive laboratory investigations devoted in particular to kwashiorkor have tended to direct attention away from the more widely prevalent milder degrees of EPM. The clinical features of EPM are a consequence of insufficient supply of energy and amino acids to the tissues necessary for protein synthesis. The result is a functional failure of different organs. Children with EPM are not only underweight but their tissues are abnormal in composition.

Intravenous anaesthetic agents such as thiopentone bind to haemoglobin and plasma protein. The free fraction is distributed to body tissues. Animals with normal levels of these blood components buffer a large amount of these drugs, leaving a small but adequate concentration to reach the brain and produce anaesthesia. The total body mass, particularly body fat, may be regarded as the 'second buffer' of intravenous anaesthetic drugs since these tissues take up a considerable amount. Undernourished individuals show a more profound level of anaesthesia than heavy individuals for a given dose of anaesthetic drug. The sleep time is likely to be increased if the results of animals given thiopentone and Althesin are extrapolated to man. Induction times are also slightly prolonged with both drugs. Although Althesin is not protein bound well-nourished individuals with their greater body mass and better production of enzymes may be better able to metabolize this drug than malnourished patients.

Profound nutritional depletion has been regarded by some as having an effect on the respiratory status of those affected. Starvation in critically ill patients makes respiratory failure quite difficult to manage. Severe starvation, of otherwise healthy subjects, often demonstrates the truth of the adage that 'death from starvation is death from pneumonia'. Chronically debilitated subjects are hypometabolic with a reduced oxygen uptake and carbon dioxide production and a proportional reduction in tidal volume although respiratory rate is unchanged. There is a marked reduction in the frequency of sighs. A reduced efficiency of gas exchange is suggested by the need to maintain an almost normal minute volume despite significantly reduced V_{O_2} and V_{CO_2}. The striking loss of periodic deep breaths in conjunction with the reduced tidal volume may lead to absence of reinflation of atelectatic areas of lung and increased susceptibility to pulmonary infection.

KWASHIORKOR

Kwashiorkor is the most prevalent and most severe form of malnutrition in the world today. It is seen mainly in the poorer people of Asia and Africa (Fig. 12.2). The name is that given to the disease by the Ga tribe living in and around Accra, Ghana. Although the disease primarily affects children in the six-months to five-year age group, the peak incidence occurs in the second and third years of life and the onset usually coincides with the discontinuance of a prolonged period of breast feeding. The disease has been called 'the sickness the older child gets when the next baby is born'. i.e. it indicates the circumstances in which the disease most commonly develops, when the demand for proteins for growth is greatest, and there is either ignorance of the best foods to give children during the weaning period or an inability to provide them.

Kwashiorkor is first and foremost a quantitative and qualitative protein deficiency disease. It may be complicated by progressively lower intakes of energy-yielding carbohydrates and further complicated by variable patterns and degrees of vitamin and mineral deficiencies. During weaning there is no supplement of milk or a totally inadequate one. Protein requirements are often increased by infections and kwashiorkor is often precipitated by outbreaks of febrile illnesses such as malaria, measles, gastroenteritis or by intestinal helminths. The first and most important sign is a failure of growth; oedema is an important sign and depends on the degree of protein deficiency, in particular the serum albumin concentration and on the amount of salt and water in the diet. Serum proteins may be very much reduced and the serum albumin may be below 10 g/l. Although there is preservation of subcutaneous fat, there is a wasting of muscles, anorexia, diarrhoea and psychomotor changes which include unhappiness or apathy.

The skin shows a dermatosis, with ulcers particularly over pressure areas and deep cracks and fissures in the skin folds, and these sites exfoliate producing areas of depigmentation; severe cases may resemble extensive burns. The hair is sparse and soft, and Negro children lose their characteristic curl. There may be changes in the colour of the hair with diffused patches or streaks of red, brown or grey colours.

Liver function is maintained and failure is unusual despite enlargement and marked structural damage. Liver biopsies show fatty changes more in the periphery than in the centre of the lobules, together with fatty cysts, and there is also cellular infiltration and evidence of fibrosis. However, the plasma bilirubin level is usually within normal

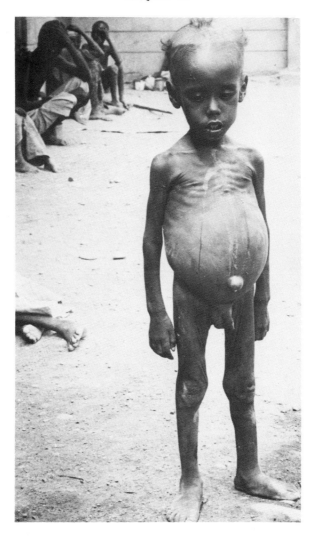

Fig. 12.2. A child suffering from severe malnutrition in the Ogaden, Ethiopia, May, 1975. (Courtesy of Stephanie Simmonds, Oxfam.)

limits—an increase is regarded as an ominous sign. The concentration of prothrombin in the blood is often reduced. Iron and folic acid are often lacking in the diet, and because there may also be impaired absorption of these and other nutrients from the intestine all varieties of anaemia may be found, the most common being a normocytic or a macrocytic anaemia. On X-ray examination the heart appears small. The electrocardiogram shows low voltage complexes and the changes due to low serum potassium concentration and there is also tachycardia. There is a deficiency of potassium in the body stores and serum potassium concentrations are markedly lowered—values below 2·5 mmol/l have been noted. The serum calcium concentration may also be lowered and muscle biopsies have shown deficiency of magnesium. The serum levels of triglyceride and cholesterol are very low and sometimes low concentrations of blood glucose are found. Death is usually due to intercurrent infections, low serum potassium levels, intractable diarrhoea or to hepatic coma. Low concentrations of serum enzymes occur, including cholinesterase, and reflect the general depletion of enzymes in tissues and organs.

MARASMUS

Marasmus is primarily a disease of infancy, within the first twelve months of life, and is due to a continued restriction of both dietary energy and protein as well as other nutrients. Marasmus means literally 'to waste' and is equivalent to starvation in adults. It is characterized by failure to thrive, irritability, and fretfulness with alternating apathy. Diarrhoea is frequent with watery or semi-solid bulky acid stools. Most infants are ravenously hungry although a few are anorexic. The infants are underweight and shrunken with little or no subcutaneous fat and they are often dehydrated. The body temperature may be subnormal. Peristalsis may be easily visible due to the thin abdominal wall and the abdomen may be shrunken or distended with gas. The muscles are weak and atrophic and limbs appear as skin and bone. The skin and mucous membranes are dry and atrophic and may reflect concomitant vitamin deficiencies. There is a marked wasting of all tissues and organs. The changes are nonspecific and show atrophy and fatty degeneration in the pancreas, kidney and some of the endocrine glands.

In marasmus, early and abrupt weaning is followed by dirty and unsound artificial feeding of infants with a very dilute milk or milk products given in inadequate amounts to avoid expense. Hence the diet is low in both energy and protein. Unsatisfactory living conditions make the preparation of clean food almost impossible so that rapid infections usually of the gastrointestinal variety develop. The mother often treats these by periods of starvation so that the infants receive only water or rice water or other non-nutritious fluids, and this in turn sets up a vicious circle of inadequate energy intake.

During anaesthesia low cardiac output and hypotensive states are liable to occur in patients with EPM who are deficient in potassium. However, the anaesthetist should not try to correct acid–base, electrolyte and fluid deficits too quickly as irreversible cardiovascular failure is likely to occur. Solutions containing glucose are useful to combat hypoglycaemia in both marasmus and kwashiorkor but may further reduce plasma potassium levels because carbohydrate administration tends to move potassium into cells. There is a reduced requirement for muscle relaxants because of the diminution in total body muscle mass; in addition, calcium and magnesium deficiencies may result in prolonged neuromuscular blockade when muscle relaxants are used.

VITAMINS

Provitamins

A provitamin is similar in structure to a specific vitamin and can be converted to it. For instance, 7-dehydrocholesterol can be converted to vitamin D_3. However, because the conversion pathway is less direct than a provitamin the amino acid tryptophan is simply called a precursor of the vitamin nicotinic acid.

Antivitamins

Antivitamins are compounds that prevent the normal function of certain vitamins, either by destroying a vitamin or by inhibiting the co-enzyme function of a vitamin.

For instance, the antivitamin thiaminase destroys thiamin. A co-enzyme is a heat stable compound that converts a protein component of an enzyme to form an active enzyme. All the water-soluble vitamins, with the exception of vitamin C, have a catalytic function, that is, they act as co-enzymes of enzymes that function in energy transfer or in the metabolism of fats, carbohydrates and proteins. Some of the fat-soluble vitamins form part of the structures of biological membranes or assist in maintaining the integrity of membranes. Some of the fat-soluble vitamins may also function at the genetic level by controlling the synthesis of certain enzymes.

Vitamin deficiencies

Since vitamins are not distributed equally in foodstuffs the more restricted the diet the more likely it is that there will be a lack of one or more vitamins. Loss of vitamins may also occur when food is cooked. For example, heat destroys vitamin A, and the water-soluble vitamins may be lost when water is extracted from food during preparation.

Vitamin deficiencies may still occur despite an adequate diet if there is interference with the absorption of the vitamin, e.g. vitamin B_{12} deficiency causing pernicious anaemia. The absence of certain digestive enzymes, for example due to pancreatic disease, can lead to failure of the digestion and absorption of fats and the fat-soluble vitamins. If the absorptive function of the intestine in gastrointestinal disease is sufficiently impaired diseases associated with severe prolonged vomiting may interfere with adequate absorption. Vitamin lack may also occur when there are increased requirements for vitamins during periods of rapid growth, i.e. childhood and pregnancy. The vitamins currently recognized are listed in Table 12.2.

Table 12.2. The vitamins.

Water soluble vitamins	Lipid soluble vitamins
Vitamin B_1 (thiamin)	Vitamin A (retinol)
Vitamin B_2 (riboflavin)	Vitamin D (ergocalciferol, D_2
Vitamin B_6 (pyridoxine and related compounds)	and cholecalciferol, D_3)
Vitamin B_{12} (cyanocobalamin and related compounds)	Vitamin E (tocopherols)
Vitamin C (ascorbic acid)	Vitamin K (phytomenadione)
Niacin (nicotinic acid, pellagra preventing factor)	
Folic acid (folacin and related compounds)	
Pantothenic acid	
Biotin	

Vitamin A

A deficiency of vitamin A may result in night blindness, xerophthalmia or keratomalacia. Permanent blindness from this cause affects approximately 20,000 children every year. Night blindness occurs because rhodopsin, the retinal pigment (visual purple) requires vitamin A for its function. A deficiency of vitamin A results in an inability of the eye to adapt in a dim light. Moreover, epithelial cells throughout the body degenerate: in the eyes, the conjunctiva and the cornea undergo changes resulting in a breakdown of the epithelium causing blindness. Other epithelial cells including the skin and the mucous membrane of the respiratory tract also degenerate resulting in hardening and drying of the skin, respiratory infections and kidney stones.

Vitamin A depletion is a long drawn-out process starting with exhaustion of the liver stores, but plasma levels of vitamin A are maintained at nearly normal levels until there is an advanced depletion. A fall in the plasma level is followed by dysfunction of the rods in the retina causing night blindness. Nearly all children with xerophthalmia have evidence of EPM. Deficiency of vitamin A results primarily from dietary lack, or secondarily to diseases causing impaired absorption or storage. Xerophthalmia affects mainly children under the age of 4 years; deprivation often begins during fetal development with inadequate liver stores, and continues throughout the first year of life with low intake from milk and cereals; requirements are high at this time because of rapid growth and infections such as measles and gastroenteritis. Thus severe deficiency of vitamin A may complicate malabsorption syndromes due to coeliac disease, sprue, fibrocystic disease or obstructive jaundice.

The vitamin B group

Vitamins B_3 and B_4 are probably the same as vitamin B_1 or thiamin. A deficiency of one member of the B group is likely to be associated with deficiencies of other members of the complex. In general these deficiencies tend to occur with excessive dependence on starches as a staple source of calories for energy production.

Vitamin B_1 (thiamin).

Takaki, a Japanese naval surgeon at the turn of the century, was the first to demonstrate that beriberi is essentially a nutritional disease arising when the proportion of polished rice in the diet is excessive. Beriberi, due to thiamin deficiency, is still an important health problem in South and East Asia. It is caused by eating diets in which most of the energy is derived from highly milled rice. Natural rice is a good source of energy but when it is highly milled, thiamin is removed with the husk and the germ of the grain. The milling of rice improves its storage properties. Beriberi is often precipitated by infection, hard physical labour, pregnancy or lactation. Although it is usually associated with the rice diet, it can also occur in groups consuming excessive amounts of highly milled wheat. Lack of thiamin can be manifested either as wet beriberi (cardiac), dry (neural), or infantile. However, it is probably unwise to consider wet and dry beriberi as separate entities as mixed syndromes can exist.

Wet beriberi. In wet beriberi (or beriberi heart disease), because of the absence of thiamin, there is a block in the decarboxylation of pyruvate and its oxidation in the citric acid cycle, and so carbohydrates are incompletely metabolized and lactic acid and pyruvic acid accumulate in the tissues and body fluids. There is a peripheral vasodilation resulting in extreme oedema and the cardiac output is increased to maintain the circulation. This eventually results in myocardial dilatation and congestive cardiac failure, which again accentuates the oedema. The signs are, therefore, of a high output cardiac failure with increased right ventricular pressure and left ventricular filling pressure associated with a low peripheral vascular resistance and increased oxygen consumption. The electrocardiogram is normal apart from showing an increased heart rate. Arterial pressure is raised and plasma and blood volumes are increased. Renal plasma flow and glomerular filtration rate are reduced and may account for the retention of sodium and water.

Dry beriberi. This is characterized by a nutritional polyneuropathy. There is a wasting of muscles with paraesthesia and impairment of sensory modalities. There may be irregularities of cardiac rhythm, dyspnoea and hypotension with bradycardia and a decreased circulation time. The electrocardiogram may show low voltage ventricular complexes, evidence of heart block or premature ventricular contractions.

Infantile beriberi. Childhood beriberi has a high incidence between the second and fourth months of life and infant mortality at this time is high. Thiamin deficiency in infants may be difficult to recognize: it may present with anorexia and vomiting, followed rapidly by neck stiffness, spasticity of the limbs, paroxysms of muscular rigidity and aphonia. There may be evidence of cardiac failure. Mothers of affected children may give a history of numbness of the feet during pregnancy and may themselves show signs of peripheral neuropathy. Thiamin 10–15 mg i.m. produces rapid clinical improvement but the neurological recovery is slow.

Thiamin deficiency occurs with the general malnutrition state encountered in chronic alcoholism. This results in varying degrees of polyneuropathy and signs of encephalopathy develop as a result of a superimposition of acute thiamin lack on the background of chronic deficiency. Acute encephalopathy is known as Wernicke's syndrome and the milder degree of this confusional state in its chronic form is known as Korsakoff's psychosis.

Cases of beriberi heart disease have obvious implications for the anaesthetist but it should also be remembered that the polyneuropathy for dry beriberi includes destruction of sympathetic fibres which may impair vasomotor responses during anaesthesia and lead to hypotension.

Riboflavin (*vitamin B₂*)

Riboflavin is the heat-stable fraction of water soluble vitamin B which remains after the antiberiberi properties have been destroyed by heat. It is widely distributed in both animal and vegetable foods but is not stored to any extent in the body although the liver and the kidney usually contain higher concentrations than other tissues. Characteristic metabolic disturbances have not been described in the deficiency state.

Riboflavin is a member of the flavoprotein group which consist of specific proteins (apoenzymes) containing either flavine mononucleotide (FMN) or flavine adenine dinucleotide (FAD) as prosthetic groups of co-enzymes. These enzymes are involved in many biological oxidation-reduction reactions. They oxidize (dehydrogenate) *l*-amino acids, *d*-amino acids, xanthine and hypoxanthine. They accept hydrogen from nicotinamide-adenine dinucleotide systems (NAD and NADP) and pass it on to the cytochrome system and thus to oxygen. The flavoproteins are relatively unstable especially when tissue protein is depleted by physiological stress, dietary deficiency or disease, when increased amounts of riboflavin are excreted in the urine. Riboflavin deficiency usually accompanies other deficiencies such as pellagra, beriberi or EPM. It can be precipitated by inadequate intake, particularly of milk, poor absorption as in diseases with chronic diarrhoea or by excessive demands as with raised metabolic rate in thyrotoxicosis, fevers or pregnancy.

Riboflavin deficiency may show itself initially as anorexia and weakness, and later as maceration of the mucosa in the angles of the mouth followed by superficial linear fissures which become crusted. The skin in the nasolabial folds, alae nasi, ears and eyelids becomes mildly erythematous, scaly and greasy. Anaemia of a nomochromic normocytic type with reticulocytopenia may also develop and responds to treatment with riboflavin. Riboflavin deficiency may also produce a magenta tongue, vascularization of the cornea, epithelial keratitis, nutritional amblyopia, scrotal dermatitis and vulvitis. In view of the importance of riboflavin in cell respiration it seems surprising that the clinical changes attributed to its deficiency are minor and do not by themselves threaten life.

Vitamin B_6 (*pyridoxine and related compounds*)

Vitamin B_6 is not a single substance but consists of three closely related chemical compounds, pyridoxine, pyridoxal and pyridoxamine, having similar physiological actions. Pyridoxine is concerned primarily in protein metabolism. Pyridoxal phosphate is concerned with the transfer of amino groups and is the co-enzyme or prosthetic group of many aminotransferases. In pyridoxine deficiency the transamination activity decreases and more nitrogen is lost from the body as urea. Another of the functions of pyridoxal phosphate is to act as coenzyme in the decarboxylation of amino acids to form special amines, e.g. serotonin from 5-hydroxytryptophan and γ-amino-butyric acid (a central inhibitory neurotransmitter) from glutamic acid. Other metabolic processes in which pyridoxal phosphate participates include the formation of melanin and in the metabolism of tryptophan.

Pyridoxine is not stored in the body to any extent; an excess is oxidized to the metabolically inert compound, pyridoxic acid. Pyridoxine deficiency may rarely arise as a result of inadequate dietary intake, but is more commonly due to some other condition that offsets an otherwise adequate intake, e.g. defective intestinal absorption, or increased renal clearance. There is evidence that pyridoxine deficiency may cause fits, particularly in infancy.

Vitamin B_6 deficiency may arise during the course of therapy with several drugs, in particular isoniazid used in the treatment of pulmonary tuberculosis, and hydralazine used in the treatment of hypertension. Rarely, cases have been described of patients with hypochromic anaemia which was refractory to iron therapy but responded dramatically to pyridoxine. Most of the cases have normoblastic erythropoiesis but in about 16 per cent of cases erythropoiesis is megaloblastic. The anaemia is usually severe, the mean haemoglobin being less than 4 g/dl and there is often iron overload and impaired liver function. It is thought that in about 30 per cent of patients an inborn error of metabolism is responsible.

Vitamin B_{12} (*cyanocobalamin*)

Vitamin B_{12} is the largest and most complicated vitamin and is synthesized almost exclusively by micro organisms; it is not found in any plants. The molecule consists of a modified metalloporphyrin with cobalt in the centre, linked to a nucleotide containing a base, ribose and phosphoric acid.

Vitamin B_{12} is present in the body in several forms including a very therapeutically effective form, hydroxocobalamin, which is retained in the body much longer than vitamin B_{12}. Vitamin B_{12} deficiency usually arises as a metabolic defect, rather than as a result of a deficiency in the diet although this possibility should be considered in undernourished populations and pure vegetarians.

Symptoms and signs of vitamin B_{12} deficiency do not usually appear until the body stores, mainly the liver, have been largely depleted. Serum levels are reduced long before this. Vitamin B_{12} deficiency may arise from dietary lack, interference with the production of intrinsic factor, and interference with the function of intrinsic factor, such as the blind-loop syndrome and jejunal diverticulosis. It can also occur in various malabsorption syndromes, particularly in patients whose ileum has been resected or bypassed and in infestation with the fish tapeworm which takes up the vitamin from the food. Excessive loss in the urine due to defective binding by serum proteins is also possible. Vitamin B_{12} deficiency may result in pernicious anaemia in which the haematological changes are identical to those due to a deficiency of folic acid. The blood picture is discussed in Chapter 11. Neurological changes may precede the haematological changes; the commonest neurological complication of vitamin B_{12} deficiency is peripheral neuropathy, but a characteristic myelopathy (subacute combined degeneration) also occurs, in which lesions of the lateral and posterior columns of the spinal cord predominate (see page 284). Although low levels of vitamin B_{12} are often encountered in tropical sprue, myelopathy is rare in this condition. Usually the myelopathic and other neurological complications of coeliac disease are not due to vitamin B_{12} deficiency.

In normal individuals the hypotensive agent sodium nitroprusside [1,2] has been shown to reduce plasma vitamin B_{12} concentration, and may be dangerous if given to patients with abnormally low levels. Sodium nitroprusside is converted in the body to thiocyanate with the formation of cyanide as an intermediate product. There is an inverse relation between plasma B_{12} and plasma cyanide levels and the administration of i.v. hydroxocobalamin may be of value as a means of minimizing cyanide accumulation.

Folic acid (folacin, pteroylglutamic acid)

Folic acid and vitamin B_{12} are intimately involved in nucleoprotein metabolism and in the maturation of erythrocytes. Folic acid deficiency is probably the most common vitamin deficiency in the Western world and is the commonest cause of megaloblastic anaemia during pregnancy. Deficiency of folic acid is also common in premature infants. The absorption of folic acid from the jejunum is reduced by sodium bicarbonate, by phenytoin, and by many gastrointestinal diseases and malabsorption syndromes. Folic acid, if heated in a neutral or alkaline medium, undergoes fairly rapid destruction and therefore can be destroyed by some forms of cooking. Several closely allied compounds have been identified in living matter and those which are biologically active are collectively known as 'folate'. Folate is converted to folic acid in the tissues, where reduction to the active form of the vitamin, tetrahydrofolic acid, readily occurs. Ascorbic acid helps to maintain the folic acid coenzymes in an active form.

Nutritional megaloblastic anaemia in adults may be due to deficiency of folate or vitamin B_{12}. The haematological distinctions between them are considered in Chapter 11. Folic acid should not be used in the treatment of pernicious anaemia because it may cause a deterioration of the neurological features of the disease.

Niacin (nicotinic acid, pellagra-preventing factor)

Pellagra means a 'rough' or 'sour' skin. It was first described in Spain in the eighteenth century after the introduction of maize from the Americas. It is a chronic and relapsing disease with a seasonal incidence due to a relative lack in the protein of maize of tryptophan, a precursor of the vitamin niacin. However, the niacin that does exist in maize is bound in an unavailable form. Pellagra is characterized by a loss of weight, increase in debility, gastrointestinal disturbances, mental changes and erythematous dermatitis which results from the exposure to sunlight and hence has a characteristic distribution. Pellagra has been called the disease of the three D's: dermatitis, diarrhoea and dementia. Alcoholism is a precipitating factor in some countries.

Features which are of particular interest to the anaesthetist are increasing debility, gastrointestinal disturbances with concomitant changes in electrolytes, glossitis and stomatitis which usually appear early in the disease, and the tongue has a 'raw beef' appearance.

Secondary niacin deficiency

Pellagra has been described in patients receiving isoniazid therapy which appears to act by replacing nicotinamide in DPN. Niacin deficiency may also occur in patients with malignant carcinoid tumours where as much as 60 per cent of the body's tryptophan is diverted to form large amounts of 5-hydroxytryptamine. Hartnup disease, a hereditary metabolic disorder, presents in childhood with pellagra and attacks of cerebellar ataxia.

Vitamin C (ascorbic acid)

In 1753 Lind, who was a Scots naval surgeon, published a *Treatise of the Scurvy* in which he showed that scurvy could be prevented and cured by fresh oranges and lemon with adequate diet and other hygienic measures. Scurvy was the scourge of mariners during long ocean voyages and its devastating effects have been immortalized in Samuel Coleridge's *The Rime of the Ancient Mariner*. In the early stages of scurvy there is swelling and bleeding of the gums and bleeding into the skin; bleeding into the muscles and under the periosteum may also occur in small children. A microcytic hypochromic anaemia develops and infants may show a megaloblastic anaemia due to combined deficiency of folic and ascorbic acids. Resistance to infection decreases. *L*-ascorbic acid is the effective antiscorbutic substance.

Vitamin C is absorbed through the buccal mucous membrane and the mucous membranes of the stomach and upper part of the small intestine. Vitamin C is a simple sugar and is the most active reducing agent known to occur naturally in living tissues; it is destroyed by oxidation, heat and strong alkalis. The concentration of ascorbic acid in the tissues appears to be related to metabolic activity. The largest concentration is found in the adrenal gland with high levels also present in liver, spleen and brain. This presence in tissues of high metabolic activity suggests a role of ascorbic acid in reactions involved in electron transfer in the cell. Vitamin C is transported from the plasma into the tissues where it plays an essential metabolic role in ovarian function, haemopoiesis, brain metabolism, corticosteroid release and liver metabolism. It is also involved in cholesterol synthesis and fatty acid metabolism, and in the synthesis of lipoproteins, plasma and tissue proteins. It influences carbohydrate metabolism by affecting the action of insulin. Vitamin C is responsible for the formation of hydroxyproline from proline and this enables normal collagen formation to occur and tissue healing to take place. Although scurvy is rare in most countries today, adult cases occur amongst elderly bachelors and widowers who cook for themselves; food faddists are especially at risk, but women even when living alone usually place a greater emphasis on fruit and vegetables in their diet.

Effects on drug biotransformation

In high doses vitamins may have pharmacological effects that are distinct from their nutritional effects and vitamin C may significantly potentiate other drugs. High doses are a not uncommon health fad and 'preventative' of the common cold.

Vitamin C is metabolized in part to ascorbic acid sulphate in man. Sulphate formation is also an important pathway for biotransformation of phenolic drugs which is of limited capacity in man and so is subject to saturation and competitive inhibition. For example, concomitant administration of vitamin C and salicylamide causes a decrease in conversion of the latter to salicylamide sulphate.

A number of drugs are extensively conjugated with sulphate and thereby inactivated in their passage through the intestinal tissues and liver following oral administration. One such drug is isoprenaline. The recommended oral dose of isoprenaline is about 100–1,000 times larger than the intravenous dose thus reflecting its inactivation by biotransformation during absorption. Salicylamide can markedly inhibit this inactivation, and similar effects may well occur when vitamin C is taken with drugs which ordinarily undergo extensive conjugation with sulphate during their initial passage across the intestinal mucosa and through the liver. This could result in a significant potentiation in the pharmacological activity of drugs so affected.

Vitamin D

Vitamin D_3 (cholecalciferol) is produced photochemically in the skin from 7-dehydrocholesterol and this forms the natural source of vitamin D_3 in man. Calciferol, or vitamin D_2, is produced in the same way from ergosterol. There is no difference in effects of vitamins D_2 and D_3 in the treatment or prevention of rickets. Both vitamin D_2 and D_3 are converted in the liver into biologically active metabolites of which 25-hydroxycholecalciferol (25-HCC) is of major importance, being somewhat more potent than vitamin D_3 itself, and this subsequently converted in the kidney into 1,25-dihydroxycholecalciferol which is many times more potent. Because vitamin D and its metabolites are formed in one part of the body and exert their effects elsewhere, they may be regarded more as hormones than vitamins.

Vitamin D and its active metabolites are necessary for the maintenance of the normal plasma calcium concentration. They promote calcium absorption from the distal part of the small intestine, promote the absorption of calcium from bone, and probably also act by increasing tubular reabsorption of calcium in the kidney. Vitamin D compounds also promote renal tubular absorption of phosphate. There are close interrelationships between vitamin D and parathyroid hormone and calcitonin. Severe vitamin D deficiency is associated with malabsorption of phosphorus and a reduced renal tubular reabsorption of phosphorus because of secondary hyperparathyroidism. (See also page 531.)

In the rachitic child the bones are softened and deformed because vitamin D deficiency has led to failure of absorption of calcium from the intestine. In adults the softening of bones is termed osteomalacia where deficiency of vitamin D produces a calcium deficiency leading to demineralization of the bones. The main factors in the genesis of these diseases are, the intake of little or no milk, lack of vitamin D and low calcium foods, cold winters and avoidance of sunlight, and pollution of the air with smog which filters ultraviolet radiation from the sun. Tetany, due to a low serum level of ionizable calcium, is a complication of rickets and more rarely of osteomalacia and is of interest to anaesthetists because it may be precipitated by overbreathing. The serum level is usually maintained due to parathyroid gland activity and is only reduced in the later stages of the disease. Serum phosphate is low as a result of diminished tubular reabsorption by the kidney. Alkaline phosphatase is normally increased although it may be unchanged in the presence of energy-protein-malnutrition. A practical guide is derived from $Ca \times P$ in mg/100 ml serum. In the normal or healing phase it is greater than 40, but in vitamin D deficiency it is less than 35.

Hypervitaminosis D was not infrequently reported after World War II and was due to mothers overdosing their children with vitamin D. The increased serum levels of calcium and phosphate result in abnormal calcification in the body and the anaesthetist should be aware of secondary effects such as hypertension and kidney damage.

Hypocalcaemia may be associated with a prolonged neuromuscular blockade following the use of muscle relaxants and particular attention should be directed to the possibility of cardiac dysrhythmias or a low cardiac output state, or both, occurring during anaesthesia.

Vitamin E

Substances which promote fertility in animals are called tocopherols and are grouped as vitamin E. There are four tocopherols, alpha, beta, gamma and delta which differ from each other in the position of the methyl groups around the ring of the molecule. They all have the same physiological properties although α-tocopherol is somewhat more potent than the others. Tocopherols protect both vitamin A and carotene from oxidation *in vitro* and this categorizes them as natural antioxidants.

The presence of vitamin E has been proven in the inner membrane of mitochondria and in the plasma membrane of erythrocytes. Vitamin E is thought to fulfil a function in the membrane by controlling membrane stability and permeability and by protecting membrane lipids against peroxides. This role as a membrane stabilizer gives the vitamin a significance as a nutrient.

Deficiency of vitamin E in premature infants may be associated with haemolytic anaemia, manifest in the 4th–6th weeks of life in infants weighing less than 1,500 g at birth. This anaemia is characterized by a haemoglobin concentration of 7–10 g/dl and an increased reticulocyte count. The red blood cells show an increased sensitivity to haemolysis in dilute solutions of hydrogen peroxide. The morphology of the red blood cells is variable but usually includes anisocytosis, poikilocytosis, irregularly contracted cells, cell fragmentation and spherocytosis. Thrombocytosis is generally present and some infants may have oedema of the feet, lower extremities and scrotal areas.

The haemolytic anaemia associated with vitamin E deficiency appears to be multifactorial and depends on a relative lack of an antioxidant (vitamin E), the presence of a substrate capable of being peroxidized (red-cell membrane poly-unsaturated fatty acid) and the presence of an agent capable of initiating free radical generation that leads to lipid peroxidation. The fatty acid complex of red blood cell membranes reflects to a large extent the fatty acid composition of the plasma, which in turn is determined by the diet. The feeding of large quantities of polyunsaturated fatty acids such as linoleic acid to infants whose capacity to absorb fat-soluble vitamins, such as vitamin E, may be limited, can lead to a relative if not absolute deficiency of this antioxidant. Because there will be an accumulation of such polyunsaturated acid in the red-cell membranes, these cells will be highly vulnerable to peroxidation causing lysis. However, iron therapy to correct the anaemia may paradoxically lead to increased lysis because of the initiation of free radical generation that leads to lipid peroxidation, i.e. the role of iron is to set the peroxidation train in motion.

Vitamin K

Vitamin K exists in nature in at least two forms, K_1 and K_2, both being derivatives of napthoquinone. The naturally occurring form of vitamin K_1 is known as phytomenadione. Vitamin K_2 is not important in medical practice. The synthetic compound menadione or menaphthone is almost as active as either of the vitamins K. Water-soluble synthetic preparations are also available for intravenous use (Synkavit). Several synthetic water-soluble preparations closely related to menadione have considerable vitamin K activity. Many species of bacteria synthesize vitamin K, including those normally present in the human intestine and this explains why adults appear to be independent of their diet for their supply of vitamin K. Vitamin K is not stored in the body.

Vitamin K is of particular interest in anaesthesia because its deficiency in the body may be associated with a tendency to bleed due to hypothrombinaemia. Since vitamin K is fat soluble, a deficiency is likely to occur whenever a failure of fat absorption develops from any cause. In surgical practice this most frequently arises in diseases of the biliary system associated with jaundice when bile salts are excluded from the intestine. Other conditions include sprue, idiopathic steatorrhoea, and ulcerative colitis. Vitamin K is necessary for the formation of prothrombin in the liver, possibly by becoming the prosthetic group of an enzyme involved in prothrombin synthesis. Prothrombin is a glycoprotein present in the blood plasma and necessary for the normal clotting of the blood. In vitamin K deficiency the time that the blood takes to clot is prolonged.

Infants in the first week of life have less prothrombin in their blood than normal adults and sometimes a prolonged prothrombin time. Deficiency of vitamin K may arise during prolonged antibiotic therapy when vitamin K-producing bacteria may be suppressed; chronic disease may have the same effect. The mode of action of all vitamin K derivatives is not identical. The action of the vitamin K analogue, menadione, against the dicoumarol anticoagulants is of little effect, unlike the naturally occurring K_1 compound.

NUTRITIONAL COMPLICATIONS OF PARENTERAL FEEDING

A formidable list of deficiencies follow massive resection of the small intestine. When only duodenum remains, permanent parenteral feeding is needed. The aim of parenteral nutrition is to supply water, calories, nitrogen, minerals and vitamins in correct proportions to achieve an anabolic state under circumstances normally asssociated with a catabolic response. Problems relating to fluid and electrolyte balance are outside the scope of this chapter and the reader is referred to reviews [13, 14, 17].

The development of long-term intravenous feeding techniques to maintain patients who have had extensive resection of the small bowel has led to recognition of the importance of minerals such as iron, calcium, chromium, magnesium, zinc, iodine, manganese, cobalt and copper. Copper deficiency can result in dimorphic anaemia with neutropenia. Experiments suggest that the elements molybdenum, vanadium, tin, nickel, silicon and possibly boron, may also be essential nutrients for mammals.

The various solutions of sugars, amino acids, fat emulsions and additives used in intravenous nutrition are capable of producing serious metabolic disturbances. Complications include hypophosphataemia, metabolic acidosis, hyperammonaemia, deficiency of essential fatty acids, hyperlipaemia and the hyperosmolar dehydration syndrome.

Hypophosphataemia results from the use of synthetic amino acid preparations in place of casein hydrolysates which contain phosphate, or failure to use fat emulsions which contain phosphate. Hypophosphataemia results in a reduction in the 2,3-diphosphoglycerate concentration of red blood cells causing a shift of the oxygen-haemoglobin dissocation curve to the left. Intralipid is a fat emulsion which provides phosphate from its phospholipid content and so prevents the hypophosphataemia which complicates amino acid infusions and in addition avoids the hyperosmolar dehydration. Intralipid is a 10 per cent emulsion of soya bean oil containing 56 g/l linoleic acid, and as much as 40 to 50 per cent of the total caloric requirement can be given in this way. Linoleic acid is the only essential fatty acid that need be provided in man. A deficiency results in a scaly rash, delayed wound healing, anaemia, increased platelet adhesiveness—which may be associated with cerebral or coronary occlusion—and a large fatty liver. Deficiencies in essential fatty acids are liable to occur in children and in long-term parenteral feeding when fat emulsions are not used.

The hyperosmolar dehydration syndrome follows the use of hypertonic carbohydrate solutions, particularly when the infusion is too rapid and there is inadequate insulin cover.

The development of metabolic acidosis is especially related to the use of fructose infusions as rates exceeding 0·5 g/kg/hr, and is particularly dangerous in children (see also page 332). Metabolic acidosis may also occur during the infusion of some modern synthetic amino acid combinations where there is an excess of the cationic amino acids (e.g. histidine, arginine, lysine) over the anionic amino acids (e.g. glutamic and aspartic acids).

Casein hydrolysates contain ammonia in appreciable quantities and hyperammonaemia may develop. This is especially liable to occur in children and patients with liver disease. The hyperammonaemia is also seen in patients given amino acid preparations which contain excess glycine and is not necessarily prevented by the addition of arginine.

Hyperlipaemia may complicate infusions of fat emulsions if the fat is not cleared by the liver. It may be detected by visually examining a centrifuged sample of blood drawn in the morning.

OBESITY

Obesity is the commonest nutritional disorder in civilized countries today. Like beauty, the concept of obesity in society depends on the eye of the beholder (see Fig. 12.3). In some parts of Africa, young girls are fattened up for marriage. The African explorer, Speke, in the last century came upon the harem of the King of Karagwe whose wives were so fat that they could not stand upright, and instead grovelled like seals on the floor of their huts. Their diet was an uninterrupted flow of milk that was sucked from a a gourd through a straw. If the young girls resisted this treatment, they were force-fed like the *pâté de foie gras* geese of Strasbourg. The commonest definition of obesity relates life expectancy to weight: this is based on pooled American life assurance

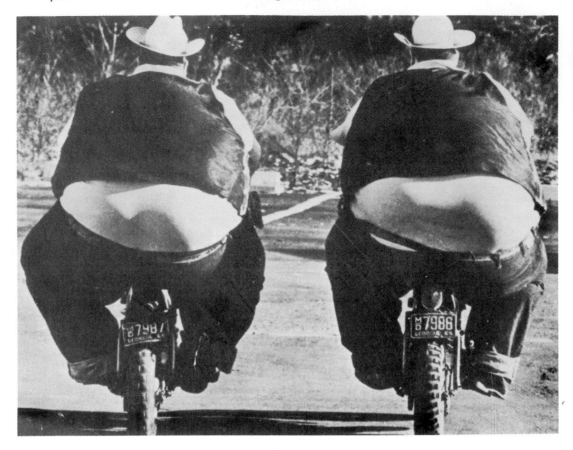

Fig. 12.3. Bill and Ben McCreary—known as the Two Man Traffic Jam. (Courtesy of *World Medicine*.)

statistics which indicate a person to be obese if he or she exceeds the ideal or expected weight, corrected for age and sex, by more than 10 per cent [35]. Objective measurements suggest that obesity exists when the fat content of the body exceeds 25 per cent in the male and 30 per cent in the female.

Associated diseases and changes in physiological functions in fat people require a careful preoperative assessment to be made: hypertension, generalized arteriosclerosis and cardiomegaly are common: diabetes mellitus may co-exist. Severe pathological changes may exist in many systems of the body in obese individuals without objective evidence of extensive disease and obesity can present one of the worst possible anaesthetic risks [18]. The factors involved in the aetiology of obesity have been reviewed [5, 19, 21, 26].

The problems of obesity related to anaesthesia have only received attention in recent years [19] and most studies have been performed on patients presenting for elective gut by-pass procedures. The anaesthetist must distinguish between two basic types of obesity. The first type is called 'simple', 'pure' or 'uncomplicated' obesity, the essential criterion of people in this category being that they do *not* have a raised arterial P_{CO_2}. The second type is the obesity–hypoventilation–syndrome (OHS) or 'Pickwickian' Syndrome (see below). OHS is as different from simple obesity as the latter is from normal; however, OHS is uncommon, accounting for only 8 per cent or less of all obese patients. The importance of distinguishing between these two groups is that the cardiopulmonary disturbances are much more severe in the OHS than in simple obesity and the consequences of operation are likely to be grave. Furthermore, weight loss in patients with OHS is associated with a reduction in arterial P_{CO_2} and an improvement in vital capacity and maximum voluntary ventilation.

RESPIRATORY FUNCTION

Important structural changes take place related to the duration and degree of obesity: the heavy enlarged abdomen tends to produce a thoracic kyphosis and lumbar lordosis, thereby raising the lower part of the sternum, limiting rib movement and producing a relative fixation of the thorax in a position of inspiration. The bellows action of the thoracic cage is reduced by the layers of fat on the chest wall and abdomen, and the diaphragm is elevated. All these factors result in an increase in the total work of breathing: ventilation becomes diaphragmatic and very prone to postural deterioration. Although there is no direct linear relation between the work of respiration and the degree of obesity the oxygen cost of breathing is increased particularly at large minute volumes.

Although the arterial P_{O_2} is lower than normal in obesity, hypoventilation characterized by a raised arterial P_{CO_2} rarely occurs. This is because those parts of the lung which remain well ventilated and well perfused can clear increased amounts of carbon dioxide because of its natural high diffusing capacity and the favourable characteristics of its dissociation curve. The response of the respiratory centre to inhalation of 5 per cent carbon dioxide is essentially normal in patients with simple obesity and normal lungs. Therefore, in the upright obese person, provided that there is no intrinsic lung disease, no fatty infiltration of muscle, and the respiratory centre is unaffected by drugs or disease, hypoventilation does not occur. The balance is, however, delicately poised and can be disturbed by simply adopting the head-down position or the establishment of general anaesthesia.

The obesity–hypoventilation (or 'Pickwickian') syndrome (OHS)

In simple obesity the increase in resting ventilation is generally appropriate to the increase in oxygen consumption and carbon dioxide production. This is in contrast to the disproportionate and insufficient increase in alveolar ventilation found in OHS. The syndrome is an association of obesity, episodic somnolence and hypoventilation, with twitching, cyanosis, periodic respiration and secondary circulatory abnormalities: polycythaemia, right ventricular hypertrophy and right ventricular failure. The primary ventilatory impairment is hypoventilation unrelated to obstructive or restrictive disease of the lung [3, 6, 22]. The adjective 'Pickwickian' relates to the fat messenger boy who kept falling asleep, described by Charles Dickens in *Pickwick Papers*, published in 1837, although introduced into the medical literature almost 120 years later [10]

The respiratory changes in OHS are more severe than those found in simple obesity: both lung and chest wall compliance are reduced, there is closure of peripheral lung units, an increased energy of breathing and a marked underventilation of the dependent regions of the lungs. In these patients weight loss is associated with a reduction in arterial P_{CO_2} and an improvement in vital capacity and maximum voluntary ventilation, but not, however, in chest wall compliance. It is suggested that OHS develops as a result of an excessive reduction in chest wall compliance which together with the inspiratory muscle weakness interact with the circulatory abnormalities in simple obesity to promote carbon dioxide retention. In OHS, alveolar hypoxia and acidaemia produce both pulmonary artery vasoconstriction and pulmonary arterial hypertension so that pulmonary arterial pressure exceeds left ventricular pressure at the end of the diastole [32].

There is some evidence that the function of the respiratory centre is altered in OHS and it is interesting that a similar syndrome occurs in nonobese patients with brain damage. Progesterone, 100 mg i.m. daily, has been used in the treatment of OHS with, in some cases, a fall of the arterial P_{CO_2} to normal values together with an improvement in arterial P_{O_2}. The therapy is likened to the mild chemical hyperventilation seen during the luteal phase of the menstrual cycle and in the hyperventilation of pregnancy.

Lung volumes

Obese subjects show a reduction in total lung capacity which is generally poorly correlated with the extent of the obesity [4]. The most consistent changes are reductions in inspiratory capacity and expiratory reserve volume (ERV) which in the sitting position may be reduced to less than 20 per cent of its predicted value and which may be obliterated in the head-down position [34]. The functional residual capacity (FRC) is reduced, that is, the resting end-expiratory position of the chest is lower than normal [23]. Closing volume (CV) is increased and this together with the decreased ERV implies underventilation of dependent lung regions during resting tidal breathing especially in the supine position, the inspired air being distributed to the upper, or nondependent, lung zones. There is a good correlation between arterial P_{O_2} and the extent of airway closure and little improvement in blood-gas exchange occurs unless patients reduce their weight to within 30 per cent of their ideal weight as calculated from height, age and sex [16].

The hypoxaemia without hypercapnia of simple obesity is related to overperfusion of the underventilated areas or to perfusion of completely unventilated areas of the lung: the resulting mismatch between air flow and blood flow in the lungs results in an increased venous admixture, a decreased arterial P_{O_2} and an increase in physiological dead space; a large increase in anatomical shunt occurs [7, 8, 33].

Lung mechanics

Obese patients who have no structural damage to their lungs have a normal airway resistance. The chest wall compliance is reduced [29], being further reduced by recumbency, and is not usually improved by a period of weight reduction. Lung compliance may be unaltered or be reduced by 25 per cent in simple obesity and 40 per cent in OHS.

In patients with OHS and right ventricular enlargement it is probable that lung compliance is further reduced by an increase in pulmonary extravascular water; this in turn increases the load on the inspiratory muscles and further impairs ventilation-perfusion relationships and pulmonary gas exchange [32]. In this connection, the importance of avoiding excessive fluid therapy during anaesthesia and in the postoperative period is emphasized. In experiments involving 'mass loading' of the lower thorax and abdomen of anaesthetized women of normal weight by means of 22·5 kg sandbags, a reduction in chest wall compliance was obtained to values observed in anaesthetized obese women; at any respiratory volume, the compliance of the obese women was about one-half that of the women of normal weights and it is suggested that the low chest wall compliance results from excess weight only [37]. This view, however, should not be accepted without considerable reservations: in the OHS there may be no change in the total compliance of the respiratory system as a result of weight loss [32]. Respiratory muscle efficiency is impaired in both types of obesity and the inspiratory muscle strength of patients with OHS is 60 to 70 per cent of normal.

CIRCULATORY FUNCTION

Obesity imposes an additional work load on a heart with an already compromised circulation in individuals with increased basal metabolism and a limited exercise tolerance [11]. Both cardiac output and blood volume are increased in obesity: the increase in blood flow is due to an increased stroke volume since the resting heart rate remains normal or low. Cardiac enlargement occurs in obese people whether or not they have hypertension. Left ventricular end-diastolic pressure may be raised in both types of obesity and pulmonary hypertension is not uncommon. Generalized atherosclerosis is two to three times more severe in obese people and there is a positive correlation between coronary artery disease and obesity.

The measurement of arterial pressure using a conventional sphygmomanometer with a standard adult arm cuff is subject to inaccuracy, usually an overestimate. Nevertheless, there is a well-established positive correlation between raised arterial pressure and an increase in body weight. The use of a thigh blood pressure cuff on the arm has been found useful—giving readings of about 20–30 mmHg higher than those recorded intra-arterially—but for long or difficult cases the continuous measurement of arterial pressure by an intra-arterial method is to be preferred. The use of a precordial, or better still an oesophageal, stethoscope and a continuous display of the ECG on an oscilloscope during the induction and maintenance of anaesthesia are highly recommended.

Dehydration and hypovolaemia are difficult to detect clinically in the obese patient and rapid infusion can prove dangerous to an already compromised circulation. The technical difficulties of surgery prolong the operation and increase blood loss. The use of central venous pressure monitoring as a guide to the adequacy of transfusion is most useful.

ANAESTHESIA

Obese patients, whose respiratory and cardiovascular functions are already compromised before operation, may be expected to react erratically to anaesthesia and surgery. The mortality figures for elective surgery for intestinal short-circuiting procedures range between 0 and 6 per cent [9] and higher figures are to be expected in more acute situations; there are reports of deaths occurring without adequate explanation in obese patients. The risks of operation are greater in the obese than in the nonobese patient [31] and obesity has been put in the Class IV physical status, or less correctly termed anaesthetic risk, category of the American Society of Anesthesiologists [18]. The problems begin, as have already been discussed, before the anaesthetic is started; the use of two operating tables side-by-side may be required to accommodate the obese patient.

The conduct of anaesthesia in the obese patient varies according to different

14

authorities. The recommended techniques include a trial of artificial ventilation before operation and performing tracheal intubation under topical anaesthesia to secure the airway before unconsciousness is produced [27]. No single technique appears to be superior to all others; the main factor which leads to a successful outcome is a comprehensive knowledge of the various problems which are involved and the skill to avoid the pitfalls. Patients with OHS may collapse on assuming the supine position before anaesthesia is started.

The preoperative period

The importance of a very thorough preoperative evaluation cannot be overstressed. Preoperative pulmonary function tests which are simple to perform, such as vital capacity, forced expiratory volume in one second and maximum expiratory flow rate, are often unremarkable in patients with simple obesity. Latent ventilatory insufficiency is a feature of average and serious obesity and will almost invariably become evident during effort. Any abnormalities of pulmonary function tests which exist in this group of patients are not usually improved by a period of weight loss. The tests should be performed with the patient $45°$ head-up as this is the position usually assumed postoperatively. Blood-gas analysis is important to provide a baseline for future measurements and invariably reveals arterial hypoxaemia: the arterial Po_2 is further reduced on changing from the sitting to the supine position. The mean arterial Po_2, in obese patients who are breathing air, in the sitting position, is reduced by 22 per cent from that predicted from their age. Although fat people generally tend to be happy and extroverted, the possibility of hidden anxiety, which itself may be related to the cause of the obesity, should be remembered when the anaesthetist makes his preoperative visit. Preoperative medication should either be omitted or be light e.g. an antisialogogue only. Adequate instruction in breathing exercises together with an explanation of certain procedures, such as awake tracheal intubation and postoperative mechanical ventilation of the lungs, should be given to the patient if necessary.

The obese patient has a potential full stomach: this applies even in elective cases. Obese patients are at even greater risk than obstetric cases. A study of 56 obese patients awaiting anaesthesia and surgery showed that 88 per cent had a gastric pH less than 2·5 units, that 86 per cent had a gastric residual volume greater than 25 ml, and that 75 per cent of the patients came into both categories. None of these patients had carbon dioxide retention [36]. Treatment with antacids should be given before the induction of either regional or general anaesthesia.

Induction of anaesthesia

The intravenous induction of anaesthesia is technically difficult because of the lack of suitable veins: there is a particular risk of accidental intra-arterial and extravascular injection. A large-blade Macintosh pattern laryngoscope should be used to facilitate tracheal intubation, preferably an instrument with a detachable handle and blade, as it may be difficult to insert the laryngoscope into the mouth because of the supra- and antesternal pads of fat; trauma to the mouth and oropharynx can easily occur. An awake tracheal intubation with topical analgesia should be considered in difficult circumstances.

The uptake and recovery time for inhalational anaesthesia is altered in the obese. The mixing times of gases in the lungs is shortened because of the low FRC and this permits a potentially rapid increase in the alveolar concentration of relatively insoluble inhalational anaesthetic agents such as nitrous oxide and cyclopropane. In practice, an inhalational induction is not easy due to intermittent upper airway obstruction and there is bucking, breath-holding and cyanosis. High pressures are often required to inflate the lungs when a face-mask is used and this may render the cardio-oesophageal sphincter incompetent with the consequent risk of the inhalation of gastric contents; hiatus hernia is also common in the obese patient. Difficulty in inflating the lungs using a face-mask in an obese patient has caused inflation of the stomach and resulted in cardiac arrest.

Maintenance of anaesthesia

Predictions of a reduction in the FRC following the induction of anaesthesia in obese patients have been confirmed, the possible causes being a loss of lung elastic recoil and premature airway closure: there is a shift of ventilation to the nondependent lung regions. The elderly obese patient with a reduced FRC may reach a state during anaesthesia where closing volume (CV) exceeds FRC. Trapped gas behind the closed airways equilibrates with venous blood and contributes to venous admixture in the pulmonary circulation. Inspired oxygen concentrations should be increased to at least 40 per cent in order to maintain arterial oxygen tension at safe levels. To maintain unconsciousness, either inhalational or intravenous anaesthetic agents are required. The uptake and storage of fat-soluble anaesthetic agents, such as the volatile anaesthetic agents, into the large fat depots during prolonged surgery is significant and will retard recovery. Methoxyflurane and enflurane are not recommended for use in obese patients because of the risk of high inorganic serum fluoride levels resulting and thus the possibility of renal tubular damage. Since methoxyflurane is very fat soluble, lengthy administration of high concentrations will result in prolonged storage, metabolism and elimination of the drug. Enflurane is capable of liberating modest amounts of fluoride but not nearly as much as methoxyflurane. Stereochemical forces hold the fluoride in enflurane fairly strongly and enflurane is not as fat soluble as methoxyflurane. Thus the amount accumulating in fat and serving as a substrate for metabolic breakdown and consequent liberation of fluorine is less. The isomer of enflurane, isoflurane, liberates even less fluorine than enflurane. When controlled ventilation of the lungs is employed, the choice of a drug to maintain unconsciousness is a potent analgesic such as fentanyl given alone or with a small dose of droperidol. However, fentanyl is not advised if the patient is not to receive elective ventilation of the lungs postoperatively as respiratory depression may well ensue as a delayed response. Pancuronium is preferred to tubocurarine as a muscle relaxant as there is less risk of hypotension occuring. Arterial oxygen tensions are severely depressed (<65 mmHg) despite inspired oxygen concentrations of 40 per cent when subdiaphragmatic packs are inserted by the surgeon or a $15°$ head-down tilt is used. Thus the prone and Trendelenburg positions should be avoided whenever possible; obstruction of the inferior vena cava may easily occur with surgical retraction. The key factor in the ability of obese patients to tolerate the supine position is that of the heart responding to an increased preload and increased work of breathing by an increase in output.

The expected improvement in arterial Po_2 during controlled ventilation of the lungs with a raised expiratory airway pressure does not always occur, and positive pressure ventilation in severe obesity may further decrease cardiac output and pulmonary blood flow and increase pulmonary vascular resistance. Correction of hypoxaemia and hypercapnia by controlled ventilation might be expected, however, to offset these effects. A tidal volume of between 10 and 15 ml/kg at a frequency of 10 to 12 a minute is recommended using a volume-preset lung ventilator. In general a positive end-expiratory pressure (PEEP) is recommended as gas distribution is improved. Uneven distribution of gas in an obese patient is due to regional differences in the pulmonary time constants as in obstructive lung disease and by airway closure. As much as 50 per cent of lung tissue may be closed off at residual volume. There is no merit, however, in adding PEEP to a technique which employs high tidal volumes. It should always be remembered that although the alveolar-to-arterial oxygen tension gradient (A–a D_{O_2}) is reduced when PEEP follows a period of IPPV the oxygen availability may be reduced because of a reduction in both $\dot{Q}s/\dot{Q}t$ and cardiac output.

Limitation of the administration of glucose solutions to 2 ml/kg/hour controls blood glucose levels during operation. Increased glucose levels may impair neutrophilic phagocytosis and wound healing while inadequate glucose availability produces lipolysis and results in increased myocardial oxygen demands.

The criteria to be satisfied before extubation is attempted are: an awake patient; a tidal volume of at least 350 ml; a vital capacity of 1,000 ml; confirmation of the termination of the effects of muscle relaxant drugs by clinical evidence such as sustained head raising, grip strength or movement of an extremity against gravity, and the use of a peripheral nerve stimulator, e.g. sustained tetanus for 5 seconds at 30 Hz, or, better still, the 'train-of-four' stimulus. A further test is the patient's ability to produce a negative inspiratory force of more than 25 cm water (2·5 kPa).

Regional anaesthesia

Spinal and extradural anaesthesia have both been recommended in the obese patient either alone or as part of a combined regional analgesia and general anaesthesia technique [12, 20, 24, 30]. The positioning of the patient, palpation of landmarks and needle location are difficult and an image intensifier is a valuable aid. Conduction analgesia is not recommended for upper abdominal surgery. Falls in cardiac output may occur while levels of regional analgesia conducive to good operating conditions further embarrass respiration and pulmonary gas exchange. Anaesthetic levels following extradural or spinal techniques may be unpredictable for unknown reasons: it is possible that the presence of fat or distended extradural veins due to pressure on the inferior vena cava may reduce the volume of the extradural and subarachnoid spaces.

The combined method mentioned above offers the benefits of abdominal relaxation and analgesia from the extradural block and airway control from the use of tracheal intubation [20]. A longer and heavier 16 gauge Tuohy needle than is usually used has been found useful in these obese patients; general anaesthesia is not induced until the level of analgesia has been verified. Higher levels of extradural block should be anticipated in obese obstetric patients in proportion to their obesity. In obese obstetric patients bupivacaine continues to anaesthetize additional segments for up to one hour in some patients. Continuous extradural analgesia has been suggested for Caesarean section in patients with morbid obesity; it is claimed that this avoids the use of lipid soluble anaesthetics which are retained in the mother's fat tissue and the metabolites of which may be fed to the neonate through breast milk. Retraction of the panniculus cephalad rather than vertically in grossly obese mothers undergoing Caesarean section can compress the inferior vena cava and lead to severe hypotension during extradural block.

Postoperative period

Meticulous monitoring of obese patients is vital. Hypoventilation due to elevation of blood buffers can further accentuate already existent hypoxaemia. Pulmonary complications are especially likely to occur after abdominal surgery and postoperative hypoxaemia has consistently been demonstrated for several days; the degree of this hypoxaemia has now been related to the degree of obesity and lung function tests do not recover to their preoperative values for at least 5 days following surgery [12, 31]. Because of the low chest wall compliance and the surgical demands for access within the abdomen, large doses of muscle relaxant drugs may be required: these in turn present problems in antagonism and the resulting residual paralysis and inefficient lung ventilation due to a painful wound often necessitate a period of postoperative lung ventilation. Careful preoperative and intraoperative management of patients with simple obesity for elective surgery may obviate the need for elective postoperative ventilation whatever choice of anaesthesia has been used. Patients with OHS, however, should be invariably considered for elective mechanical ventilation of the lungs in the postoperative period in order to maintain oxygenation and alveolar ventilation and to provide adequate analgesia.

Whenever possible patients should be nursed in the semi-sitting position to gain maximum diaphragmatic excursion and arterial oxygenation provided that the circulatory system is stable [25]. The problem of providing pain relief to obese patients who are breathing spontaneously receives scant attention in the literature; the proponents of techniques involving an extradural catheter to provide regional analgesia have an undisputed advantage for operations involving the lower extremities and abdomen. Transverse, in contrast to longitudinal abdominal incisions are less painful as a rule.

The potential dangers of obesity in the postoperative period are not confined to the respiratory system. Wound infection is more than twice as common due to the longer incisions, the protracted time of operation, the trauma due to excessive surgical retraction, the difficulty in obliterating tissue dead space and the inability of adipose tissue to resist infection. There is a twofold increase in the incidence of postoperative pulmonary embolism: the incidence of deep vein thrombosis is increased for operations lasting over an hour.

REFERENCES

1 ADAMS AP. Techniques of vascular control for deliberate hypotension during anaesthesia. *Br J Anaesth* 1975; **47**: 777–92.
2 ADAMS AP. Drugs in elective arterial hypotension. In: C Prys-Roberts, ed. *The Circulation in Anaesthesia. Applied physiology and pharmacology*. Oxford: Blackwell Scientific Publications, 1980: 491–508.
3 ALEXANDER JK, AMAD KH, COLE VW. Observations on some clinical features of extreme obesity, with particular reference to cardiorespiratory effects. *Am J Med* 1962; **32**: 512–24.
4 ALEXANDER JK, GUTHRIE AE, SAKAGUCHI H, CRAWFORD HW, COLE VW. Lung volume changes with extreme obesity. *Clin Res* 1959; **7**: 171.
5 ANDERSON J. Obesity. *Br Med J* 1972; **1**: 560–3.
6 AUCHINCLOSS JH Jr, GILBERT R. The cardiorespiratory syndrome related to obesity: clinical manifestations and pathologic physiology. *Prog Cardiovasc Dis* 1959, **1**, 423.

7 BARRERA F, REIDENBERG MM, WINTERS WL, HUNGSPREUGS S. Ventilation—perfusion relationships in the obese patient. *J Appl Physiol* 1969; **26**: 420–6.

8 BARRERA F, HILLYER P, ASCANIO G, BECHTEL J. The distribution of ventilation, diffusion, and blood flow in obese patients with normal and abnormal blood gases. *Am Rev Respir Dis* 1973; **108**: 819–30.

9 Leading article: Surgery for severe obesity. *Br Med J* 1974; **2**: 575.

10 BURWELL CS, ROBIN ED, WHALEY RD, BICKELMANN AG. Extreme obesity associated with alveolar hypoventilation: a Pickwickian syndrome. *Am J Med* 1956; **21**: 811–18.

11 BUSKIRK E, TAYLOR HL. Maximal oxygen intake and its relation to body composition, with special reference to chronic physical activity and obesity. *J Appl Physiol* 1957; **11**: 72–8.

12 CATENACCI AJ, SAMPATHACHAR KR. Ventilatory studies in the obese patient during spinal anesthesia. *Anesth Analg: Current Researches* 1969; **48**: 48–54.

13 CATTELL WR. The physiological basis of fluid and electrolyte balance. *Hosp Med* 1967; **1**: 1130–7.

14 CATTELL WR. The assessment and management of fluid and electrolyte balance. *Hosp Med* 1968; **2**: 419–24.

15 DAVIDSON S, PASSMORE R, BROCK JF, TRUSWELL AS. *Human Nutrition and Dietetics*. 6th ed. London: Churchill Livingstone, 1976.

16 FAREBROTHER MJB, MCHARDY GJR, MUNRO JF. Relation between pulmonary gas exchange and closing volume before and after substantial weight loss in obese subjects. *Br Med J* 1974; **3**: 391–3.

17 FARIS I, LE QUESNE LP. Assessment and replacement of body fluid deficits. *Br J Hosp Med* 1972; **7**: 465–7.

18 FEINBERG GL. Obesity. Class IV anesthesia risk. *N Y J Med* 1971 **71**: 2200–1.

19 FISHER A, WATERHOUSE TD, ADAMS AP. Obesity: its relation to anaesthesia. *Anaesthesia* 1975; **30**: 633–47.

20 FOX GS. Anaesthesia for intestinal short circuiting in the morbidly obese with reference to the pathophysiology of gross obesity. *Can Anaesth Soc J* 1975; **22**: 307–15.

21 GARROW JS. Metabolic aspects of obesity. *Br J Hosp Med* 1973: **10**: 24.

22 HACKNEY JD, CRANE MG, COLLIER CC, ROKAW S, GRIGGS DE. Syndrome of extreme obesity and hypoventilation: studies of etiology. *Ann Intern Med* 1959: **51**: 541–52.

23 HOLLEY HS, MILIC-EMILI J, BECKLAKE MR, BATES DV. Regional distribution of pulmonary ventilation and perfusion in obesity. *J Clin Invest* 1967; **46**: 475–81.

24 JACOBS LL, BERGER JC, FIERRO FE. Obesity and continuous spinal anesthesia: a case report. *Anesth Analg: Current Researches* 1963; **42**: 547–9.

25 LOURENCO RV. Diaphragm activity in obesity. *J Clin Invest* 1969; **48**: 1609–14.

26 MCCRACKEN BH. Etiological aspects of obesity. *Am J Med Sci* 1962; **243**: 99–111.

27 MCINTYRE JWR. Problems for the anaesthetist in the care of the obese patient. *Can Anaesth Soc J* 1968; **15**: 317–24.

28 MCLAREN DS. *Nutrition and its disorders*. London: Churchill Livingstone, 1972.

29 NAIMARK A, CHERNIACK RM. Compliance of the respiratory system and its components in health and obesity. *J Appl Physiol* 1960; **15**: 377–82.

30 NOBLE AB. The problem of obesity in anaesthesia for abdominal surgery. *Can Anaesth Soc J* 1962; **9**: 6–14.

31 POSTLETHWAIT RW, JOHNSON WD. Complications following surgery for duodenal ulcer in obese patients. *Arch Surg* 1972; **105**: 438–40.

32 ROCHESTER DF, ENSON Y. Current concepts in the pathogenesis of the obesity-hypoventilation syndrome. Mechanical and circulatory factors. *Am J Med* 1974; **57**: 402–20.

33 SAID SI. Abnormalities of pulmonary gas exchange in obesity. *Ann Intern Med* 1960; **53**: 1121–9.

34 SIEKER HO, ESTES EH Jr, KELSER GA, MCINTOSH HD. A cardiopulmonary syndrome associated with extreme obesity. *J Clin Invest* 1955; **34**: 916.

35 SOCIETY OF ACTUARIES. *Build and blood pressure study*. Vol I. Chicago: Society of Actuaries, 1959.

36 VAUGHAN RW, BAVER S, WISE L. Volume and pH of gastric juice in obese patients. *Anesthesiology* 1975; **43**: 686–9.

37 WALTEMATH CL, BERGMAN NA. Respiratory compliance in obese patients. *Anesthesiology* 1974; **41**: 84–5.

38 WILLIAMS CD. Malnutrition. *Lancet* 1962; **2**: 342–4.

39 WORLD HEALTH ORGANISATION. Energy and protein requirements. Report of a joint FAO/WHO Ad Hoc Expert Committee. *Technical Report Series No.* 522. Geneva: World Health Organisation, 1973.

Chapter 13
Pituitary Disease

J. G. WHITWAM AND K. MASHITER

Hormones produced in the pituitary gland affect many tissues, directly or indirectly, by regulating the activity of other endocrine glands. The hypothalamus has many functions including the control of pituitary function, water and calorie balance, body temperature and sexual activity. It provides a mechanism for the endocrine system to respond to changes in activity of the central nervous system which may be caused by drugs, environmental, psychological and physical factors and trauma.

Disorders of the pituitary gland cause a wide variety of clinical conditions which have been well documented. Those of the anterior pituitary gland which can present major anaesthetic problems are caused either by excessive secretion of growth hormone (acromegaly) or adrenocorticotrophic hormone (Cushing's disease) or by an unsuspected decrease in the production of adrenocorticotrophic hormone causing a reduction in cortisol secretion by the adrenal gland and the development of hypotension.

ANATOMY

The adult gland is approximately 1 cm by 1·3 cm by 0·6 cm and weighs about 0·5 g. The anterior part accounts for 75 per cent of the total weight. It is larger in parous females and enlarges (up to 1 g) and becomes much more vascular during pregnancy.

NOMENCLATURE

The terminology recommended by the International Commission on Anatomical Nomenclature is shown in Table 13.1. In man the *pars intermedia* is virtually absent and the *pars tuberalis* is a thin layer of cells on the anterior surface of the stalk. Thus in man the terms adenohypophysis and *anterior pituitary gland* are virtually synonymous and refer to the anterior lobe of the gland.

In contrast the term *neurohypophysis* includes three components, i.e. the median eminence, the infundibular stem and the infundibular process or neural lobe. The *posterior pituitary gland* is the neural or posterior lobe of the gland within the *sella turcica* although some authors use the term to include the appropriate hypothalamic nuclei and the connecting stalk.

In the present discussions the terms anterior and posterior pituitary will be used to refer to the two parts of the gland.

DEVELOPMENT

The anterior part of the pituitary gland arises from Rathkés pouch which is an upward evagination of the stomodaeum. The posterior part develops from a down-growth of the floor of the diencephalon, the cells of which become modified to form pituicytes. Nerve fibres from the hypothalamus grow into the posterior pituitary gland via the

Table 13.1. Divisions of pituitary gland.

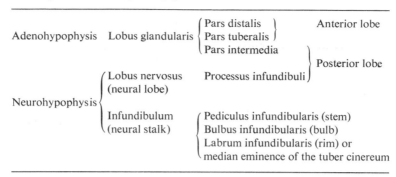

pituitary stalk. Thus the two parts of the gland have separate origins and they function independently.

By the end of the first trimester several pituitary hormones can be detected in the fetal pituitary. The age at which hormone secretion under feedback control is initiated in man has not been definitely established, but there is some evidence that a cortico-trophin control system may be present by the twelfth week.

RELATIONS

The gland lies in the *sella turcica* which is enclosed above by a layer of dura mater the *diaphragma sella,* through which the pituitary stalk passes to connect the gland with the hypothalamus. Its superior relations include the hypothalamus, third ventricle and the optic chiasma. More laterally lie the optic tracts and cavenous sinuses which contain within their walls the internal carotid arteries, the first division of the trigeminal nerve and the third, fourth and sixth cranial nerves. The third nerve lies lateral to the edge of the pituitary fossa and can be damaged by treatment of the gland with radio-therapy. Posteriorly are the *dorsum sella* and posterior clinoid processes, while below and in front are the sphenoid sinuses.

BLOOD SUPPLY

The anterior pituitary receives its blood supply from two sources. The superior hypophyseal arteries arise from the internal carotid arteries in the middle cranial fossa and provide arterial blood. In addition venous blood enters the gland by a portal system which originates in specialized vascular structures, the gomitoli in the median eminence. These are short straight terminal arterioles surrounded by a dense capillary network. Blood from these capillaries is collected into a series of parallel veins which run down the anterior part of the pituitary stalk and drain into the sinusoidal capillaries of the anterior lobe. *These vessels transport the various releasing factors from the hypothalamus to the anterior lobe.* The posterior pituitary is supplied by the inferior hypophyseal arteries which arise from the internal carotids in the cavernous sinuses. Hence the blood supply of the two lobes is largely separate. Venous blood from both lobes drains into the cavernous sinuses.

ANTERIOR PITUITARY

MICROSCOPIC STRUCTURE AND CELL TYPES

The glandular cells are arranged in columns separated by wide vascular channels which are lined by reticuloendothelial cells. Using simple stains such as haematoxylin and eosin, the cells are divided into acidophil, basophil and chromophobe types. Histochemical staining methods, electron microscopy and immunofluorescent techniques have shown that each major hormone is secreted by a distinct cell type. The three principal groups of pituitary hormones are summarized in Table 13.2. The acidophils

Table 13.2. Anterior pituitary hormones.

Type	Hormone	Site of action	Hormone released or effect
Somatrophin	Growth (GH)	Bone, viscera, soft tissue	Metabolic effects Protein synthesis Fat breakdown Hyperglycaemia Insulin antagonism Liver somatomedins (growth of tissues)
	Prolactin	Prepared breast	Lactation
Corticotrophin	Adrenocorticotrophic (ACTH)	Adrenal cortex	Cortisol (hydrocortisone)
	LPH (lipotrophin)		Generation of endorphins
Glycotrophin	Thyroid stimulating (TSH)	Thyroid gland	Thyroxine Triiodothyronine
	Follicle stimulating (FSH)	Ovarian follicle Seminiferous tubules	Oestrogens Spermatozoa
	Luteinizing (LH) or interstitial cell stimulating (ICSH)	Ovarian follicle Interstitial cells	Ovulation Corpus luteum ↓ Progesterone Testosterone

include cells which secrete growth hormone (GH somatotrophin) and prolactin. The basophils are the source of thyroid stimulating hormone (TSH) and follicle stimulating hormones (gonadotrophins GT). The chromophobe cells are believed to secrete adrenocorticotrophic hormone (ACTH) and melanocyte stimulating hormone (MSH) although these may also be reproduced by certain types of basophils. Corticotrophic cells are found in the anterior part of the posterior pituitary (*pars intermedia*, i.e. the posterior rim of Rathkés pouch) and also the *pars tuberalis*. At any one time about one quarter of the pituitary cells appear to be nonsecretory.

HORMONES

The hormones secreted by the pituitary gland consist of combinations of amino acids, referred to as amino acid residues, and hence are peptides or proteins.

GROWTH HORMONE

The serum levels of growth hormone (mol.wt. 21,500) in nonfasting adults are usually less than 5 μg/l. Its plasma half life is 20–25 min, and its secretion normally occurs in short bursts during 1–2 hours mainly in the early part of the night during sleep. Its output can be stimulated by stress, e.g. trauma or surgery, severe hypoglycaemia and exercise. Human chorionic somato-mammotrophin (placental lactogen HCS or HPL) is a protein produced in the placenta which has similarities in structure and action to both prolactin and growth hormone.

Clinical effects

Hypersecretion causes excessive body growth affecting both the soft tissues and skeleton leading to gigantism and acromegaly before and after fusion of the epiphyses respectively.

Growth hormone deficiency may be congenital or acquired (see below). Congenital deficiency causes pituitary dwarfism which does not become obvious for several months after birth. Growth hormone deficiency in the fetus does not affect its growth but the reason for this is not clear.

PROLACTIN

Normal plasms levels of prolactin (mol. wt. 21,000) vary due to its pulsatile secretion, but are normally less than 25 μg/l. There is an increased secretion at night, associated with sleep and levels fall during the morning; however its secretion rhythm is independent of other pituitary hormones. It is secreted in response to stimulation of the breast and by stress, even of a minor nature such that a rise in plasma level may occur in response to venepuncture.

Although a wide variety of functions have been ascribed to prolactin, in man only its role in lactation and gonadal function have been established. It causes milk secretion in mammary glands which have been prepared by other hormones (oestrogen, progesterone); while lactation continues prolactin remains elevated and suppresses gonadal function, at least during the early post partem period.

Clinical effects

Hyperprolactinaemia is probably the most common hypothalamic–pituitary disorder seen in nonpregnant subjects in clinical practice. 13–30 per cent of female patients presenting with amenorrhoea and infertility are suffering from hyperprolactinaemia, of whom approximately 30 per cent complain of galactorrhoea. Males suffer from impotence and a loss of libido. They tend to present relatively late with a prolactinoma and symptoms and signs of a space occupying lesion in the pituitary. In addition to micro- or macro-adenomata of the pituitary, hyperprolactinaemia may be caused by disruption of the hypothalamic-hypophyseal portal system and by irritation of thoracic spinal nerves (e.g. trauma, herpes zoster). Very commonly drugs which either

Dopamine
→ inhibition of prolactin

block dopaminergic receptors or cause dopamine depletion in the brain, and other drugs which antagonize the effects of dopamine at pituitary level and hence do not have to cross the blood–brain barrier, may cause hyperprolactinaemia.

Additional causes of hyperprolactinaemia are primary hypothyroidism and chronic renal failure.

Underproduction of prolactin is relatively rare and leads to failure of normal lactation but otherwise does not appear to have any serious consequences.

CORTICOTROPHIN (ACTH)

This is a polypeptide (mol.wt 4,500). It promotes the synthesis of corticosteroids in the adrenal cortex—mainly cortisol (hydrocortisone) and to a lesser extent corticosterone. It also increases the blood flow through the adrenal gland. Its output has a circadian rhythm which causes a parallel variation in the level of plasma cortisol. The lowest level is about the time of retiring, the concentration begins to rise about 0300 hr and reaches a maximum about the time of awakening. In man the normal plasma level of ACTH between 0800 hr and 1000 hr ranges from 22 to 154 μmol/l. The half-life of ACTH in the circulation is less than 40 minutes. Factors which increase its release from the pituitary are stress, e.g. trauma and surgery, pain, anxiety, hypoglycaemia, vasopressin and pyrogens.

It is now clear that ACTH is one of a number of intcrrelated peptides comprising β-lipoprotein (β-LPH, amino acid residues -91), λ lipoprotein (λLPH, amino acid residues 1–58), and so on, e.g. βMSH (41–58), ACTH (1–39), αMSH (1–13) cortico-trophin like intermediate peptide (CLIP 18–39) as well as the enkephalins and endor-phins (e.g. β and λ). Although all these peptides occur in vcrtebrate pituitaries, αMSH, βMSH and CLIP are found predominantly in spccics having a distinct middle lobe (pars intermedia). Whereas such a lobe is present in the human fetal pituitary it becomes vestigial in adult life.

Clinical effects

Overproduction of ACTH causes Cushing's syndrome which may arise from either pituitary or ectopic secretion (see below). When plasma levels of ACTH are very high (e.g. above 1000 μmol/l) skin pigmentation occurs, which has been attributed to the concurrent secretion of βMSH (see below). However activity attributed to βMSH in man is probably due to an extraction artefact and is most probably caused by βLPH or possibly λLPH which both contain its amino acid sequence. βLPH is released at the same time as ACTH. The increased skin pigmentation is therefore not the result of βMSM secretion, as in lower animals, but from the βMSH present in βLPH. Under-production causes a decreased secretion of cortisol (and also androgens) and is associated with a reduction in βMSH production. In pituitary disease ACTH produc-tion is often relatively well maintained, and hence when its level starts to fall there is usually a deficiency of gonadotrophin, growth hormone and thyroid stimulating hormone. ACTH deficiency is associated with weakness, hypoglycaemia, weight loss and hypotension.

THYROID STIMULATING HORMONE (TSH)

Thyroid stimulating hormone (TSH) is a glycoprotein with a molecular weight of

27,000. Its secretion has a circadian rhythm. Maximal levels occur between 2115 and 0530 hr and minimal between 1020 and 1840 hr. Human plasma contains less than 10 mU/l and in 10 per cent of normal individuals TSH is undetectable with current radio immunoassay techniques. Its mean half-life in the circulation is approximately 50 minutes. Unlike ACTH, growth hormone and prolactin, its release is not stimulated by hypoglycaemia and pyrogens and in this respect it is similar to the gonadotrophins.

Clinical effects

TSH increases practically all aspects of thyroid function and its vascularity. It increases the height of the follicular epithelium and reduces the amount of colloid. However, most cases of hyperthyroidism are due to dysfunction of the thyroid gland itself rather than the pituitary. A reduction in TSH production causes a reduction in the secretion of thyroid hormones which contributes significantly to the picture of panhypopituitrism.

GONADOTROPHINS

Follicle stimulating hormone FSH is a glycoprotein (mol.wt about 30,000). It stimulates the development of the primary follicle of the ovary. It also stimulates proliferation of granulosa cells and the production of oestrogens. In the male it increases spermatogenesis and the development of the seminiferous tubules.

Luteinizing hormone (LH) or interstitial cell stimulating hormone (ICSH)

This is a glycoprotein (mol.wt about 30,000) which induces ovulation and initiates and maintains the corpus luteum. In the female it stimulates oestrogen production by the theca interna. In the male LH (ICSH) stimulates the interstitial cells of the testis to produce androgens.

At the menopause following failure of the ovaries, the secretion of gonadotrophins increases. Preparations of extracted urinary gonadotrophin have been used to stimulate ovulation in certain types of infertility. Placental gonadotrophin is similar to LH.

HYPOTHALAMIC CONTROL OF THE ANTERIOR PITUITARY

It seems likely that synthesis of the various regulatory hormones takes place in distinct groups of cells in the hypothalamus which have yet to be defined. These hormones are stored in the median eminence and are released as required, to pass down the portal system into the anterior pituitary to cause the release of the pituitary hormones. The known hypothalamic regulatory hormones, some of which are called releasing factors, are summarized in Table 13.3.

The circulating target gland hormones provide negative feedback which in the case of growth hormone, prolactin and ACTH occurs principally at the hypothalamic level. In contrast thyroid hormones inhibit TSH by a direct action on the anterior pituitary. The hypothalamus provides mechanisms whereby neural influences—e.g. circadian periodicity, stress, trauma, surgery, hypoglycaemia and exercise can influence the output of anterior pituitary hormones. Some of these ideas are summarized in Fig. 13.1.

Table 13.3. Hypothalamic regulatory hormones which affect anterior pituitary function.

Anterior pituitary hormone	Hypothalamic hormone or factor
Growth (GH)	Growth hormone releasing factor GHRF (somatotrophin releasing factor SRF)
	Growth hormone release inhibitory hormone GRI (somatostatin) (somatotrophin inhibitory factor SIF)
Prolactin	Prolactin releasing factor (PRF)
	Prolactin inhibitory factor (PIF)
Adrenocorticotrophic (ACTH)	Corticotrophin releasing factor (CRF)
Melanocyte stimulating (MSH)	Melanocyte hormone releasing factor (MRF)
	Melanocyte hormone inhibitory factor (MIF)
Thyroid stimulating (TSH)	Thyrotrophin releasing hormone (TRH)
Follicle stimulating (FSH)	Follicle stimulating releasing hormone (FSH—RH)
Luteinizing (LH or ICSH)	Luteinizing hormone releasing hormone (LH—RH)

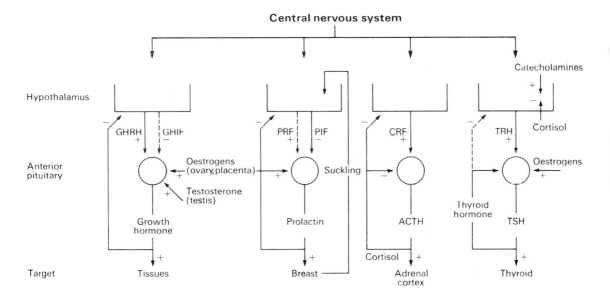

Fig. 13.1. Schema of control of the secretion of growth hormone, prolactin, cortisol and thyroid hormones.

Growth hormone

The hypothalamus controls growth hormone synthesis principally by means of growth hormone releasing hormone and growth hormone release inhibitory hormone (somatostatin). The releasing factor for somatostatin in the hypothalamus remains to be identified although there is considerable experimental evidence to support the existence of such a substance. Somatomedins are substances produced in bone and the liver which appear to inhibit growth hormone secretion. All the metabolic and other factors (e.g. trauma, stress, hypoglycaemia, pyrogens) which affect growth hormone release are believed to act at the hypothalamus.

Prolactin

Secretion of prolactin by the anterior pituitary, unlike all other hormones, is under tonic inhibition. There is now considerable evidence to suggest that this prolactin inhibitory factor is dopamine.

Prolactin levels are higher in females than males and this difference is correlated with breast development. Prolactin levels increase during pregnancy as a result of higher circulating oestrogen levels; the highest levels occur in the last 3 months of pregnancy. The predominant influences which affect prolactin secretion are neural (suckling, emotional stress). As in the case of growth hormone there is a negative feedback mechanism regulating its secretion.

ACTH. Production is stimulated by corticotrophin releasing factor (CRF). Cortisol, produced in response to ACTH production acts on the hypothalamus to reduce the production of CRF. It also probably acts at the anterior pituitary to reduce directly the secretion of ACTH.

Gonadotrophins

The mechanisms controlling the release of the gonadotrophins and the mid-cycle circulatory L.H. surge is still poorly understood. There is no circadian periodicity to their secretion except at puberty. The sex steroids from the gonads act upon sites in the hypothalamus where they exert some of their feedback action. They also have some action on the pituitary itself. Oestradiol, rather than progesterone, seems to be responsible for the major negative feedback effect, although progesterone may have a synergistic action. The situation is complicated by the fact that on occasion, oestradiol can have a positive feedback effect.

TSH. Thyroid stimulating hormone secretion by the anterior pituitary is now recognized to be under hypothalamic dopaminergic control which regulates the production of thyrotrophin releasing hormone. The thyroid hormones appear to inhibit TSH production principally by an action on the pituitary gland itself. However, the normal setting of TSH secretion seems to be under the control of the hypothalamus which regulates the output in response to heat and cold and integrates thyroid activity with mechanisms for the control of body temperature. Thyroid hormones block the pituitary response to TRH. Animal experiments suggest that inhibition of deiodination of T_4 to T_3 prevents blocking by T_4 on TRH mediated TSH release, which implies that T_4 is relatively inert and the feedback mechanisms is provided by T_3.

Oestrogens can cause an increase in TSH secretion. Glucocorticoids inhibit the production of TRH in the hypothalamus and may also act on the pituitary depending on dose. It is now thought that, although psychological factors may play a part in the production of Graves' disease, they do not act through the pituitary thyroid axis since, in general, emotional stress inhibits the production of TRH and TSH.

TESTS OF HYPOTHALAMIC-PITUITARY FUNCTION

Measurements of normal basal values of pituitary hormones produced by target glands can be made in blood and in urine. Some of these are shown in Table 13.4.

Table 13.4. Normal basal values[1] for hormone assays.

Hormone	Normal range	Notes
Pituitary		
GH	< 5 mIu/l*	Normal levels often undetectable. The stress of venepuncture during a period of spontaneous release can cause values found in acromegaly. Dynamic tests (in fasting subjects), suppression —GTT., stimulation—ITT, Bovril, Glucagon.
TSH	< 4 mu/l**	Useful in differentiating primary from secondary hypothyroidism.
LH follicular/luteal	3–8 u/l***	
midcycle	22–25 u/l	
FSH follicular/luteal	2–8/l***	
midcycle	9–12 u/l	
Prolactin	5–25 ng/l†	Unique among anterior pituitary hormones in being predominantly under inhibitory control (by the hypothalamic hormone PIF). Elevated in pregnancy and suckling. Inhibited by dopamine like drugs, e.g. l-dopa and bromocriptine. Increased by a large number of drugs (e.g. phenothiazines) that affect dopamine production. Disorders usually associated with hyper-prolactinaemia (unless gland infarcts). Causes amenorrhoea, infertility and galactorrhoea.
ACTH 9.00 am	< 80 ng/l	Useful in establishing the aetiology of Cushing's syndrome. Undetectable levels in one or two morning samples indicate an adrenal adenoma or carcinoma. Values above 200 ng/l suggest ectopic ACTH secretion by a broncial or other neoplasm. Basal ACTH determinations are of value in predicting those patients likely to develop Nelson's syndrome following bilateral adrenalectomy. Differentiates between primary and secondary adrenal insufficiency.
12 mid	< 10 ng/l	
Thyroid		
T_4	50–150 nmol/l	—Total circulating T_4. Most used in the diagnosis of hypothyroidism.
T_3	1·5–3·0 nmol/l	—In hypothyroidism there is some overlap with the normal range, but in hyperthyroidism levels are usually elevated above the normal range.
Adrenal		
Plasma		
Cortisol 9·00 am	0·1–0·5 μmol/l	Pregnancy 9·00 am—0·5–1·75 μmol/l. In Cushing's syndrome midnight values are elevated.
12.00 midnight	< 0·2 μmol/l	
Urinary		
Cortisol	< 0·27 μmol/ 24 hr	Pregnancy 0·23–0·67 μmol/24 hr. In Cushing's syndrome >0·27 μmol/24 hrs. Urinary free cortisol reflects circulating free (unbound) cortisol levels and its assay provides a high degree of discrimination between Cushing's syndrome and conditions which simulate it such as obesity.
17 oxosteroids (OHCS)	6–18mg/24 hr	Age dependent
17 oxogenic steroids (OGS)	5–20mg/24 hr	Age dependent.

* WHO 1st International reference preparation (66/217)

**Preparation 68/38

*** MRC 69/104

†Friesen 72–4–9

[1] The values given are representative only and can vary between laboratories depending on the method used and the standard.

Stimulation tests

Insulin tolerance test. This tests the hypothalamic-pituitary adrenal axis. The patient is starved at night. Hypoglycaemia is induced by a dose of intravenous insulin. The sensitivity to insulin, and therefore the dose, depends on the type of patient. Patients with hypopituitarism are the most sensitive and the dose of insulin used is 0·1 units/kg. To test a normal patient, for example one who has had corticosteroids in the past, a dose 0·15 units/kg is used. Patients with suspected Cushing's disease or acromegaly are insulin-resistant and need a dose of 0·3 units/kg. For an adequate hypoglycaemic response, the patient should sweat, and the blood sugar should fall to less than 2·2 mmol/l. If this does not occur by 1 hour a further dose of insulin is given. In response to this stimulus, plasma ACTH, corticosteroids, growth hormone, prolactin and catecholamines should rise. In normal subjects, plasma flurogenic corticosteroids (cortisol and cortisone measured by the Mattingly method) should rise by at least 0·5 μmol/l to over 1·0 μmol/l and growth hormone levels increase to over 20 μg/l.

Metyrapone test is useful in the diagnosis of Cushing's disease. The drug inhibits 11 β-hydroxylation and blocks the final step in cortisol synthesis causing an accumulation of cortisol precursors. Because the plasma cortisol level is reduced, the normal negative feedback at hypothalamic level is reduced and there is an increased secretion of CRF and plasma ACTH. This stimulates the adrenal gland causing a rise in the production of cortisol precursors (11-deoxycortisol) which can be measured directly in plasma or in the urine as 17-oxogenic steroids. Metyrapone has a short half-life and is a relatively weak drug. For an adult the normal dose is approximately 750 mg and is administered 4 hourly for at least one or more days. It may cause dizziness and nausea. In normal subjects, after administration for 24 hours, the subsequent 24 hour urinary 17-oxogenic steroids should rise to more than double the basal value. In patients with Cushing's disease (i.e. pituitary dependent) there is an exaggerated response. Patients with Cushing's syndrome due to adrenal adenoma or carcinoma or ectopic ACTH production, show an impaired or absent response.

Hypothalamic releasing factors LH-RF and TRF can be administered to test pituitary reserve in combination with an insulin tolerance test to form a combined pituitary

Table 13.5. Pituitary test responses—combined test.

Normal responses to 200 μg TRH, 100 μg LH- RF and 0·1 unit/kg Insulin

Time	LH–RF		TRH		Hypoglycaemia	
Minutes	LH u/l	FSH u/l	TSH mu/l	Prolactin μg/l	Cortisol μmol/l	GH mIu/l
0	3–4	2–8	< 1–4	5–25	0·1–0·5	< 5·0
30	4–34	2–11	4·5–20	20–45	Peak >0·5–1·0	Peak > 20
60	5–34	2–11	4–20	10–32		
90	—	—	—	—		
120	—	—	—	—		

function test, the normal responses to which are summarized in Table 13.5. These tests have replaced the use of lysine and arginine vasopressin to stimulate ACTH and GH secretion by the pituitary.

The clomiphene stimulation test is used to assess gonadotrophin reserve.

Screening test for growth hormone deficiency in children. Oral Bovril 20 g per 1·5 m² surface area in 100 ml of water should increase serum growth hormone levels above normal.

Suppression tests

Various suppression tests related to target organ function may indicate abnormal pituitary function. The administration of dexamethasone 2 mg 6 hourly for 2–3 days should cause a 50 per cent reduction in plasma cortisol to less than the lower range of normal (0·1 μmol/l) and does so in patients with pituitary dependent Cushing's syndrome but not in those patients with ectopic ACTH syndrome or adrenal adenoma or carcinoma. A low dose dexamethasone test—2 mg between 2200 and 2400 hours followed by a 0900 hours blood sample—shows suppression of cortisol in normal subjects, but not in those with Cushing's syndrome (pituitary dependent).

Oral glucose tolerance test. During the performance of a glucose tolerance test (50 g of glucose in water), in normal subjects the serum growth hormone levels should suppress to virtually undetectable levels at some stage of the test. Patients with acromegaly or gigantism fail to show this response and 10 per cent demonstrate a paradoxical increase. Failure of suppression is also seen in patients with severe liver or renal disease, in heroin addicts or patients receiving l-dopa.

Table 13.6. Aetiology of hypopituitarism.

Primary	*Secondary to:*

1 Tumours:
    (a) Anterior pituitary. Principally chromophobe and eosinophil adenomas in adults and craniopharyngiomas in children
    (b) Secondary carcinomas principally from breast and lung
    (c) Local intracranial tumours, e.g. meningiomas, gliomas
	1 Hypothalamic disease—suprasella tumours (e.g. craniopharyngiomas, optic gliomas) meningiomas:

2 Vascular disease causing infarction, e.g. postpartum necrosis (Sheehan's syndrome), sickle-cell anaemia, severe diabetic degenerative vascular disease, arteritis, cavernous sinus thrombosis, carotid aneurysms, severe hypotension	2 Trauma 3 Infections (e.g. encephalitis) 4 Hydrocephalus 5 Congenital malformations 6 Granulomas (e.g. sarcoid) 7 Functional disorders secondary to malnutrition (starvation, anorexia nervosa and malabsorption syndromes)
3 Trauma, head injuries	
4 Granulomatous disease. Sarcoidosis, nontuberculous giant cell granulomas may sometimes affect the thyroid and adrenal glands as well as the pituitary causing a multiple glandular syndrome. Hand-Schüller-Christian disease. Haemachromatosis	
5 Iatrogenic—surgical removal or irradiation of the gland. Selective failure of TSH or ACTH production following prolonged therapy with thyroid or steroid hormones respectively	
6 Infections—Tuberculosis, syphilis, mycoses, brucellosis	
7 Empty sella syndrome	

HYPOPITUITARISM

Primary hypopituitarism may be caused by a variety of lesions such as surgical removal or radiation ablation of the gland, tumours both primary and metastatic, trauma, infarction and various infective and granulomatous processes which are summarized in Table 13.6. At present the commonest cause is a pituitary tumour (chromophobe adenoma in adults and craniopharyngioma in children), while Sheehan's syndrome accounts for the majority of non-neoplastic cases.

Deficiency of the posterior pituitary does not often occur in diseases confined to the pituitary fossa unless there is associated damage to the hypothalamus or pituitary stalk (e.g. following surgery). In contrast, disease of the hypothalamus often presents with a deficiency of vasopressin.

Clinical manifestations of hypopituitarism do not usually occur until approximately 75 per cent of the gland is destroyed. Although deficiencies of single hormones can occur, during progressive destruction of the anterior pituitary it is more usual for clinical evidence of hormonal deficiency to occur in this order—gonadotrophins, growth hormone, thyroid stimulating hormone, adrenocorticotrophic hormone, prolactin, and finally failure of the posterior pituitary. However, there are frequent exceptions to this sequence. In many cases of hypopituitarism (i.e. secondary to hypothalamic disease), prolactin secretion is increased. This is probably due to the fact that the hypothalamus normally exerts a tonic inhibition on prolactin secretion.

CLINICAL FEATURES OF PAN HYPOPITUITARISM

The clinical features depend on the degree of failure of the gland, the pattern of failure of the different hormones and on associated features of any underlying disease causing the failure. They are outlined in Table 13.7.

Total failure of the anterior pituitary is incompatible with life in man. The causes

Table 13.7. Principle features of anterior pituitary hormone deficiency.

ACTH:	Features of corticosteroid deficiency Weakness, nausea, vomiting, meningism, hypoglycaemia, hyperthermia (above 41 °C is common) coma, hypotension which eventually causes death, reduction in the voltage of the ECG
LPH:	Pallor. Depigmentation of breast areolae, failure to pigment in response to sunlight
GH:	Dwarfism in children In adults, growth hormone deficiency may contribute to a change in the skin texture, which becomes very fine. Increased sensitivity to insulin
Prolactin:	Failure of lactation may be first sign of postpartum pituitary necrosis
TSH:	Features of hypothyroidism. *In children*—retardation of growth. *In adults*—Lassitude with intolerance to cold, dryness of skin, prolongation of tendon reflexes and other features similar to primary thyroid deficiency (myxoedema)
Gonadotrophin:	*In children*—hypogonadism. In selective failure, without growth hormone deficiency, height may be normal or increased because puberty is delayed. Anosmia is an associated symptom. In adult males—loss of libido, impotence, aspermia, testicular atrophy, decrease of body and facial hair *In adult females*—decreased libido, amenorrhoea, atrophy of uterus and vagina, reduced body hair. Menopausal symptoms do not occur. In both sexes the skin acquires a fine texture with excessive wrinkling which is very marked in the face

of *coma* when it occurs vary but include hypoglycaemia, water intoxication and hypo-osmolarity, hypotension, hypothyroidism and hypothermia.

Hypoadrenocorticism occurs 4–14 days after withdrawal of maintenanc theerapy in someone who has undergone total hypophysectomy. Adrenal insufficiency is the most important element in the acute hypopituitary syndrome and the symptoms include nausea, vomiting and hypotension causing death. The hypophysectomized patient is able to conserve sodium better than the patient with Addison's disease because aldo-sterone secretion is relatively unimpaired. *Hyponatraemia* when it occurs is due to water retention since water clearance is impaired by cortisol deficiency, but whether this is entirely due to the loss of a direct effect of cortisol on the renal tubules or whether cortisol lack causes ADH secretion is uncertain. Thus *hypo-osmolarity* without *hypo-volaemia* can occur within a few days of removal of the anterior pituitary gland. In patients with disease of the hypothalamus or posterior pituitary and *diabetes insipidus* anterior pituitary failure decreases its severity. The apparent improvement of diabetes insipidus caused by anterior pituitary failure is thought to be due to the reduced glomerular filtration caused by growth hormone and steroid deficiencies and the increased tubular reabsorption of water due to cortisol deficiency. Thus in patients with total pituitary ablation associated with diabetes insipidus, cortisol replacement therapy will increase the severity of the diabetes insipidus (e.g. from 5–6 litres of urine per day to between 7 and 15 litres per day which occurs in patients with primary failure of the posterior pituitary whose anterior pituitary is intact).

Hypothyroidism takes more than four weeks to become severe following hypophy-sectomy. In patients with spontaneous hypopituitarism (e.g. pituitary adenoma) thyroid hormone deficiency may take over five years to develop. The symptoms may be indistinguishable from primary thyroid deficiency (i.e. myxoedema). Basal metabolism falls, the serum protein bound iodine reaches extremely low levels and the serum cholesterol is elevated. Iodine uptake by the thyroid gland is grossly reduced. Thyroid function is restored by TSH administration. Exceptionally some patients do not develop hypothyroidism. The usual explanation is the presence of primary hyperthyroidism (e.g. due to nodular goitre) and in several documented cases this has been associated with plasma long acting thyroid stimulating hormone (LATS).

Carbohydrate metabolism may not change much after hypophysectomy because of a compensatory decrease in insulin release, although fasting blood sugar levels are lower than normal. However, in patients who were previously diabetic and who are receiving insulin, the reduction in insulin requirements increases the possibility of hypoglycaemia even in spite of cortisol therapy. This suggests that growth hormone deficiency is a major cause of the reduced insulin requirement.

Anaemia is not as severe as the pallor of the skin suggests. It is normocytic, normo-chromic and may be due to the effect of pituitary and target gland hormones (e.g. thyroid and adrenal) on either the secretion or the action of erythropoietin.

The weight of patients with chronic hypopituitarism is usually normal and the nutritional state is good. Severe weight loss should suggest either an alternative diagnosis (e.g. anorexia nervosa) or malignant disease.

DIAGNOSIS OF HYPOPITUITARISM

This depends on clinical and laboratory evidence of hormone deficiency and evidence of a possible cause of pituitary damage. The patient may present with obvious clinical signs associated with pituitary hormone deficiency. There may be a visual field defect, suggesting pressure on the optic chiasma. Occasionally there may be evidence of damage to the ocular nerves, e.g. the third.

The hormone secretion tests have been outlined above. In general, deficiency of pituitary target organ secretion can be accepted if a lesion of the target organ is excluded by its response to trophic hormone (e.g. ACTH—tetracosactrin and TSH). Raised levels of pituitary trophic hormones indicate the presence of pituitary tumours or disease of the target organs with loss of the appropriate feed-back mechanism.

One of the major problems is that the basal levels of hormone secretion may be relatively well maintained, and it is only when dynamic tests are applied to test the pituitary reserve that deficiencies are revealed.

Further tests are then directed at finding a cause of damage to the hypothalamic-pituitary system. X-rays of the skull may reveal evidence of enlargement of the pituitary gland, e.g. a 'double floor' of the sella turcica on lateral X-ray, enlargement of the sella and erosion of the posterior clinoids. There may be evidence of calcification in the region of the pituitary which may be due to a craniopharyngioma or old tuberculosis. A chest X-ray, and in women examination of the breasts, are essential to exclude common sources of metastatic tumours. If a tumour of the pituitary gland is suspected as a cause of the hypopituitarism, air encephalography will confirm the diagnosis and also reveal its site and extent. Modern scanning procedures will eventually replace air encephalography.

Differential diagnosis

A number of conditions may present a similar picture. *Chronic malnutrition* may simulate hypopituitarism with a decreased secretion of ACTH, TSH and gonadotrophins although GH secretion may be increased. *Anorexia nervosa* is the most often confused diagnosis; however, severe weight loss is unusual in hypopituitarism and should suggest an alternative diagnosis. The gonadotrophins are the most consistently reduced hormones in emaciated patients and their output increases rapidly on refeeding. Insulin sensitivity is increased in anorexia nervosa; growth hormone levels respond normally to hypoglycaemia and the pituitary-adrenal response to metyrapone is normal. In *Addison's disease* there is an increased output of ACTH and β-MSH by the pituitary causing increased skin pigmentation, which contrasts with the pallor and loss of pigmentation seen in hypopituitarism. In *myxoedema* there is sometimes a smaller loss of body hair, the skin is thicker, rougher and dryer with a yellowish tinge and possibly peripheral cyanosis. There is an intolerance to cold and a tendency to hypothermia. Raised serum TSH levels indicate primary hypothyroidism. To distinguish primary hypothyroidism from hypopituitarism it is necessary to test the response of the thyroid to TSH administration (3 daily injections of 10 units of TSH after which the serum thyroxine, protein bound iodine and iodine uptake by the gland are redetermined). Plasma cortisol levels are usually normal in myxoedema and reduced in secondary hypothyroidism (i.e. pituitary dependent).

A premature menopause may suggest hypopituitarism, but the body hair remains normal, steroid hormone levels are normal, and the presence of other symptoms (e.g. hot flushes) gives the clue to diagnosis. *Hypogonadism* due to gonadal disease can be distinguished by measurement of the gonadotrophins. Hypopituitarism may also be suspected when testicular atrophy and general debility occur in men with severe *liver disease*. In most cases the diagnosis can be established by routine laboratory procedures.

Treatment

Treatment is directed to the underlying disorder when present. In some patients where there is no detectable cause it is important to determine the pattern of hormone deficiency. Once a diagnosis is established, for example following pituitary ablation, appropriate hormone replacement therapy is initiated.

With the exception of the gonadotrophins and growth hormone, replacement of pituitary hormones, although theoretically sound, has little practical use because of the expense and the discomfort of the injections. It is more usual to replace the target organ hormones.

Deficient *cortisol output* must be replaced but relatively small doses are required, e.g. 12 mg–40 mg of cortisone acetate per day. Most commonly patients require cortisol in a dose of 20 mg on waking and 10 mg in the evening. It is important to monitor the levels achieved. Plasma cortisol reaches a peak 30–60 minutes after oral administration and ideally the concentration should peak between 0·5 and 0·9 μmol/l after the morning dose and then fall slowly to 0·15–0·2 μmol/l before the evening dose, after which a peak of 0·4–0·5 μmol/l is reached. Mineralocorticoids such as fludrocortisone are not required since aldosterone secretion is maintained in the absence of ACTH.

Experience shows that it is important to correct thyroid deficiency but this should not be done until cortisol therapy has been initiated. On average a dose of *thyroxine* of 0·1–0·2 mg/day is required. In middle-aged patients or those with heart disease, the initial dose should be reduced to 0·05 mg daily, and even such small doses may induce angina in patients with ischaemic heart disease. The use of propanolol may be indicated to control cardiac symptoms and thus allow correction of the thyroid deficiency.

The administration of *androgens* in men restores general strength and vigour, libido and potency. Methyltestosterone 20–30 mg orally per day is sufficient. Alternatively testosterone injections every 3–4 weeks may be preferred. *Gonadotrophin* therapy with human FSH and HCG (chorionic gonadotrophin extracted from urine) can induce ovulation and allow pregnancy to occur, and in males this therapy may restore fertility. When ovulation is induced by clomiphene, HCG may help to prolong the span of the corpus luteum. In young women, substitution therapy cyclically with *oestrogens* and *progesterone* can induce withdrawal bleeding, improve breast size, skin texture, mental state and protect the bones from oesteoporosis. *Growth hormone* is used to treat pituitary dwarfism together with other target hormones as required.

With replacement of all target hormone deficiencies the patient can be restored to normal active life, and if provision is made to increase corticosteroid therapy during periods of stress, e.g. surgery, life expectancy is relatively normal.

Pituitary coma

It is advisable to have made a diagnosis based on clinical findings and measurement of plasma levels of both pituitary and target organ hormones. Baseline measurements of the state of the patient should include blood pressure, heart rate, oesophageal and rectal temperature, depth of coma, blood sugar, haematocrit, electrolytes (Na^+, K^+, Cl^-, HCO^-_3) urea and arterial pH, Po_2 and Pco_2.

Emergency treatment should include the i.v. administration of dextrose—saline and hydrocortisone hemisuccinate—500 mg immediately and then 100 mg every 6–8 hours which will restore blood pressure. Plasma electrolytes may require correction. Oxygen therapy should be routine and artificial ventilation may be considered desirable to reduce muscle activity and hence the tendency to acidosis during treatment and rewarming if the patient is hypothermic.

Although acute cortisol deficiency may be associated with hyperthermia, patients with hypopituitarism associated with myxoedema may not be able to maintain body temperature so that as with myxoedema, in a cold environment, hypothermic coma may occur. However, elderly patients in a cold environment often become hypothermic without either hypopituitarism or myxoedema.

Rewarming should proceed gradually (e.g. from 30°C to 37°C during 24 hours) otherwise ventricular fibrillation may occur. The patient should be placed in an unheated bed in a warm room and wrapped in foil. Thyroid replacement therapy is important but should proceed with caution along with other measures. Tri-iodothyronine 2·5–5·0 μg every six to eight hours would be appropriate and should be administered in a suspension by stomach tube. After 24 hours the dose may be doubled and again after 48 hours. Large parenteral doses of T_3 are dangerous since they may precipitate heart failure or ventricular fibrillation. Infection should be treated vigorously. The art of management is to correct the severe hypotension relatively rapidly and then to 'titrate' the patient gradually back to normality. In the past, overzealous rewarming and the use of thyroid hormones in hypothermia in the elderly and patients with panhypopituitarism and myxoedema has probably accounted for the relatively high mortality rate. Too rapid correction of any one factor may precipitate circulatory failure. Once therapy is under way, it may be thought desirable to treat a severe anaemia with whole blood. If evidence of cardiac failure appears, this should be treated with appropriate measures. When the patient is restored to consciousness measures should be undertaken to determine the cause of the hypopituitarism if this is not known.

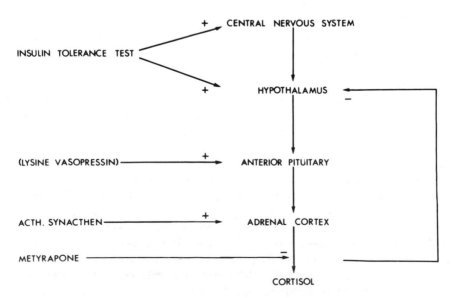

Fig. 13.2. Summary of tests of hypothalamic pituitary-adrenal function.

Assessment of patients with suspected hypopituitarism for surgery under anaesthesia

These patients fall into two groups, patients with pituitary tumours which require pituitary surgery or ablation procedures under anaesthesia; patients with pituitary disease or who have been on prolonged steroid therapy who require incidental surgery.

Assuming that adequate diagnostic criteria have been fulfilled, the important system to assess is the hypothalamic-pituitary-adrenal axis and its potential response to stress. Basal plasma cortisol levels may be relatively normal and the most important test is the insulin tolerance test. If the cortisol response to hypoglycaemia is below normal then the patient will almost certainly become hypotensive during surgical stress and steroid replacement must precede surgery. If the insulin tolerance test is normal, it does not necessarily mean that the patient will not become hypotensive in response to surgery, but experience suggests that this is unlikely and routine steroid therapy is unnecessary. The principal tests used in the assessment of pituitary adrenal function are summarized in Fig. 13.2.

PITUITARY TUMOURS

Anterior pituitary adenomas account for 10 per cent of all intracranial tumours. They are classified by the staining properties of their secretory granules into chromophobe, which account for 79 per cent, cosinophilic (15 per cent) and basophilic (6 per cent), but these staining characteristics do not necessarily correlate with their hormone production. Chromophobe adenomas are the commonest cause of 'spontaneous' hypopituitarism in adult life. They may be very large and locally invasive but rarely metastasize. They are rare in childhood and are distributed equally between the sexes. Eosinophilic adenomas have a similar age and sex distribution. Basophil adenomas are only rarely large enough to expand the pituitary fossa.

Pituitary adenomas, particularly chromophobe, may be part of a syndrome of multiple endocrine adenomatosis involving principally the parathyroids, adrenal glands, pancreatic islets and occasionally the thyroid. In addition, multiple lipomas, bronchial adenomas and intestinal carcinoids, may occur. The syndrome is inherited as an autosomal dominant trait with high penetrance. The islet cell tumours may be either insulin-or gastrin-secreting giving rise respectively to hypoglycaemia or the Zollinger–Ellison syndrome. The latter syndrome is associated with severe multiple peptic ulceration which involves the third part of the jejunum as well as the more usual sites (duodenum stomach and distal oesophagus), there may be a profuse diarrhoea (7–8 l/day) associated with considerable potassium loss.

Posterior pituitary tumours are rare.

Craniopharyngiomas are the most important nonpituitary tumours in the sella turcica region. They are believed to arise from remnants of Rathké's pouch which are usually situated above the sella and account for 4 per cent of intracranial tumours. They vary in size, may be very large, cystic or solid, are often calcified, and are the commonest tumours in the pituitary area in children and adolescents. Symptoms arise before 15 years in half the patients and they are the commonest cause of 'spontaneous' hypopituitarism in this age group. *Tumours* of the optic chiasma, hypothalamus, third ventricle, midbrain and pineal gland may all affect this region. They may consist of meningiomas, chordomas, teratomas and metastatic tumours from many sources.

LOCAL EFFECTS OF PITUITARY TUMOURS

The clinical manifestations of pituitary tumours are caused by local effects of the tumour and by the hormonal changes which usually occur.

Headaches are common, presumably due to distortion of the dura and blood vessels.

Visual field defects are common due to pressure on the optic chiasma causing typically a bitemporal hemianopia. This often starts as a defect of vision in the upper temporal quadrant associated with enlargement of the blind spot and disturbances of colour vision, especially for red. The tumour may expand asymetrically so that the types of visual field disturbance vary considerably. The optic nerves may be compressed, and while optic atrophy is common, papilloedema is rare. Haemorrhage into a tumour may cause acute loss of vision.

Cranial nerve palsies are rare and most commonly affect the IIIrd nerve. The IVth and VIth nerves and the olfactory nerves and tracts can be affected.

The hypothalamus may be compressed or infiltrated by large tumours, causing a variety of syndromes, the commonest of which is diabetes insipidus. There may be disturbances in appetite (associated with either obesity or weight loss), sleep and temperature regulation. Focal seizures of uncinate type have been reported. Damage to the area of the hypothalamus in which the releasing factors are produced, or to the pituitary stalk, can cause anterior pituitary failure. If the tumour is very large, internal hydrocephalus with raised intracranial pressure can occur.

Haemorrhage into a tumour causes 'pituitary apoplexy' which may be associated with headache, sudden loss of vision and acute pituitary failure causing hypotension and hypothermia. Removal of the clot and control of bleeding is a matter of extreme urgency if vision is to be saved.

Empty sella syndrome. This is believed to be due to small infarcts of tumours of the pituitary leading to cystic degeneration which may produce the appearance of an empty fossa with air encephalography since the air passes into an enlarged pituitary fossa which contains very little pituitary tissue. There may be surprisingly normal pituitary function and these patients are often discovered during radiological examination for other indications.

X-rays of the skull may show enlargement and erosion of the walls of the fossa. The anterior and posterior clinoid processes may become eroded and thin. Almost half the patients with adenomas may show a double floor to the fossa in lateral X-rays, due to asymmetrical expansion of the tumour, and this is often the first abnormality to be seen. Calcification may indicate a craniopharyngioma. Further examination may include tomograms and air encephalography, but modern scanning techniques should be available.

HORMONAL CHANGES

These are caused either by excess or deficient production of the pituitary hormones. Clinical syndromes have been described in association with pituitary neoplasms due to overproduction of growth hormone (gigantism and acromegaly), prolactin, and adrenocorticotrophic hormone (Cushing's disease) which is often associated with excessive release of melanocyte stimulating hormone. Only extremely rarely are thyrotrophin or gonadotrophins secreted by pituitary tumours.

GROWTH HORMONE—ACROMEGALY

The tumours which cause this condition are usually eosinophilic. There is no recognizable hereditary factor but men are affected more than women. Its course is extremely variable and often the disease 'burns out'. The reasons for this are not clear. Rarely the tumour infarcts; more usually growth hormone levels are maintained but tissue proliferation is arrested presumably by some process of adaptation.

Clinical features

The major clinical features of acromegaly can be divided into three groups related to the effects of growth hormone, i.e. (a) tissue growth and (b) intermediary metabolism and (c) to the presence of a pituitary tumour.
The typical progression of the appearance of a patient with acromegaly is illustrated in Fig. 13.3.

Skeletal system

Before puberty, growth is excessive and continues longer because epiphysial closure may be delayed by associated hypogonadism which is a feature of the disease. Giants who survive to adult life have long limbs and mildly acromegalic features. After puberty there is little increase in height, but there is a general increase in periosteal bone formation. The *skull* deformities are most striking (Fig. 13.4). The mandible increases in thickness and length ('Lantern Jaw') so that the dental occlusion may be reversed with the lower incisors protruding beyond the upper ones by up to 2 cm. Often the teeth are abnormally separated. The frontal, malar and nasal bones, the supraorbital ridges and muscle attachments are overgrown, which adds to the coarsening of the features (Fig. 13.3). The paranasal sinuses are often grossly enlarged. The pituitary fossa may be enlarged and because the eosinophilic cells lie anteriorly there may be excessive erosion of the anterior clinoid processes. Most of these changes are illustrated in Fig. 13.4.

The bones of the hands and feet are also affected with thickening of the cortical bone and tufting of the distal phalanges. To a lesser extent the whole skeleton is involved with thickening of bones and in the vertebrae this is most marked on the anterior surface.

Arthritis is common due to joint distortion, with thickening of the capsule and ligaments and this may be crippling. Initially the articular cartilages proliferate but later they may become eroded so that eventually the picture is similar to osteo-arthritis.

Muscle size and strength may be increased at first, but eventually there is a generalized myopathy and weakness.

Soft tissues

There is an increase in connective tissue throughout the body. In spite of this the increase in weight may not be great and only about 40 per cent of acromegalic patients show a marked increase in total body mass. The combination of soft tissue and bone growth causes a coarsening of the features and large spade-like hands.

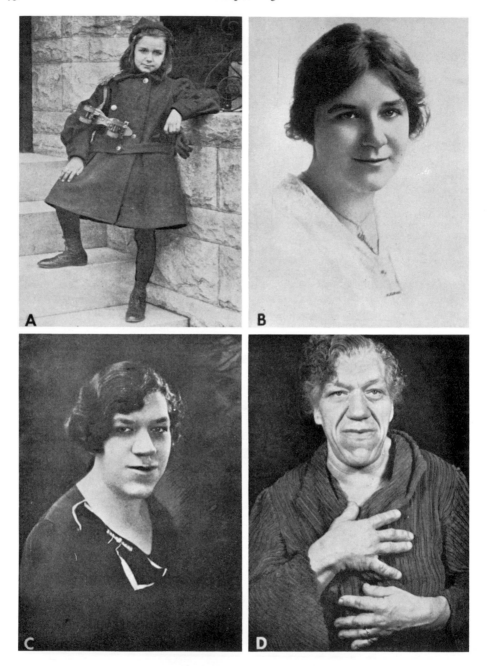

Fig. 13.3 Typical progression of a patient with acromegaly. (*American Journal of Medicine* 1956; **20**: 133.)

Skin

This appears coarse and leathery, body hair is increased and coarse, moderate melanosis occurs in about half the patients, fibroma mulloscum occurs in 27 per cent of patients and in active phases of the disease most patients complain of excessive sweating.

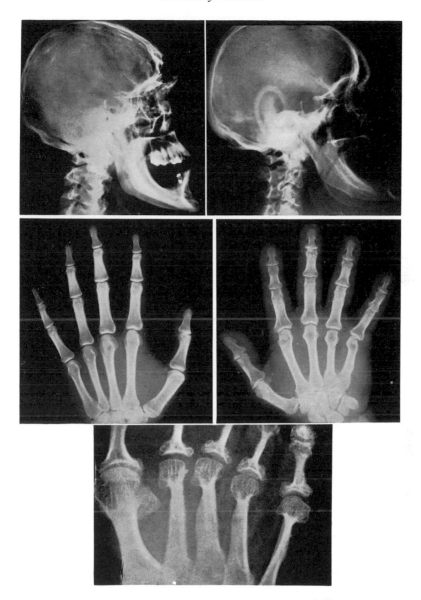

Fig. 13.4. Skulls, hands and foot, showing typical changes of acromegaly. (*Quarterly Journal of Medicine* 1952; **27**: 405.)

Cardiorespiratory system

Cardiac enlargement is usual and hypertension is common. In some, a true cardio-myopathy develops. Eventually progressive congestive failure may develop and some patients have presented in acute pulmonary oedema [9]. In middle-aged patients degenerative cerebrovascular changes occur. Patients with acromegaly have large lung volumes and altered ventilation-perfusion ratios. They are prone to chest infections [1]. One of the major problems is an overgrowth of the tissues of the upper airways and larynx which may cause respiratory obstruction requiring a tracheotomy. Marked voice changes indicate laryngeal involvement [6]. During sleep, episodes of hypoxia and hypercarbia can occur due to respiratory obstruction and failure of the medullary respiratory mechanism, damaged by cerebrovascular disease and previous episodes of hypoxia, to respond to the rise in Pa_{CO_2}.

Cerebral function

Increasing age, cerebrovascular degeneration and repeated hypoxic episodes may make the patient very sluggish and sensitive to the effects of hypnotic and narcotic drugs so that even small doses of opiates may cause respiratory arrest.

Renal function

There is a very large increase in the size of the kidneys with increased glomerular filtration, glucose and phosphate reabsorption causing a mild hyperphosphataemia. Provided the parathyroid glands are intact, calcium excretion increases and in over 50 per cent of patients exceeds 300 mg per day on a normal diet.

Other organs

There is enlargement of all the organs of the body including the gut, liver, spleen, thyroid, parathyroids, pancreas and kidneys.

Function of other endocrine glands

Although many patients appear hyperthyroid and about 25 per cent have a goitre, thyroid function tests are normal but as the tumour increases in size TSH production may fall. Similarly adrenal function is normal until ACTH production decreases as the tumour enlarges. Many patients have increased prolactin secretion and persistent galactorrhoea may precede other signs of the disease by many years. Decreased gonadotrophin production is a fairly common feature of the disease.

Metabolism

Many patients have a high metabolic rate. Overt diabetes mellitus occurs in about 12 per cent of patients and in about an equal number there is evidence of impaired glucose tolerance. It has been suggested that those patients who develop diabetes have a hereditary predisposition to the disease.

Nervous system

Involvement of peripheral nerves is common due to trapping by bone (e.g. the vertebrae) and soft tissue overgrowth. A carpal tunnel syndrome sometimes occurs. Because of the proliferation of the connective tissue in the peripheral nerves they may become clinically enlarged. Encroachment of the vertebrae on the spinal canal may lead to cord symptoms and long tract signs.

DIAGNOSIS

Because of the slow progression of the disease, it is often many years before the patient seeks advice and by then, in most patients, the diagnosis is obvious. During previous years the patient may have noticed a progressive increase in glove, ring, hat and shoe sizes. Serial photographs may be useful (Fig. 13.3) for observing slowly progressive changes in the features. X-rays, urinary calcium excretion, impaired glucose tolerance may all assist diagnosis. However, the final confirmation is a high *serum growth hormone level* (normally less than 5·0 μg/l) which does not fall during an oral glucose tolerance test.

PROGNOSIS

Patients with untreated acromegaly have twice the expected mortality rate, and usually die from cardiovascular complications. Although the disease may become static, in patients where the growth hormone levels remain elevated the potential complications remain since spontaneous cure by infarction of the tumour is rare.

TREATMENT

Until relatively recently treatment has been either by surgery or irradiation. Recently a drug, bromocriptine, has become available which may be of value in some patients [7]. It is an ergot alkaloid and is a dopamine receptor stimulant. It is also used in the treatment of parkinsonism. Its side-effects include nausea, dizziness and swelling of the ankles. Its role in the treatment of the disease is being evaluated.

ADRENOCORTICOTROPHIC HORMONE CUSHING'S DISEASE

'Cushing's syndrome' is a generic term applied to all those clinical and chemical abnormalities which are caused by chronic excess of cortisol and these are described elsewhere (p. 469). The more specific term 'Cushing's disease' is applied to those patients whose illness is caused by inappropriate secretion of ACTH by the anterior pituitary. When iatrogenic and ectopic groups are excluded pituitary dependent Cushing's disease accounts for about 70–80 per cent of patients presenting with Cushing's syndrome. The disease was originally described by Harvey Cushing in 1932 who attributed it to the presence of small basophilic tumours in the anterior pituitary.

It seems likely that in the majority of patients with Cushing's disease the main defect lies in the hypothalamus so that the control of ACTH secretion is abnormal. 40–64 per cent of patients with pituitary dependent Cushing's disease have radiological or histological evidence of a pituitary tumour. Rarely they may be malignant.

The possible breakdown of normal hypothalamus-pituitary adrenal central system in Cushing's disease and the various forms of Cushing's syndrome are illustrated in Fig. 13.5. High levels of trophic hormone continue to be produced in spite of a high level of circulating cortisol. Much higher doses of dexamethasone are required to reduce ACTH production as compared with normal subjects. The response of the hypothalamus to a fall in plasma cortisol is retained since metyrapone which blocks its synthesis, causes a rise in ACTH output. In Cushing's disease the response to the insulin tolerance test is lost.

Pituitary dependent Cushing's disease differs from Cushing's syndrome caused by the overactivity of the adrenal cortex in the following respects.

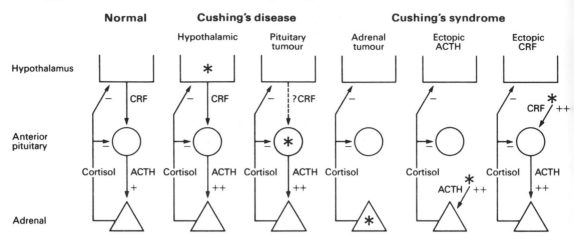

Fig. 13.5. Points of breakdown of normal hypothalamic-pituitary-adrenal control system in Cushing's disease and the various forms of Cushing's syndrome. The asterisk indicates point of breakdown or source of hormones.

1 There is a high level of plasma ACTH associated with increased skin pigmentation.

2 Plasma cortisol levels are partially suppressible by dexamethasone.

3 There is a vigorous pituitary adrenal response to metyrapone.

4 Normalization of plasma cortisol by adrenalectomy and replacement therapy is associated with high levels of ACTH, intense pigmentation and a rapid increase in the size of the pituitary gland (Nelson's syndrome).

DIAGNOSIS

This is made on the following criteria.

1 Clinical symptoms and signs associated with excessive steroid production (see p. 469) especially if this is associated with increased skin pigmentation.

2 High plasma cortisol levels with a loss of rhythm (the most consistent finding is a high midnight value) which undergoes suppression by dexamethasone.

3 Vigorous response to metyrapone.

4 A high plasma ACTH level particularly at midnight. This is the most important finding but can also be caused by ectopic sites of hormone production.

5 Radiological and clinical evidence of a pituitary tumour. Approximately 20 per cent of patients have an enlarged pituitary fossa when they are first seen.

Differential diagnosis

Most patients referred with suspected Cushing's disease are suffering from simple obesity. It must not be forgotten that the most common cause of Cushing's syndrome is iatrogenic due to the administration of exogenous steroids. Ectopic sites of ACTH production can cause considerable difficulty and all patients should have a chest X-ray to exclude a lung tumour, and in the case of women a pelvic examination as certain ovarian tumours can produce steroid hormones (Table 13.9).

It is important to differentiate pituitary from adrenal dependent cortisol secretion since incorrect removal of the adrenal glands will produce Nelson's syndrome (rapid enlargement of the pituitary associated with local signs, excessive ACTH production associated with gross generalized pigmentation).

Treatment

Irradiation or surgical removal of the pituitary gland is required. ACTH secreting tumours appear to be particularly sensitive to radiation. One of the problems is that in some patients it requires only a small number of active ACTH secreting cells to remain in the fossa for the disease to continue.

PROLACTIN

The syndrome of nonpuerpural lactation unassociated with acromegaly (Forbes–Albright syndrome) was first described in 1954. The tumours contain chromophobe cells but a few are eosinophilic.

Clinical features

Patients with prolactinomas may present in a wide variety of ways to a number of medical disciplines, with features relevant either to a pituitary tumour (e.g. headache, or visual field defects) or to prolactin secretion, e.g. amenorrhoea, galactorrhoea, infertility, irregular or absent menstruation, impotence [3].

Diagnosis

Although many dynamic tests have been used to establish hyperprolactinaemia and its differential diagnosis, the single most important finding is a high plasma prolactin level. Multiple sampling (e.g. 4 hrly, for 24 hr) may be helpful in borderline cases since many patients with prolactinoma's lost their rhythm and additional samples may remove spurious elevation due to the stress of venepuncture.

Differential diagnosis

The major pathological causes of hyperprolactinaemia are:
1   drug therapy with dopamine receptor blocking or depleting drugs, which include phenothiazines (chlorpramazine, perphenazine, trifluoperazine) haloperidol, metoclopramide, reserpine, methyldopa, oestrogens in oral contraceptives and TRH;
2   hypothalamic or pituitary stalk lesions—trauma, granulomas (sarcoidosis, tuberculosis), tumours (craniopharyngioma, glioma);
3   pituitary tumours—prolactinomas, mixed tumours secreting ACTH or GH;
4   miscellaneous: hypothyroidism, chronic renal failure including patients on haemodialysis, ectopic secretion (e.g. lung cancer), idiopathic.
    Physiological changes in prolactin levels are associated with sleep, stress, pregnancy and suckling.

TREATMENT OF ANTERIOR PITUITARY HYPERSECRETION

Drugs which affect activity of the hypothalamus may be used increasingly in the future but at present therapy still depends on destruction of the gland. Ablation or removal of the anterior pituitary gland is performed on the following groups of patients.

1 Those with a primary pituitary pathology:
  (i) acromegaly,
  (ii) cushing's disease,
  (iii) other pituitary tumours either secreting (e.g. prolactin) or nonsecreting.
2 Patients with metastatic carcinoma of breast and prostate.
3 Some patients with diabetic retinopathy.

This discussion will be restricted to the first of these groups. The aims of therapy are to prevent extension of the tumour and to correct the particular hormone excess. Ideally this should be done without affecting other functions of the gland sufficiently to require maintenance therapy. These aims can be achieved in a fair number of patients and there are several reports of successful pregnancy in patients who have undergone pituitary ablation for prolactin secreting tumours and Cushing's disease.

RADIOTHERAPY

Destruction of the pituitary can be achieved with implantation of [^{90}Y] yttrium or [^{198}Au] gold seeds into the pituitary gland via a transnasal or transethmoidal approach. Narrow introducing cannulae are used, one for each side of the gland, and these are driven into position using biplane image intensification. Destruction can also be achieved with external irradiation, either using conventional methods or accelerated proton beams.

SURGERY

There are basically three different methods. The gland can be approached by a transnasal anterior transphenoidal approach, by a classical neurosurgical transfrontal approach, or by employing cryosurgery. As with the implantation of radioactive seeds, a probe, which can be cooled with liquid nitrogen, is introduced using biplane image intensification and the gland can then be destroyed by freezing.

In general, very large tumours which extend beyond the sella will require either external irradiation or some form of surgery. Conventional X-ray therapy is more difficult to regulate than the implantation of radioactive seeds, and in many cases it is not entirely satisfactory as there is the risk of damage to surrounding tissues when doses adequate to control the hypersecretion of the gland are used. Proton beams have caused a high incidence (up to 30 per cent) of oculomotor paralysis which in some patients is persistent. It is difficult to quantify and regulate cryosurgery, but good results have been reported in acromegaly. For tumours confined to the sella, implantation of radioactive seeds can give excellent results.

For Cushing's disease implantation of ^{90}Y (which is a pure β-emitter) in a dose of 100–500 grays (1 gray (Gy) = 100 rads) probably gives the best results. For some large tumours ^{198}Au may be preferred because this also emits γ-radiation which has a greater penetration and hence is less likely to leave active cells at the periphery of the sella, only a few of which are necessary to continue excessive secretions of ACTH. Implantation techniques are also satisfactory for prolactin secreting tumours [5]. In acromegaly the best results have been obtained with surgery using the anterior transphenoidal approach to the gland, but the implantation of ^{90}Y also gives satisfactory results. A craniotomy is performed only when the tumour is inaccessible to other techniques and when alternative methods of treatment are not available.

Surgery and implantation are usually performed under general anaesthesia. It is not germane to the present discussion to review the details of surgical techniques and complications. However, from the viewpoint of the effects of the hormones secreted by the pituitary gland, certain general considerations are relevant. These have been reviewed in more detail previously [8].

ANAESTHETIC CONSIDERATIONS IN PATIENTS WITH ANTERIOR PITUITARY DISEASE

PREOPERATIVE ASSESSMENT

A full assessment of pituitary function will have been made by the referring physician. The most important aspect is the pituitary-adrenal reserve and, except in Cushing's disease, this should be assessed by the insulin tolerance test. It must be emphasized that although subnormal cortisol and a poor response to hypoglycaemia indicate that during the stress of surgery, evidence of steroid deficiency will amost certainly occur (Fig. 13.6), occasionally the converse may not be true. In the final analysis, the only real test is the response of each individual patient to the surgical stress.

ACROMEGALY

Hypertension is frequent and sometimes cardiac failure may be present [9] so that the patient may be receiving digitalis, diuretics and antihypertensive drugs. Diabetes mellitus is fairly common. A major problem is overgrowth of the tissue of the upper airways and larynx. This may cause respiratory obstruction which may reverse after treatment [2]. Marked voice changes may indicate laryngeal involvement. Occasionally enlargement of the thyroid gland may be present, which may be retrosternal and cause narrowing and distortion of the trachea so that the outline of the upper airways should be visualized on X-rays.

INDUCTION AND INTUBATION

Because of their size and muscular development, patients with acromegaly may require a dose of thiopentone of 500 mg to ensure loss of awareness during intubation and while transferring to maintenance drugs. However, some have an unstable cardiovascular system and require care during the administration of the induction agent, which should be given slowly until the patient is asleep. Owing to the large body mass of some patients and hence the possible rapid reduction in brain level due to redistribution of the induction agent, the need for further thiopentone and suxamethonium should be anticipated, particularly if intubation proves difficult. Factors which make intubation difficult in patients with acromegaly include the following:

15

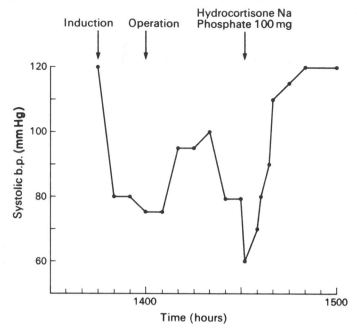

Fig. 13.6. Blood pressure in a steroid deficient patient. Male patient aged 34 years, wt. 75 kg. Diagnosis—acromegaly. Previous pituitary implant with [⁹⁰Y] yttrium. Very poor plasma cortisol response to insulin (ITT). At second pituitary implant: premedication—papaveretum 20 mg, hyoscine 0·4 mg. After induction of anaesthesia with thiopentone 350 mg and intubation using suxamethonium 75 mg followed by *d*-tubocurarine 30 mg and intermittent positive pressure ventilation with a nitrous oxide oxygen mixture (70/30), the systolic blood pressure stabilized at approximately 80 mmHg (10·7 kPa) rising by approximately 20 mmHg (2·6 kPa) in response to the onset of surgical stimulation. After this the systolic blood pressure fell to 60 mmHg (8 kPa) at which the plasma cortisol level was extremely low. The blood pressure rapidly returned to normal values in response to the intravenous administration of 100 mg of hydrocortisone phosphate.

1 The distance from the teeth to the larynx is greatly increased.
2 The lips and particularly the tongue are large, which combined with the general thickness of the tissues in the upper airways, and in some patients a very large epiglottis, cause a tendency to respiratory obstruction as soon as narcosis is induced.
3 Due to hypertrophic overgrowth of the respiratory and laryngeal mucosa, the surface anatomy of the region may be difficult to interpret. It is very easy to produce oedema and swelling in this mucosa and it is possible to distort further the superficial appearance with a laryngoscope thereby preventing a view of the laryngeal aperture.
4 The general thickening of tissues in some patients may produce narrowing of the glottic opening.
5 In some patients it is difficult to rotate the laryngeal aperture anteriorly to secure a view of the vocal cords [4].

CUSHING'S DISEASE

These patients may be diabetic and hypertensive and they may progress to cardiac failure. Hypokalaemia, perhaps made worse by diuretics, may occasionally be a feature. They are susceptible to infections. One of the most important problems is the severe

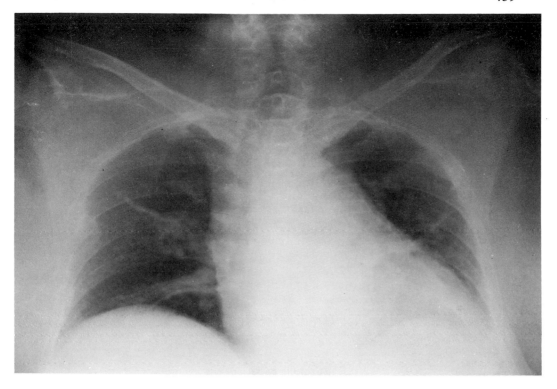

Fig. 13.7. Chest X-ray (supine P-A) of a female patient with severe Cushing's disease (wt 78 kg) showing reduction in size of the thoracic vertebrae, rib fractures, a high diaphragm, enlargement of the heart, distortion of the main airways and areas of atelectasis in the lungs.

degree of osteoporosis which may be present in patients with long-standing disease. Patients with severe osteoporosis require careful handling during positioning on the operating table to avoid causing fractures. Also, owing to osteoporosis there is a considerable shortening of the thoracic spine. The end result is that there is a small thoracic cavity, a high diaphragm and a tendency for collapse of the basal segments of the lower lobes (Fig. 13.7). These patients may also have a general myopathy and muscular weakness which is proximal in its distribution. It is advisable to measure the FEV_1 and to perform arterial blood-gas analysis in those patients with severe disease. The superficial appearances of patients with Cushing's disease may be deceptive, and they require very careful appraisal to assess the extent of potential respiratory insufficiency. Untreated Cushing's disease is a lethal condition having a high incidence of myocardial infarction, hence once the diagnosis has been made, provided the patient is not suffering from an active respiratory infection, treatment must be instituted as soon as possible.

CHROMOPHOBE ADENOMA OR OTHER FUNCTIONLESS PITUITARY TUMOURS

The major complication is hypopituitarism of which the most relevant feature is ACTH deficiency associated with low basal steroid secretion and an abnormal insulin tolerance test.

Corticosteroid cover

The aim of treatment is partial pituitary ablation, and in a large number of patients, when the overactivity of the gland is treated with implantation of ^{90}Y, it is possible to restore normal activity to the pituitary gland without the subsequent need for maintenance therapy with target organ hormones (cortisol, thyroxine, testosterone). Patients with large tumours or optic tract compression are given steroid therapy to reduce local tissue reaction to treatment in an attempt to reduce pituitary swelling. Patients with a gross reduction of pituitary function, or in whom total ablation of the gland is being performed also need steroids. One recommended regime is as follows.

Day 1 (day of operation) Cortisone hemisuccinate 100 mg intramuscularly at the time of premedication. Hydrocortisone 300 mg intravenously (by infusion during 24 hr)

Day 2 and 3 Prednisone 60 mg/day (20 mg × 3) administered orally

Day 4 and 5 Prednisone 40 mg (10 mg × 4)

Day 6 and 7 Prednisone 10 mg (2·5 mg × 4)

Day 8 onwards Prednisone 7·5 mg (2·5 mg × 3).

In tumours exerting pressure on the optic nerves, the dose of prednisone may be continued at 20 mg/day (starting with the doses outlined above) until the tenth day, or even later, if the hazard of local swelling is not judged to have passed, after which the dose is gradually reduced.

POSTOPERATIVE MANAGEMENT

Several considerations dictate that the anaesthetic technique should ensure that the patient is awake at the end of the procedure. Acromegalics may obstruct when unconscious and the airway must be secure. Patients with Cushing's disease must have the best chance of spontaneous ventilation if one is to avoid artificial ventilation in the postoperative period. After pituitary implantation, cryosurgery or the anterior surgical approach to the pituitary, there may be bleeding into the nasopharynx with the possibility of inhalation of blood clots and tissue debris in an unconscious patient. Except in very advanced disease, or a preterminal state, there should be no need for either a tracheoctomy in acromegalics or artificial ventilation in patients with Cushing's disease.

Postoperative recovery is usually uneventful but the following complications may occur. In *diabetic patients* there may be a two- to threefold increase in insulin requirements during steroid therapy. However, when the ablative effect begins, and the excessive steroid cover has finished, the insulin requirement usually falls to below initial values usually by the fifth postoperative day in the case of ^{90}Y implantation. The insulin requirements of successfully treated Cushing's syndrome may fall within a few days of implantation and almost invariably within three months, whereas in acromegalic patients with diabetes an early reduction in insulin requirement is less likely. In patients who have undergone surgical removal of the gland, which is much more difficult to regulate than X-ray therapy, there may be total loss of pituitary function and a gross reduction in insulin requirements.

Steroid deficiency

This may occur in a few patients with pituitary disease undergoing partial ablation with radiotherapy or ^{90}Y when the need for steroid cover was not anticipated.

It is always a probable occurrence following surgical removal of the gland. Anorexia, nausea, tachycardia and pyrexia may indicate cortisol deficiency, which may often, but not always, be confirmed by the electrocardiogram, which shows flattening or inversion of the T-waves. If steroid deficiency is suspected, a blood sample is taken for estimation of the plasma cortisol level. The clinical response to steroid therapy is apparent within a few hours (oral prednisone 5 mg, hourly for 6 doses and then a maintenance dose of 2·5 mg three times daily). If the patient is severely nauseated, treatment is initiated with hydrocortisone 100 mg given intramuscularly hourly until symptoms improve. Meningism may be a feature of cortisol deficiency and can be mistaken for meningitis. The rapid response to steroid therapy will confirm the diagnosis, but sometimes a lumbar puncture is desirable.

Disturbances of fluid balance

These are rare, usually mild and occur several days postoperatively.

Diabetes insipidus is indicated by polyuria, possibly associated with weight loss, and a rising serum level of sodium and urea. It is confirmed by the inability to concentrate the urine after a period of fluid restriction. When severe it may be controlled by an injection of pitressin tannate in oil or by oral administration of chlorpropamide 500 mg daily, although this needs a few days to take effect. Continuing severe diabetes insipidus requires treatment with DDAVP,* pitressin tannate in oil (intramuscularly) or lysine vasopressin contained in a nasal spray.

Acute water retention occasionally occurs from drinking continually in excess of need which has been minimized by the excessive release of vasopressin caused by pituitary radiation. This causes headache, nausea and fatigue and can be recognized by a weight gain of 1–2 kg and the finding of hyponatraemia. The syndrome is treated by restricting fluid intake to $\frac{1}{2}$–1l over 24 hours until the weight and serum sodium return to normal. In more severe cases, where a disturbance of consciousness occurs, an osmotic diuretic such as oral urea or intravenous mannitol is used and may be combined with hypertonic saline administered intravenously.

Infection

This is uncommon. Localized pituitary sepsis may cause headache and neck stiffness but the cerebrospinal fluid is clear. Such infection is treated with broad spectrum antibiotics, usually a combination of chloramphenicol, cloxacillin and sulphadiazine. Gentamycin may be added to the regimen to cover the possibility of infection by pseudomonas pyocyaneus, or when other therapy appears ineffective.

Cerebrospinal fluid rhinorrhoea may occur after implantation of the gland or surgery. The CSF leak may be mild and cease spontaneously. If the leak is persistent it may have to be treated surgically. By the time treatment is undertaken the pituitary gland may have subnormal activity and steroid cover is required. Because of the presence of a communication between the nasopharynx and the subarachnoid space, inflation of the lungs by facepiece could theoretically displace infected material into the CSF. These patients are preoxygenated and intubated without prior inflation.

---

* Desamino-cys^1-*d*-arginine^8-vasopressin.

On discharge from hospital, patients who have undergone treatment of the pituitary gland carry a card which indicates:
1 that partial or total ablation of the pituitary gland has been performed;
2 the steroid therapy needed, if any; with instructions when needed to increase the dosage of steroids in the presence of infection or trauma;
3 whom to contact in the event of late problems or complications.
The patient's family physician is also provided with this information.

Pituitary function should be reassessed 3 and 12 months after treatment and thereafter as thought desirable.

POSTERIOR PITUITARY

The neurohypophysis consists of three parts. The median eminence of the hypothalamus, the infundibular stalk and the neural lobe or posterior pituitary which is composed of nerve cells and their fibres, neuroglia, blood vessels and connective tissue.

Nerve fibres from the supraoptic and paraventricular nuclei of the hypothalamus travel via the stalk to enter the posterior lobe where they end in juxtaposition to capillaries.

The hormones are synthesized by the cells in the hypothalamus and pass down their axons to enter the posterior pituitary where they are released. In other words, these cells act rather like peripheral nerve fibres except that the effector substance which is released enters the circulation as opposed to exerting its effect directly on the receptors and cells of an innervated tissue. The stimulus for release of the hormones arises in the hypothalamic nuclei. Action potentials arriving at the nerve terminals in the neural lobe cause release of hormone and, as with other 'neurotransmitters', calcium plays an important role in linking deplorization to secretion.

POSTERIOR PITUITARY HORMONES

Vasopressin

Antidiuretic hormone is a cyclic octapeptide (mol.wt about 1,000). Arginine vasopressin is the antidiuretic hormone in all mammals with the exception of the pig, hippopotamus, hog and peccary where lysine vasopressin is found. The latter is more stable and, since its synthesis, has been used in the treatment of diabetes insipidus. It has also been used for testing the reserve of the anterior pituitary, since it causes the release of ACTH, but it is unpleasant for the patient and other tests are now used as described above.

Oxytocin

This is similar to vasopressin in structure, leucine being substituted for arginine and isoleucine for phenylalanine (Fig. 13.8).

Neurophysin

This is a substance with a large molecular weight (approximately 30,000) and it is a protein carrier. Its function is unknown but it may play a role in the storage of the

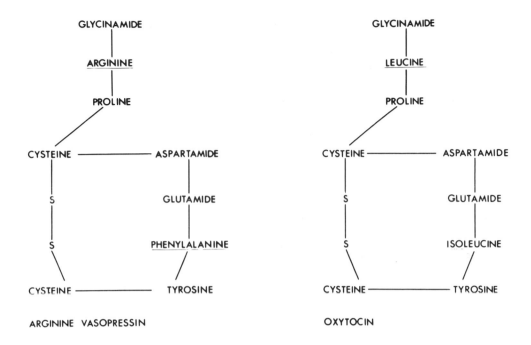

Fig. 13.8. Structural formulae of vasopressin and oxytocin.

hormones. Whether it is released into the circulation to act as a transport mechanism is not known.

Control of posterior pituitary secretion is summarized in Fig. 13.9. The principal physiological factor causing vasopressin release appears to be osmoreceptors in the hypothalamus. These combined with thirst centres are the principal factors concerned in the maintenance of water balance as summarized in Fig. 13.10. The other important physiological factor regulating ADH is the blood volume. A reduction in blood volume stimulates ADH release even when the plasma is hypotonic. Thus the volume control appears to override the osmotic control. The mechanism is probably a loss of pressure in the venous system with decreased afferent activity from the various receptors which are situated in the great veins and atria. However, there are rich connections between the nuclei of the hypothalamus and the rest of the nervous system and a variety of other stimuli will affect the release of antidiuretic hormone. Stimulation of peripheral nerves, pain, trauma and emotional factors will cause increased ADH secretion. Alcohol has a weak effect inhibiting ADH release while other drugs increase its release, e.g. opiates, barbiturates, anaesthetic agents, nicotine and acetylcholine.

VASOPRESSIN DEFICIENCY—DIABETES INSIPIDUS

Aetiology

This syndrome is most commonly associated with vasopressin deficiency. Apart from a rare familial syndrome, the majority of cases (45 per cent) are idiopathic. The deficiency may also be secondary to tumours of the pituitary and hypothalamus both

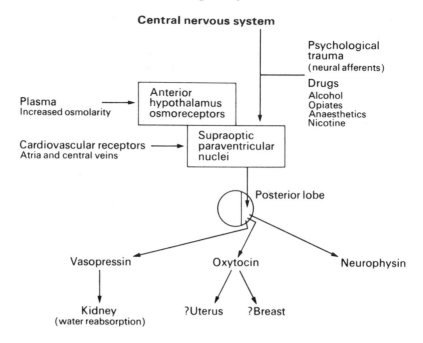

Fig. 13.9. Principal factors concerned with the regulation of the activity of the posterior pituitary. The various hormones are synthesized in the hypothalamus and travel along the axons of the pituicytes to reach the gland.

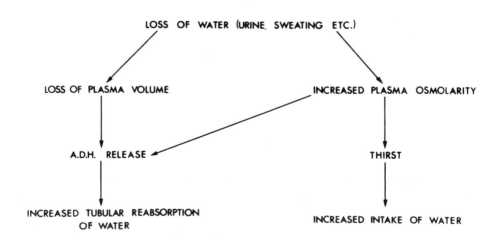

Fig. 13.10. Principal factors concerned in the conservation of water by the body.

primary and secondary and at one time this was the next most common aetiology. However, with the increasing number of road accidents and neurosurgical procedures, a traumatic group is becoming more significant. Birth injury may also be a traumatic cause. Chronic granulomatous and infective lesions, including tuberculosis and syphilis are rare possible aetiologies.

Renal diabetes insipidus is unresponsive to vasopressin and is caused by a sexlinked recessive genetic defect affecting male infants. Polyuria occurs within eight weeks of birth.

The polyuria due to potassium depletion, hypercalcaemia, amyloidosis and some other forms of renal disease is also unresponsive to vasopressin.

Clinical features

These include polyuria and polydipsia with urine volumes of 6 l to 15 l per day, which has a low specific gravity (e.g. 1·001–1·005, i.e. 50–200 mmol/kg). Sleep is often disturbed.

Adequate circulating corticosteroids are necessary to excrete a larger water load, and if the disease process also produces anterior pituitary deficiency, there will be a reduction in the urine volume. Patients with suspected diabetes insipidus should be tested for cortisol deficiency.

Diagnosis

This may be obvious on clinical history. The differential diagnosis includes:

1 Renal disease—if chronic the urine osmolality is often fixed at about 285 mmol/kg whereas in diabetes insipidus the osmolality is much lower and less than 200 mmol/kg. Examination of the urine for albumin, casts, cells and organisms, measurement of the plasma urea, creatinine clearance and IVP are all indicated.
2 Diabetes mellitus—the urine has a high specific gravity and there is impaired glucose tolerance.
3 Hypokalaemia and hypercalcaemia are associated with a diuresis.
4 Psychogenic (compulsive water drinking).

Eight hour fluid deprivation test. Since vasopressin cannot be routinely assayed in blood, the most valuable test is water deprivation. The principle is to establish that the patient cannot concentrate the urine in response to a rise in plasma solute concentration (intravenous hypertonic saline could be used but is potentially dangerous).

The patient should start well hydrated because those with ADH deficiency can become severely dehydrated during the test. Close supervision is necessary not only for safety but also to prevent compulsive water drinkers from obtaining water during the test.

Treatment with antidiuretic substances should have been stopped for 72 hours. The patient is weighed at the start and then at 4, 6, 7 and 8 hours. If more than 3 per cent of weight is lost the test should be stopped. In response to the withdrawal of fluid and food for eight hours a *normal subject* will elaborate urine with an osmolality of 600 mmol/kg or more while the plasma osmolality will not rise above 300 mmol/kg because water will be retained, i.e. the urine to plasma osmolality ratio is in excess of 2 and the urine flow rate falls to less than 0·5 ml/min.

In patients with *diabetes insipidus* the plasma becomes abnormally concentrated with an osmolality in excess of 300 mmol/kg whereas the urine remains dilute— osmolality < 270 mmol/kg—and the urine volume remains relatively high. The urine to plasma osmolality ratio does not rise above 1·9. *Psychogenic water drinking* can usually be differentiated, the main problem is preventing the patient obtaining access to water. Unlike patients with diabetes insipidus the plasma osmolality is relatively normal or low (i.e. 273–293 mmol/kg) and concentration of the urine occurs during the test.

15*

Cranial and nephrogenic diabetes insipidus can be differentiated by the response to antidiuretic hormone.

Therapy

1 Pitressin (soluble extract of pig or bovine pituitary). By injection in oil (pitressin tannate) intramuscular or subcutaneously. Dose 5–10 units; duration of action, 1–3 days. It is unpleasant for the patient.

2 Lysine vasopressin nasal spray contains the synthetic polypeptide in a concentration of 10 units/ml. Two sprays up each nostril (each approximately 5 units) are given as often as necessary. Duration of action, 4 hours. It can cause nasal irritation.

3 DDAVP (see footnote, page 441) is now the drug of choice. It is a synthetic analogue of arginine vasopressin. Its antidiuretic activity is much greater than the natural hormone and the pressor effect is less, so that side-effects (pallor, hypertension, abdominal cramps and diarrhoea) are reduced. Its rate of destruction is much slower and it is active when administered nasally. Dose—nasal administration—adults 10–20 μg and children 5 μg once or twice daily.

Chlorpropamide is normally used as an oral hypoglycaemic drug but it also appears to cause a marked increase in the sensitivity of the renal tubules to vasopressin. Hence patients in whom only small amounts of vasopressin are being secreted by the pituitary, respond dramatically to chlorpropamide and there may be no need for vasopressin therapy. In patients who are not fully controlled by chlorpropamide only small intermittent doses of vasopressin will be required. The drug takes 2–3 days to become fully effective. There must be an adequate carbohydrate intake throughout the day to prevent hypoglycaemia which is most likely to occur in children or in patients with associated dysfunction of the anterior pituitary, hence it is important to ensure that cortisol and growth hormone levels are normal. Patients receiving chlorpropamide do not tolerate alcohol which causes flushing and a severe headache (cf. Antabuse).

The normal dose is 100–350 mg once daily but in the presence of diabetes mellitus this may be increased to 500 mg daily.

VASOPRESSIN EXCESS

Hyponatraemia due to water retention will occur if the hypothalamic osmoreceptor system fails or if there is ectopic production of vasopressin. Many patients with severe illness and the 'sick cell syndrome' have inappropriate secretion of ADH. Ectopic vasopressin production most commonly occurs with oat cell carcinoma of the bronchus.

Clinical findings. The urine volume may be small, and its osmolality is at least twice that of the plasma. The serum sodium is less than 120 mmol/l. If the serum sodium falls below 100 mmol/l symptoms of hyponatraemia appear, e.g. anorexia, somnolence, depression, confusion, coma and convulsions. Oedema is rare.

Treatment is simple. The patient's water intake is restricted to less than the urine volume, e.g. 500 ml/day. In an emergency associated with coma and convulsions, hypertonic saline (500 ml containing 15 g of NaCl) may be given intravenously.

The presence of pigmentation suggests that an ectopic source of ADH is also producing ACTH and GH. Hypercalcaemia associated with malignant disease may cause a diuresis, so that the ADH effect will only become apparent when the serum calcium is reduced with treatment.

OXYTOCIN

The precise role of this hormone in man has yet to be determined. It appears to have roles in the contraction of the uterus and ejection of milk from the breast. As yet there have been no disease states associated with oxytocin excess or deficiency.

ECTOPIC SECRETION OF PITUITARY HORMONES

Many nonpituitary tumours acquire the capacity to produce pituitary hormones but the reasons for this are not clear.

The pituitary hormones most commonly involved are listed in Table 13.8. ACTH

Table 13.8. Pituitary hormones produced by nonendocrine tumours in order of frequency.

Hormone	Clinical syndrome or effects
1 ACTH (occasionally with CRF) ? LPH	Cushing's syndrome
2 Gonadotrophins	None or gynaecomastia or precocious puberty
3 Vasopressin	Water retention
4 TSH	Hyperthyroidism
5 CRF	Cushing's syndrome
6 Prolactin	Amenorrhoea, galactorrhoea
7 Growth hormone	None or hypertrophic pulmonary osteoarthropathy

and MSH are by far the most common and the tumours most frequently involved are tumours of the lung, thymus and pancreas. Both bronchogenic and renal carcinomas have been associated with prolactin secretion in men. Chorionepitheliomas and testicular tumours have both caused syndromes due to release of a thyrotrophic substance. Gonadotrophin secretion often occurs in association with teratomas.

ECTOPIC ACTH SYNDROME

This is the most important of these syndromes and was first formally described by Liddle in 1962 although the first case report of Cushing's syndrome in association with bronchial carcinoma was by Brown in 1928. The syndrome is characterized by explosive

Table 13.9. Neoplasms associated with ectopic ACTH syndrome.

Tumours	Approximate % cases
Bronchial carcinoma	50
Thymic carcinomas	10
Pancreatic carcinomas including islet cell and carcinoid	10
Neoplasms of neural crest tissue, i.e. phaeochromocytoma, neuroblastoma, ganglioneuroma	5
Thyroid, medullary carcinoma	5
Bronchial adenoma (including carcinoid)	2
Miscellaneous (ovary, prostate, breast, thyroid, kidney, salivary glands, testes, stomach, colon, gall-bladder, oesophagus, appendix)	2

Modified from Williams (1974).

Table 13.10. Cushing's syndrome compared with ectopic ACTH syndrome.

	Cushing's syndrome	Ectopic ACTH syndrome
Sex incidence	Predominantly female	Predominantly male
Onset	Slow	Explosive
Pigmentation	Uncommon	Common
Oedema	Rare	Common
Weight loss	Uncommon	Common
Course	Years	Short–weeks
Cause of death	Complications of hypertension, cardiovascular degeneration. Heart failure and infection	Carcinoma

Modified from Hall *et al.* (1980).

onset, extremely high plasma ACTH and cortisol levels, pigmentation, a low serum potassium and alkalosis. Only a few patients show the typical features of Cushing's syndrome when they present, despite the high levels of cortisol, because it usually takes many months for the classical features of Cushing's syndrome to develop in response to excess cortisol production or administration. The tumours principally involved are listed in Table 13.9. Cortisol production is extremely high and the plasma levels are almost diagnostic and cause a hypokalaemic alkalosis. The principal clinical features are summarized in Table 13.10 and the principal investigations in Table 13.11.

Unlike Cushing's disease, during ectopic ACTH production plasma cortisol levels cannot be suppressed by dexamethasone nor is there any response to metyrapone and in this respect the syndrome is similar to patients with adrenal dependent Cushing's syndrome. However, when the syndrome is produced by bronchial carcinoids, dexamethasone does cause suppression of cortisol production. The explanation is that in

Table 13.11. Findings and investigations in patients with Cushing's disease and syndromes

	Normal	Cushing's disease Hypothalamic	Adrenal tumours	Ectopic ACTH	Ectopic CRF
Plasma cortisol	$0\cdot1$–$0\cdot5\mu$mol/l	High no rhythm	High no rhythm	Very high no rhythm	Very high no rhythm
Plasma ACTH (8–10 am)	22–154μmol/l	High	Low or absent	Very high	Very high
Urinary free cortisol/24 hr	$< 0\cdot27\mu$mol	High	High > 100	Very high e.g. $> 1,000$	Very high
Urinary 17 OHCS* response to ACTH	Increase	Increase	Only small increase or no response	Increase	Increase
Urinary 17 OGS† in response to metyrapone	Increase	Increase	May fall	May fall	May fall
Dexamethasone suppression	Fall	Partial fall (i.e. at 2 mg, 6 hourly not at $0\cdot5$ mg 6 hourly)	No suppression	No suppression	No suppression
Hypokalaemic alkalosis	—	Rare	Common	Usual	Usual
Hyperglycaemia	—	Common	Common	Usual	Usual

* 17 OHCS i.e. hydroxycorticosteroids include cortisol (hydrocortisone) and cortisone.
† 17 OGS oxogenic steroids are the metabolites of corticosteroids, i.e. cortisol precursors which accumulate in the presence of metyrapone which blocks the final stage in the production of cortisol.

some of these tumours a peptide with the ability to release ACTH is produced, i.e. a corticotrophin-releasing hormone similar to CRF. In CRF-producing tumours not only does suppression of cortisol by dexamethasone occur but also there is an increase in 17-urinary oxogenic steroids in response to metyrapone, i.e. the syndrome is very similar in some respects to Cushing's disease.

DIAGNOSIS

The most important clue to diagnosis of this syndrome is the hypokalaemic alkalosis. Any patient who has a neoplasm associated with hypokalaemia, abnormal glucose tolerance, and increased pigmentation should be appropriately investigated. The principle findings of investigations in the various forms of Cushing's syndrome are shown in Table 13.11. If the ectopic syndrome is diagnosed, it is then necessary to search for a tumour. Chest X-rays, including tomography, bronchoscopy, sputum cytology, urine tests and IVP, tests for occult blood in faeces and barium studies etc. may all be necessary.

PROGNOSIS AND TREATMENT

Patients with carcinoma who develop this syndrome usually have a poor prognosis. However, some tumours are amenable to surgical removal and the patients do well (e.g. bronchial carcinoid). The patients may require considerable amounts of potassium during preparation for surgery, but once the nonmetastasizing tumour is completely removed the condition remits. In patients who are unsuitable for surgery, radiotherapy or chemotherapy, cortisol production can be reduced by treatment with metyrapone (750 mg 6–8 hourly) and aminoglutethimide (250–500 mg 8 hourly). Over zealous treatment with these drugs can lead to acute cortisol deficiency. It is necessary to monitor the plasma cortisol levels at frequent intervals and some authorities recommend administering prednisone while the dose of the drugs is adjusted.

REFERENCES

1 BRODY JS, FISHER AB, COCMEN A, DUBOIS AB. Acromegalic pneumomegaly: lung growth in the adult. *J Clin Invest* 1970; **49**: 1051–60.

2 CASSAR J, MCKECLINE P, JOPLIN GF. Reversal of laryngeal obstruction following treatment of acromegaly. *Laryngal Otol* 1979; **93**: 403–4.

3 CHILD DF, GORDON H, MASHITER K, JOPLING GF. Pregnancy, prolactin and pituitary tumours. *Br Med J* 1975; **2**: 87–9.

4 EDGE WG, WHITWAM JG. Chondro-calcinosis and difficult intubation in acromegaly. *Anaesthesia* 1981; **36**: 677–80.

5 KELLY WF, MASHITER K, DOYLE FH, BANKS LM, JOPLIN GF. Treatment of prolactin secreting pituitary tumours in young women by needle implantation of radioactive yttrium. *Quart J Med* 1978; **47**: 473–93.

6 KITAHATA LM. Airway difficulties associated with anaesthesia in acromegaly: three case reports. *Br J Anaesth* 1971; **43**: 1187–90.

7 Leading article. Bromocriptine—a changing scene. *Br Med J* 1975; **4**: 667–8.

8 WHITWAM JG, TUNBRIDGE WMG, FULLER WI. Management of patients for yttrium 90 implantation of the pituitary gland. *Br J Anaesth* 1973; **45**: 1121–9.

9 WRIGHT AD, HILL DM, LOWY C, FRASER TR. Mortality in acromegaly. *Quart J Med* 1970; **39**: 1–16.

FURTHER READING

WILLIAMS RH, ed. *Textbook of endocrinology.* 5th ed. Philadelphia: WB Saunders, 1974.

HALL R, ANDERSON J, SMART GA, BESSER M. *Fundamentals of endocrinology.* 3rd ed. London: Pitman Medical, 1980.

MARTINI L, BESSER GM, eds. *Clinical neuroendocrinology.* London: Academic Press, 1977.

Chapter 14
Adrenal Disease

G. W. BLACK AND D. A. D. MONTGOMERY

The adrenal glands, although forming an anatomical entity, consist of two parts which differ in their origin, structure and function. The outer cortex, derived from the embryonic coelomic epithelium, secretes steroid hormones under the control of anterior pituitary adrenocorticotrophin (ACTH) and is essential for life. The inner medulla is derived from the neural crest, forms a specialized part of the sympathetic nervous system and is not essential for survival.

THE ADRENAL CORTEX

ANATOMY AND HISTOLOGY [56]

The two adrenal glands, each weighing about 4 to 5 g, are situated directly above and close to the upper pole of each kidney. They receive a rich arterial blood supply from small vessels from the abdominal aorta, the phrenic and renal arteries. The adrenal vein is usually single. It is short and drains directly into the inferior vena cava on the right side, while on the left it joins the left renal vein.

The cortex consists of three zones of cells. The outer, the *zona glomerulosa*, which produces aldosterone, is not prominent and has a focal distribution. The inner two zones, the *zona fasciculata* and *zona reticularis* function as a single unit, the latter (the innermost zone) producing all the steroid hormones, except aldosterone, while the *zona fasciculata* (the middle zone) acts as a storehouse for steroid precursors. Under ACTH secretion the clear cells at the junction of the two zones are converted into compact cells and the *fasciculata* shrinks as the *reticularis* increases in thickness and becomes rich in enzymes and RNA.

The structure of the cortex varies with age and functional activity. In fetal life the glands are large and at birth consist of a larger *fetal zone* and a small outer layer from which the adult cortex develops. The fetal zone, which is concerned with the production of oestrogen precursors for oestrogen synthesis by the placenta, atrophies within a few weeks of birth and the true cortex continues to grow throughout childhood. At puberty the *zona reticularis* enlarges and the whole gland matures rapidly. Thereafter, growth diminishes until late middle adult life, after which the gland gradually decreases in size. ACTH is responsible for maintaining the structural integrity and responsiveness of the inner zones and atrophy of these follows hypophysectomy or pituitary inhibition with glucocorticoid therapy. Atrophic adrenal glands secrete less steroid in response to a given dose of ACTH than intact glands and it may take months for them to recover normal responsiveness. Conversely, glands which have been exposed to prolonged exposure to ACTH, as in Cushing's syndrome, show an enhanced response to exogenous ACTH.

PHYSIOLOGY

The adrenal cortex is essential for life and its secretions are in large part regulated by ACTH from the pituitary gland. Adrenocortical hormones consist of three groups: *mineralocorticoids*, which control sodium and potassium metabolism; *glucocorticoids*, which exert their effect mainly on carbohydrate and protein metabolism; and *sex hormones*, which supplement but cannot take the place of the hormones of the gonads.

ADRENOCORTICOTROPHIN (ACTH)

ACTH controls the secretion of the glucocorticoid and sex hormones. It supports the secretion of aldosterone and may temporarily promote an increase in aldosterone output during stress, but it does not provide the main stimulus. After hypophysectomy or inhibition of ACTH secretion the inner zones atrophy, but the *glomerulosa* is relatively unaffected and aldosterone secretion continues largely unaltered. ACTH stimulates steroidogenesis by activating cyclic AMP which promotes the conversion of cholesterol into pregnenolone.

$ACTH_{1-39}$ is a straight chain polypeptide. It has been synthesized and human ACTH is available for clinical use. It is secreted by the basophil cells of the anterior pituitary largely under the control of corticotrophin releasing hormone (CRH). Adrenergic, cholinergic and serotoninergic pathways all appear to play a part in the central nervous system regulation of ACTH release. The secretion of CRH and ACTH is governed by three mechanisms, an inherent circadian rhythm, stress and negative feedback both at the hypothalamic and at the pituitary level. The system responds with exquisite sensitivity to appropriate stimuli. For example, during surgery the concentration of ACTH rises appreciably within a few minutes of starting the operation.

CRH and ACTH are subject to indirect (and possibly direct) negative feedback mechanism involving cortisol. In effect CRH and ACTH are secreted when they are needed and inhibited when they are not. Since no other adrenal hormone has this action cortisol controls the secretion of all adrenal steroids except aldosterone. The inhibitory effect can, however, be overcome by an increased drive for ACTH secretion when necessary, so that the response to stress is not self-limiting.

Normally there is a low basal rate of ACTH secretion which is at its lowest level at about midnight reaching a peak between 0700 and 0900 hours. Thereafter, secretion decreases irregularly until the next cycle of activity commences. The secretion of cortisol follows that of ACTH closely with a time-lag of a few minutes. This pattern of hypothalamic-pituitary-adrenal function may be modified by changes in bodily activity, stress or sleeping habits, and it takes several days to readjust after a rapid journey into a different time zone (so-called jet lag). Absence of a circadian rhythm indicates an abnormality of the system which may be functional or organic.

SYNTHESIS OF ADRENAL CORTEX HORMONES [42, 48]

The early synthetic steps are common to all steroids and involve the formation of cholesterol and then, by removal of its side chain, of pregnenolone. From then onward the pathways of the different steroids diverge.

The *zona glomerulosa* possesses all the enzymes necessary to convert cholesterol to aldosterone, including the essential enzyme necessary to produce the aldehyde group

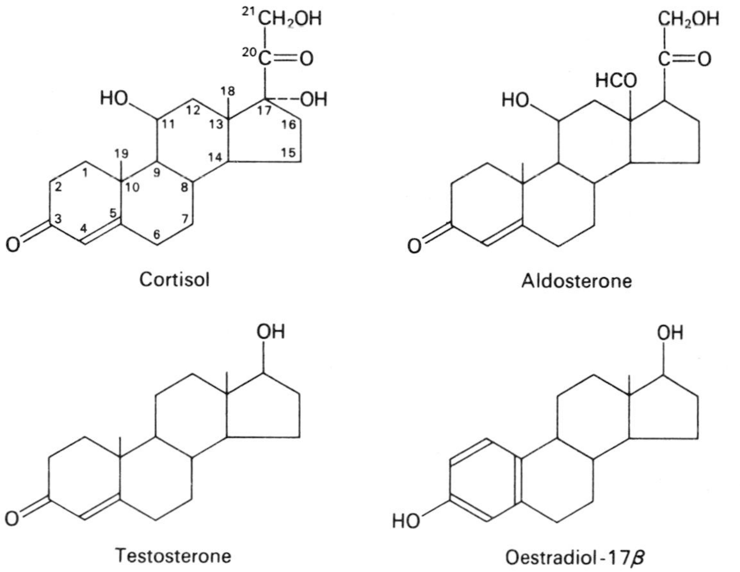

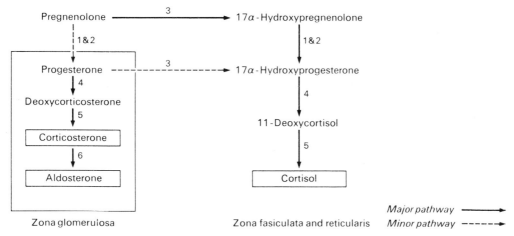

Fig. 14.1. Principal steroid hormones (the numbers indicate the position of the carbon atoms).

at position 18 (Fig. 14.1 and 14.2) but it lacks 17α-hydroxylase. Thus it secretes corticosterone and aldosterone but normally no 17-hydroxylated steroids or sex hormones. Conversely, the *zona fasciculata* and *reticularis* possess 17α-hydroxylase but lack the enzymes active at position 18. Hence, aldosterone cannot be produced but large amounts of cortisol and sex hormones are secreted instead.

The C$_{21}$ steroids which include cortisol, corticosterone and aldosterone (the major glucocorticoids and mineralocorticoids) are synthesized in the manner shown in Fig. 14.2.

Fig. 14.2. Steroid biosynthesis of principal C$_{21}$ steroids (in boxes) and enzymatic steps (numbers).
1 and 2 3 β-hydroxysteroid dehydrogenase and Δ$^{5-4}$ isomerase.
3 17 α-hydroxylase
4 21-hydroxylase
5 11 β-hydroxlase
6 18-hydroxylase and 18-hydroxysteroid dehydrogenase.

The synthesis of the C_{19} steroids (dehydroepiandrosterone (DHA) and testosterone) and C_{18} oestrogens in the adrenal cortex depend on other pathways which are also fully worked out.

The main hormones of the adrenal and their site of origin are thus as follows:

Type	Main hormone	Zone of origin
Mineralocorticoid	Aldosterone (deoxycorticosterone)	Glomerulosa (all three zones)
Glucocorticoid	Cortisol Corticosterone*	
Sex-androgenic†	Dehydropiandrosterone Androstenedione 11-hydroxyandrostenedione	Fasciculata and Reticularis
(Oestrogenic)†	(Oestradiol-17β) (Oestrone)	
Progestogenic	Progesterone	

* Secreted in small amounts by *glomerulosa*.
† Variable small amounts of testosterone and oestradiol may be secreted also, but ordinarily production is minimal [1].

ALDOSTERONE

Aldosterone is the most powerful natural mineralocorticoid and controls the metabolism of sodium and potassium. It shares, in weak manner, some of the activities of cortisol. Aldosterone is secreted in small amounts when the intake of sodium is normal (100 mmol daily) [46]. Its secretion is regulated by three mechanisms: The renin-angiotensin system (the major factor); electrolyte metabolism; and ACTH. These may operate together or independently.

Renin–angiotensin system [58]

Renin, a proteolytic enzyme is secreted and stored in cells of the juxta-glomerular (JG) apparatus. This structure consists of a composite group of cells believed to be derived from modified smooth muscle cells of the afferent arteriole and specialized cells at the origin of the distal tubule that form the *macula densa* (Fig. 14.3). A fall in blood pressure or blood volume and sodium depletion increase renin release, while expansion of the blood volume inhibits it. These changes are probably mediated through a JG stretch-receptor mechanism. Renin release, independent of perfusion pressure, is also thought to be mediated by changes in the sodium content in the distal tubule, but it is uncertain whether renin responds to an increase or decrease in the sodium concentration. The autonomic nervous system and catecholamines also play a part. For example, patients with autonomic insufficiency and those treated with chronic β-adrenoceptor blockade with propranolol may show impaired renin secretion to appropriate stimuli. Antidiuretic hormone (ADH) also inhibits renin release probably by a direct effect on JG cells.

Mechanism of renin action (Fig. 14.3)

Once released into the circulation, renin converts renin substrate peptide, an α_2 globulin synthesized in the liver, to an inactive decapeptide, angiotensin I (a pro-

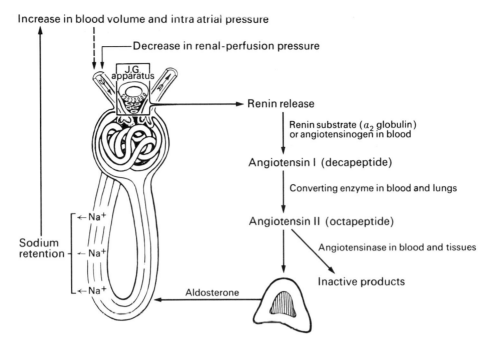

Fig. 14.3. Regulation of aldosterone secretion (Renin-Angiotensin system).

hormone). A converting enzyme, found mainly in the lung, but also in plasma and other organs, converts angiotensin I to the active octapeptide angiotensin II. Angiotensin II is a potent vasoconstrictor and the main stimulus for aldosterone secretion by cells of the *zona glomerulosa*. It is rapidly destroyed by circulating enzymes. Renin release is subject to a feedback control by angiotensin II directly, and indirectly through effects mediated via aldosterone on blood volume, blood pressure and sodium balance. Angiotensin II plays a major role in bodily homeostasis through a direct effect on arteriolar smooth muscle contraction and aldosterone stimulation. Although it is the most potent pressor substance known in man it is not normally required for blood pressure regulation except in the presence of plasma volume depletion. Recently inhibitors of the renin–angiotensin system have been synthesized [12, 28]. These include a competitive inhibitor for angiotensin II receptors (saralasin, 1-sar-8-ala-angiotensin II) and a converting enzyme inhibitor (S.Q. 14225, D-3-mercapto-2-methylpropanoyl-L-proline, Captopril) which block the conversion of angiotensin I to angiotensin II after oral administration. Both cause a fall in blood pressure and may prove to be effective in the treatment of hypertension.

Electrolyte metabolism

A potassium load increases aldosterone secretion, while potassium depletion diminishes it. These effects are probably independent of changes in the volume of body fluids and favour an intrarenal mechanism. Aldosterone secretion is also closely related to sodium metabolism being increased during sodium restriction and diminished during sodium retention. These changes are probably mediated through alterations in the extracellular fluid volume and perfusion pressure. However, it is likely that renin secretion depends also on the concentration of sodium in the distal renal tubules, but the relative importance of these two mechanisms is uncertain.

Effect of ACTH

Pharmacological doses of ACTH increase aldosterone secretion, although doses sufficient to increase cortisol output effectively do not do so. Pathological states in which ACTH secretion is increased, do not increase aldosterone, and it has beeen suggested recently that prolonged treatment with ACTH reduces rather than enhances *zona glomerulosa* responsiveness.

Hypophysectomy and hypopituitarism are associated with some impairment in aldosterone production, which can be restored by ACTH. Thus, ACTH may support the secretion of aldosterone, but it is not the main stimulus.

Actions of aldosterone

Aldosterone controls sodium retention and potassium excretion in a variety of tissues, particularly the kidney, but also in the sweat and salivary glands, muscle, and intestinal mucosa. It promotes the absorption of sodium in the distal renal tubule after a latent period of several hours, by increasing active sodium transport (the sodium pump theory) or by increasing the permeability of the cells to sodium (permease hypothesis). Secondarily aldosterone increases potassium, hydrogen, and magnesium ion excretion, possibly on an ion exchange basis for sodium. However, actions on sodium retention and potassium excretion may be dissociated in time, so that other factors such as variations in the availability of either ion, may be involved. The overall effect of aldosterone is to increase the amount of sodium in the body, but as this would increase the plasma osmolality ADH is released which inhibits water excretion. As a consequence the plasma volume is increased and the osmolality remains unaltered.

The administration of aldosterone to normal subjects consuming a normal salt intake leads to sodium retention for several days. Thereafter, sodium excretion increases until it reaches the level of the intake. This 'escape' mechanism involves decreased reabsorption of sodium in the proximal tubule which allows sufficient sodium to pass into the distal tubule. Here, despite an increased sodium and potassium exchange, sufficient sodium is lost eventually to restore the sodium balance.

Aldosterone-receptor proteins are found in all tissues responsive to the hormone and they can be blocked by drugs of the spironolactone series.

When aldosterone is present in excess, the serum sodium level rises, potassium is lost from the kidney and hypokalaemia develops. This is associated with a metabolic alkalosis because hydrogen ions migrate from the extracellular fluid into the cells in place of potassium ions which have been lost. Conversely, lack of aldosterone leads to sodium loss and a rise in serum potassium. A metabolic acidosis develops as the potassium ions displace hydrogen ions from the tissue cells. Aldosterone may play an indirect role in blood pressure regulation since hypotension follows when it is absent (Addison's disease) and hypertension results from its excess (hyperaldosteronism).

CORTISOL

Cortisol is the principal glucocorticoid hormone of the adrenal in man; corticosterone provides only about 10 per cent of the total glucocorticoid output. Cortisol production is related to surface area and increases steadily from birth to adult life to reach about $40-55$ $\mu mol/24$ hr. It is secreted episodically in phase with ACTH.

Cortisol is discharged in a free state into the circulation. About 95 per cent is rapidly bound to corticosterone binding globulin (CBG), an α_1-globulin, where it remains in equilibrium with free cortisol. CBG while having a high affinity for cortisol has a relatively low capacity. When the level of cortisol exceeds 700 nmol/l CBG becomes saturated and a higher proportion of cortisol circulates in a free form or becomes loosely attached to albumin which has a low affinity but a high capacity. CBG levels are increased by oestrogen therapy, some anabolic steroids and during pregnancy, while the level falls in hypoproteinaemic states.

Actions of cortisol

Cortisol (hydrocortisone) is the only steroid hormone which is essential for life. Its actions are widespread: it promotes hepatic gluconeogenesis and protein synthesis in the liver; it has a catabolic action on protein synthesis elsewhere, especially in skeletal muscle; there is a mechanism whereby it influences the distribution of fluid across cell membranes; it has a lytic action on lymphoid tissue and eosinophils, an anti-inflammatory and antiallergic action, and an effect on the function of cells in the CNS.

Carbohydrate and protein metabolism

Cortisol promotes the breakdown of protein throughout the body and the formation of glucose from the liberated aminoacids by stimulating enzymes in the liver. At the same time it raises the blood glucose, inhibits its peripheral utilization and stimulates the formation of glycogen in the liver. The term glucocorticoid is derived from these 'diabetogenic' actions. Cortisol is an important member of a group of hormones (growth hormone, insulin, glucagon, adrenaline and thyroxine) whose actions control intermediary metabolism. Associated with these changes there may be a negative nitrogen balance and creatinuria, signifying muscle breakdown; increased uric acid due to lysis of lymphoid and other tissue may also be found in the urine. In excess, cortisol causes wasting of skeletal muscle and muscular weakness. Loss of protein from the bone causes osteoporosis, an effect which is aggravated by the inhibitory action of cortisol on calcium absorption from the gut (antivitamin D action).

Fat metabolism

Cortisol promotes the deposition of fat in the body but its mode of action is not clear. In excess, as in Cushing's syndrome, it causes a redistribution of fat so that it is laid down in the cheeks, trunk, shoulders and abdomen, while fat in the arms and legs is decreased.

Water and electrolyte metabolism

Cortisol has actions similar to, but much weaker than those of aldosterone. It promotes sodium retention and potassium excretion by the kidney and facilitates the excretion of a water load, by increasing glomerular filtration and diminishing its reabsorption by the tubules.

Blood cells

Cortisol appears to increase the total mass of red cells and neutrophil polymorphs and to diminish the number of lymphocytes and eosinophils. In addition, it reduces the fixed mass of lymphoid throughout the body. This destructive process involves the inhibition of protein synthesis in the affected cells but the reason for the action is not known.

Miscellaneous effects

Some actions of cortisol, as in stress, are *'permissive'* so that while cortisol does not initiate the activity, the activity cannot be effective in the absence of cortisol. For example, cortisol is necessary for the proper function of the central nervous system. Cortisol is concerned in the maintenance of the blood pressure by facilitating the action of noradrenaline on the arterioles, and in the secretion of gastric juice by the stomach. Three further actions which may be pharmacological rather than physiological are inhibition of inflammatory reactions, suppression of allergic responses and reduction in fibroblastic activity.

SEX HORMONES

Adrenal *androgens* are all weak in comparison to testosterone. In the male they cannot promote or maintain normal sexual activity after castration. In females, they may assist in the growth of sexual hair and the skeleton at puberty. In both sexes they may encourage protein anabolism and other metabolic responses.

Adrenal *oestrogens* are secreted in very small quantities and cannot be important physiologically.

The adrenal *progestogens* provide essential precursors for the biosynthesis of important steroids (cortisol and aldosterone), but are probably unimportant otherwise.

THE ADRENOCORTICAL RESPONSE TO ANAESTHESIA SURGERY AND STRESS [32, 59]

In recent years there has been increasing interest in the response of the adrenal cortex to anaesthetic agents mainly because of the availability of newly introduced techniques of hormone assay, and several well-documented studies have now been reported [60].

Plasma concentrations of aldosterone are found to be significantly raised and plasma renin action is increased during anaesthesia with ether, halothane, methoxyflurane and enflurane, further increases being noted after the start of surgery. A significant decrease in urinary Na/K ratio with all inhalational agents accompanies these rises in the plasma concentration of aldosterone. Increases in plasma ACTH concentrations are noted during the inhalation of halothane and enflurane and these are much more pronounced during surgery. It is suggested that the marked increase in ACTH secretion or increased plasma serum activity or both account for the elevations of plasma aldosterone found during anaesthesia and surgery. Aldosterone plays some role in homeostasis and serum electrolyte balance during anaesthesia and surgery but since there are no substantial differences in the plasma concentrations of aldosterone with different inhalational anaesthetics any may be used in the management of adrenalectomy for primary aldosteronism although methoxyflurane should be avoided as it is nephrotoxic [61].

Preoperative apprehension may induce an increase in adrenocortical activity and effective preanaesthetic sedation results in a fall in plasma cortisol levels. Changes in plasma cortisol concentration associated with the use of intravenous anaesthetics are related more to the extent of the operation and appear to reflect the degree of stress caused by surgery [16].

The inhalation of ether and cyclopropane produces significant elevations in plasma cortisol levels in man; in contrast, halothane and more particularly methoxyflurane are largely devoid of such activity. It would appear that those inhalational anaesthetics which provoke the greatest increase in adrenocortical activity are those whose administration is associated with elevations in circulating plasma catecholamines. Operative stress, however, is a more important factor in stimulating the adrenal cortex, and surgery is capable of inducing marked rises in plasma cortisol concentrations even during halothane or methoxyflurane anaesthesia.

It is clear that the operative procedure plays a much greater part in influencing adrenocortical activity than does anaesthesia, the extent of the surgery being all important in determining the magnitude of the response. Intra-abdominal operations, especially those associated with pain-eliciting traction of the viscera, appear to provoke the greatest response by the adrenal cortex, although this is a process which may be blunted to some extent by general anaesthesia and appropriate regional analgesia.

Increased aldosterone secretion during surgery is probably due to a stress-induced release of ACTH, although other factors associated with the injurious process such as changes in blood volume and the release of cellular potassium are also capable of producing this response. It is likely that the increased production of aldosterone accounts mainly for the changes in fluid, sodium and potassium which occur in the post-injury period. The increased production of aldosterone matches the extent of the rise in plasma cortisol level and is more pronounced following major surgery.

Increased liberation of corticosteroids occurs during conditions of stress such as major surgery, trauma, severe infections, blood loss and circulatory collapse. This increase in cortical function is also manifested by elevations of free fatty acid concentrations and by hyperglycaemia, and is part of the general metabolic and endocrine response to the injurious process.

Peak levels of plasma cortisol concentrations occur within six hours of the commencement of surgery and normal values are usually regained during the next twelve hours. These increases may be partly due to a reduction in the conjugation of cortisol by the liver brought about by the diminished hepatic blood supply which often accompanies major surgery and other forms of trauma. It is probable that the adreno-cortical response to a major surgical procedure is maximal because the intraoperative administration of ACTH produces no additional increase in plasma cortisol concentration, although such a reaction can be evoked by giving ACTH 24 hours after operation. The responsiveness of the adrenal cortex to stress may be dependent on blood flow, and the low plasma cortisol levels found in patients with shock often rise to normal following resuscitation.

The most important trigger-mechanism producing the typical metabolic-endocrine response to surgery appears to be mediated by apparent neurogenic stimuli arising from the operative site and passing to the hypothalamus. Extensive studies have shown that blockade of these afferent neurones from the surgical area by epidural analgesia modifies the endocrine response to surgery, the usual increases in cortisol, growth hormone, aldosterone, renin and adrenaline which accompany surgery being significantly inhibited [35]. Also, there is evidence that the intra- and postoperative metabolic profiles of patients receiving general anaesthesia reflect substrate mobilization (increased glucose, lactate and 3-hydroxybutyrate) whereas epidural analgesia prevents these changes, probably because of an inhibited response of adrenaline to surgery. Free fatty acid and glycerol levels are also substantially reduced by epidural blockade, indicating inhibition of lipolysis [36]. These unwanted effects of the metabolic response to surgery are also modified by the use of intravenous morphine and fentanyl [23].

DISORDERS OF THE ADRENAL CORTEX [68]

Lesions of the adrenal glands are important for they frequently cause disturbance of endocrine function. Surgery may be necessary to correct lesions causing increased function so that anaesthetists must be familiar with all aspects of their management. Conversely, lesions which impair function increase the hazards of surgery so that effective treatment must be prescribed before operative treatment. The lesions and syndromes may be classified as in Table 14.1.

Table 14.1. Lesions and syndromes of the adrenal cortex.

With disturbance of endocrine function

INCREASED SECRETION	DECREASED SECRETION
Lesions	*Lesions*
Hyperplasia	Hypoplasia
Adenoma	Atrophy
Carcinoma	Destruction (haemorrhage, infarction, infective process, infiltration)
	Surgical removal
Syndromes	*Syndromes*
Excess of glucocorticoids causes Cushing's syndrome	Chronic deficiency causes Addison's disease
Excess of mineralocorticoids causes aldosteronism	Acute deficiency causes acute adrenal failure (adrenal crisis)
Excess of androgens causes virilization	
Excess of oestrogens causes feminization	
Mixed syndromes	

Without disturbance of function

Lesions

Adenoma
Carcinoma
Cysts, rare tumours, etc

PATHOLOGY OF ADRENAL DISORDERS

Hyperplasia is usually bilateral. Hyperplasia of the *zona glomerulosa* is found in secondary hyperaldosteronism and in most patients with primary hyperaldosteronism. Hyperplasia of the inner zones affecting the *reticularis* with corresponding shrinkage of the *fasciculata* is found in Cushing's syndrome, congenital adrenal hyperplasia, and exogenous stimulation with ACTH. *Hypoplasia* results from agenesis or hypoplasia of the pituitary. It also occurs as a congenital recessive disorder. *Atrophy* is usually bilateral but may be unilateral if there is a functionally active tumour in the opposite gland. Atrophy with impaired adrenal function is found with: (a) hypopituitarism and hypophysectomy; (b) inhibition of ACTH secretion by therapeutic administration of corticosteroids; (c) glucocorticoid-secreting tumours cause atrophy of the opposite gland and of the uninvolved portion of the affected gland; and (d) autoimmune disease. Tumours which secrete mainly androgens and aldosterone do not cause atrophy. *Tumours* include benign adenomas and carcinomas. *Adrenocortical* nodules are not true tumours. *Cortical micronodules* are commonly associated with hyperplastic glands. In more extreme form the condition is known as *nodular hyperplasia*.

INVESTIGATION OF ADRENOCORTICAL DISORDERS

Investigations that are of help in the diagnosis of adrenocortical disorders include the following:

Radiological examination [67]

Radiology of the adrenal glands is often helpful but, unless the indications for highly specialized methods are present, the patient may be exposed unnecessarily to procedures which are potentially dangerous and which are expensive and time consuming for the radiologist. The same methods are applicable to both cortex and medulla. For the latter special precautions are necessary (see below). *Plain radiographs* may show a soft tissue shadow with displacement of the kidney due to an adrenal carcinoma. Patchy calcification is seen in some cancers and neuroblastomas. 'Egg-shell calcification' is found occasionally in phaeochromocytomas and adrenal cysts. Calcification of the adrenal now occurs rarely in Addison's disease (10 per cent). With larger tumours, *intravenous urography* combined with tomography will show displacement of the kidney. However, the method is not accurate enough to visualize the average sized adenoma or bilateral hyperplasia.

When gas (oxygen, nitrous oxide or carbon dioxide) or air is introduced into the retroperitoneal space it dissects tissues around the kidney and adrenal glands and enables them to be visualized on plain films or tomograms. Retroperitoneal pneumography is not without risk of gas or air embolism. Tumours larger than 2 or 3 cm in diameter are usually seen but smaller lesions are frequently missed. Retroperitoneal pneumography has now been superseded by arteriography and venography. Adrenal carcinomas and phaeochromocytomas are vascular so that they are easily demonstrated by arteriography but cortical adenomas are rarely seen because of a poor blood supply. Venography and venous sampling are more helpful. With retrograde injection of the adrenal vein with contrast media it is possible to outline quite small adenomas. It is the most sensitive method of demonstrating small tumours. At the same time blood samples can be obtained from various sites for estimation of the blood levels of cortisol, aldosterone and catecholamines which assist in the location of the lesion.

Radioisotope visualization of the adrenal with radioactive iodocholesterol, or derivatives of it such as 75-selenomethyl-19-norcholesterol (Scintadren, Amersham) is helpful in some cases but is slow to carry out. The technique is probably of greatest value in distinguishing unilateral adrenocorticol dysfunction from bilateral disease in Cushing's syndrome and for localizing other steroid secreting tumours and ectopic adrenal tissue. Ultrasound and CAT scan localization of tumours may also be of value.

Indirect tests of adrenocortical function

Plasma electrolytes

The measurement of plasma sodium and potassium may be useful in the investigation of adrenal disorders. The changes that may be expected are described under the individual disorders.

Water load test

A simple test has been devised to check cortisol secretion. Water (20 ml per kg of body weight) is taken by mouth over 15 to 20 minutes, after an 8-hour fast, and the urine is collected for 4 hours. Normally, 90 per cent or more of the water is excreted in 4 hours, whereas in those with adrenocortical failure less than 55 per cent is excreted. The oral administration of hydrocortisone 40 to 80 mg 2 hours before the test improves the diuresis in those with adrenal insufficiency, but not in those with other lesions causing impaired water excretion (hepatic disease, hypothyroidism and dehydration).

Direct measurement of adrenocortical steroids and their metabolites

Measurements of adrenal steroids and their metabolites in blood and urine are essential for diagnosis of the adrenocortical disorders. Normal values are shown in Table 14.2. The secretion rates of aldosterone, cortisol and some other steroids can be estimated accurately by isotopic dilution methods but, because of technical problems these are not generally available.

Aldosterone

Aldosterone in the urine (10–55 nmol/24 hr) plasma (100–500 pmol/l) and production rate (190–550 nmol/24 hr) can all be measured. It is essential to relate the aldosterone secretion to the sodium intake, so that a diet containing, at least, 100 mmol of sodium chloride daily for a week is necessary before the initial measurement is made. As normal values have been found occasionally in patients with hyperaldosteronism, the estimation should be repeated several times. Special techniques are available for measuring the components of the renin–angiotensin system. Ideally, the simultaneous determination of aldosterone and renin enhances the diagnosis of primary hyper-aldosteronism because the level of the former will be higher than normal and the latter will be low or totally suppressed.

Cortisol

Urine. The 11-hydrocorticosteroid (11-OHCS) and free cortisol methods provide a sensitive index of adrenal activity and correlate well with cortisol secretion. Other measurements of urinary steroids, 17-hydroxycorticosteroids (17-OHCS), 17-oxogenic steroids (17-OGS) and total 17-oxogenic steroids (total 17-OGS) are less reliable and are being gradually phased out.

Blood. Plasma cortisol is best measured by radioimmunoassay rather than by the fluorogenic method of Mattingly [44].

Table 14.2. Basal urinary excretion and blood plasma levels of steroids under normal conditions and in states of cortisol excess and deficiency. Ranges (and means).

| | Urine (per 24 hours) | | | | Blood plasma (per litre) | | | | Cortisol secretion rate (mg/24 hours) [18, 19] |
| | Free cortisol (μg) [2, 14] | Free 11-OHCS (μg) [43] | Total 17-OGS or 17-OGS (mg) | 17-OHCS (mg) | 11-OHCS (nmol) | | 17-OHCS (nmol) [24] | | |
					0700–1000	Midnight	0700–1000	Midnight	
Normal Male	0–95 (40)	115–340 (230)	4–20 [7] (9)	4–14 [62] (7)	160–700 [44]	0–160 [44]	160–650	0–200	6–28 (16)
Normal Female		70–280 (175)	3–18 [7] (7)	4–10 [62] (6)					
Cushing's syndrome — Pituitary / Adrenal adenoma	110–1,000 (300)	400–3,000	7–70 [43]	10–60 [45]	275–2000 [18]	275–1400 [18]	140–1000	100–525	35–120 (64)
Adrenal carcinoma	(very high)	>2,000	>100 [43]	(very high)	(very high)	(very high)			>120
Ectopic ACTH	4000	3,000	40–120 [43]	(very high)	(very high)	(very high)	(very high)	(very high)	>400
Addison's disease	0–12	19–56	0–5 [45]	0–5 [45]	0–160 [44]	0–160 [44]	(low)	(low)	0·5–19
Hypopituitarism	(very low)	(very low)	0–5 [45]	0–5 [45]	(low)	(low)	(low)	(low)	0·5–2

References [2] Beardwell et al. [7] Borth et al. [14] Burke & Beardwell [18] Cope [19] Cope & Pearson [24] Ernest [43] Mattingly & Tyler [44] Mattingly & Tyler [45] Mills [62] Peterson

Note: The values in this table are obtained from references which antedate the introduction of S.I. units and have not been converted. The converted values are used in the text.

Measurements should be made at least twice in the 24 hours because of the circadian variation in blood levels; 0800 and 2300 hours or midnight are convenient. A single low morning cortisol level must not be taken as conclusive evidence of adrenal insufficiency. ACTH measurements taken at the same time add greatly to the knowledge of pituitary-adrenal interrelationships. A loss of the circadian response is usually a sign of disordered adrenal function, but it may be lost in blind subjects, in patients with a variety of cerebral diseases and in those with lesions in the neighbourhood of the hypothalamus. It may also be disturbed by drugs, among which are chlorpromazine, other phenothiazines, phenytoin, reserpine and morphine and its analogues. Prolonged glucocorticoid therapy inhibits ACTH secretion and the circadian response and, following withdrawal of treatment, many months may elapse before normal hypothalamic-pituitary-adrenal function recovers. The practical application of this for anaesthetists is discussed later. Under basal (nonstressed) conditions measurement of urinary free cortisol or 11-OHCS and plasma 11-OHCS will distinguish between normal adrenal secretion and hyper- and hyposecretion. However, they rarely elucidate the cause of the abnormal secretion, so that other methods of stimulating and inhibiting higher centres must be used.

Stimulation and suppression tests

Stimulation tests using ACTH (in the form of tetracosactrin) are not commonly performed now in the routine assessment of adrenal function. Tetracosactrin (250 μg) is injected intramuscularly and the plasma level of 11-OHCS is measured before and exactly 30 minutes later. If the response is normal the 11-OHCS rise by 190 to 750 nmol/l with a peak response of 550–1150 nmol/l. In Addison's disease the rise and peak values are less than 195 nmol/l [63]. Should it be necessary to distinguish between primary and secondary adrenocortical insufficiency, a larger dose of tetracosactrin (1 mg) is necessary and the response is tested at 4 or 6 hours later. In primary adrenal failure there is little or no response, while in hypopituitarism the response is subnormal [26]. An indirect test using *metyrapone* [49] performs the same function and tests the hypothalamic-pituitary integrity at the same time. Metyrapone inhibits the enzyme 11β-hydroxylase (Fig. 14.2) so that when it is given by mouth in a dose of 4·5 g daily the secretion of cortisol falls, while that of 11-deoxycortisol rises. The latter does not inhibit the release of CRH and ACTH which respond to the impairment of cortisol secretion. Provided that the hypothalamus and pituitary are normal, all these hormones increase greatly. The metabolites of 11-deoxycortisol can be measured in the 17-hydroxycorticosteroids in the blood and urine, and in the oxogenic steroids in the urine. A positive response indicates integrity of the whole hypothalamic-pituitary-adrenal axis. Insulin hypoglycaemia also stimulates the hypothalamus to release CRH and ACTH and the plasma 11-OHCS rise significantly within 2 hours [29]. The simultaneous measurement of the plasma ACTH during stimulation and also suppression tests (below) improves their reliability and ease of interpretation.

Suppression (by inhibition of pituitary ACTH production) tests are performed with dexamethasone, a synthetic glucocorticoid, which is about 35 times more potent than cortisol. It can be administered in two doses, 0·5 mg and 2 mg 6-hourly. With the former, normal subjects show a fall of the urinary 17-OHCS to less than 2·5 mg [38] and the urinary-free cortisol to less than 75 nmol/24 hr on the second day [14]. Patients with Cushing's syndrome fail to suppress with the smaller dose but many do so with the higher dosage. The test is used mainly to differentiate between the various forms of Cushing's syndrome. If there is unequivocal suppression the patient has pituitary-dependent Cushing's syndrome. If there is no suppression an adrenal tumour or an ectopic tumour secreting ACTH should be suspected.

An overnight oral dexamethasone test is useful in excluding Cushing's syndrome. The plasma 11-OHCS and ACTH are measured at 2300 hours and 2 mg of dexamethasone are given by mouth. The blood tests are repeated next morning at 0800 hours. If the second plasma cortisol value does not exceed 180 nmol/l [41] and the ACTH does not show its expected rise, Cushing's syndrome can be virtually excluded.

Androgens

The 17-oxosteroids reflect mainly the output of androgenic steroids. In the male, the testes account for about one-third, but in the female they are derived mainly from the adrenal cortex, the ovary making a small contribution. High values are found in virilizing syndromes and in some patients with Cushing's syndrome. Very high values usually indicate an adrenal cancer or testicular tumour. Low levels are found in adrenal insufficiency. Dexamethasone suppression will help to differentiate pituitary dependent lesions (hyperplasia) from autonomous tumours of the adrenal or elsewhere.

PRIMARY ALDOSTERONISM (CONN'S SYNDROME)

In 1955, shortly after the discovery of aldosterone, Conn described the condition in which the adrenal gland produces an excess of aldosterone independent of the normal physiological control mechanism. The condition is called primary aldosteronism or Conn's syndrome and it is a well established, though rare, clinical entity [17]. It must be distinguished from secondary aldosteronism in which aldosterone is stimulated by increased renin secretion.

CAUSATIVE LESIONS AND PATHOLOGY

In just over two-thirds of the cases a single, small benign and well-encapsulated cortical adenoma is found. Most are less than 3 cm in diameter and some measure only a few millimetres. In the remainder the adrenal glands show either hyperplasia, often with nodular changes, or no obvious abnormality. The kidneys show vacuolation and distortion of the distal (and occasionally of the proximal) tubular cells as a result of loss of potassium. An associated chronic pyelonephritis is common, and hypertensive changes in the arterioles are usual. The juxtaglomerular cells are decreased in number and show a loss of granularity.

CLINICAL FEATURES

Conn's syndrome is approximately twice as common in women as in men, and very rare in childhood. The clinical features are caused by the metabolic effects of aldosterone, and vary in their severity. Retention of sodium expands the blood volume and causes hypertension. Loss of potassium is responsible for the other features. The main findings are as follows.

Hypertension which is constant, varying from mild to severe. Grade 3 and 4 retinal changes of accelerated hypertension are rare. Chronic hypokalaemia impairs the normal baroreceptor regulation of the blood pressure, so that postural hypotension may develop. Oedema is rare, probably as the result of the sodium escape mechanism.

Deficiency of potassium causes episodes of generalized or localized muscular weakness which may proceed to flaccid paralysis of the lower limbs and occasionally of the whole body. Hypokalaemia is usual but may be intermittent. Rarely, normal potassium levels may be found, so that the condition may be overlooked.

Hypokalaemic alkalosis reduces the amount of ionized, but not the total amount, of calcium in the blood. This results in tetany and paraesthesia which is not relieved by calcium intravenously. Low serum magnesium is found sometimes and may also contribute to the tetany.

Renal lesions (hypokalaemic nephropathy) may cause polydipsia and polyuria, with nocturia. The urine osmolality is low and the polyuria is resistant to vasopressin and deprivation of water.

INVESTIGATION

These can be divided into routine investigations and more specialized tests, some of which can only be undertaken in special centres.

Routine

Estimation of the *plasma electrolytes* confirms the hypokalaemia but it needs to be repeated several times as normal values may be found occasionally. The plasma sodium and bicarbonate are often raised slightly. The blood urea and NPN are usually elevated. The *glucose tolerance* is mildly impaired in about half the patients (effect of K^+ depletion on insulin release) but the fasting plasma glucose is usually normal. The *urine* is alkaline, of low osmolality and contains a modest amount of protein. The urinary potassium is increased (>25 mmol/24 hr). The *ECG* may show the changes typical of hypokalaemia, hypertension or both. *Routine X-rays* of the chest may show the features of hypertension. Special investigations are necessary to demonstrate small tumours.

Special

Urinary and plasma hormone estimations are usually confined to special centres. The excretion of aldosterone in the urine and the aldosterone secretion rate are high in the presence of a normal sodium intake (100 mmol per day at least). The other urinary steroids are normal. The plasma level of aldosterone is high while those of renin and angiotensin II are low [11]. The renin output remains low (suppressed) even in the presence of severe salt restriction (10 mmol daily) and the maintenance of the upright posture. In normal circumstances these stimuli cause renin and angiotensin to increase.

Deoxycorticosterone (DCA) suppression inhibits the secretion of aldosterone in normal subjects and in secondary aldosteronism [4] but not in Conn's syndrome.

Adrenal angiography, radioisotope visualization of the gland and *venous sampling* are the best means of identifying small tumours, while the latter may indicate the presence and location of a tumour which is too small to be seen.

DIAGNOSIS AND DIFFERENTIAL DIAGNOSIS

Primary aldosteronism, although a rare disease, is a curable form of hypertension. It should be considered in any hypertensive patient with a plasma potassium below 3·5 mmol/l provided that thiazide diuretics have not been taken in the previous two weeks. Confirmation of the diagnosis depends on proving that the hypokalaemia is secondary to urinary loss of potassium, that aldosterone secretion is increased, and that it is primary and not secondary. The first step is relatively simple if the daily loss of potassium exceeds 25 mmol/day when the plasma value is less than 3·5 mmol/l or less. The second can be demonstrated by measurement of aldosterone in blood and urine. The third may be very difficult unless an adrenal adenoma can be demonstrated by angiography. The finding of *low* levels of renin and angiotensin in the blood and the result of the DCA test are most helpful. In *secondary aldosteronism* the plasma renin, angiotensin and aldosterone levels are high. If there is good reason to suspect primary aldosteronism surgical exploration of the adrenals may give final confirmation.

The distinction between an adrenal adenoma and hyperplasia cannot always be made with confidence, even with venography and venous sampling. A computer-assisted analysis using data from hormone and electrolyte investigations appears to separate the two groups reliably [10].

TREATMENT

Hypertension is the most serious feature of the disease so that early diagnosis and treatment are important. In those with an adrenocortical adenoma, removal of the tumour is the treatment of choice. The beneficial effect of spironolactone suggests that it may be used successfully for patients with bilateral adrenal hyperplasia, who would otherwise require total adrenalectomy [25]. However, it is undesirable in those with tumours, most of whom are cured by operation. Should surgery be refused or contra-indicated, spironolactone therapy is an acceptable alternative.

Preoperative management includes the correction of metabolic disturbances, especially the depletion of potassium by means of spironolactone and potassium supplements. Operation may be undertaken as soon as the hypokalaemia is corrected. The blood pressure falls with spironolactone therapy and the extent is an indication of the likely response to surgery. Hydrocortisone is not normally required for removal of an adenoma, but if both glands need to be mobilized or if total adrenalectomy is necessary for adrenal hyperplasia, its use is advised for the former and it is essential for the latter.

Postoperative complications, apart from those associated with any major surgery, are unlikely if preoperative treatment has been adequate. However, temporary hypo-aldosteronism may follow removal of an adenoma and can be quickly corrected by fludrocortisone 0·1 or 0·5 mg orally twice or three times daily. Renal function may beome worse temporarily as a result of the fall in blood pressure but improves when the blood pressure is stabilized and as the hypokalaemic nephropathy recovers.

SECONDARY ALDOSTERONISM

This results from excessive stimulation of the *zona glomerulosa* by angiotensin. Plasma renin, angiotensin and aldosterone levels are all raised and the *glomerulosa* undergoes hyperplasia. Secondary aldosteronism leads to the retention of sodium and to the aggravation of pre-existing hypertension and oedema. On other occasions the plasma volume expands until sodium escape occurs and oedema is avoided. There is a concomitant progressive renal loss of potassium with hypokalaemia and muscle weakness. When oedema is present hypertension and hypokalaemia are less prominent than when it is absent.

Causes

Overproduction of angiotensin may be brought about in three ways (Table 14.3).

Table 14.3. Classification of aldosteronism and comparison of types.

Type	Blood pressure	Oedema	Plasma renin and angiotensin
PRIMARY ALDOSTERONISM	High	Absent	Low
SECONDARY ALDOSTERONISM			

A *Diminished plasma volume*
  1 *Without oedema*
    (i) Low sodium intake and diuretic therapy
    (ii) Sodium- and potassium-losing renal disease
    (iii) Excessive loss of alimentary secretions
    (iv) ? Pregnancy
	Variable	Absent	High

2 *With oedema*
    (i) Hepatic cirrhosis with ascites
    (ii) Nephrotic and hyponatraemic syndromes
    (iii) Cardiac failure
    (iv) ? Cyclical oedema
	Variable	Present	High

B *Increased renin production*
  1 *Renal ischaemia*
    (i) Renal artery stenosis
    (ii) Accelerated and malignant hypertension
    (iii) ? Congenital aldosteronism
  2 *Other causes*
    (i) Renin-secreting renal tumour
    (ii) Increased renin substrate (oestrogen therapy)
	High	Absent	High

C *Insensitivity to angiotensin* Bartter's syndrome	Low	Absent	High

Diminished plasma volume. This activates the renin–angiotensin system in a compensatory manner so that aldosterone secretion is increased, sodium is retained and potassium is excreted. Hypertension is not a prominent feature and oedema occurs only in conditions which favour it.

Direct stimulation of renin. Production of renin may be stimulated directly without alteration in the blood volume. Hypertension is usually a prominent feature and oedema is absent.

Juxtaglomerular hyperplasia (Bartter's syndrome) [40]. This probably results from insensitivity of the blood vessels to angiotensin. Elevated renal prostaglandin levels are thought to be responsible for this and other major features of the syndrome. Despite the aldosteronism and raised levels of plasma renin and angiotensin II the blood pressure is low or normal because of the resistance to the pressor action of angiotensin. Treatment with potassium and triamterene, with or without spironolactone to block the action of aldasterone and propranolol to inhibit the secretion of renin, is usually unsatisfactory. Better results can be achieved with indomethaciri and other prostaglandin synthetase inhibitors.

CUSHING'S SYNDROME [3, 51]

The clinical manifestations of this uncommon disease result from the excess production of cortisol by the adrenal cortex. Hypersecretion of cortisol may arise as a result of excessive secretion of ACTH or by the autonomous secretion of an adrenal tumour. Similar effects may be produced by the administration of pharmacological doses of ACTH or glucocorticoids.

CAUSATIVE LESIONS AND PATHOLOGY OF PITUITARY AND ADRENAL GLANDS

ACTH may be secreted by the pituitary under the influence of CRH, by an autonomous pituitary adenoma or by a tumour of some other tissue. In the former, the essential defect appears to be due to lack of sensitivity of the hypothalamic feedback system, the circadian rhythm is lost and CRH and ACTH are secreted continuously throughout the 24 hours. Pituitary adenomas are found in at least half the patients and two-thirds of these are chromophobe while the remainder are basophil. Most are very small and only 10 to 15 per cent of patients show enlargement of the pituitary fossa when the condition is diagnosed. The commonest finding is bilateral adrenal hyperplasia (found in about 70 per cent of cases) sometimes with cortical nodules as a result of continuous overproduction of ACTH. Benign adenomas are found in 10 per cent and malignant carcinomas are also found in about 10 per cent. Many other tumours, oat cell carcinoma of the bronchus, secrete large quantities of ACTH. Most are highly malignant but a few are caused by benign carcinoid tumours of bronchus or gut.

METABOLIC AND CLINICAL FEATURES

The features of the syndrome depend to some extent on the nature of the causative lesion, especially in those with pituitary or ectopic tumours. It occurs two or three times more often in women than in men, and while all ages may be involved, it occurs most commonly between 20 and 50 years. Excessive cortisol production affects all the tissues of the body so that patients with Cushing's syndrome present with a variety of symptoms. Usually they complain of tiredness, alteration in their appearance, obesity, menstrual irregularity or impotence, symptoms referrable to the associated hypertension, mental changes, oedema of ankles, purpura and ecchymoses, muscle wasting and weakness, and polyuria and polydipsia. Symptoms and signs can be related to the physiological actions of cortisol and to the inhibition that excessive levels have on anterior pituitary gonadotrophin secretion (amenorrhea or impotence). The main features may be summarized as follows.

Fat metabolism. Changes in fat deposition lead to centripetal obesity and thin arms and legs.

Protein metabolism. Catabolism of protein leads to muscle weakness and wasting, striae atrophicae and oestoporosis.

Carbohydrate metabolism. Altered carbohydrate tolerance occurs in about 20 per cent and definite diabetes mellitus in about 10 per cent of cases.

Electrolyte metabolism. Plasma electrolytes are usually normal but hypokalaemic alkalosis is found in some, especially if plasma cortisol levels are very high, as with ectopic ACTH syndrome, or with excessive secretion of deoxycorticosterone.

Cardiovascular system. Hypertension is found in over 90 per cent of patients, and complications (myocardial or cerebral ischaemia, retinopathy or cardiac failure) are found in nearly half the patients after the age of 40.

Mental changes. Mental disturbance, sometimes amounting to frank psychosis is found in about 20 per cent of patients.

Sexual function. Amenorrhoea and sterility are common in women. In men, loss of libido and impotence is usual and the testes may be atrophied.

Skin and hair. Livid striae atrophicae, hirsutism, patchy cyanosis, acne, greasiness of skin, telangiectases and melanin-pigmentation may all occur.

Cushing's syndrome varies from a mild and transient disease to one which is severe and progressive. In general, 50 per cent of those with benign disease die within five years from cardiovascular lesions and infection if untreated. The advent of cortisone in the early 1950s rendered adrenalectomy and hypophysectomy relatively safe and has improved the prognosis of those with benign lesions so that two-thirds of patients are alive and in remission up to 20 or more years after operation.

INVESTIGATIONS

Two main questions need to be answered: is Cushing's syndrome present and what is the nature of the underlying lesion?

Diagnosis is usually suggested by the clinical features, while urine and plasma steroids (Table 14.1) provide objective evidence of cortisol excess. The plasma 11-OHCS are frequently normal in the morning but the circadian rhythm is lost and the midnight value is elevated and corresponds fairly closely to the morning level. Lack of overnight suppression with dexamethasone indicates the presence of Cushing's syndrome.

The nature of the underlying lesion may be suggested by the clinical features. Age, length of history and clinical findings are all important. In children under 10 years the lesion is nearly always an adrenal carcinoma. A history of a few months is suggestive of an adrenal carcinoma, and one of a few weeks of an ectopic ACTH-secreting carcinoma. Adrenal cancers are often palpable or visible on plain X-rays, while pituitary tumours cause characteristic neurological signs and enlarge the pituitary fossa.

Estimation of the urinary and plasma steroids do not differentiate between pituitary-dependent adrenal hyperplasia and adrenal adenomas. Very high values are found with adrenal cancers and with the ectopic ACTH syndrome. Stimulation with metyrapone and tetracosactrin and suppression with dexamethasone are usual in pituitary-dependent lesions but adrenal adenoma are usually, and carcinomas and ectopic tumours are completely autonomous in their behaviour. Plasma ACTH levels are raised in adrenal hyperplasia, greatly elevated in the ectopic ACTH syndrome and very low in adrenal tumours.

Treatment with potassium and triamterene, with or without spironolactone to block the action of aldosterone and propranolol to inhibit the secretion of renin is usually unsatisfactory. Better results can be achieved with indomethacin and other prostaglandin synthetase inhibitors.

TREATMENT

Medical measures may be required for cardiac failure, hypokalaemia, diabetes, psychosis or infections. No satisfactory drug is yet available for the long-term inhibition of cortisol secretion. However, metyrapone, aminoglutethimide or 1,1-dichloro-2-(*o*-chlorophenyl)-2-(*p*-chlorphenyl)-ethane (O,*p*'DDD) may be useful preoperatively in poor risk patients.

The object of treatment is to reduce or abolish the production of cortisol by the adrenals. This can be achieved by total adrenalectomy or removal of an adenoma but treatment for the individual depends on the underlying cause and other features. In pituitary dependent Cushing's syndrome without signs of a pituitary tumour irradiation of the pituitary either by conventional external radiation, with proton beam therapy, by ^{90}Y implant or pituitary microdissection by the trans-sphenoidal route may be tried. If there are signs of a pituitary tumour hypophysectomy combined with irradiation, cryosurgical destruction, or proton beam therapy may be employed. (See Chapter 13.) However, the predictable and permanent control of the syndrome makes bilateral adrenalectomy the treatment of choice for many patients and the necessity for permanent replacement therapy must be accepted. The evidence that irradiation of the pituitary gland will prevent further progression of a small pituitary adenoma suggests that some form of pituitary irradiation should be used also. Without irradiation about 10 to 15 per cent of patients develop signs of a pituitary tumour for the first time relatively soon after operation with very high ACTH values (Nelson's syndrome). Treatment of this is the same as for tumours presenting initially.

Adrenal tumours

Surgical removal of an adrenal adenoma is curative. Removal of adrenal carcinoma should be attempted. Residual or recurrent tumour may be treated, sometimes with temporary palliation, with O,*p*'DDD. However, the ultimate prognosis is bad.

Ectopic ACTH syndrome

Most patients are in the terminal stage of their disease and only palliation is possible. Occasionally, resection of the primary lesion or cure of the syndrome by total adrenalectomy is possible. Removal of a benign carcinoid tumour cures the syndrome without the necessity for adrenalectomy.

PRE- AND POSTOPERATIVE MANAGEMENT

Preoperative care of the patient with Cushing's syndrome includes the treatment of any hypertension or congestive heart failure with a salt free diet, diuretics and digitalis

Table 14.4. Steroid replacement for adrenalectomy in Cushing's syndrome.

Day	Steroid dosage	Route	Total daily dose of hydrocortisone (or cortisone)
1 (night before)	Cortisone acetate-100 mg into each buttock	i.m.	200 mg
0 (day of operation)	Hydrocortisone sodium succinate 25 mg hourly for 4 hours during and after operation, then 10 mg hourly for 20 hours	i.v.	300 mg
+1	Hydrocortisone 50 mg per 6 hours	i.v.	200 mg
+2	Hydrocortisone 25 mg per 6 hours+ hydrocortisone 20 mg 12-hourly	i.v.	140 mg
+3	Hydrocortisone 25 mg 6-hourly+fludrocortisone 0·1 mg daily	oral	100 mg
+4 to 7	Hydrocortisone 20 mg 6-hourly+fludrocortisone 0·1 mg daily	oral	80 mg
+8 to 10	Hydrocortisone 20 mg 8-hourly+fludrocortisone 0·1 mg daily	oral	60 mg
+11 to 14	Hydrocortisone 10 mg 6-hourly+fludrocortisone 0·1 mg daily	oral	40 mg
+15 onwards	Hydrocortisone 10 mg 8-hourly+fludrocortisone 0·1 mg daily	oral	30 mg

together with the correction of any potassium depletion. Anaemia and intercurrent infections will require appropriate attention.

Adrenalectomy and hypophysectomy for Cushing's syndrome must be covered by larger doses of hydrocortisone than for other conditions. The regimen shown in Table 14.4 is satisfactory, although the dose of hydrocortisone must be altered according to requirements. A rapid fall of the blood pressure to below 100 mmHg necessitates the immediate intravenous infusion of 100 mg hydrocortisone.

The dose of hydrocortisone is reduced as rapidly as possible in the hope of preventing infection and breakdown of the wound, but it must not be forgotten that infection increases the need for steroid replacement. Adrenal insufficiency itself causes tachycardia and fever but no leucocytosis. *Subacute adrenal insufficiency* develops if hydrocortisone is withdrawn too quickly. It may be expected in mild degree in most patients, since the correct dosage of hydrocortisone can be determined only by trial and error. Signs include weakness, tachycardia, low grade fever, hypotension, vomiting and a scaly desquamation of the skin at the hair margins which spreads to the rest of the skin. All the symptoms and signs respond to an increase in the dose of hydrocortisone.

Anaesthetic management

Patients with Cushing's syndrome are often obese and thick set so that there may be problems with venepuncture and the insertion of an endotracheal tube. The presence of osteoporosis may increase the susceptibility to pathological fractures. Anaesthetics of choice include thiopentone, nitrous oxide, halothane or methoxyflurane because these are agents which in the main do not cause significant stimulation of adrenocortical function. Ether and cyclopropane are best avoided since they cause increases in plasma cortisol levels, and, of course, they are not now commonly used in clinical practice. Mechanical ventilation should be provided during anaesthesia as obesity and surgical manipulation may otherwise impede free diaphragmatic movement. Monitoring of the heart rate and the arterial pressure is necessary during surgery since exploration of the adrenal gland may produce cardiac dysrhythmia and hypertension.

Postoperative stabilization

After bilateral adrenalectomy or hypophysectomy, patients vary greatly in the time necessary to achieve replacement therapy equilibrium. A steroid dose that achieves a peak plasma cortisol level between 550 and 800 nmol/l is satisfactory. Most adults require 30 mg of hydrocortisone daily, either 20 mg on waking and 10 mg in late afternoon, or 10 mg 8-hourly. It is usually advisable to give fludrocortisone acetate (a mineralocorticoid) 0·1 mg daily to maintain a normal electrolyte metabolism. The usual precautions for patients on steroid therapy must be taken and the patient must fully understand the need for lifelong replacement. After removal of an adrenal adenoma the remaining atrophic tissue will recover after a varying interval, which can only be discovered by trial reduction in the dose of hydrocortisone.

Remission of Cushing's syndrome follows rapidly after total adrenalectomy or hypophysectomy and is usually complete in 6 to 12 months. It does so much more slowly after pituitary irradiation. After adrenalectomy plasma levels of ACTH increase greatly, at least for a time and may be accompanied by pigmentation of the skin and operation scars. The pituitary fossa should be X-rayed regularly after adrenalectomy to detect pituitary tumours; treatment is the same as for tumour presenting initially (Nelson's syndrome). The first sign of this may be widespread melanin pigmentation.

CONGENITAL ENZYMATIC DISORDERS OF THE ADRENAL CORTEX [30, 52]

Hereditary inborn errors of metabolism may affect the adrenal cortex and result in defects in the biosynthesis of cortisol or aldosterone. Six varieties are recognized, the first of which (21-hydroxylase deficiency) is relatively common and the remainder are very rare. Most are associated with deficiency of cortisol and, as a result, the secretion of CRH and of ACTH is increased and the adrenal cortex undergoes hyperplasia, (congenital adrenal hyperplasia: CAH).

The hyperplastic adrenals secrete actively, elaborating hormones and precursors of those hormones whose synthesis is not blocked. Several of these are androgenic and cause virilization and two (corticosterone and deoxycorticosterone) which are mineralocorticoids cause hypertension. Deficiency of cortisol causes adrenocortical insufficiency and that of aldosterone causes electrolyte disturbances. It is important for the anaesthetist to recognize that all may show features of adrenal insufficiency so that patients must be protected by suitable treatment from the stress of surgery and anaesthesia.

The six varieties can best be understood by reference to Fig. 14.2.

Deficiency of 21-hydroxylase

This is the commonest defect. The clinical features are due to adrenal androgens which cause female pseudohermaphroditism in girls and isosexual precocity in boys.

Deficiency of 11-hydroxylase

11-Hydroxylase is essential for the final formation of cortisol and corticosterone, so that in its absence, increased amounts of deoxycortisol and deoxycorticosterone are formed. The mineralocorticoid effects of the latter add hypertension to the above clinical features.

Deficiency of 20, 22-hydroxylase/desmolase and 3 β-hydroxysteroid dehydrogenase

These very rare enzyme defects impair the synthesis of cortisol, aldosterone as well as androgens in both the adrenal and testis. Adrenal insufficiency is severe and most affected infants have died.

Deficiency of 17-hydroxylase

Corticosterone and deoxycorticosterone, which do not require 17-hydroxylation, accumulate in excess and cause hypertension whilst cortisol, androgen and oestrogen synthesis is impaired. The condition may be mistaken for primary aldosteronism.

Deficiency of 18-hydroxylase/hydroxysteroid dehydrogenase

The production of aldosterone is impaired and patients present with hyponatraemia, hyperkalaemia, deficiency of aldosterone and raised levels of renin and angiotensin. The production of cortisol is normal and there is neither virilization nor adrenal hyperplasia.

THE ADRENOGENITAL SYNDROME

This syndrome results from an excess of adrenal androgens and causes virilism in women and girls and precocious sexual development in boys. It is not a clearly established identity in men. Bilateral adrenal hyperplasia, the biochemical defects of which have been described, is the commonest cause. Adrenal tumours, both benign adenomas and carcinomas, secreting androgens predominantly are occasionally implicated.

The effects of androgens on tissues vary with the age and sex of the patient and hence different varieties of the syndrome are found.

Virilizing hyperplasia can be managed satisfactorily by the administration of hydrocortisone, which inhibits the formation of ACTH and consequently the increased production of androgens, while at the same time providing a proper substitute for cortisol which is deficient. In growing children it is important to regulate therapy in response to the rate of growth and skeletal development. Adult patients with mild postpubertal adrenal hyperplasia and disturbed sexual function can often be treated successfully by a synthetic steroid administered in a single dose each night (e.g. 5 or 7·5 mg of prednisolone at 2300 hours).

Such patients may suffer from acute adrenocortical insufficiency unless given additional amounts of hydrocortisone to carry them over an operation. Even untreated patients who reach adult life without overt adrenal insufficiency may develop a crisis after a minor surgical operation.

Infants with the salt-losing form of congenital adrenal hyperplasia usually need additional salt to maintain normal salt balance. Should the child require any form of surgery the danger of postoperative vomiting must be remembered, and intravenous salt supplementation together with 0·05 to 0·1 mg fludrocortisone acetate may be indicated.

ADRENOCORTICAL INSUFFICIENCY [31]

When insufficient amounts of cortisol and aldosterone are produced to meet metabolic needs adrenal failure develops. This may be acute, subacute or chronic. The latter may become acute in the face of stress. Adrenal insufficiency is of great importance to anaesthetists, for mild degrees may go unrecognized and become apparent only under conditions of stress.

ACUTE AND SUBACUTE ADRENOCORTICAL INSUFFICIENCY

This is encountered most frequently in patients on long-term steroid treatment (suppressive or replacement therapy) who have had their treatment reduced too quickly, had it stopped or who have not had their dose increased sufficiently to meet the needs of a stressful situation.

Clinical features

The features are those of an adrenal crisis which is indistinguishable from oligaemic shock. The patient is seriously ill, collapsed, and in danger of dying. Pigmentation is present only when there has been chronic deficiency (Addison's disease) previously. Features of the subacute form are less severe and resemble those of the steroid withdrawal syndrome seen after adrenalectomy for Cushing's syndrome. Laboratory tests show a low plasma sodium and a raised plasma potassium and blood urea. Plasma cortisol values are low whereas they are raised in most other forms of stress.

Causes

Adrenalectomy

An acute crisis may follow adrenalectomy for Cushing's syndrome if steroid cover is inadequate.

Acute destruction of the adrenals

Traumatic injury to the adrenals may cause haemorrhagic destruction of the glands so that oligaemic shock merges into acute adrenal failure. Adrenal apoplexy in the newborn may follow prolonged and difficult labour. Similar haemorrhagic destruction of the adrenals occurs in septicaemia, which is frequently meningococcal.

Impaired adrenal reserve

It is important that Addison's disease should be recognized in surgical patients otherwise minor trauma or infection may precipitate a crisis. A low blood pressure, patches of pigmentation and thinning of the pubic and axillary hair, should arouse suspicion. An adrenal crisis is most likely to be confused with oligaemic shock and it should be suspected at once (and confirmatory evidence sought) if the blood pressure fails to respond to adequate replacement of blood. Long-term steroid and ACTH therapy also results in a diminished adrenal reserve and prophylactic measures must be taken to avoid adrenal crisis. These are by far the commonest causes of acute or subacute adrenal failure and are all avoidable.

Secondary adrenal failure (primary pituitary failure) is rarely so acute or sudden in onset as primary adrenal failure because of the continuation of aldosterone production. Nevertheless, these patients withstand stress poorly.

Treatment

An adrenal crisis must be treated promptly if life is to be saved. The principles of treatment are:

1 provision of sufficient hydrocortisone;
2 correction of fluid and electrolyte imbalance;
3 prevention of hypoglycaemia;
4 treatment of infection.

An intravenous injection of hydrocortisone sodium succinate (100 mg) or hydrocortisone sodium phosphate ester (100 mg) or prednisolone 21-disodium phosphate (20 mg) is given. At the same time an intramuscular injection of hydrocortisone (100 mg) is given to provide a depot for absorption. An infusion of 5 per cent dextrose, containing 100 mg of hydrocortisone, is run in during the first 2 to 4 hours. This may be repeated with higher dosage if the response is inadequate, or continued more slowly if the patient's condition improves. If the fall in blood pressure is profound, or if it has failed to reach 100 mmHg after hydrocortisone has been started, aldosterone 0·5 mg or angiotensin amide 0·5 mg can be added to the infusion fluid. Hydrocortisone is continued after the initial treatment at the rate of 25 to 50 mg intramuscularly every six hours, until the patient is able to swallow, when it is given by mouth. Thereafter, the amount is gradually reduced to a maintenance dose of 30 to 40 mg daily, as in the treatment of Addison's disease. Aldosterone 0·5 mg intramuscularly is given at the start of treatment and twice daily for the first 2 or 3 days. It may be omitted thereafter if there is no sodium deficiency, or changed to fludrocortisone 0·1 to 0·5 mg once or twice daily by mouth if there is hyponatraemia. The amount and composition of fluid and electrolyte replacement are determined from the results of biochemical investigation. Patients with acute adrenal insufficiency are liable to hypoglycaemia and this must be corrected by glucose infusion.

CHRONIC ADRENOCORTICAL INSUFFICIENCY

Chronic primary adrenocortical failure occurs in Addison's disease, after a too radical partial or subtotal adrenalectomy, as well as in the congenital forms mentioned above. It may be secondary to a primary pituitary failure following pituitary destruction or hypophysectomy or as a result of inhibition by cortisone of pituitary secretion of ACTH.

ADDISON'S DISEASE [31]

This is adrenocortical insufficiency resulting from primary disease or destruction of the adrenal cortices. It is characterized by the features of cortisol deficiency and ACTH and β-MSH excess.

Causative lesions

Tuberculous destruction which used to be the commonest cause now accounts for less than a third of the cases. An autoimmune adrenal necrosis of the glands can occur and antibodies to adrenal antigen can be detected in about 60 per cent of cases. Patients with this form of adrenal destruction are prone to have associated autoimmune disease of other endocrine glands (thyroid, parathyroid and gonads) and pernicious anaemia. Rare forms of Addison's disease are secondary to infiltration of the cortex by carcinoma, amyloid, granulomas, mycoses and haemochromatosis.

Clinical features

The disease may occur in both sexes and at all ages, although it is very rare in childhood. The onset is often insidious but in a third, the first indication of the disease may be a crisis. Most patients present with signs and symptoms which point directly to Addison's disease, but in some the presentation is atypical, so that adrenal insufficiency is discovered only after admission to hospital for other complaints, or as the result of a crisis precipitated by a surgical operation.

Early complaints are of tiring easily, loss of weight, distaste for food and malaise. These symptoms increase gradually until the patient is constantly tired with muscular weakness and unable to work. Gastrointestinal symptoms of anorexia, nausea and diarrhoea occur with increased frequency as the disease progresses. Pigmentation is an important and characteristic sign. It is caused by increased deposition of melanin, under the influence of β-MSH and ACTH. Pigmentation develops mainly in areas subjected to pressure, light and irritation and around scars. It is seen characteristically as brown or blue-black patches in the mouth, on the tongue, lips, gums, palate and buccal mucous membrane. Sometimes areas of depigmentation or leukoderma (vitiligo) may occur in those with the autoimmune form of the disease.

Hypotension is almost invariable and reflex maintenance of the blood pressure is impaired so that dizziness and faintness are common complaints. The loss of aldosterone secretion allows sodium to be excreted inappropriately in the urine. Loss of sodium and water leads in turn to dehydration, hypotension and muscle cramps. The plasma potassium increases and there is a metabolic acidosis. These changes are greatest in a crisis. Many patients complain of inertia, mental fatigue and depression. Rarely a confusional state may result from the effects of hypoglycaemia, dehydration and electrolyte changes or from actual deficiency of cortisol. Loss of body hair is more severe in women than in men because in the latter the testes continue to produce androgens. Amenorrhoea or oligomenorrhoea is common at the onset before treatment is started.

A mild normochromic anaemia is often present and there is an increase in the total lymphocytes and eosinophils. Pernicious anaemia sometimes occurs in autoimmune Addison's disease.

Investigations

Laboratory tests are helpful in diagnosis and treatment. The electrolytes are usually normal when the disease is mild but when it is severe, and in a crisis, the plasma sodium is low, the potassium and urea are high and the urine contains large amounts of sodium. The plasma steroid levels are low, and the circadian rhythm is impaired or lost. The urinary excretion of steroids is low (Table 14.2). There is no significant increase of urinary or plasma steroids after stimulation with ACTH. Plasma levels of ACTH, renin and angiotensin are increased. The cortisol secretion rate is usually low while the water load test reveals impaired diuresis.

16*

Radiology is rarely of help as adrenal calcification is present in only about 10 per cent of cases, and extensive adrenal calcification may be found in the presence of normal adrenal function.

The presence of adrenal antibodies confirms the diagnosis of autoimmune adrenal disease, but the test is frequently negative, especially in men. A search for antibodies to other tissues should be carried out in appropriate cases.

Differential diagnosis

Other forms of pigmentation, which may be mistaken for Addison's disease, are found in hyperthyroidism, pernicious anaemia, haemochromatosis, intra-abdominal malignancy, steatorrhoea, scleroderma, Cushing's syndrome with a pituitary tumour, Peutz–Jegher's syndrome, neurofibromatosis and poisoning with heavy metals. Long-continued treatment with drugs of the phenothiazine group, busulphan, mepacrine, oestrogens for contraception, or psoralen may increase melanin deposition in the skin.

Adrenocortical insufficiency secondary to pituitary failure can be distinguished easily from Addison's disease by the lack of pigmentation, absent or very low levels of ACTH and negative response to metyrapone.

Inhibition of ACTH secretion

Hydrocortisone and its analogues, even in physiological doses, inhibit CRH and ACTH, and thus cause atrophy of the adrenal cortices. As a result, the endogenous secretion of cortisol ceases. Serious inhibition of the hypothalamic-pituitary-adrenal function is usual after 12 to 18 months' continuous treatment, but in some patients it occurs much sooner. In some, normal function may take months to recover after steroid treatment has been stopped, and during this period there may be relative adrenal insufficiency. If a patient is subjected to stress while receiving steroids (or within 12 to 18 months of doing so) he may not respond with a normal increase in cortisol and may develop acute adrenal insufficiency.

The likely response of the hypothalamic-pituitary-adrenal axis to the stress of surgery in such a patient can be assessed preoperatively by studying the cortisol response to exogenous ACTH (250 μg of tetracosactrin i.v.)[33]. The plasma 11-OHCS should increase by 330 nmol/l and exceed 700 nmol/l at 30 minutes.

Treatment of chronic adrenocortical insufficiency

Hydrocortisone and a normal or increased intake of salt will restore nearly all patients to full health, maintain them in normal electrolyte balance and enable them to withstand stress. The synthetic glucocorticoids, which lack mineralocorticoid action, are unsuitable. The usual dose, which must be established by trial and error, is 30 to 40 mg hydrocortisone daily by mouth. The dose is divided; the larger (20 mg) being given on rising and the smaller (10 mg) in the late afternoon or early evening. A dose that achieves a morning peak plasma cortisol of 550–800 nmol/l is usually satisfactory. A few patients who lose salt excessively require additional salt or fludrocortisone (0·1 mg daily or more often as required). Those taking a potent mineralocorticoid must be watched carefully for signs of hypertension or oedema for the margin of safety with fludrocortisone is much less than that with hydrocortisone. Replacement therapy must be thorough and lifelong and the patient must be made aware of the nature of the disability and the danger of stopping hydrocortisone. Every patient should have a steroid card or bracelet giving details of the condition from which he is suffering.

Anaesthesia and adrenal insufficiency

Patients suffering from untreated Addison's disease are poor subjects for anaesthesia as they are likely to be anaemic, debilitated and hypovolaemic because of electrolyte disturbances and the neoplastic or tuberculous nature of their illness. Loss of sodium chloride and large amounts of urine, possibly with diarrhoea and vomiting, may produce a degree of dehydration, which, if untreated, may well lead to intra- or post-operative circulatory collapse. Adequate preoperative treatment with blood trans-fusion, electrolytes and fluid, dextrose and hydrocortisone greatly reduces this hazard. The patient with Addison's disease is often susceptible to the effects of barbiturates, general anaesthetics and narcotics. Only minimal amounts of thiopentone should be given and a light plane of anaesthesia maintained if hypotension is to be avoided, while care in the use of pethidine and morphine as analgesics will reduce the danger of respiratory depression in the postoperative period. The stress of anaesthesia and surgery may result in an excessively low systolic blood pressure and the degree of hypotension may well be out of proportion to the degree of blood loss.

There have been many reports of collapse during or following surgery in patients treated with glucocorticoids, and this has been presumed to be due to adrenocortical insufficiency. Of special importance to anaesthetists is the fact that a proportion of patients treated with glucocorticoids, who do not receive steroid supplementation before surgery, may develop hypotension during the intraoperative period. However, it has not always been found possible to correlate such falls in pressure with biochemical evidence of cortical insufficiency and plasma cortisol levels are often within normal limits. Thus the plasma concentration of cortisol may not be the major factor in maintaining the level of the blood pressure during and after surgery in steroid treated patients. It is known that cortisol secretion is necessary for the conversion of nor-adrenaline to adrenaline and impaired catecholamine activity, secondary to impaired cortisol secretion, has been thought to be responsible for circulatory instability. However, this is unlikely to be a factor since the concentrations of noradrenaline and adrenaline in unsupplemented glucocorticoid treated patients were found to be similar to normal subjects [34]. Although cardiovascular responses to catecholamines in the presence of glucocorticoid deficiency are not clearly understood, at least one study suggests that the secretion of catecholamines and their cardiovascular effects are unchanged in unsupplemented glucocortical treated patients, even where plasma cortisol levels are reduced. Clearly the reason for the collapse which sometimes occurs in these circumstances is as yet unknown.

In order to avoid the possibility of adrenocortical insufficiency the following patients should receive steroid therapy before and during surgery.

1   Those who have been on treatment with steroids for more than 2 weeks at the time of surgery.

2   Those who show an inadequate response to ACTH stimulation or insulin hypo-glycaemia.

3   Those who have received steroid treatment for longer than one month in the 12 months prior to operation. If time permits the response of the hypothalamic-pituitary adrenal axis to stress should be tested preoperatively.

4   Patients who have had or who are to have adrenal or pituitary surgery.
5   Patients with adrenocortical insufficiency.

Any operation, even the most trivial, is a potential hazard to patients being treated for adrenal insufficiency (either primary or secondary). For dental extraction under local analgesia, they should be given twice their normal dose of hydrocortisone on the day of extraction. Normal treatment is continued the next day provided there are no complications. For operations of any severity necessitating anaesthesia, the patient should be admitted to hospital three or four days in advance of the day of operation, for preoperative assessment and correction of any fluid or electrolyte imbalance that may be present. Replacement therapy does not need to be of the magnitude required for adrenalectomy in Cushing's syndrome but the following regime is satisfactory:

Day	Steroid dosage	Route	Total daily dose of steroid
− 1	Hydrocortisone 50 mg 8-hourly	i.m.	150 mg
0 (day of operation)	Hydrocortisone sodium succinate* 100 mg to cover operation and 25 mg 6-hourly thereafter	i.v. infusion	175 mg
+ 1	Hydrocortisone sodium succinate 25 mg 6-hourly	i.v. infusion	100 mg
2–4	Hydrocortisone 20 mg 6-hourly	By mouth	80 mg.

Thereafter, the dose of hydrocortisone is tapered off gradually in accordance with the rate of the patient's recovery and presence or absence of complications.

THE ADRENAL MEDULLA [53]

The adrenal medulla is a specialized part of the sympathetic nervous system which is derived from the neural crest. Sympathetic fibres enter the medulla and form synapses with the medullary cells and stimulate them to release hormones into the blood stream. The tissue is composed mainly of chromaffin cells (phaeochromocytes). These contain dense core vesicles, which surround secretory granules. Similar but smaller vesicles are found at the sympathetic nerve endings throughout the body. The cells of the medulla share the APUD† characteristics of many other derivatives of the neural crest [55]. Similar aggregations of chromaffin tissue are distributed widely throughout the body and are known as paraganglia. One at the origin of the inferior mesenteric artery is known as the organ of Zukerkandl. Most of the paraganglia disappear in childhood but some persist and may give rise to tumours. At three sites they persist and form structures of physiological importance, namely the carotid body, the glomus jugulare and the aortic body.

---

* During operation a fall in blood pressure must be considered likely to be due to adrenal insufficiency and larger doses of hydrocortisone i.v. may be necessary.

† APUD is an acronym which recalls the histochemical characteristics of such cells, viz. a high **A**mine content, **P**recursor **U**ptake and amino acid **D**ecarboxylase.

PHYSIOLOGY

The hormones of the adrenal medulla and the amines of the sympathetic nervous system are known as catecholamines. The active secretions are dopamine, noradrenaline and adrenaline, which are formed in the neural tissue from the amino acid tyrosine. *Dopamine* serves as a precursor of noradrenaline and as a neutrotransmitter in the hypothalamus and other areas of the brain. *Noradrenaline* (*norepinephrine*) is present mainly in the sympathetic nerves of the peripheral and central nervous systems, and acts locally as a neurotransmitter on effector cells throughout the body. *Adrenaline* (*epinephrine*), which is synthesized almost entirely by the medulla, acts principally on distant target organs.

The biosynthesis of the catecholamines involves the following steps (Fig. 14.4).

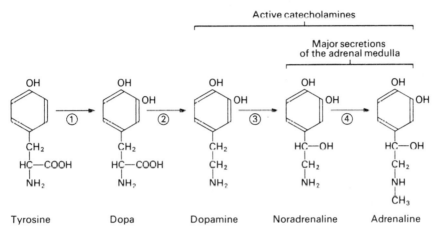

Fig. 14.4. Biosynthesis of catecholamines. Numbers in circles indicate enzymes responsible for biosynthetic steps as follows.

(1) Tyrosine hydroxylase (this reaction is the rate-limiting step in catecholamine synthesis).
(2) Dopa decarboxylase.
(3) Dopamine β-hydroxylase (DBH).
(4) Phenylethanolamine-N-methyltransferase.

Tyrosine from the blood enters the cells and is converted to dihydroxyphenylalanine (DOPA) by the enzyme tyrosine hydroxylase, and thence, in the cytoplasm to dopamine (dihydroxphenylethylamine) by the enzyme dopa decarboxylase. Inhibitors of this enzyme, such as methyldopa, are available for clinical use. Dopamine enters the dense core vesicles, where it is converted to noradrenaline by dopamine β-hydroxylase (DBH). Noradrenaline and DBH are stored in the nerve endings, but in the medulla much of the noradrenaline is converted into adrenaline by the enzyme phenyl-ethanolamine-N-methyltransferase.

Adrenaline passes directly into the blood and is secreted rapidly and in large amounts as a result of stress, including fear, hypotension, hypoxia, hypoglycaemia, trauma and haemorrhage. It prepares the body for fright, flight or fight.

Noradrenaline is immediately available in its storage vesicles for direct local stimulation of tissues. Sympathetic nerve stimulation releases noradrenaline into the synaptic cleft where it acts on its effector cell. A small amount enters the blood stream. It is concerned largely with vascular homeostatis and regulation of the blood pressure.

The synthesis of adrenaline and noradrenaline is limited by an internal negative feedback. Excess of either in the tissues inhibits the action of tyrosine hydroxylase, which is essential for their formation. The approximate concentrations of catecholamines in the blood in the absence of stress, are adrenaline 0·25 nmol/l and noradrenaline 1 nmol/l.

Action of the catecholamines

Adrenaline prepares the body in an emergency to respond to many forms of stress. It redistributes the blood flow by constricting blood vessels in the skin and gut and dilating those in skeletal muscle, the heart and brain. It diminishes the total peripheral resistance and increases the heart rate, the cardiac output and pulse pressure. The pupils dilate, the upper lids retract and there is a feeling of panic. It raises the blood glucose level and stimulates metabolism. Other actions which are made use of therapeutically, include dilatation of the bronchi and the inhibition of sensitivity reactions to foreign protein.

Noradrenaline is concerned with maintenance of the blood pressure to continually changing needs. It constricts all blood vessels (except those in the heart), increases the peripheral resistance and raises the systolic and diastolic blood pressure. It has little or no effect on metabolism.

To explain the varying actions of the catecholamines, some of which are excitatory and some inhibitory, Ahlquist in 1948 proposed the existence of α and β receptors (adrenoceptors) in sensitive tissues which mediate their physiological effects. The adrenoceptors have not been identified anatomically, but there is good physiological and pharmacological evidence for their existence. They are important therapeutically because different drugs block α and β receptors selectively. The catecholamines stimulate both types of receptor, but noradrenaline is predominantly an α stimulator, whereas adrenaline affects both equally. Dopamine receptors are found in the renal and mesenteric vascular bed and in the brain. The presence of cortisol and thyroid hormones is necessary for the catecholamines to exert their optimal effects.

METABOLISM AND EXCRETION OF CATECHOLAMINES

Catecholamines are mainly taken up and metabolized at sympathetic nerve endings, in effector cells and by the liver. At nerve endings they are converted by monoamine oxidase to dihydroxymandelic acid. In effector cells and in the liver, catechol-*o*-methyltransferase, and monoamine oxidase convert the catecholamines largely to dihydroxymandelic acid, metadrenaline and normetadrenaline and finally, largely to vanilmandelic acid (VMA) and 4-hydroxy-3-methoxyphenylglycol (Fig. 14.5). Homovanillic acid (HVA) is the major metabolite of dopamine.

Small amounts of the catecholamines (up to 5 per cent of those secreted) are excreted in the urine both free and conjugated. Larger quantities (about 25 per cent) are found as 'meta' derivatives while the largest fraction consists of VMA and HPMG. The normal 24-hour urine values are:

Catecholamines	$<0.65\ \mu$mol
'Meta' derivatives	$<8\ \mu$mol
VMA	$<0.35\ \mu$mol
HMPG	$<15\ \mu$mol

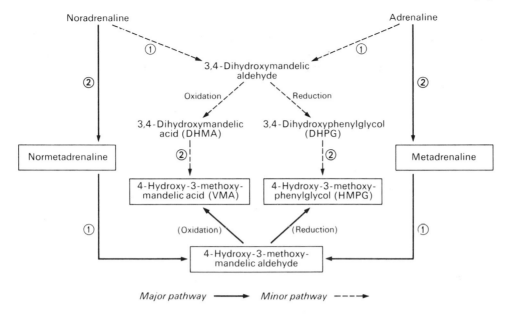

Fig. 14.5. Catabolic pathways of the catecholamines. Main excretion products (methoxy derivatives) in boxes. Numbers in circles indicate enzymes responsible.
(1) Monamine-oxidase.   (2) Catechol-*o*-methyltransferase.

PHARMACOLOGY

Many drugs influence the function of the sympathetic nervous system and adrenal medulla causing either stimulation or inhibition. The adrenoceptor blocking drugs are playing an increasingly important role in clinical therapeutics. Drugs which affect the release of catecholamines are of special importance to anaesthetists (Table 14.5).

Table 14.5. Mechanisms by which drug action can influence sympathetic nervous activity.

Stimulation of adrenoceptors
α: e.g. noradrenaline, phenylephrine and adrenaline
β: (i) both β_1 and β_2, e.g. isoprenaline, orciprenaline and adrenaline
   (ii) mainly β_2 receptors, e.g. salbutamol, terbutaline

Blockade of adrenoceptors
α: e.g. phentolamine, phenoxybenzamine
β: (i) both β_1 and β_2, e.g. propranolol, oxprenolol
   (ii) mainly β_1 receptors, e.g. practolol, metoprolol

Enhancement of transmitter substance release, e.g. amphetamine, ephedrine and tyramine

Reduction of transmitter substance release
  (a) by depletion of noradrenaline stores, e.g. reserpine and other rauwolfia compounds
  (b) by blocking the release of noradrenaline, e.g. guanethidine, bethanidine and debrisoquine
  (c) by the formation of a false neurotransmitter, e.g. methyldopa which forms alpha-methyl-noradrenaline

Alterations in catecholamine metabolism
  (a) inhibition of monoamine oxidase, e.g. tranylcypromine, phenelzine
  (b) inhibition of catecholamine uptake, e.g. amitriptyline, imipramine and chlorpromazine

Note: β_1 receptors are located in the cardiovascular system and β_2 receptors in the respiratory tract.

DISEASES OF THE ADRENAL MEDULLA

The only important diseases of the adrenal medulla are tumours. Nearly all are phaeochromocytomas; but one-third of the benign ganglioneuromas and malignant neuroblastomas arise in the adrenal medulla. There is no recognizable syndrome of adrenal medullary insufficiency.

INVESTIGATIONS [69]

This necessitates the estimation of excessive excretion of catecholamines, their precursors and their metabolites in blood and urine and X-rays to locate tumours or their metastases.

Urinary catecholamines and their excretion products (Table 14.6)

Adrenaline and noradrenaline. These may be increased separately or together. Salicylates, antibiotics, methyldopa, MAO inhibitors and coffee cause false high readings. Adrenaline is excreted mainly, but not solely, from phaeochromocytomas in the adrenal itself, whereas noradrenaline is secreted by both adrenal and extra-adrenal tumours.

Vanilmandelic acid (VMA). This is perhaps the commonest test used for the investigation of phaeochromocytomas. The consumption of large quantities of fruit (bananas or citrus fruits), coffee, tea or several drugs (nalidixic acid, aspirin, sulphonamides or antibiotics) may cause false high readings. False low readings are caused by clofibrate and MAO inhibitors.

Increased levels of excretion are found in the majority of patients with phaeochromocytomas and in most forms of stress.

Metadrenalines. This estimation is more difficult to perform than that of VMA but may provide a more specific diagnostic index of secretory medullary tumours. Chlorpromazine, MAO inhibitors and methyldopa may cause falsely high readings.

Other metabolites. Dopamine, HVA and other substances formed in the biosynthesis and catabolism of catecholamines can be measured in special centres but are not usually available for routine investigations.

Plasma catecholamines

The estimation of plasma catecholamines is technically difficult and not every hospital

Table 14.6. Urinary excretion of catecholamines and related substances (upper limits of normal).

Age	VMA μmol/24 hr	μmol/mmol creatinine	Metadrenalines μmol/ 24 hr	μmol/mmol creatinine	Adrenaline and noradrenaline nmol/ 24 hr A	NA	A+ NA	Dopamine μmol/ 24 hr	HVA μmol/ 24 hr	μmol/mmol creatinine
—1 yr	6	8·3	—	2·6	20	100	120	0·7	—	22
—5 yrs	10	4·1	—	1·7	45	190	235	1·3	—	8
—15 yrs	20	1·8	—	1·1	55	415	470	2·0	—	7·5
Adults	35	1·9	7	0·7	75	480	550	3·2	30	1·5

laboratory possesses the necessary facilities. Nevertheless, when available it provides a most useful indication of sympathoadrenal activity. The trihydroxyindole (THI) method based on a fluorometric principle is commonly used for differential determinations of plasma adrenaline and noradrenaline [39]. Upper limits of normal with this technique are usually considered to be about 2·7 nmol/l adrenaline and 8·2 nmol/l noradrenaline.

Radiological investigation

Special precautions are necessary for investigations involving the use of contrast media as a hypertensive crisis may be provoked. Since the purpose of radiology is to localize the tumour it should be postponed until all the biochemical investigations have been completed and the patient is ready for surgery. The patient should be prepared for X-ray studies and operation by α-receptor blockade. An intravenous catheter should be in place and the pulse rate and blood pressure must be monitored continuously. Phentolamine (5 mg) must be available for immediate injection if the blood pressure rises significantly. Venography is less successful than arteriography in demonstrating medullary tumours but selective venous sampling with estimation of the plasma catecholamines may be helpful in locating lesions in unusual sites.

PHAEOCHROMOCYTOMA

These tumours are usually benign and most arise in the abdomen where 80 per cent are located in one or other adrenal. The right adrenal is involved more commonly than the left. Multiple tumours, either in the adrenals or elsewhere are found in about 20 per cent. Tumours may arise in extra-adrenal chromaffin tissue in the abdomen, chest, neck, in the bladder, wall of the heart or even within the brain. Malignant cases with metastases to para-aortic nodes, liver, lungs and skeleton are rare.

Histologically, the tumour resembles adrenal medullary tissue, but the cells may vary considerably in size, shape and definition. A chromaffin reaction is always present but varies in intensity.

Many phaeochromocytomas secrete large amounts of noradrenaline or a mixture of noradrenaline and adrenaline in which the former usually predominates. Tumours in which the secretion of adrenaline exceeds that of noradrenaline are rare and usually arise in the adrenal itself. Catecholamines are responsible for the clinical manifestations. Stimulation of the α-receptors results in hypertension and central nervous excitation, while the effects on the heart (tachycardia) and metabolism are mainly due to β-receptor stimulation. The mechanism of sweating (under the control of cholinergic sympathetic nerves) which is a common feature, especially during paroxysms of hypertension, is not known.

CLINICAL FEATURES

Phaeochromocytomas are equally common in both sexes, and occur from infancy to old age. Most are diagnosed between the ages of 20 and 50 years. In 5 per cent the condition is familial and inherited through a dominant gene. Affected families frequently exhibit associated lesions (see later) and the tumours are often multiple.

The symptoms are variable, depending on the relative proportion of the two catecholamines and whether their secretion is continuous or intermittent. Two main hypertensive syndromes are recognized but patients may show features of both while others have quite unusual manifestations. Phaeochromocytomas has been described as the great 'mimic'.

Paroxysmal hypertension is the most characteristic, but not the commonest, clinical manifestation. Paroxysms of hypertension (200/100 mmHg) occur at intervals and may last for a few minutes only, or for up to a week. They may arise spontaneously or be precipitated by exercise, emotion, hypoglycaemia or abdominal palpation. Associated features include headache, tachycardia, sweating, pallor, nervousness and tremor. Less commonly, patients complain of vertigo, dyspnoea, chest pain, paraesthesiae, vomiting, blurring of vision and abdominal pain. Weakness, exhaustion and hypotension may follow an attack. Hyperglycaemia and glycosuria are frequently present if sought. In some severe attacks, the blood pressure swings from very high to very low levels every few minutes. Death from cerebral haemorrhage, pulmonary oedema, or circulatory collapse may occur.

Between attacks, the blood pressure may be normal but in longstanding cases some degree of hypertension is often found. The condition must be differentiated from hyperinsulinism, anxiety neurosis, paroxysmal tachycardia, thyrotoxicosis and cerebral tumour.

Sustained hypertension is the commoner though less spectacular finding. The blood pressure may rise progressively from the onset or become fixed after a previous labile period. The clinical features and complications are the same as those of benign, or in very severe cases, of accelerated hypertension. Moderate or severe retinopathy is found in over half the patients. The fasting blood glucose is high in 70 per cent and glycosuria is common. The BMR is frequently raised but thyroid function is normal. The condition must be distinguished from other forms of hypertension, thyrotoxicosis and diabetes. Drugs which block adrenergic neurones and sympathetic ganglia have the paradoxical effect of raising the blood pressure in patients with phaeochromocytoma (at least in the recumbent position). Such an unusual response to drug therapy in a hypertensive patient should raise the suspicion of a medullary tumour.

Unusual manifestations are often found. In some the metabolic effects of adrenaline outweigh the circulatory action of noradrenaline so that the patient exhibits symptoms which simulate hyperthyroidism or diabetes mellitus (*metabolic syndrome*). *Paroxysmal hypotension*, without preceding hypertension, occurs rarely and is found in tumours which secrete a high proportion of adrenaline. Occasionally a phaeochromocytoma arises in the wall of the bladder and paroxysmal hypertension may be precipitated by micturition. *Von Recklinghausen's* disease may be associated with a phaeochromocytoma. In the syndrome of *multiple endocrine adenopathy* type II (MEA II) multiple submucous neuromas, medullary cell carcinoma of the thyroid and hyperparathyroidism may be associated with phaeochromocytoma. *Polycythaemia* is found quite often and usually reflects haemoconcentration due to the action of noradrenaline in constricting the veins; very rarely it is due to the secretion of an erythropoietin-like substance by an associated cerebellar tumour. *Cushing's syndrome* which results from the ectopic secretion of ACTH by a phaeochromocytoma is very rare. Very occasionally, tumours secrete DOPA in addition to the other catecholamines. Affected patients may be normotensive since DOPA appears to antagonize some of the peripheral actions of noradrenaline. *Circulatory collapse at operation or after injury* has been observed in patients with unsuspected phaeochromocytoma and some deaths have occurred from cardiac arrest or peripheral circulatory failure. Induction of anaesthesia may provoke a hypertensive attack, and if the condition is suspected the operation should be abandoned.

The main conclusions drawn from a recent study of 72 patients with phaeochrome tumours are that many phaeochromocytomas remain undiagnosed until after death; appropriate investigation of patients in which this diagnosis is suspected would probably bring more tumours to light; some 90 per cent of tumours are benign; after appropriate preparation, surgical removal carries a very low operative mortality; although hypertension may persist it is amenable to medical therapy and no longer constitutes a threat to life; the long term prognosis is excellent [47].

Investigation

Since approximately half a per cent of patients with hypertension probably harbour a phaeochromocytoma, the possibility of one being present must be considered in every patient with hypertension. The presence of one or more tumours can nearly always be confirmed by chemical and pharmacological tests, and their location determined radiographically.

Pharmacological tests

Phentolamine is a short-acting α-blocker which has been adapted as a pressor-inhibiting test for phaeochromocytoma. Drugs are withheld beforehand and the blood pressure is recorded (in both arms) for half an hour at rest. Phentolamine 5 mg is injected rapidly intravenously. When positive, the systolic pressure falls at least 35 mmHg, and the diastolic 25 mmHg for 3 to 5 minutes. Normal people and other hypertensives usually sustain a much smaller fall, but false positives are known to occur. *Pressor agents* (histamine, tyramine and glucagon) cause phaeochromocytomas to release catecholamines and raise the blood pressure rapidly and have been used extensively as provocative tests. However, as they are potentially dangerous and not reliable their use is not recommended.

Chemical tests

Urinary collection of catecholamines, VMA or metadrenaline should be measured on three occasions over 24 hours. Occasionally high levels may be found immediately after a paroxysm when they are normal at other times. In such circumstances a 24-hour urine collection should be started immediately after the attack.

TREATMENT

Surgical removal of a phaeochromocytoma is the most effective treatment. Medical measures are, however, necessary for the control of hypertensive crises, for preoperative preparation and for the few patients whose tumour cannot be located or removed.

Hypertensive crises

Most are short-lived so that treatment is not usually required. For attacks persisting for hours or days, immediate α-adrenoceptor blockade is necessary. Phentolamine (5 to 10 mg) injected intravenously will lower the blood pressure for some minutes and should be tried initially. If the pressure rises again, an infusion of phenoxybenzamine (1 mg/kg body weight) in 5 per cent dextrose may be given over a period of 1 to 2 hours. The dose may need to be adjusted up or down according to the response. At the same time, phenoxybenzamine is given by mouth in a dose of 10 mg 8-hourly; the dose being increased later as required. Tachycardia develops in patients treated by α-blockade, so that if the heart rate becomes excessive (over 140/minute) or causes symptoms, the β-blocker propranolol should be started in a dose of 10 mg 6-hourly. Propranolol should never be given to a patient with a phaeochromocytoma who has not previously been given an α-blocker, since the α-adrenergic effects of the circulating catecholamines will then cause a dangerous increase in the blood pressure.

Preoperative preparation

Patients undergoing surgery for removal of a phaeochromocytoma require meticulous care before and during surgery if hazards such as extreme alterations in arterial pressure and heart rate and rhythm are to be minimized.

There may be impairment of cardiovascular homeostasis and since plasma levels of both adrenaline and noradrenaline are frequently elevated, preoperative differential measurements of these two amines may be of great value in predicting the responses of the circulation to anaesthesia and surgery.

There may be pronounced peripheral vasoconstriction caused by the increased concentration of noradrenaline acting on the α-adrenoceptors in the blood vessels of skin and muscle, which overcomes any increase in β vasodilatory action in muscle produced by adrenaline. The marked rise in peripheral vascular resistance leads to a reduction in plasma and total blood volumes. If α-adrenoceptor blockade is not carried out in the preoperative period dangerously high levels of arterial pressure may be reached during surgery, especially with handling of the tumour. In contrast, precipitous falls in arterial pressure may follow removal of the tumour because of the sudden withdrawal of α-adrenergic stimulation on the vascular bed. Phenoxybenzamine, an α-adrenergic blocking agent, is the most suitable drug for use in combating these unwanted responses. It is given orally in a dose of 10 mg 8-hourly, this being increased by 10 mg increments until the recumbent diastolic pressure is 90–100 mmHg, and there is no disabling postural hypotension. This treatment should be continued for one week before any special radiological investigations or surgery are undertaken.

The use of β-adrenoceptor blocking drugs is less frequently indicated in the pre-operative period and only when undue sympathoadrenal effects on the heart, such as tachycardia and ventricular dysrhythmia, are in evidence. Propranolol 40 mg given orally every eight hours may be effectively used for this purpose but it can cause depression of myocardial contractility and may produce bronchospasm particularly in the asthmatic or bronchitic patient. Practolol is more cardioselective in its action and has some intrinsic sympathomimetic activity. However, in some patients it produces an oculomucocutaneous syndrome and oral preparations have been withdrawn. α-methyl-para-tyrosine (AMPT), which acts by reducing the synthesis of noradrenaline by inhibiting tyrosine hydroxylase, has been used to minimize the undersirable side effects associated with elevated levels of circulating catecholamines, the dose being 250 mg orally every 8 hours. Treatment with oral chlorpromazine 50 mg every 6 hours for the 3 days before surgery causes the patient to be mildly sedated. This phenothiazine compound has adrenergic blocking, antidysrhythmic and sedative properties which are beneficial in this clinical situation.

A suitable preanaesthetic medication regime consists of pethidine 50–100 mg, chlorpromazine 25–30 mg, promethazine 25–50 mg and hyoscine 0·4 mg, given by intramuscular injection one hour before surgery. Such a combination ensures that the patient comes to operation adequately sedated, thereby reducing the likelihood of apprehension with its attendant risk of elevation in heart rate and arterial pressure [5]. Atropine may induce a substantial degree of tachycardia because of its vagolytic action and is best avoided.

Anaesthetic management

Intravenous infusion lines should be in place before anaesthesia is commenced, two for blood and other fluid therapy and one inserted centrally for the measurement of central venous pressure. Arterial pressure is measured by placing a catheter in the radial artery and connecting this to a strain gauge, the tracing being displayed on either a direct writer recorder or screen during the operation. Equipment utilizing the Doppler ultrasonic principle provides a suitable noninvasive alternative for the measurement of arterial pressure.

The stimulation caused by intubation and laryngoscopy may cause a reflex sympathomimetic effect with increases in arterial pressure and the appearance of cardiac irregularities. These disturbances may be obviated by intravenous injection of 5 mg phentolamine, given immediately prior to the induction of anaesthesia together with the antidysrhythmic drug lignocaine 25–50 mg. Propranolol 2 mg intravenously may be effective and can be repeated provided continuous monitoring of heart rate and arterial pressure is available.

There is clear evidence that halothane suppresses sympathetic activity since it does not increase plasma catecholamine levels [22], and consequently it has been advocated as a suitable inhalational agent for the patient with a phaeochromocytoma. However, as is the problem with all halogenated hydrocarbons, it sensitizes the myocardium to the effects of catecholamines and for this reason halothane should not be used in the management of these patients.

Methoxyflurane is a halogenated ether and although it resembles halothane in not causing increases in circulating sympathetic amines [22], it produces only minimal myocardial sensitization and dysrhythmia is not a feature of its use. It would appear to be a safer choice for use in patients with phaeochromocytomas. Only minimal inhaled concentrations of 0·2–0·5 per cent are acceptable, however, because of the danger of the dose-related nephrotoxicity which has been found to follow the use of this agent and is best avoided in those patients who may have disturbed renal function.

Enflurane, a more recently introduced halogenated ether, has been recommended as the anaesthetic of choice for the surgical removal of phaeochromocytoma tumours because it is less likely to induce cardiac dysrhythmias than halothane and because the danger of nephrotoxicity is less pronounced than with methoxyflurane. In one case report, normal sinus rhythm persisted during enflurane anaesthesia while a phaeochrome tumour was being removed, in spite of a tenfold increase in plasma catecholamine concentrations [37]. Total sympathetic epidural blockade has also been advocated for the intraoperative management of phaeochromocytoma [20].

When considering the choice of muscle relaxant the undesirable tachycardia associated with gallamine and the possibility of histamine release when using tubocurarine should be remembered. Pancuronium is a preferable alternative.

The patient undergoing surgery for removal of a phaeochromocytoma is subject to extreme fluctuations in the capacity of the vascular bed, and it is vital to maintain an adequate blood volume during the operation and in the postoperative period. Quantitative determinations of plasma volume are not usually required and hypovolaemia is detectable by continuous monitoring of central venous and arterial pressure, and urinary output. Brock has recently drawn attention to the value of the gradient between central and peripheral temperature as an accurate and early guide to the presence of the hypovolaemic state [9]. He also emphasizes that the maintenance of an adequate arterial pressure following removal of a phaeochrome tumour is not dependent on the administration of pressor amines but on prompt intravenous replacement therapy.

It is important to avoid hypertensive crises during surgery in these patients. Sodium nitroprusside (SNP), a potent peripherally acting hypotensive drug with an extremely evanescent action, has been successfully used for the intraoperative management of phaeochromocytoma, being effective even in the presence of high plasma catecholamine concentrations [21]. These authors suggest that a simple and reliable regime for surgery may be based on oral adrenoceptor-blocking medication to provide basal hypotensive and antidysrhythmic cover. Intravenous SNP is then used as the main hypotensive agent, dysrhythmias being controlled with intravenous propranolol.

Sudden haemorrhage during surgery can be hazardous because the compensatory reflexes of the circulation may be in abeyance. In the presence of combined α- and β-adrenoceptor blockade not only is there a lack of vasoconstriction in response to blood loss but the warning sign of tachycardia may also be absent. [66].

Postoperative care

Although the arterial pressure may remain labile for the first 24 hours it usually then becomes more stable, with plasma and urinary catecholamine levels returning to within normal limits in a few days. If the arterial pressure and the plasma catecholamine levels rise again after being normal then the presence of a second tumour should be suspected. A recurrent tumour or the functional metastases of a malignant phaeochromocytoma can often be controlled with phenoxybenzamine and propranolol should further surgery be contraindicated.

NEUROBLASTOMA AND GANGLIONEUROMA [54]

Neuroblastomas probably arise from primitive sympathogonia and are highly malignant. The tumour, although rare, is one of the commonest malignant tumours of infancy and early childhood. In contrast, the benign ganglioneuroma is very rare, and occurs most often later in childhood or early adult life. Symptoms are usually nonspecific. Both tumours (especially ganglioneuroma) may cause diarrhoea, and occasionally hypertension and other features associated with phaeochromocytomas occur. These tumours secrete large amounts of DOPA, dopamine and noradrenaline but not adrenaline because they lack the enzyme necessary for the latter's formation. The excretion of catecholamines and their metabolic products is increased in three-quarters of cases. Characteristically the excretion of DOPA, dopamine and HVA is high.

Ganglioneuromas can usually be excised satisfactorily. Radical removal of neuroblastomas should be attempted. Preparation for operation should be the same as that for phaeochromocytomas because the effects on the blood pressure may be identical. The prognosis for ganglioneuromas is excellent, whereas that for neuroblastomas is bad. However, new combined chemotherapeutic regimes have prolonged the lives of some patients with metastatic spread.

SYMPATHOADRENAL RESPONSES
TO ANAESTHESIA AND SURGERY

Sympathoadrenal and adrenocortical activity are closely related and many stressful situations bring about increased liberation of both cortisol and catecholamines. It is probable that cortisol can readily pass from the adrenal cortex to the medulla by means of rich vascular connections, adequate concentrations of glucocorticoids being necessary for the proper functioning of the chromaffin cells and for the conversion of noradrenaline to adrenaline.

A wide variety of emotional and physical stimuli are capable of evoking augmented sympathoadrenal activity and this is reflected by the raised levels of urinary and plasma catecholamines which occur in these situations.

Inhalational anaesthetics exert differing effects on the sympathoadrenal system, and it is probable that the magnitude of the response which an anaesthetic elicits determines many of its pharmacological features. The arterial pressure, stroke volume and cardiac output are related to changes in sympathetic neuronal activity. Anaesthetic agents may induce such changes by acting at autonomic ganglia, postsynaptic nerve terminals and at receptors in the heart and in the peripheral vessels. It has been suggested that other circulatory, respiratory and metabolic changes which occur during anaesthesia may also be the result of alterations in plasma noradrenaline concentrations [6].

Although most general anaesthetics cause depression of isolated heart-lung preparations such experiments do not take into account the homeostatic reflexes of the sympathoadrenal system, and in the intact animal the arterial pressure is usually well maintained when anaesthetics known to produce increases in plasma catecholamines are being inhaled. The importance of a properly functioning sympathoadrenal system for the preservation of normal circulatory function during anaesthesia was unequivocally shown by ingenious studies carried out some 25 years ago by Beecher and his group in Boston [8]. They found that there was an increase in cardiac output in intact dogs, a peak value of 240 per cent being reached at arterial ether levels of 100 mg per cent. When ether was administered to adrenalectomized dogs with total sympathetic blockade the cardiac output failed to rise above control values, and instead there was an average decrease of 40 per cent. During ether anaesthesia in man there is a substantial rise in plasma noradrenaline concentration with only a slight increase in adrenaline levels [6]. This increase in circulating noradrenaline persists in patients with bilateral adrenalectomy, and this is a finding which suggests that the sympathetic nervous system rather than the adrenal medullae is important in maintaining circulatory homeostasis during ether anaesthesia. In the intact animal and in man the maintenance of arterial pressure and the increase in cardiac output is the result of the counterbalance between the direct myocardial depressant effect of ether and the catecholamine-induced stimulation of α- and β-adrenoceptors. In deep levels of ether anaesthesia, in spite of the increases in the concentrations of circulating amines, the vasoconstriction seen during lighter levels of narcosis disappears and the blood pressure falls. This may be due to the fact that ether interferes with the ability of noradrenaline to constrict vascular smooth muscle, and indeed there is considerable evidence to suggest that this occurs.

Cyclopropane anaesthesia in man is also associated with increases in stroke volume and cardiac output, and with elevations in plasma catecholamines [64]. In contrast to ether, however, cyclopropane enhances the responsiveness of vascular smooth muscle to noradrenaline so that vasoconstriction is pronounced and the arterial pressure is well maintained even where high concentrations of gas are inhaled.

Although it is probable that the increases in circulating catecholamine levels which occur during the inhalation of ether and cyclopropane reflect augmented sympatho-adrenal activity, factors such as impaired uptake and binding of the amines and inhibition of catechol-*o*-methyl transferase (COMT) may be partly responsible [27].

Studies of plasma catecholamine levels during halothane anaesthesia indicate that there is no increase in sympathoadrenal activity but because of the limitations of the sensitivity of the widely used fluorometric method it was not possible to determine if actual reductions in catecholamine concentrations occurred. Recently, however, it has been demonstrated that in rats the total plasma catecholamine concentrations during 1 per cent halothane anaesthesia were only about 12 per cent of those in awake animals [65]. Also, as the concentration of inhaled vapour was increased the level of plasma catecholamine fell further, paralleling the drop in arterial pressure. These decreases appear to be due to the diminished release of noradrenaline from the sympathetic nerve endings as well as adrenaline from the adrenal medullae. Such findings may help to explain the reductions in mean arterial pressure, cardiac output and myocardial contractility, which occur during halothane anaesthesia.

Plasma catecholamines are not elevated during the inhalation of methoxyflurane and this is in keeping with the observation that cardiovascular depression is a feature of the use of this anaesthetic. Recent animal studies have shown that methoxyflurane inhibits catecholamine release from the adrenal medullae, an effect which is at least partially due to a direct action on the chromaffin cell; it also diminishes the pressor induced effect of splanchnic nerve stimulation by inhibiting the secretion-stimulating effect of acetylcholine [22]. Other studies by the same workers show that halothane and methoxyflurane both act in the same manner as regards spontaneous catecholamine liberation and catecholamine output during splanchnic nerve stimulation.

Enflurane probably inhibits the release of noradrenaline at sympathetic nerve endings throughout the body. Increases in plasma catecholamine concentrations are not a feature of enflurane anaesthesia and since myocardial sensitization is minimal, the appearance of spontaneous cardiac dysrhythmia is uncommon.

Few studies have been made of the influence of surgery on sympathoadrenal activity although a group in Helsinki found that, contrary to what might be expected, potentially stressful and painful procedures, such as upper abdominal surgery, did not evoke higher titres of circulating catecholamines than superficial operations [57]. They also found that elevations in heart rate and arterial pressure during operative stress were invariably accompanied by substantial rises in plasma noradrenaline and that the return of pain during recovery was associated with elevations in both adrenaline and noradrenaline.

Persistent hyperglycaemia and glycosuria may follow the surgical procedure, and are a reflection of the derangement of carbohydrate metabolism produced by trauma. As part of the response to the injurious process gluconeogenesis and glycogenolysis from protein sources are increased in order to sustain blood glucose concentrations. As with other endocrine changes the degree of hyperglycaemia appears to be related to the duration and magnitude of the operative procedure. The liberation of cortisol, ACTH, growth hormone and glucagon is increased as the result of trauma and all may contribute to the production of hyperglycaemia. However, the interrelationship between sympathomimetic activity and insulin may well be a more important influence. The suppression of the normal insulin response associated with surgical and other trauma may be the result of increased adrenaline liberation. It has been postulated that in the fasting state basal insulin secretion takes place from the larger or two pools or compartments situated in the cells of the pancreas (Fig. 14.6). Secretion of insulin from

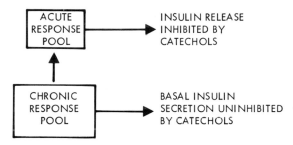

Fig. 14.6. Mechanism of release of insulin (after Porte & Bagdade [63]).

this compartment may be important for the regulation of the metabolic response to surgery. Unlike the acute insulin response to hyperglycaemia (small pool release) basal insulin secretion is relatively insensitive to sympathetic activity [63].

It has been shown that the raised blood sugar which follows surgery can be reduced by intra- and postoperative regional blockade [13]. This suggests that the reduction of sympathetic activity resulting from the regional blockade allows the storage pool of insulin to respond to the hyperglycaemia.

With these considerations in mind it is of interest to examine the influence of anaesthetic agents on the level of the blood sugar. Uncomplicated ether anaesthesia in man does not usually produce hyperglycaemia. In contrast, ether anaesthesia associated with metabolic acidosis such as may occur during major surgery, may give rise to elevations in blood sugar concentrations. In the former situation it is noradrenaline which is mainly liberated in increased amounts and this is an amine which has little effect on carbohydrate metabolism. In the latter situation adrenaline is released in addition to noradrenaline and may well be the factor responsible for inducing hyperglycaemia. Likewise the inhalation of cyclopropane in man does not cause raised blood sugar levels unless there is an associated acidosis. Hyperglycaemia is not normally present during the administration of halothane and this is to be expected in view of the suppressed sympathoadrenal response associated with this anaesthetic. During methoxyflurane anaesthesia blood sugar levels in man are within normal limits, findings which again are in keeping with diminished sympathetic nervous activity. Intravenous anaesthetics apparently have little effect on blood sugar levels and it may well be that any changes which occur merely reflect their differing abilities to diminish the response to surgical stress [15].

REFERENCES

1 BAIRD DT, HORTON R, LONGCOPE C, TAIT JF. Steroid dynamics under steady-state conditions. *Recent Prog Horm Res* 1969; **25**: 611–64.

2 BEARDWELL CG, BURKE CW, COPE CL. Urinary free cortisol measured by competitive protein binding. *J Endocrinol* 1968; **42**: 79–89.

3 BESSER GM, EDWARDS CRW. Cushing's syndrome. *Clin Endocrinol Metab* 1972; **1**: 451–90.

4 BIGLIERI EG, SLATON PE, KRONFELD SJ, SCHAMBELAN M. Diagnosis of an aldosterone-producing adenoma in primary aldosteronism. *JAMA* 1967; **201**: 510–14.

5 BINGHAM W, ELLIOTT J, LYONS SM. Management of anaesthesia for phaeochromocytoma. *Anaesthesia* 1972; **27**: 49–60.

6 BLACK GW, McARDLE L, McCULLOUGH HELEN, UNNI VKN. Circulating catecholamines and some cardiovascular, respiratory, metabolic and pupillary responses during diethyl ether anaesthesia. *Anaesthesia* 1969; **24**: 168–79.

7 BORTH R, LINDER A, RIONDEL A. Urinary excretion of 17-hydroxy-corticosteroids and 17-keto-steroids in healthy subjects in relation to sex, age, body weight and height. *Acta Endocrinol* 1957; **25**: 33–44.

8 BREWSTER WR Jr, BUNKER JP, BEECHER HK. Metabolic effects of anaesthesia; mechanism of metabolic acidosis and hyperglycemia during ether anesthesia in the dog. *Am J Physiol* 1952; **171**: 37–47.

9 BROCK LORD. Hypovolaemia and Phaeochromocytoma. *Ann R Coll Surg Engl* 1975; **56**: 218–21.

10 BROWN JJ, CHINN RH, DAVIS DL, *et al*. Plasma electrolytes, renin and aldosterone in the diagnosis of primary hyperaldosteronism. *Lancet* 1968; **2**: 55–9.

11 BROWN JL, FRASER R, LEVER AF, LOVE DR, MORTON JJ, ROBERTSON JIS. Raised plasma angiotensin II and aldosterone during dietary sodium restriction in man. *Lancet* 1972; **2**: 1106–7.

12 BRUNNER HR, GAVRAS H, LARAGH JH, KEENAN R. Angiotensin-II blockade in man by Sar¹-Ala⁸-Angiotensin-II for understanding and treatment of high blood pressure. *Lancet* 1973; **2**: 1045–8.

13 BUCKLEY FP. *Effects of autonomic blockade on metabolism* II. Symposium: 'Problems of metabolism in anaesthesia and intensive therapy', Royal College of Surgeons of England, November 1974.

14 BURKE CW, BEARDWELL CG. Cushing's syndrome. An evaluation of the clinical usefulness of urinary free cortisol and other urinary steroid measurements in diagnosis. *Quart J Med* 1973; **42**: 1975–204.

15 CLARKE RSJ, BALI IM, ISAAC M, DUNDEE JW, SHERIDAN B. Plasma cortisol and blood sugar following minor surgery under intravenous anaesthetics. *Anaesthesia* 1974; **29**: 545–50.

16 CLARKE RSJ, JOHNSTON H, SHERIDAN B. The influence of anaesthesia and surgery on plasma cortisol, insulin and free fatty acids. *Br J Anaesth* 1970; **42**: 295–9.

17 CONN JW. The evolution of primary aldosteronism 1954–67. *Harvey Lect* 1967; **62**: 257–91.

18 COPE CL. The adrenal cortex in internal medicine. Pt 1. *Br Med J* 966; **2**: 847–53.

19 COPE CL, PEARSON J. Clinical value of the cortisol secretion rate. *J Clin Pathol* 1965; **18**: 82–7.

20 COUSINS MJ, RUBIN RB. The intraoperative management of phaeochromocytoma with total epidural sympathetic blockade. *Br J Anaesth* 1974; **46**: 78–81.

21 DAGETT P, VERNER I, CARRUTHERS M. Intraoperative management of phaeochromocytoma with sodium nitroprusside. *Br Med J* 1978; **2**: 311–13.

22 DRYER C, BISCHOFF D, GOTHERT M. Effects of methoxyflurane anesthesia on adrenal medullary catecholamine secretion. *Anesthesiology* 1974; **41**: 18–26.

23 Editorial (Hall GM) Fentanyl and the metabolic response to surgery. *Br J Anaesth* 1980; **52**: 561–2.

24 ERNEST I. Steroid excretion and plasma cortisol in 41 cases of Cushing's syndrome. *Acta Endocrinol* 1966; **51**: 511–25.

25 FERRISS JB, BROWN JJ, FRASER R, *et al*. Results of adrenal surgery in patients with hypertension, aldosterone excess and low plasma renin concentration. *Br Med J* 1975; **1**: 135–8.

26 GALVAO-TELES A, BURKE CW, FRASER TR. Adrenal function tested with tetracosactrin depot. *Lancet* 1972, **1**: 557–60.

27 GARDIER RW, ENDAHL GL, HAMELRERG W. Cyclopropane: effect on catecholamine biotransformation. *Anesthesiology* 1967; **28**: 677–9.

28 GAVRAS H, BRUNNER HR, LARAGH JH, SEALEY JE, GAVRAS I, VUKOVICH RA. An angiotensin converting enzyme inhibitor to identify and treat vasoconstrictor and volume factors in hypertensive patients. *N Engl J Med* 1974; **291**: 817–21.

29 GREENWOOD FC, LANDON J, STAMP TCB (1966) The plasma sugar, free fatty acid, cortisol and growth hormone response to insulin. I. In control subjects. *J Clin Invest* 1966; **45**: 429–36.

30 HAMILTON W. Congenital adrenal hyperplasia. *Clin Endocrinal Metab* 1972; **1**: 503–47.

31 IRVINE WT, BARNES EW. Adrenocorticol insufficiency. *Clin Endocrinal Metab* 1972; **1**: 549–94.

32 JOHNSTON IDA. The endocrine response to trauma. *Adv Clin Chem* 1972; **15**: 255–85.

33 KEHLET H, BINDER C. Value of an ACTH test in assessing hypothalmic-pituitary-adrenocortical function in glucocorticoid treated patients. *Br Med J* 1973; **2**: 147–9.

34 KEHLET H, NIKKI P, JAATTELA A, TAKKI S. Plasma catecholamine concentrations during surgery in unsupplemented glucocorticoid-treated patients. *Br J Anaesth* 1974; **46**: 73–7.

35 KEHLET H. Influence of epidural analgesia on the endocrine-metabolic response to surgery. *Acta Anaesthesiol Scand* (Suppl) 1978; **70**: 39–42.

36 KEHLET H, BRANDT MR, HANSEN PRANGE A, ALBERTI KGMM. Effect of epidural analgesia on metabolic profiles during and after surgery. *Br J Surg* 1979; **66**: 543–6.

37 KREUL JF, DAUCHOT PJ, ANTON AH. Hemodynamic and catecholamine studies during pheochromocytoma resection under enflurane anesthesia. *Anesthesiology* 1976; **44**: 265–8.

38 LIDDLE GW. Tests of pituitary-adrenal suppressibility in the diagnosis of Cushing's syndrome. *J Clin Endocrinal Metab* 1960; **20**: 1539–60.

39 MCCULLOUGH H. Semi-automated method for the differential determination of plasma catecholamines. *J Clin Pathol* 1968; **21**: 759–63.

40 MCGIFF JC. Bartter's syndrome results from an imbalance of vasoactive hormones. *Ann Intern Med* 1977; **87**: 369–72.

41 MCHARDY-YOUNG S, HARRIS PW, LESSOF MH, LYNE C. Single dose dexamethasone suppression test for Cushing's syndrome. *Br Med J* 1967; **2**: 740–4.

42 MAKIN HLJ, TRAFFORD DJH. The chemistry of the steroids. *Clin Endocrinal Metab* 1972; **1**: 333–60.

43 MATTINGLY D, TYLER C. (1972) Plasma 11 hydroxycorticosteroid levels in surgical stress. *Proc RS Med* 1965; **58**: 1010–12.

44 MATTINGLY D, TYLER C. Simple screening test for Cushing's syndrome. *Br Med J* 1967; **4**: 394–7.

45 MILLS IH. *Clinical aspects of adrenal function.* Oxford: Blackwell Scientific Publications, 1964: 95–113.

46 MILLS IH. Primary aldosteronism. *Clin Endocrinol Metab* 1974; **3**: 593 608.

47 MODLIN IM, FARNDON JR, SHEPERD A, *et al.* Phaeochromocytomas in 72 patients: clinical and diagnostic features, treatment and long term results. *Br J Surg* 1979; **66**: 456–65.

48 MONTGOMERY DAD, WELBOURN RB. *Medical and surgical endocrinology.* London: Edward Arnold, 1975: 69.

49 Ibid. 26.

50 Ibid. 99.

51 Ibid. 100.

52 Ibid. 119.

53 Ibid. 143.

54 Ibid. 157.

55 Ibid. 490.

56 NEVILLE AM, MACKAY AM. The structure of the adrenal cortex in health and disease. *Clin Endocrinol Metab* 1972; **1**: 361–95.

57 NIKKI P, TAKKI S, TAMMISTO T, JAATELA A. Effect of operative stress on plasma catecholamine levels. *Ann Clin Res* 1972; **4**: 146–51.

58 OPARIL S, HABER E. The renin-angiotensin system. *N Engl J Med* 1974; **291**: 389–401.

59 OYAMA T. *Anesthetic management of endocrine disease.* Berlin: Springer-Verlag, 1973.

60 OYAMA T. Endocrine responses to anaesthetic agents. *Br J Anaesth* 1973; **45**: 276–81.

61 OYAMA T, TANIGUCHI K, ISHIHARA H. *et al.* Effects of enflurane anaesthesia and surgery on endocrine function in man. *Acta Anaesthesiol, Scand* (Suppl) 1979; **71**: 32–8.

62 PETERSON RE. The influence of the thyroid on adrenocortical function. *J Clin Invest* 1958; **37**: 736–43.

63 PORTE D Jr, BAGDADE JD. Human insulin secretion: an integrated approach. *Annu Rev Med* 1970; **21**: 219–40.

64 PRICE HL, LINDE HW, JONES RE, BLACK GW, PRICE ML. Sympatho-adrenal responses to general anaesthesia in man and their relation to haemodynamics. *Anesthesiology* 1950; **20**: 563–75.
65 ROIZEN MD, MOSS J, HENRY DP, KOPIN IJ. Effects of halothane on plasma catecholamines. *Anesthesiology* 1974; **41**: 432–9.
66 ROSS EJ, PRICHARD BNC, KAUFMAN L, ROBERTSON AIG, HARRIES BJ. Preoperative and operative management of patients with phaeochromocytoma. *Br Med J* 1967; **1**: 191–8.
67 STARER F. The radiology of suprarenal masses. *Br J Hosp Med* 1970; **4**: 207–12.
68 STEINBECK AW, THEILE HM. The adrenal cortex. *Clin Endocrinol Metab* 1974; **3**: 557–91.
69 WOLF RL. Phaeochromocytoma. *Clin Endocrinol Metab* 1974; **3**: 609–21.
70 WOOD JB, FRANKLAND AW, JAMES VHT, LANDON J. A rapid test of adrenocortical function. *Lancet* 1965; **1**: 243–5.

FURTHER READING

ALTURA BM, ALTURA BT. Effects of local anesthetics, antihistamines, and glucocorticoids on peripheral blood flow and vascular smooth muscle. *Anesthesiology*, 1974; **41**: 197–214.
BURKE CW. *The adrenal cortex in practical medicine*. London: Gray-Mills, 1973.
CLARKE RSJ. Anaesthesia and carbohydrate metabolism. *Br J Anaesth* 1973; **45**: 237–43.
GANONG WF, ALPERT LC, LEE TC. ACTH and the regulation of adrenocortical secretion. *N Engl J Med* 1974; **290**: 1006–11.
GLENN TM. Steroids and shock. London: University Park Press, 1974.
HOELDTKE R. Catecholamine metabolism in health and disease. *Metabolism* 1974; **23**: 663–86.
MORRIS DJ, DAVIS RP. Aldosterone: current concepts. *Metabolism* 1974; **23**: 473–94.
O'BOYLE A, GANNON D, HINGERTY D. Sympatho-adrenal response to stress. *J Ir Med Assoc* 1973; **66**: 699–000.
PEART WS. Renin-angiotensin system. *N Engl J Med* 1975; **292**: 302–6.
THOMPSON EB, LIPPMAN ME. Mechanism of action of glucocorticoids. *Metabolism* 1974; **23**: 159–202.

Chapter 15
The Endocrine Pancreas

T. M. HAYES

ANATOMY AND HISTOLOGY

The body of the pancreas lies in front of the bodies of the second and third lumbar vertebrae. The head is encompassed by the duodenum and the tail extends laterally to lie in close relationship to the spleen. The exocrine secretions travel by the pancreatic duct which joins the common bile duct and then drains into the second part of the duodenum via the ampulla of Vater.

Sympathetic fibres carrying pain are limited to the greater splanchnic nerves (T5–T10). Parasympathetic fibres reach the gland through the vagus nerves and terminate in the intrinsic pancreatic ganglia. Although the islets are richly innervated the nervous control of insulin secretion is probably not of great importance.

The endocrine parts of the human pancreas, the islets of Langerhans, are irregularly distributed throughout the pancreatic parenchyma. Although it has been estimated that the pancreas of an adult human may contain 1×10^6 islets, their total weight is only 2–3 g and they represent only 2–3 per cent of the volume of the whole gland. The average size of an islet is between 100 and 200 μm. Each islet is highly vascularized.

There continues to be discussion amongst histologists but the present concensus is that there are 4 basic types of cell recognizable by their ultra-structure. α cells (20 per cent), some of which (type A2) secrete glucagon, β cells (75 per cent) which secrete insulin, δ cells which secrete somatostatin, and PP cells (or D1) which, probably, secrete pancreatic polypeptide. Immunofluorescence studies have also detected VIP (vasoactive intestinal polypeptide) in the nerve fibres within the pancreas, and cells which secrete GIP—gastric inhibitory peptide (K cells), motilin, 5HT and substance P—the last three from enterochromaffin cells which are the cells involved in carcinoid tumours.

Since the gut and the pancreas share a common embryological origin it is perhaps not surprising that some of the endocrine cells of the pancreas may also be found in the gut mucosa—notably D and PP cells. Gastrin secreting cells do not occur in the normal pancreas, even though gastrin secreting tumours may arise in the pancreas.

The pancreas is a common source of endocrine tumours, insulinoma and gastrinoma being the commonest. Glucagonomas, vipomas and stomatostatinomas have also been described, though they are extremely rare.

No pathognomonic features can be identified in the pancreas of diabetics, though atrophic and hypertrophic changes are sometimes recognized; hyaline changes are frequently found in elderly diabetics and an inflammatory infiltrate may be found in newly diagnosed insulin dependent diabetics coming to postmortem.

PHYSIOLOGY

Insulin is produced by cleavage from the larger precursor molecule, proinsulin. Small quantities of proinsulin are present in the peripheral circulation but they have little biological activity. The secretion of insulin from the normal pancreas is provoked by a variety of stimuli, including the amino acids arginine and leucine and hormones such as glucagon, but the most important stimulus is glucose. The secretion of insulin into the portal vein has important actions in the liver; glycogen and fatty acid synthesis are stimulated and glycogenolysis, gluconeogenesis and ketogenesis are inhibited; insulin therefore has an important role in regulating hepatic glucose output. Peripherally, insulin stimulates the cellular uptake of glucose and inhibits adipose tissue lipolysis. Glycerol and fatty acid synthesis are stimulated in adipose tissue, whilst in muscle, protein and glycogen synthesis are stimulated. Insulin is not required for glucose utilization by the brain, red cells or the renal cortex; insulin has no effect on intestinal absorption.

Glucagon stimulates hepatic glycogenolysis, thereby rapidly raising blood glucose levels. Hepatic gluconeogenesis from amino acids, lactate and pyruvate is also stimulated. By a direct effect on the β-cells, glucagon stimulates insulin release and in pharmacological doses it stimulates the adrenal medulla. Other effects of pharmacological, but not physiological doses, include an inotropic action on cardiac muscle and a stimulation of renal electrolyte secretion.

Other hormones are produced by the endocrine pancreas but the detailed physiology of many of these is still unclear. Gastric inhibitory peptide (otherwise known as glucose dependent insulinotrophic peptide or GIP), is also secreted by the upper intestinal mucosa and it inhibits both acid secretion and motor activity by the stomach. This hormone also stimulates the secretion of insulin and glucagon leading to the suggestion that it might be the mediator of the enteroinsular axis, whereby the presence of food in the duodenum stimulates insulin secretion.

Pancreatic polypeptide (PP) is secreted in response to food, but the details of its function are uncertain. It appears to be concerned in the regulation of exocrine pancreatic secretion and bile flow. High plasma levels of PP are found in some islet cell tumours and carcinoids with no obvious effects, but when they are found in asymptomatic members of families with multiple endocrine neoplasia type I, they suggest the presence of an islet cell tumour.

Somatostatin is a widely distributed hormone found in the brain, gut and pancreas. It inhibits the release of a variety of hormones—insulin, glucagon, growth hormone, gastrin and motilin, and it also inhibits gastric acid secretion.

Vasoactive intestinal polypeptide (VIP) is a vasodilator which also stimulates both the exocrine pancreas and the flow of intestinal juice, whilst inhibiting gastric acid secretion.

DIABETES

Diabetes is a common disorder; prevalence rates in the United Kingdom range between 1.2 per cent and 14 per cent depending upon the diagnostic criteria used and throughout the world they range between 0.03 per cent (Greenland Eskimos) and 45 per cent (Pima Indians). Many diabetics are elderly and obese and this, plus the morbidity associated with the disease, makes diabetics more likely to need surgery than the rest of the population: it has been estimated that 50 per cent of diabetics will need an operation at some time during their life. The vascular and renal complications of diabetes with the metabolic problems produced by the disease and its treatment generally increase the potential for surgical and anaesthetic problems. The mortality for diabetics undergoing surgery has been reported within the last decade as being about 4 per cent.

A further dimension to the problem arises because diabetes often presents *de novo* on surgical wards. This may be the serendipidous discovery of asymptomatic maturity onset diabetes, or it may be the stress of either the surgical illness or its treatment that have made latent diabetes overt. Diabetic ketoacidosis may mimic an acute abdominal emergency in many respects and it is, therefore, incumbent on all concerned with the management of surgical cases to screen their patients for diabetes before surgery, otherwise the results could be disastrous. As many as 25 per cent of all diabetics in surgical wards will be newly diagnosed.

As long as diabetes is recognized and treated correctly the hazards of surgery can be greatly reduced. Many systems for the management of these patients have been described, but in this chapter only a single, logical and practical system is described. For those who wish to review alternative systems a list of key references is given at the end of the chapter [1, 2, 7, 8].

Classification and presentation

The current classification of diabetes is shown in Table 15.1.

The old division of diabetes into juvenile onset and maturity onset is of limited value since, although the majority of maturity onset diabetics will not need insulin, a significant minority do: conversely, a few young people who develop diabetes will not

Table 15.1. Classification of diabetes.

Type I   Insulin dependent
    A Transient islet cell antibodies
    B Persistent islet cell antibodies associated with other organ specific antibodies

Type II   Noninsulin dependent
    A Obese
    B Nonobese

Gestational
Diabetes starting in pregnancy and disappearing after delivery. This is associated with an increased frequency of subsequent glucose intolerance and diabetes

Stress induced
Diabetes induced by steroids, burns, etc., returning to normal on removal of the stress

Genetic syndromes
Many rare syndromes are described, but they account for a very small proportion of diabetic patients

Potential abnormality
Patients who because of obstetric (e.g. the previous delivery of a baby weighing over 4·5 kg), or genetic (having a first degree relative with diabetes) have an increased risk of developing diabetes

Impaired glucose tolerance
Borderline abnormalities of glucose tolerance associated with an increased frequency of atherosclerosis but not of diabetic microangiopathy

need insulin, particularly those with so called MODY—maturity onset diabetes of the young.

All truly insulin dependent diabetics will have islet cell antibodies at the onset of the disease, but only in those with an autoimmune diathesis will these still be present after one year. These latter patients may give a history of other endocrine disease, especially thyroid or adrenal disease, or this may be present in their family, and antibodies against adrenal, thyroid and parietal cells may be found even before overt disease of these other organs. Evidence of these other deficiencies (hypothyroidism or Addisons disease) may come to light with stress, such as surgery.

Untreated insulin dependent diabetics lose weight and develop ketonuria, even when well fed. They are almost invariably symptomatic at the time of presentation and do not develop the important microvascular complications of diabetes until the disease has been present for at least 5, and usually, 10 years.

The classical symptoms of diabetes—thirst, polyuria and genital pruritus—may be present in either group. In the noninsulin dependent diabetic the symptoms will have been present for very many months, but even in the newly diagnosed insulin dependent diabetic child, the symptoms may have been present for some weeks before diagnosis. Reversible visual impairment is common in the newly diagnosed diabetic due to osmotic changes in the lens and cornea. These correct themselves within a few weeks of controlling the diabetes. A polyneuropathy may also be present at the time of diagnosis but this does not always improve with treatment.

It is now recognized that there is not a clear distinction, at least in terms of glucose tolerance, between nondiabetics and diabetics, and this has led to the concept of borderline or impaired glucose tolerance. Epidemiological studies have shown that patients with this type of glucose tolerance curve have an increased risk of developing atherosclerosis, but unless they become truly diabetic at a later date, do not develop diabetic microangiopathy with the associated renal and retinal problems [4].

The diagnostic criteria for diabetes and impaired glucose tolerance are shown in Table 15.2.

Table 15.2. Diagnostic criteria.

Diabetes

    1 Classical symptoms and a random blood glucose over 12 mmol/l

    or

    2 In a 50 g oral glucose tolerance test—

       (i) a fasting venous blood glucose over 7 mmol/l

       (ii) plus a 2 hour venous blood glucose over 10 mmol/l

       (iii) plus one intervening value at or above the 2 hour value

Impaired glucose tolerance

    In a 50 g oral glucose tolerance test—

       (i) a fasting venous blood glucose less than 7 mmol/l

       (ii) and a 2 hour venous blood glucose over 7 mmol/l *BUT* less than 10 mmol/l

Plasma glucose values are approximately 1 mmol/l higher than venous blood levels.

COMA IN DIABETES

The three commonest ways in which a diabetic patient may present in coma are with ketoacidosis, in a hyperosmolar state and as a consequence of hypoglycaemia. The principle differences between them are set out in Table 15.3.

Table 15.3. Diabetic comas.

	Onset	Dehydration	Ketosis	Acidosis
Ketoacidosis	Hours or days	+++	+++	+++
Hyperosmolar	Hours	+++	+	—
Lactic acidosis	Variable	+	+	+++
Hypoglycaemia	Minutes	—	—	—

If a patient is deeply unconscious he should be assumed to be hypoglycaemic until proved otherwise and should be immediately given 50 ml of 50% dextrose i.v.

Ketoacidotic coma

The presenting features of ketoacidosis include not only thirst and polyuria, but central abdominal pain, nausea and vomiting. On examination, bowel sounds may be absent or sparse and there will be abdominal tenderness. The picture may easily be confused with an acute abdominal emergency. However, surgery without recognition and correction of the ketoacidosis will often be fatal. Therefore, it is imperative that any patient presenting with an acute abdomen, no matter how florid the symptoms appear, must have the urine tested before going to theatre. Any established diabetic thought to have had an acute abdominal catastrophe but with hyperglycaemia and ketosis, must have these corrected before going to theatre. The insulin, fluid and electrolyte replacement, nasogastric suction and circulatory support which are needed to correct the ketoacidosis will buy time with regard to any abdominal emergency. Surgery without metabolic correction will usually be fatal and correction of the metabolic disturbance frequently cures the 'acute abdomen'. However, the tenderness may persist for 48 hours after the treatment is started and plasma amylase levels are frequently elevated, sometimes to very high levels in uncomplicated keotacidosis. The converse of painless peritonitis in a diabetic with autonomic neuropathy is very rare.

Management

Insulin (Actrapid or Soluble) should be given by continuous intravenous infusion, ideally using a syringe pump at a rate of 5–6 u/hour. (Less ideally—because it is more difficult to vary the infusion rate independently of fluid replacement, and because insulin will stick to the large areas of plastic with which it will be in contact—it may be added to the infusion fluids or given by burette.) The rate may be adjusted according to the blood sugar response but an increasing insulin requirement above this rate in the absence of technical problems with the infusion is an ominous prognostic sign; it may imply either serious underlying disease or a complication such as the development

17

Table 15.4. Basic principles of treating ketoacidosis.

Insulin	*Actrapid*—continuous i.v. infusion 5–6 u./hour or hourly deep intramuscular injections 5–10 u. Dose adjusted according to hourly blood sugars
Fluids	Isotonic saline 1l first 30 minutes, then 1 litre in 1 hour 1 litre in 2 hours 1 litre 6 hourly Average deficit 6 litres
Potassium	13 mmol in first litre of saline then according to hourly plasma levels

of lactic acidosis. An alternative regime is to give 5–10 u by deep i.m. injection hourly (see Table 15.4).

Intravenous fluids. This should be almost exclusively isotonic saline. The average fluid deficit is 6l; the first litre of replacement should be given rapidly, the second in 2 hours and subsequent fluid should then be given more slowly. There is no place for the use of intravenous bicarbonate in uncomplicated diabetic ketoacidosis: even patients with a profound metabolic acidosis respond satisfactorily to insulin and fluids. Bicarbonate is not only usually unnecessary, but is potentially dangerous; it provides a large sodium load which will induce excessive falls in the plasma potassium and possibly result in the late development of alkalosis when sufficient insulin has been given to clear the ketones. If the pH is less than 7, a small amount of bicarbonate (50 mmol) plus potassium may be given. Dextrose 4 per cent 1/5 normal saline or 5 per cent dextrose may be used when the blood sugar falls below 12 mmol/l.

Potassium. This is needed in all patients with ketoacidosis. Often the administration may be delayed until the blood glucose begins to fall, but since this happens early with present day treatment regimes, it is as well to add potassium to the infusion fluid from the beginning and only withdraw it if the initial plasma potassium is over 4.5 mmol/l. Large quantities of potassium may be needed. Traditionally potassium chloride is used. The theoretical benefits of using potassium phosphate have not been confirmed in recent studies.

Circulatory support with plasma or dextrans is sometimes needed, as is *nasogastric suction,* since the patients have gastric atony and may be vomiting.

When the blood glucose is stable between 5 and 10 mmol/l, the acidosis has been corrected, bowel sounds have returned and the patient has stopped vomiting, a light diet may be started and subcutaneous insulin given before meals according to the blood sugar (not urine sugar which is too imprecise for this purpose). Intravenous insulin infusions should not be withdrawn before subcutaneous insulin has been started since the half-life of intravenous insulin is less than 5 minutes.

Hyperosmolar coma

Hyperosmolar coma presents with gross dehydration and may mimic a variety of disorders. There is gross hyperglycaemia, but no ketones in either urine or plasma. It usually occurs in older patients and is often produced by the combination of a febrile illness and attempts to assuage thirst by drinking sugar-containing drinks. It may be the presenting feature of diabetes in this age group. It has been reported as a cause of nonrecovery of consciousness from anaesthesia: needless to say, there must have been immoderate overdosage with glucose in such cases.

Treatment consists of liberal fluid replacement with saline. It is possible to treat the patient entirely with 'normal' saline, since this will be hypotonic compared to their plasma. However, it is often advisable to reduce the sodium load by alternating isotonic saline with N/2 saline. Insulin is needed in smaller doses than for ketoacidosis.

Hypoglycaemia

Hypoglycaemia can occur in either insulin-treated diabetics or in those taking sulphonylureas. It does not occur in diabetics treated with diet alone, or with biguanides. The typical onset is rapid with a classical warning which consists of agitation, sweating, circumoral parasthesiae, palpitations, etc. A period of confusion follows, in which the patient may resist therapy; the final stage is coma and sometimes grand mal convulsions. However, in some patients, especially those with autonomic neuropathy or those taking β-adrenergic receptors blocking drugs, the warning symptoms may be absent. There is no convincing evidence that diabetics develop hypoglycaemic symptoms at higher blood glucose levels than nondiabetics.

The treatment consists of oral glucose, 10–20 g if the patient can still take oral fluids: alternatively, i.v. glucose 25 g will be effective in immediately correcting the majority of hypoglycaemic attacks. An alternative used by the relatives of some unstable diabetics is glucagon 1 mg. i.m. In an occasional patient consciousness is not regained even though the blood sugar is corrected. These patients may have developed cerebral oedema and i.v. mannitol or dexamethasone may be indicated. Patients on long-acting sulphonylureas such as chlorpropamide who become hypoglycaemic may relapse over many hours unless additional carbohydrate is given orally or intravenously.

MANAGEMENT OF DIABETES

Insulin dependent

These patients require a diet which controls the carbohydrate intake, omitting rapidly absorbed concentrated carbohydrate and spreading its intake throughout the day to cover the insulin. They will usually be taught a carbohydrate exchange system to allow them to vary the diet to fit in with their personal preferences. A restriction in the total intake of carbohydrate is not necessary.

The insulins available and their durations of action are shown in Table 15.5. In most centres the purified insulins, 'monocomponent' (Novo) or 'rarely immunogenic' (Nordisk) have become the standard treatment for newly diagnosed diabetics; however, many diabetics remain well controlled on the older 'dirty' insulins. ('Dirty' in this sense refers to contamination of the insulin with proinsulin, insulin dimers or other pancreatic peptide hormones, etc. The 'clean' insulins are highly purified and as a consequence are of very low antigenicity.) Recently, British insulin manufacturers have produced a series of cleaner insulins and it seems likely that in due course the older insulins will be replaced. Random changes between the purified and 'dirty' insulins should be avoided since this can lead to loss of diabetic control. A patient controlled on purified insulin and given a 'dirty' insulin in the same dosage will become hyperglycaemic and will probably develop local reactions at the injection sites. A patient

Table 15.5. Insulins.

Type	Duration of action	Purity	Minimum frequency of injection
Soluble	Short	Low	
'Nuso'	Short	Low	
'Actrapid'	Short	Very high	TWICE DAILY
'Leo neutral'	Short	High	
Semitard	Short/intermediate	Very high	
Isophane	Intermediate	Low	USUALLY TWICE
'Rapitard'	Intermediate	Very high	BUT SOMETIMES
'Retard'	Intermediate	Very high	ONCE/DAY
Monotard	Intermediate	High	
Lente	Long	Low	
'Lentard'	Long	Very high	ONCE DAILY
'Ultratard'	Very long	Very high	

controlled on 'dirty' insulin given purified insulin in the same dose will become hypoglycaemic.

Insulin dependent diabetics, apart from the very young (less than 5 years old) or the elderly, are nowadays treated with insulin twice daily and are often given mixtures of short and intermediate acting insulin which they give in a single injection and the proportions of which they adjust according to their need.

Noninsulin dependent

Correct diet is the cornerstone of treatment. If the patient is obese one should restrict all calorie-containing foods to induce weight loss: if the patient is not obese, its aim is to avoid rapidly absorbed concentrated carbohydrate.

Oral hypoglycaemic agents are only used for the patient who cannot be adequately controlled with diet alone. There are two types of agent, the sulphonylureas which mainly act by stimulating insulin secretion, and the biguanides which do not increase insulin secretion and whose exact mode of action is uncertain. Various preparations of sulphonylureas are available (Table 15.6), and they may produce hypoglycaemia which may be prolonged with long acting drugs such as chlorpropamide. Only one biguanide, metformin, is in common use in the U.K. Phenformin has largely fallen into disuse because of the risk of producing lactic acidosis. Metformin also produces a rise in plasma lactate levels, but much less so than phenformin. The only cases of lactic acidosis discovered to date in association with metformin therapy have been in patients who also had other causes of hyperlactaemia, such as pulmonary embolus or renal failure.

It is essential to stop all oral hypoglycaemic drugs at least 24 hours and preferably 48 hours before elective surgery. This removes the risk of hypoglycaemia in those taking suphonylureas and hyperlactaemia in those taking biguanides.

Assessment of control

The ideal result of treatment is the restoration of normal glucose tolerance but in the

Table 15.6. Oral hypoglycaemic drugs.

Sulphonylureas	Maximum daily dose
Chlorpropamide (Diabinese)	
100 mg & 250 mg tabs	375 mg
Glibenclamide (Glucagon or Daonil)	
2·5 mg & 5 mg tabs	20 mg
Glipizide (Glibenese or Minodiab)	
5 mg tabs	20 mg
Tolbutamide (Rastinon)	
0·5 mg tabs	3 mg
Glibonuride (Glutril)	
25 mg tabs	75 mg
Gliquidone (Glurenorm)	
30 mg tabs	180 mg
Biguanides	
Metformin (Glucophage)	
500 g & 850 g tabs	1750 mg
Phenformin (Dibotin)	
25 mg & 50 mg tabs	100 mg

insulin-dependent diabetic this is not possible. In all adult diabetics the aim should be to keep them at, or slightly below, the normal weight for their age, sex and height. Growth in diabetic children is a useful measure of good control. The levels of blood glucose to be aimed for are shown in Table 15.7. Haemoglobin A_{1C}, a glycosylated haemoglobin, has been shown to be a useful guide to longer term (2–6 weeks) control*. Raised levels indicate poor control during that period (the normal upper limit varies somewhat with the assay technique but is around 7·5 per cent).

Table 15.7. Aims for diabetic control.

	Insulin dependent	Noninsulin dependent
Blood glucose		
Fasting	5·0 mmol/l	5·0 mmol/l
2 hr postprandial	7·0 mmol/l	6·0 mmol/l
Preprandial	6·0 mmol/l	6·0 mmol/l
Haemoglobin A_{1C}	5·5–8·0%	5·5–8·0%
Urine glucose	90% Negative	All Negative
plus	No unexplained hypoglycaemic attacks	

COMPLICATIONS OF DIABETES

Atherosclerosis

Diabetics are at risk from developing premature atheroma and, therefore, have a greatly increased frequency of peripheral, coronary and cerebral arterial disease.

* Many laboratories only measure HbA_1: the correlation with diabetic control is broadly similar.

Myocardial infarction is more hazardous in the diabetic than the nondiabetic, particularly during the first 48 hours, presumably due to an increased frequency of dysrhythmias. Silent or painfree myocardial infarctions occur in diabetics who may present with cardiac failure, dysrhythmias or cardiogenic shock.

Renal disease

The classical renal disease of diabetics, glomerulosclerosis, presents with albuminuria, initially intermittent, but progressing to the nephrotic syndrome and renal failure. It takes a number of years to progress from the first recognition of albuminuria to full blown renal failure and the typical patient is a diabetic who develops the disease during childhood and goes into renal failure in his thirties. By the time renal failure occurs the patient has usually had diabetes for at least 15 years. The condition, which is a form of diabetic microangiopathy, is associated with that other form of diabetic small vessel disease, retinopathy, and the absence of retinopathy would make it unlikely that albuminuria was due to diabetic glomeruloscelerosis.

The treatment of early phases of diabetic glomerulosclerosis is with an increased protein diet, diuretics and hypotensive agents. When uraemia develops then renal transplantation may be considered. Dialysis, usually peritoneal because of the problems of arterial access, is only undertaken if transplantation is thought possible since it appears that many diabetic complications worsen on long-term dialysis.

There is uncertainty as to whether pyelonephritis occurs more commonly in diabetics, but necrotizing papillitis is a recognized hazard of diabetes which may complicate pyelonephritis or diabetic ketoacidosis.

Eye complications

Diabetes is the commonest cause of blindness in the U.K. in the age group 30–60 years. It is estimated that of the 10,000 blind diabetics, 3,000 are due to cataract and 7,000 to retinopathy.

Cataracts. Juvenile cataracts may occur particularly in poorly controlled young diabetics but are, fortunately, not common. Senile cataracts occur more commonly and at an earlier age in diabetics than in nondiabetics. As long as there is no retinal disease they may be satisfactorily treated in standard ways.

Retinopathy. There are two types. Background retinopathy consisting mainly of microaneurysms and hard exudates does not damage vision unless the macula is involved. Proliferative retinopathy with new vessel formation and subsequently large retinal and vitreous haemorrhages is associated with blindness. Early treatment with photocoagulation delays or may halt its progress. At later stages vitreous surgery may offer hope for a few blind diabetics. If proliferative retinopathy is present elevation of the blood pressure, even transiently, must be avoided since it may precipitate vitreous haemorrhages.

Neurological complications

Symmetrical polyneuropathy with absent tendon reflexes and stocking and glove anaesthesia is common and in its minor form often asymptomatic. It may be present at the time of diagnosis.

Diabetic amyotrophy is a motor neuropathy affecting particularly the pelvic girdle and most obviously the quadriceps. There is muscle wasting, absent ankle jerks and commonly pain around the knees. It may be associated with poor diabetic control and often improves if the blood glucose levels are brought to normal.

Mononeuritis multiplex affecting single large nerves often in succession and with improvement over a period of weeks may occur in diabetes. A similar syndrome may affect the oculomotor nerves. Typically a IIIrd nerve palsy in a diabetic is painful, associated with sparing of the pupil and improves in a few weeks.

Autonomic neuropathy is a widespread disorder with serious implications for anaesthetists. The gastrointestinal tract may be involved with diabetic diarrhoea which is paroxysmal and often nocturnal. Gastric atony may occur and such patients will have delay in gastric emptying and possibly troublesome vomiting. Bladder disturbances are often asymptomatic and acute retention only occurs with florid autonomic neuropathy. There may be testicular anaesthesia, impotence and altered oesophageal motility. Disorders of sweating with dry hands and feet, sometimes gustatory facial sweating and rarely paroxysms of nocturnal sweating are features of the disorder. There may be disturbed temperature regulation. The most serious manifestations are however cardiovascular. Postural hypotension is troublesome and may become evident only after the patient has been put to bed for some days. Cardiac denervation may be associated with dysrhythmias [6], particularly during anaesthesia: it may be recognized by some simple tests which should be carried out in all diabetics prior to anaesthesia (see Table 15.8) [3]. Painless myocardial infarction and lack of warning of hypoglycaemia are both hazards of autonomic neuropathy.

Table 15.8. ECG test for autonomic neuropathy.

The ECG is run whilst the patient moves from the lying to the standing position and the R–R intervals for the 15th and 30th complexes after standing are measured.

Ratio (*15th to 30th*)

> 1·11	Normal
1·04–1·11	Borderline
< 1·04	Pathological

Evidence of autonomic neuropathy should be looked for in every diabetic prior to elective surgery. If it is present, continuous ECG monitoring is essential throughout anaesthesia and until full recovery; the patient should also be mobilized early to minimize problems from postural hypotension. Respiratory tract infections and respiratory depressant drugs are both particularly hazardous in these patients.

Diabetes and the feet

Lower limb problems are a common cause of surgery in diabetics. Intermittent claudication or ischaemic changes may necessitate vascular surgery and neuropathic lesions may need debridement. Lesions are commonly mixed with ischaemic changes being painless because of neuropathy and compounded by infection.

PREGNANCY

Pregnancy holds special hazards for the diabetic women. Her diabetes will tend to become unstable and unless it is very well controlled the chances of her producing a healthy child are greatly reduced. In the days before insulin, perinatal mortality was over 60 per cent and for many years after the discovery of insulin it did not fall below 30 per cent. Nowadays when excellent control of diabetes is achieved, the perinatal mortality should be around 2 per cent.

To achieve these results close collaboration is needed between physician, obstetrician and the patient. Frequent monitoring, often with the patient measuring her own blood sugar, ensures that the blood sugar is kept within the normal range. Any obstetrical problems such as urinary tract infections or pre-eclampsia need prompt treatment and unless the patient's diabetes is perfectly controlled, she should be admitted to the obstetric ward for assessment during the last few weeks of pregnancy.

All (except the mildest gestational diabetic whose blood glucose and Hb A_{1C} levels are normal on diet alone) are treated with insulin and a twice daily regime, usually of insulin mixtures, is the rule.

Delivery is now usually at about term. Many patients are allowed to go into spontaneous labour. Epidural anaesthesia is often of value in vaginal delivery, since it avoids the unpredictable swings of blood sugar produced by a painful normal delivery. Operative delivery is still needed more frequently than for normal women, but less so than in the past.

Whatever the method of delivery, it is essential to maintain normoglycaemia until the baby is delivered. This means that the obstetrician and anaesthetist cannot have the luxury of maintaining hyperglycaemia so as to avoid the risks of hypoglycaemia during anaesthesia.

The most satisfactory method of managing the delivery of a diabetic is to provide a continuous insulin infusion, ideally from a syringe pump (Actrapid 1–3 u/hour), with a 5 per cent dextrose infusion, 1 litre every 8 hours. Blood glucose is measured hourly and the insulin rate adjusted as necessary: it rarely needs adjusting beyond the stated limits. If operative delivery is needed, then the insulin and dextrose infusion are simply maintained. The anaesthetist can monitor the blood sugar before and during anaesthesia using one of the simple systems mentioned below. Throughout delivery by either method, the blood glucose should be kept within the range 3–7 mmol/l. Higher levels will stimulate the fetal pancreas producing the risk of neonatal hypoglycaemia: too low a figure may induce both maternal and fetal hypoglycaemia.

EFFECTS OF SURGERY AND ANAESTHESIA ON NORMAL CARBOHYDRATE METABOLISM

The degree of metabolic upset produced by surgery (and trauma) depend upon the extent of the injury: minor, superficial operations have minimal effects but major surgery, particularly intraperitoneal surgery or surgery complicated by sepsis or shock, has far reaching consequences. The changes include glucose intolerance, protein breakdown and an increased metabolic rate. Catabolism is dominant.

The first metabolic effects of elective surgery include the elevation of various hormones, ACTH, cortisol and catecholamines, before the operation probably as a consequence of anxiety. Insulin secretion is suppressed during surgery and this combined with the hormonal changes results in a rise in the blood glucose. Post-operatively, insulin secretion is increased but insulin resistance develops so that glucose intolerance persists.

Fasting, both pre- and postoperatively, exacerbates the catabolic response. During short-term starvation the brain and red cells require the supply of 180g of glucose a day and this is met initially by breakdown of hepatic glycogen, but this does not last long and subsequently muscle glycogen is used and protein is broken down to supply aminoacids for gluconeogenesis. To supply energy for other tissues, lipolysis occurs with the liberation of free fatty acids. Some of these will be used directly as an energy source whilst some will be converted by the liver to ketone bodies, another useful energy source. If starvation persists 'ketoadaption' occurs with an increase in the use of free fatty acids and ketone bodies, and a reduction in the need for glucose, even by the brain. At this stage there is a smaller need for protein breakdown to supply energy needs and the plasma ketone bodies may be high enough to induce a slight acidaemia and for ketonuria to occur.

Anaesthesia itself has an effect on carbohydrate metabolism though not usually of a great magnitude. Spinal and extradural anaesthesia have virtually no direct effect at all. Ether and chloroform, by inducing ACTH stimulation and catecholamine release, induce hyperglycaemia and lipolysis. Halothane has only minor effects.

ANAESTHESIA AND SURGERY—THEIR EFFECTS ON DIABETES

Insulin dependent diabetics (type I diabetes) are effectively totally insulin deficient and if untreated metabolic chaos will ensue. Most peripheral tissues, particularly muscle and adipose tissue, cannot utilize glucose and gluconeogenesis and glycogenolysis are freed from the normal restraining action of insulin, hence hyperglycaemia occurs. There is protein breakdown with the liberation of gluconeogenic precursors and lipid mobilization is increased with elevated fatty acid levels. Ketogenesis is markedly increased and ketone body supply exceeds the level at which they can be used resulting in ketoacidosis.

In insulin independent diabetes (type II diabetes) plasma insulin may be increased, though a relative deficiency is present. There is a failure of the peripheral tissues to take up glucose leading to hyperglycaemia though enough insulin is present to control adipose tissue metabolism and prevent ketoacidosis.

The diuresis induced by hyperglycaemia induces loss of electrolytes, sodium, calcium, magnesium, phosphate and potassium in the urine and when ketoacidosis is present this will further increase the loss of intracellular potassium.

Surgery or injury will worsen the metabolic upset of diabetes. The usual increase in insulin levels induced by stress cannot occur and severe hyperglycaemia will result. This will be most severe in type I diabetes but will also occur to a lesser extent in type II. The extent of these changes will also depend, as in the nondiabetic, upon the severity of the surgery or injury.

PREOPERATIVE ASSESSMENT IN DIABETES

The preoperative evaluation of a diabetic should include an assessment of the quality
17*

of diabetic control (see Table 15.7), and a search for relevant diabetic complications. These include the following.

Autonomic neuropathy—which increases the risks of cardiorespiratory arrest and may produce various hazards such as delayed gastric emptying and postoperative urinary retention.

Proliferative retinopathy—even transient increases in blood pressure may produce vitreous haemorrhage.

Atherosclerotic changes—especially evidence of previous myocardial ischaemia or infarction, which may have been painless and of impaired peripheral or cerebral circulation.

Nephropathy—usually associated with hypertension and retinopathy and which would increase the metabolic problems and may affect the excretion of many drugs.

It is obviously important to consider the other drugs which a diabetic may well be taking for associated diseases and also the effects on the patient's diabetes of drugs which may be used during anaesthesia and in the postoperative period such as steroids, catecholamines and β-blockers.

MANAGEMENT OF DIABETES DURING SURGERY

Insulin dependent diabetes

Preoperatively

For elective surgery, long and intermediate acting insulins should be stopped 24 hours preoperatively and the patient changed to a short-acting insulin. Whilst soluble insulin is satisfactory for those previously controlled on 'dirty' insulins, for those treated with monocomponent or highly purified insulins, Actrapid or Leo Neutral insulins should be used and given at least twice a day. It is important to ensure that the patients take their normal carbohydrate intake, even though they may be apprehensive.

When the first meal is missed because of preoperative fasting a 5 per cent dextrose infusion delivering 1l/ 8 hr (this will provide 150 g of carbohydrate in 24 hours) is set up with an insulin infusion delivering 1–3 u/hour of the appropriate short-acting insulin. The insulin infusion should be separate from the glucose infusion so that the rates of the two infusions may be adjusted independently, an ideal solution being to deliver the insulin via a syringe pump. Although some authorities recommend the addition of albumin or other protein to the insulin infusion to prevent the insulin sticking to the infusion equipment, this is not usually necessary. The rate of the insulin infusion is adjusted to ensure that the blood glucose level remains between 7 and 11 mmol/l. Blood glucose measurements will be needed at least 2 hourly.

During surgery

The glucose and insulin infusions are maintained as above with measurement of blood glucose level at induction and every 30 minutes thereafter. Instantaneous results can be obtained using the simple systems described below. There is no need to maintain hyperglycaemia in order to avoid the risks of hypoglycaemia during surgery: indeed the practice is to be strongly deprecated. If surgery is prolonged it may be advantageous to add potassium to the infusion, 13 mmol/l of glucose (1 g Kcl).

Postoperatively

The glucose and insulin infusions are maintained until the patient can eat: the infusions can then be discontinued and the insulin given as subcutaneous doses before the three main meals of the day. Initially 12–16 u at each dose will probably suffice and the doses can then be adjusted according to blood glucose levels. These should be measured 4–6 hourly whilst the intravenous infusion is running and then before meals and last thing at night when the patient is eating. 'Sliding scales' based on urine tests should not be used, since they are too imprecise and result in wildly surging blood glucose levels.

Potassium can be added to the i.v. glucose with advantage whilst the insulin infusion is running. A dose of 13 mmol per litre of glucose is usually adequate. Plasma potassium levels should be measured at least 12 hourly.

Noninsulin dependent diabetes

The management of these patients will depend upon whether or not they were well controlled preoperatively and the nature of the operation they are about to undergo. A well-controlled diabetic managed by diet alone about to undergo a minor surgical procedure needs no special metabolic management.

Preoperatively

In order to assess diabetic control, blood glucose measurements will be necessary. If these are higher than 12 mmol/l, then the patient's diabetic control can be classified as poor and unless a very minor operation is planned, insulin will be needed and the patient should be treated during the operation as though they were insulin dependent using Actrapid or Leo Neutral insulins (not Soluble insulin). An obese patient will be relatively insulin resistant and may need increased insulin dosages.

Long acting sulphonylureas, chlorpropamide in particular, needs to be discontinued 3 days preoperatively and the patient changed to a short acting sulphonylurea, such as glipizide. Short and intermediate acting sulphonylureas should be discontinued on the morning of the operation. Biguanides, phenformin and metformin, must be avoided since they increase plasma lactate levels. They are best discontinued 24 hours preoperatively.

Diabetics well controlled on diet alone or treated with sulphonylureas will not require any additional treatment unless major surgery is planned or if it is expected that the patient will not be able to eat for more than 24 hours postoperatively. Under these circumstances infusions of glucose and of insulin should be set up and the patient treated as though they were insulin dependent.

During surgery

If the patient is having glucose and insulin intravenously then they should be treated as though they were insulin dependent; otherwise all that is necessary is to avoid infusions which may induce hyperglycaemia, i.e. dextrose, Hartmanns and other lactate solutions, and fructose. If these become necessary then insulin will also have to be given.

Postoperatively

If the patient is having glucose and insulin infusions, these should be continued until he is eating, when oral hypoglycaemic agents may be restarted. It is often advisable to continue insulin until any postoperative problems such as sepsis have been resolved.

If the patient has not had insulin during the operation then monitor blood glucose levels 4–8 hourly and reintroduce oral hypoglycaemic agents, if previously used, when the patient has started eating.

PARENTERAL FEEDING

Should this be necessary either pre- or postoperatively in a diabetic, the following basic considerations should be noted:

1 Glucose remains the carbohydrate of choice and its administration should be spread continuously throughout the period of feeding; glucose feeding should not stop whilst the patient is receiving an alternative infusion such as lipid.

2 A continuous intravenous insulin infusion should be used as discussed above, though the dose needed may be much higher.

3 Fructose, sorbitol and lactate should all be avoided. Lactate solutions such as Hartmanns (Ringer lactate) induce hyperlactaemia and push up the blood glucose by stimulating gluconeogenesis [9]. Lactate disposal may be impaired in diabetics. Fructose will be converted to lactate and glucose [10].

Sorbitol levels may already be elevated in a poorly controlled diabetic and these may be implicated in the development of complications such as cataracts and some forms of neuropathy.

4 Electrolyte loss, particularly potassium and phosphate, may be particularly marked in diabetics.

BEDSIDE BLOOD GLUCOSE MONITORING

Various systems are available based upon test strips that can be used with capillary blood samples; they are relatively cheap and simple to use but will only give accurate results if the makers' instructions are adhered to fully. Strips that are at present available in the United Kingdom include—Dextrostix (Ames), Reflotest (Boehringer) and BM 20–800 (Boehringer). All can be read visually against charts supplied with the bottles, but the BM 20–800 is recommended if they have to be used in this way. This uses two adjacent test areas which change different colours at different rates, thereby increasing their accuracy when read directly. The other two strips can be read in meters which give accurate results as long as they are properly maintained and used correctly. It is advisable to make regular checks on their accuracy by checking the blood glucose reading against simultaneous samples sent to the laboratory. Fresh strips only should be used, Dextrostix in particular giving grossly inaccurate results if they have been exposed to the air, even for only a few mintues. Any person using this equipment must be fully trained or the results will be inaccurate.

More sophisticated equipment is available for giving rapid results, such as the Yellow Springs Blood Glucose Analyser but they are expensive and need special training in their use. It is likely that sophisticated equipment giving rapid results at the bedside will become available over the next few years.

SPONTANEOUS HYPOGLYCAEMIA

Although this diagnosis is often considered, it is rarely confirmed. Proof of the diagnosis requires the demonstration of hypoglycaemia (a whole blood glucose less than 2·2 mmol/l or a plasma glucose less than 2·5 mmol/l), coinciding with symptoms of neuroglycopenia. The symptoms in these patients are not usually those which initially affect the diabetic taking too much insulin: spontaneously hypoglycaemic patients do not usually complain of the symptoms of catecholamine secretion but rather present with the neurological symptoms—neuroglycopenia—of confusion, bizarre behaviour, fits and unconsciousness.

Many causes for spontaneous hypoglycaemia have been described but clinically they be may be divided into two broad groups—fasting hypoglycaemia and stimulative hypoglycaemia (Table 15.9).

Table 15.9. Causes of spontaneous hypoglycaemia.

Fasting hypoglycaemia
Insulinoma and islet cell hyperplasia
Idiopathic hypoglycaemia of childhood
Glycogen storage disease
Nonpancreatic tumours—especially
retroperitoneal sarcoma
Hepatic failure

Stimulative
Postgastrectomy
'Pre-diabetes'
Sensitivity to leucine, fructose or galactose
Alcohol

Insulinoma is the commonest cause of excess endogenous insulin. These are rare tumours and most are benign. The symptoms are of fasting hypoglycaemia or hypoglycaemia induced by exercise. The patients may be obese because of their excessive sugar consumption. The diagnosis depends on the recognition of inappropriate insulin levels with low blood sugars. The diagnosis is often difficult to prove (or disprove) and a number of specialized tests—glucagon tests, insulin suppression of C-peptide secretion, etc., have been described but the details of these are beyond the scope of this chapter. Those needing more information are referred to a review [5] by Marks and Rose. Confirmation of the diagnosis of endogenous hyperinsulinism leads to attempts at localizing the tumour by means of coeliac axis arteriography or transhepatic portal venography. The treatment is surgical removal. A glucose infusion will be needed during preoperative fasting and until the tumour is removed. Following removal a transient diabetes is common. Permanent diabetes develops in some patients in later years.

Tumour induced hypoglycaemia is another important, though rare, cause of fasting hypoglycaemia. The most usual tumour is a retroperitoneal fibrosarcoma. The tumours are usually large, but if resection is possible a cure is achieved.

Reactive hypoglycaemia is an extremely rare disorder and most patients so labelled have a neurotic disorder. Hypoglycaemia after carbohydrate-containing meals in patients who have gastric surgery is well recognized. A glucose tolerance test will show an initial high peak followed by a hypoglycaemia phase. The symptoms may sometimes be severe enough to require reconstructive surgery.

ENDOCRINE SECRETING PANCREATIC TUMOURS

These are rare tumours, the commonest being the insulinomas described above.

Zollinger–Ellison syndrome

Although the normal pancreas contains no gastrin-secreting cells, it is the commonest site (60 per cent) for the gastrin-secreting tumours which give rise to this syndrome.

The clinical findings in patients with this syndrome are recurrent peptic ulceration with gastric acid hypersecretion and less commonly, diarrhoea, steatorrhoea and multiple endocrine abnormalities (up to 40 per cent in some cases—hyperparathyroidism being the most common). The diagnosis is confirmed by the detection of raised serum gastrin levels; stimulation tests using calcium infusions or secretin injections may have to be employed in equivocal cases.

Glucagonomas

These rare tumours produce a syndrome consisting of a typical rash (migratory necrolytic erythema), stomatitis and glossitis, diabetes mellitus, low plasma aminoacids and anaemia. The tumours are slow-growing and ideally should be treated by resection; however, they have not infrequently metastasized by the time of diagnosis when streptozotocin (an antimitotic agent also used for malignant insulinoma) or embolization of the hepatic artery may be of value.

Somatostatinomas

These very rare tumours produce a syndrome of diabetes mellitus, gallstones and malabsorption.

Carcinoid tumours are dealt with elsewhere.

REFERENCES

1 ALBERTI KGGM, THOMAS DJB. The management of diabetes during surgery. *Br J Anaesth* 1979; **51**: 693–710.
2 BARNETT AH, ROBINSON MH, HARRISON JH, WATKINS PJ. Mini-pump: a method of diabetic control during minor surgery under general anaesthesia. *Br Med J* 1980; **1**: 78–9.
3 CLARKE BF, EWING DJ, CAMPBELL IW. Diabetic autonomic neuropathy. *Diabetologia* 1979; **17**: 195–212.
4 KEEN H, JARRETT RJ. Diabetes and atherosclerosis. In: Keen H, Jarrett RJ, eds. *Complications of diabetes*. London: Edward Arnold, 1975.
5 MARKS V, ROSE FC. *Hypoglycaemia*. 2nd ed. Oxford: Blackwell Scientific Publications, 1981.
6 PAGE MMcB, WATKINS PJ. Cardiorespiratory arrest and diabetic autonomic neuropathy. *Lancet* 1978; **1**: 14–16.
7 ROSSINI AA, HARE JW. How to control the blood glucose in the surgical diabetic patient. *Arch Surg* 1976; **3**: 945–9.
8 TAITELMAN U, REECE EA, BESSMAN AN. Insulin in the management of the diabetic surgical patient. *JAMA* 1977; **237**: 658–60.
9 THOMAS DJB, ALBERTI KGMM. Hyperglycaemic effects of Hartmann's Solution during surgery in patients with maturity onset diabetes. *Br J Anaesth* 1978; **50**: 185–8.
10 WOODS HF, ALBERTI KGMM. Dangers of intravenous fructose. *Lancet* 1972; **2**: 1354–7.

Chapter 16
Thyroid and Parathyroid Disease

R. F. FLETCHER

THYROID DISEASE

With the exception of diabetes and infertility, the thyroid diseases are by far the commonest group of endocrine disorders. They are much more common in females than in males, the ratio being about 9:1 for hypothyroidism and 4:1 for hyperthyroidism. All ages are affected with perhaps peaks of incidence of hyperthyroidism in early adult life and old age, while hypothyroidism is relatively more common in the elderly. A familial incidence is also common.

It is important to distinguish between size and function. Although a correlation may be seen, exceptions are common and very large goitres may produce normal levels of thyroid hormones while gross hormone excess may come from a gland which appears virtually normal.

EXAMINATION OF THE THYROID

The physical examination of a goitre is important. The shape of the neck should be observed while the patient swallows some water. Palpation from the front and also from behind using the fingers of both hands, during swallowing, is helpful. The isthmus of the normal gland across the trachea can be felt in most persons but the lateral lobes are masked by the sterno-mastoid muscles, and moderate enlargement in the lobes may be difficult to detect. An attempt should be made to define the size, shape, consistency and mobility of the gland.

If the gland does not move on swallowing or if the finger cannot be inserted below it there may be a retrosternal extension. The goitre may be hard and immobile if it is the site of a malignant tumour infiltrating into the adjacent tissues. Plain radiographs of the thoracic inlet will show if there is tracheal distortion or compression and may reveal a retrosternal goitre (Fig. 16.1).

THYROID PHYSIOLOGY

Tests of thyroid function are easier to understand if the principal features of thyroid physiology are recalled. The total amount of free iodine in the body is normally quite small (about 250 μg) and the thyroid tissue takes up iodine avidly from the blood passing through it. The acinar cells iodinate tyrosine to mono- or diiodo-tyrosine and these molecules are then coupled to form either triiodothyronine (T3) or thyroxine (T4) with, respectively, three or four iodine atoms in the molecules. The hormones are stored in association with globulin in the acinar colloid from which they are released into the circulation. All four main steps, the trapping of iodine, its organification, storage and release in thyroid hormones, are stimulated by thyrotrophin (thyroid stimulating hormone, TSH) from the anterior pituitary. The secretion of TSH is controlled by thyrotrophin releasing hormone (TRH) from the hypothalamus. There

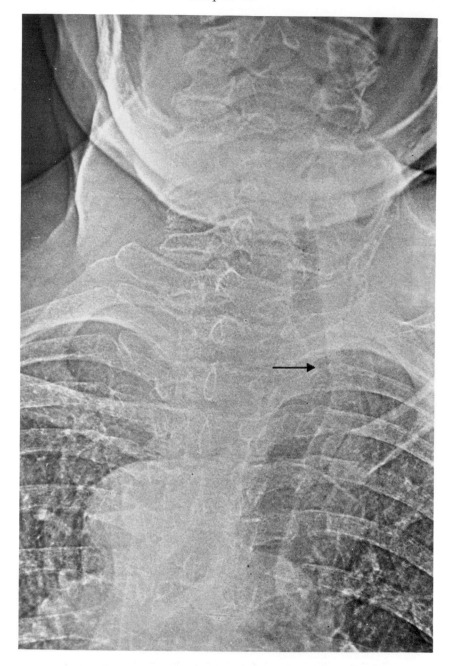

Fig. 16.1. Photograph of Xerograph of thoracic inlet showing deviation and compression of trachea (arrowed).

is a feedback modulating system involving the circulating thyroid hormones (both T3 and T4) acting on the hypothalamus and/or anterior pituitary.

Both T3 and T4 are released from the gland but some T3 is formed peripherally by de-iodination of T4. The normal plasma level of T3 is much lower than that of T4 but as T3 has a much faster turnover (half-life of about 12 hours compared to about six days for T4) and is more potent than T4, approximately half the thyroid hormone effect on the tissues is exerted by each of the two hormones. Thyroid hormones act on cells via the adenyl cyclase system to produce complex changes resulting in increased oxygen consumption and energy production.

Another thyroid hormone called reverse T3 (rT3) has been identified. It is similar to ordinary T3 (3, 5, 3') but the three iodine atoms are arranged in a different pattern (3, 3', 5') and this slight change makes rT3 almost inert. The plasma level of rT3 is known to fluctuate, e.g. with changes in calorie intake, but its physiological role is unknown.

Over 99 per cent of the thyroid hormones in the plasma is bound to carrier proteins, mostly to thyroxine binding globulin (TBG) and yet it is presumably the free hormone which is in equilibrium with the tissues and metabolically active. Direct measurements of the free hormones are difficult and available at present only for research.

TESTS OF THYROID FUNCTION [3, 5]

These can be considered conveniently at three levels:

1 indications of tissue effects of thyroid hormones;
2 measurement of thyroid activity;
3 circulating thyroid hormones.

Tissue effects

The prime example of a test of tissue effects of thyroid hormones was the 'Basal Metabolic Rate' (BMR) in which body oxygen consumption at rest was compared with that expected for a person of that age, sex, height and weight. The test has been largely abandoned because of its technical difficulty and unreliability. Simple recording techniques for the speed of contraction and relaxation of the tendon reflexes (usually the ankle jerk) have also been used. This method utilizes the fact that the speed of the tendon reflexes is dependent on thyroid hormone action—fast in hyperthyroidism and slow in hypothyroidism. This test is simple and fast but like the BMR is not sufficiently accurate for reliable, routine diagnosis. Potentially, such tests could be ideal as they indicate exactly what one needs to know, i.e. the level of effect of thyroid hormones in the tissues.

Thyroid activity

Most of these tests use radioactive isotopes of iodine. After the introduction of the isotope by mouth or intravenously, the radioactive iodine mixes with the inert isotopes of iodine present in the body and is taken up proportionately by the thyroid tissue which does not discriminate between the iodine isotopes. The radio-iodine can be measured by its emissions using radiation detectors near the thyroid gland. The measurements may be used in two ways. As the 'tracer' of radioactive material labels the body pool of iodine and behaves as part of it, relative movements of the tracer indicate how the body pool is changing and what effect the thyroid gland is having, e.g. by taking up iodine avidly (in hyperthyroidism) or only sluggishly (in hypothyroidism). The radiation dose is negligible but the tests are relatively expensive, and inconvenient for outpatients. The tests are susceptible to interference from contamination of the patient by iodine. Organic iodides such as those in radiographic contrast media

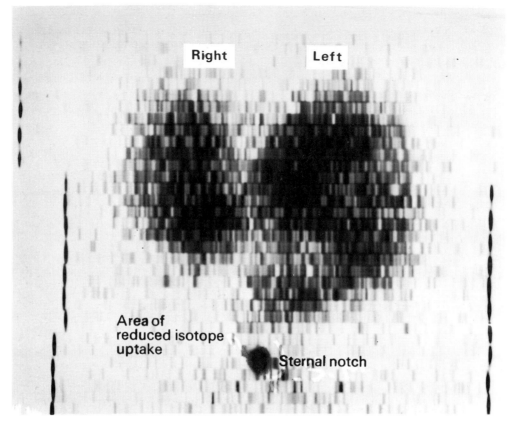

Fig. 16.2. Thyroid scan using Technetium 99^m showing asymmetrical uptake in the two lobes and an area of deficient uptake to the right lower lobe.

used in cholecystograms, pyelograms, myelograms, etc., are particularly troublesome as they persist in the body, and slowly release iodine, for months or years.

If a somewhat larger dose of radio-iodine is given (e.g. 50 μCi) there should be sufficient radiation from the gland to permit detailed localization of the isotope using a collimated crystal detector or a gamma camera. These 'scans' are helpful in determining whether nodules in the gland are taking up iodine or not and delineating aberrant thyroid tissue behind the sternum or elsewhere (Figure 16.2). [^{99}Tc^m] technetium is a radioactive isotope which is taken up by the thyroid and can be used for thyroid scanning but it is not organically bound and cannot be used for other measurements of thyroid function.

In general, as thyroid hormone assays have improved, tracer methods have tended to go out of use although scanning is still valuable in a few patients.

Hormones in blood

Plasma T4

The measurement of plasma T4 is now the standard test of thyroid function. The normal range is approximately 50–150 nmol/l*. Various methods of immunoassay or

* Alternatively, 4.0–11.5 μg/100 ml (T4 mol.wt = 777).

competitive binding, often in 'kit' form, are available. In general the results are of satisfactory reliability and are not affected by iodine contamination.

An increase in binding proteins in the plasma increases the level of T4 but not its physiological effect so that in this circumstance a high result is misleading. The commonest causes of increase in binding proteins are pregnancy and oestrogen-containing tablets as used in combined oral contraceptives and hormonal treatment of the menopause. Clofibrate and perphenazine have a similar effect while binding proteins tend to be depressed by androgens, anabolic steroids and corticosteroids.

The difficulty can be overcome by combining the measurement of T4 with an estimation of the binding proteins with the 'T3 binding test' (see below) or a direct measurement of TBG, in a ratio. The result is called the Free thyroxine index (FTI) and corrects for the level of binding proteins. The FTI is probably the best single index of thyroid function available at present but nevertheless may be influenced by drugs such as phenothiazines, salicylates, sulphonylureas and phenytoin. A careful history of drug ingestion is important in the interpretation of thyroid function tests.

Plasma T3

This can be measured and the test is coming into general use. The normal range is approximately 1·5–3·0 nmol/l*. In the majority of patients known or suspected of having thyroid disease it is not necessary to measure plasma T3 as well as plasma T4. The double measurement may be useful in demonstrating an abnormality in patients with thyroid glands damaged by treatment because in such patients the normal ratio of plasma T3 to T4 may be disturbed. The measurement of T3 is necessary also for the diagnosis of T3 'toxicosis' (see below). Like T4, the plasma level of T3 is affected by the level of the binding proteins.

T3 binding test (T3B)

This test, also sometimes called the 'T3 uptake test' (T3U) is unfortunately named because it gives no information about the level of T3 in the sample. Radio-iodine labelled T3 is equilibrated in a test-tube between the thyroid hormone binding proteins in the patient's plasma and some kind of artificial binding material such as Sephadex. The distribution of the labelled hormone between the two kinds of binding sites is then determined. The result is influenced by the amount of T4 present and by the level of binding proteins. As a single test it is of limited value but is useful in calculating the FTI (see above).

Protein bound iodine (PBI)

The normal range is approximately 300 nmol/l (3·5 μg/100 ml) to 600 nmol/l (7·0 μg/100 ml). The PBI is now obsolete having been replaced by the measurement of plasma T4.

Thyroid antibodies [3]

In many kinds of thyroid disease, and also in some normal people, circulating antibodies against thyroglobulin, second colloid antigen, and thyroid microsomes may be

---

* Alternatively, 100–200 ng/100 ml (T3 mol.wt = 651).

detected using various methods. The ability to form these antibodies is probably under genetic control which relates presumably to the common familial incidence of thyroid disease. The presence of thyroid antibodies is not diagnostic of any particular disorder but high titres are almost invariable in lymphadenoid goitre.

Serum TSH

This can be measured by an immunoassay and the normal range is about 1·0 to 3·0 i.u/l. A raised level is a reliable diagnostic test for primary hypothyroidism and also is a good indicator of inadequate replacement therapy. The TSH response to intravenous thyrotrophin releasing hormone (TRH) is exaggerated in hypothyroidism and absent in hyperthyroidism.

GOITRE [3, 8]

The types of goitre in approximate order of decreasing frequency of occurrence are
    'Simple' goitre
    Adenoma (single or multiple)
    Toxic (Graves' disease)
    Lymphadenoid
    Acute thyroiditis
    Carcinoma.
(There are other extremely rare forms including septic thyroiditis and dyshormono-genetic goitre.)

'Simple' goitre

The 'simple' goitre (sometimes equally misleadingly called 'colloid' goitre) is of un-known aetiology. Goitre from iodine deficiency is now very rare in this country. Usually the patient is euthyroid and therapy is dictated by cosmetic and pressure considerations. Treatment with thyroxine to suppress thyrotrophin release is recom-mended by some but the results are disappointing.

Adenoma

These benign neoplasms are usually multiple even if this is not apparent on palpation. Single or multiple adenomas may retain the capacity to secrete hormone, i.e. 'hot nodules'. These escape from physiological control and produce hyperthyroidism. If the nodule is 'cold', i.e. nonfunctioning, it may be cystic and this can be revealed readily by ultrasound examination. With the 'cold' nodule the possibility of carcinoma arises (see below).

The solitary thyroid nodule [1, 8]

The management of the solitary thyroid nodule is a common and difficult problem. If the nodule is 'hot', that is takes up radio-isotope and is causing hyperthyroidism, it is accepted that surgery or radio-iodine therapy will be required. If however the nodule is 'cold', i.e. inactive, as is usually the case, the management is debatable. The problem is the risk of malignancy and this is uncertain because it rests on histological opinion which is quite variable in this condition. Some authorities consider that 10 per cent or more of these nodules are malignant but this is not reflected in clinical experience. Many patients are known to harbour these nodules for many years because surgery is never offered or is refused and yet later spread is most uncommon.

Some risk undoubtedly exists and so most surgeons recommend that all cold nodules should be removed. This view is being challenged and perhaps practice will change. The significance of the finding of a cystic nodule in this context remains to be seen.

Toxic goitre

This is typically a moderate sized, fairly soft, smooth, symmetrical, mobile goitre over which there is a systolic bruit. It is accompanied by the features of hyperthyroidism with eye changes (see below). The management is that of the hyperthyroidism.

Lymphadenoid goitre (Hashimoto's disease)

This is a sterile inflammatory condition of the gland produced probably by an auto-immune process. It leads to a moderate sized firm goitre which may be asymmetrical. There may be a hyperthyroid stage at first but later, and more typically, the patient is euthyroid and, later still, hypothyroid as the gland is destroyed progressively. Surgery is unnecessary and should be avoided if possible. However, the diagnosis often is uncertain and the condition is revealed histologically after operation. High levels of thyroid antibodies are very suggestive of this condition. Drill biopsy would seem particularly useful in this condition but is not in general use because the small specimens obtained are difficult to interpret.

Acute thyroiditis

This uncommon condition of unknown aetiology (perhaps viral) presents as an acute sterile inflammation of the gland which enlarges over a few days or weeks and becomes tender. There may be some systemic response with malaise and fever. Uusally, thyroid function is normal. The condition resolves spontaneously but corticosteroids may assist recovery.

Carcinoma

Thyroid carcinoma is unusual but not rare. It is suspected clinically if a goitre enlarges rapidly, is hard, tethered to adjacent structures, lacks mobility, affects the voice or is associated with enlarged lymph nodes. Four types are recognized.

Papillary. This is the commonest form. It occurs in children and before middle age. It spreads to adjacent lymph nodes but is relatively benign. Local resection is usually successful and the prognosis is good.

Follicular. This is the next commonest form, tends to occur later in life and has a fair prognosis. Mixed papillary and follicular tumours occur.

Anaplastic. This is less common and tends to occur in the elderly. It is a highly malignant tumour with a bad prognosis.

Medullary. This rare tumour occurs in young adults, usually as part of the syndrome of multiple endocrine adenomatosis type II. The associated tumours are parathyroid adenoma and phaeochromocytoma. The tumour, arising from parafollicular cells in the thyroid, secretes calcitonin which constitutes a useful marker in the plasma.

HYPERTHYROIDISM [5, 9]

Aetiology

The occurrence of hyperthyroidism implies that the hormone secretion is no longer thyrotrophin dependent. In the inflammatory thyroid disorders this is due to tissue destruction and release of preformed hormone. In an adenoma the neoplastic tissue is presumably biochemically incomplete in that although hormone synthetic capacity is present the normal control pathways are not. In the more common forms of hyper-thyroidism, in which the gland is diffusely involved, Graves' disease, the process is more difficult to understand.

It is likely that 'thyroid stimulating immunoglobulins' (TSI) in the plasma are involved in Graves' disease as part of an auto-immune process. The term 'TSI' includes substances variously reported before as long-acting thyroid stimulator (LATS), LATS protector and thyroid stimulating antibodies. Despite many efforts the significance of these substances is still uncertain and their measurement is not used currently in routine diagnosis or treatment.

Population studies have implicated an increased intake of iodine in the aetiology of Graves' disease. The possible role of stress is uncertain.

Diagnosis

In many patients the diagnosis is obvious from the clinical features (below) and a single measurement of plasma T4 will suffice for confirmation. In the borderline case an FTI and perhaps a TRH test will be needed. A variant of hyperthyroidism called 'triiodothyronine thyrotoxicosis' (T3 toxicosis) has been defined and constitutes 2–3 per cent of cases. The clinical features are identical with other forms of hyperthyroid-ism but the level of plasma T4 is normal while the level of plasma T3 is raised. Obviously a measurement of plasma T3 is necessary to confirm the diagnosis.

Clinical features

These are many and vary considerably between patients, particularly in the elderly. The most useful guides are in the patient's behaviour, the eyes and the cardiovascular system. In the patient's history, weight loss with retention of appetite is usual, and changes in mentality with irritability and insomnia are common. Diarrhoea may occur. The patient's behaviour is often significant, with heightened awareness, quickness of speech and movement, and restlessness.

On examination the thyroid gland is almost always palpable although it may be surprisingly small. Tremor of the hands is often present and although a fine tremor is typical a gross, coarse tremor may occur. The pulse is fast and the skin warm and moist. Atrial fibrillation is common in the elderly patient. Proximal muscle weakness is common.

Eye changes

Some eye changes occur in most patients with hyperthyroidism, except the elderly, but the severity of the changes is very variable and correlates poorly with the severity of the hyperthyroidism. The biochemical causes of the changes are still uncertain; thyroxine is not a major factor but may cause some lid retraction. Typical eye changes may occur in individuals who are euthyroid, and sometimes precede the development of hyperthyroidism. The changes may be strikingly asymmetrical or even unilateral.

The present terminology of the eye changes is unsatisfactory. The phrase 'endocrine exophthalmos' is employed but is inadequate and it is perhaps better to use descriptive terms. Four features may be noted and they can occur largely independently of each other except in the more severe forms, when all are usually present.

Lid retraction

This is the commonest manifestation and accounts for the so-called 'thyrotoxic glitter' which many patients show—a sort of bright-eyed, alert look. It is due to increased tone in the palpebral muscles. In more severe degree, the palpebral fissure is much widened. When the patient looks down the lowering of the upper lid lags behind the movement of the eyeball.

Conjunctivitis

This is a sterile inflammation with injection of the conjunctivae without pus formation and produces a 'gritty' sensation in the eyes. It may extend to produce marked oedema of the eyelids. For the patient, it can be one of the more troublesome features of hyperthyroidism.

Exophthalmos

In most instances this is slight and the protrusion of the eyeball amounts only to 2–3 mm when measured. Lid retraction gives the appearance of greater exophthalmos than is actually present. The condition is due to an increase in bulk of the retro-ocular tissues and muscles by oedema and a deposition of fat and mucopolysaccharide. The combination of exophthalmos and lid retraction may be of such a degree that the eyelids can no longer cover the cornea during blinking. Dryness of the cornea may lead to dangerous ulceration and secondary infection.

Paresis of the external ocular muscles

Some weakness of these muscles is common leading to a complaint of diplopia, perhaps only in certain directions of gaze. Rarely, an external ophthalmoplegia with fixed eyes occurs but accommodation is not affected.

Management of eye changes

The treatment of the eye changes is unsatisfactory. Correction of the level of thyroid function, which is relatively easy, brings little benefit to the eyes, except for an easing of the lid retraction. Indeed, the eye changes may become more severe, particularly, it is said, if thyroid function is corrected too quickly. The patient should be warned of the prognosis but reassured that the eye changes will probably eventually remit spontaneously although this may take several years and some degree of exophthalmos may be permanent. Local and systemic corticosteroids have been of little help but very large systemic doses have been recorded as effective in severe disease. Similarly, both β-adrenergic blockade and guanethidine locally do not seem to be effective. The use of methyl cellulose eye drops, to ease discomfort in the eyes is a useful symptomatic remedy. If the cornea is in danger because of inadequate lubrication lateral tarsorrhaphy is a simple, reversible and effective operative treatment. Orbital decompression, a more difficult procedure with possible danger to sight may be necessary to preserve the eye in the most severe cases.

Management of hyperthyroidism

Natural history

A discussion of the management of hyperthyroidism should follow an understanding of its natural history. A 'toxic' adenoma is unlikely to remit spontaneously but the diffuse 'toxic' goitre will revert to normal after 12–24 months in about 50 per cent of patients. Such goitres rarely cause serious pressure symptoms. If the original hyperthyroidism is due to an auto-immune thyroiditis, hypothyroidism is likely to be the end result, whichever treatment is employed.

Selection of treatment

In the management of hyperthyroidism there are three options—drugs, radioactive iodine and surgery. To some extent the choice between them is a matter of opinion, but some general guides can be set down. Surgery is the treatment of choice for a toxic adenoma, a large gland or if there are marked pressure effects. In the patient with a small goitre, thiocarbamides are preferred with resort to surgery if control is difficult or relapse occurs later. Radio-iodine is particularly useful in the elderly or infirm.

Drugs

β-adrenergic blockade [10]

The advent of drugs with this action has added a new dimension to the management of hyperthyroidism. Thyroid function is little affected but many of the clinical features such as tremor and tachycardia are suppressed quickly. This is particularly helpful in the acutely distressed patient and provides symptomatic relief until more definitive therapy becomes effective. It is uncertain whether these drugs alone provide adequate preparation for surgery.

Thiocarbamides

These are the main stay of drug treatment of hyperthyroidism; carbimazole is the drug of choice at present but the thiouracils are still used. Potassium perchlorate is a useful alternative if the patient cannot tolerate a thiocarbamide. The dose needs to be related to the individual and usually requires adjustment as treatment proceeds. The effect is fairly slow and it may be three to six weeks before the patient is euthyroid. Although the antithyroid drugs are supposedly goitrogenic, the gland usually slowly diminishes in size. If long-term drug treatment is to be used it is necessary to continue for two years to ensure the lowest possible relapse rate. Side-effects are uncommon but gastric upsets or a generalized nonspecific pruritic macular or papular rash may occur and, very rarely, agranulocytosis. Patients should be warned of the possibility of adverse reactions, and asked to stop treatment at once and report any untoward features. Routine white cell counts are not helpful. If an adverse reaction occurs an alternative antithyroid drug or other form of treatment will be needed.

Surgery [2]

For the hyperactive adenoma hemiresection of the gland is the usual procedure. For diffuse goitre, partial thyroidectomy (7/8ths) is normal. It is considered best that the patient be made euthyroid before surgery with thiocarbamides but many surgeons prefer to discontinue this treatment and change to oral iodine for 10–14 days before operation in the belief that this will maintain the patient in the euthyroid state until surgery and reduce the vascularity of the gland. The iodine is sometimes given as 'Lugol's solution' but a 60 mg tablet of potassium iodide once a day is more convenient and fully effective.

Operative complications are few and the outcome is usually satisfactory. For unknown reasons the remnant of the gland usually returns to physiological control although sometimes the remnant hypertrophies and hyperthyroidism recurs. More commonly, although the incidence varies widely in different series, the remnant fails completely and permanently.

Radioactive iodine

Because of possible radiation damage hazards (particularly to the gonads) it is usual in the U.K. to restrict the use of therapeutic radioactive iodine to men over 45 years of age and postmenopausal women. The main hazard is the late development of hypothyroidism. The incidence is substantial and continues to rise over many years without evidence of reaching a plateau. To minimize this danger current dosage is quite low (e.g. ^{131}I, 3 to 5 mCi) and the effect correspondingly slow; treatment with thiocarbamide is used until the radio-iodine takes effect. Repeated doses of radio-iodine may be needed.

Special situations

Hyperthyroidism in pregnancy

This provides special problems. If thiocarbamides are used they may cause goitre and hypothyroidism in the newborn infant but if the patient can be managed on low doses, with a change to iodine in the last three weeks of pregnancy, the danger is minimized. Subtotal thyroidectomy in the third trimester seems to be safe for the fetus and is recommended by some. The value and safety of β-adrenergic blockade in pregnancy is not yet established.

'Thyroid storm' (thyrotoxic crisis)

This condition is a severe exacerbation of hyperthyroidism with fever, prostration and, usually, cardiac arrythmias. It may occur in neglected hyperthyroidism or after subtotal thyroidectomy in a patient who has not been adequately prepared. The condition may be fatal and calls for immediate vigorous treatment with rehydration, oxygen and drugs for heart failure. Full intravenous doses of β- adrenergic blocking drugs are recommended combined with a large oral dose of carbimazole. Other therapies which have been employed include cooling for hyperpyrexia, corticosteroids and intravenous iodine.

Preparation for anaesthesia in the acute situation

There are occasional circumstances, such as incipient respiratory obstruction, some stages of pregnancy, or severe reaction to antithyroid drugs in which it may be necessary to operate on a patient who is not euthyroid.

Adrenergic blocking agents are highly effective in ameliorating most peripheral manifestations of hyperthyroidism. Many studies have shown benefits by β-blockade with propranolol 40 mg orally four times a day leading to a reduction in cardiac output and a fall in pulse rate, though not necessarily to normal. In the more urgent situation, intravenous administration may be required. The dose required is that necessary to bring the heart rate to near the normal range. Propranolol must be used with considerable caution in patients in heart failure.

There are other logical pharmacological approaches. Reserpine, by depleting stores of noradrenaline, and guanethidine by diminishing its release, have both been shown to be effective. However, they are prone to more side-effects and may present the anaesthetist with greater problems. Methyldopa also slows the pulse but generally has less effect on the other clinical manifestations of the disease. The addition of α-blockade with phenoxybenzamine appears to lead to a concomitant reduction in oxygen consumption and is indicated if systolic hypertension is present. If time allows, potassium iodide should be given orally as recommended above. In an acute situation, sodium iodide 10 mg can be given intravenously.

Opinions differ as to the wisdom of discontinuing propranolol therapy prior to anaesthesia. To do so inevitably carries the risk of precipitating a thyroid crisis with cardiac decompensation. If an anaesthetic technique is chosen which does not rely on sympathetic compensation to overcome myocardial depression, β-blockade is not incompatible with surgery and anaesthesia. The anaesthetist must, however, be aware that the compensating response, for example, to haemorrhage, may be masked.

Anaesthesia in the presence of hyperthyroidism

Adequate premedication is obviously essential and benzodiazepines such as diazepam appear to be effective and without adverse effects. Drugs which can stimulate the sympathoadrenal axis are best avoided; liver function may be abnormal, and this must also be borne in mind in choosing a sedative. Atropine is best omitted as it may aggravate tachycardia and prevent sweating.

For induction, thiopentone remains the agent of choice, and indeed the thiobarbiturates possess specific antithyroid activity which lasts for some days in animals.

The choice of inhalation agent (if indeed one is indicated at all), requires some care. Ether and cyclopropane which stimulate the sympathoadrenal system are contra-indicated, as is any technique which may cause hypercarbia. Methoxyflurane depresses this system but also unfortunately has a negative inotropic effect on the myocardium which is dose-dependent and which would potentiate the action of some β-blocking drugs. Another theoretical possibility is that the metabolism of this agent might be raised in the hypermetabolic state and this could enhance its nephrotoxicity. Some of the same arguments apply also to halothane. A balanced technique using muscle relaxants, nitrous oxide, controlled hyperventilation supplemented if necessary by analgesics, would seem the most appropriate choice.

HYPOTHYROIDISM [3]

Aetiology

Histological evidence suggests that primary hypothyroidism is usually the end result of an autoimmune process which destroys the gland. It is presumably related to, or a variant of lymphadenoid goitre, and the incidence of thyroid antibodies is high. However, at the time of diagnosis there is usually no thyroid tissue palpable and no history of a goitre. Because of the failure of the thyroid remnant hypothyroidism is a common late sequel of subtotal thyroidectomy. It is even more frequent after treatment with radioactive iodine. In the newborn, hypothyroidism may be due to agenesis of the gland or to failure of the gland, which may be ectopic, in late pregnancy.

Clinical features

Most of these can be understood as results of the reduction in metabolic activity and consequent slowing of function of most organs in the body leading to a diminution in both mental and physical activity. The clinical features vary widely in their severity depending on the degree of thyroid failure. In the later stages the patient is lethargic and slow in thought and movement, sleeps excessively and becomes constipated. There may be a preference for warm weather. The pulse is slowed, the heart enlarged and the peripheral circulation poor so that the skin is cool and dry, and may become coarsened and scaly. The hair greys and thins; the facial appearance is dull and the eyelids may be swollen. The speed of the tendon reflexes is slowed, particularly during the relaxation phase. Deterioration in mental function may lead to depression and even psychosis. An increase in body weight, despite a reduced appetite, is almost invariable.

Cretinism is hypothyroidism arising at birth or shortly afterwards. Often the condition is not apparent clinically at birth but later the infant is dull and apathetic with coarse facies and a hoarse cry. An umbilical hernia and constipation are usual. Development is retarded and there may be permanent brain damage if treatment is not started promptly. Because of this and the difficulty of early diagnosis neonatal screening may be introduced. The incidence is about 1:3,500 live births.

Management

Treatment with oral l-thyroxine sodium should always be satisfactory. Because of the danger of precipitating heart failure or myocardial infarction thyroid hormone levels must be restored slowly. In the severe case it is preferable to begin with 25 μg of T4 a day for several days but in the average case 50 μg per day can be used. Thereafter, the dose is increased by 50 μg steps each week up to a dose of 150 μg per day. The very slow metabolism of thyroxine means that a steady plasma level is not reached until a particular dose has been maintained for several weeks. Thus if 150 μg per day does not lead immediately to a satisfactory clinical response the same dose should be persisted with for some time.

The well-being of the patient is the best guide to the level of permanent replacement dose that is required, and there is still no entirely satisfactory test to supplement clinical observation, although measurements of plasma TSH may help. It is to be expected that the patient will lose weight to their previous level, lose the previous symptoms and find themselves back to their own 'normal'. Long-term dosage is usually in the range 100–200 μg per day with 150 μg per day being suitable for most patients. It is important to emphasize to the patient, and perhaps their relatives, the importance of continued regular medication (even when they have apparently returned to normal), and the lifelong nature of the condition. Thyroxine is still prescribed quite frequently in divided doses but this is unnecessary and the patient should take the whole daily dose at whichever time is convenient. The thyroxine tablets should be continued during intercurrent illness and should be taken in combination with any other medication.

The results of treatment are usually most gratifying although occasionally the appearance of angina prevents complete replacement. The combination of β-adrenergic blockade and thyroxine may be helpful. The prognosis with regular treatment is the same as for a person with normal thyroid function.

'*Myxoedema coma*'

This is often associated with hypothermia which calls for the usual slow spontaneous warming. It is still uncertain as to whether large or small doses of thyroid hormones are indicated. With either regime the mortality is high.

Anaesthesia and hypothyroidism

Patients receiving treatment for known hypothyroidism present no special problems. If a patient is remaining in normal health whilst receiving substantially less than the normal maintenance doses quoted above, the diagnosis must be in question. In the assessment of the adequacy of therapy, the history and clinical examination are more reliable than laboratory tests but a raised plasma TSH indicates undertreatment. If a patient has been without replacement therapy for a few days prior to surgery the slow turnover of T4 will ensure that an adequate blood level is still present.

It is the patient with obvious hypothyroidism that is chiefly at risk. Immediate administration of replacement hormone, though logical, takes a considerable time to produce a detectable effect, ranging from 1 to 4 days. Administration of large doses is not more effective; it is positively dangerous and may induce arrhythmias or severe angina, or cardiac arrest. The mortality associated with anaesthesia and surgery is said to be high, although this opinion is based on a relatively small amount of modern clinical experience. It is clearly desirable to delay surgery until the hypothyroid state has been corrected, if this is possible. Intensive oral therapy takes some days to be effective and is not without risk. Parenteral therapy with T3 should restore the situation in 72 hours but is likewise somewhat hazardous. 100 μg of T3 may be added to 1 litre of 5 per cent dextrose and given at a rate of about 20 drops/minute, observing the ECG for signs of flattening of the T waves and depression of the S-T segment.

If delay is not possible there are several aspects of technique to be borne in mind. Adrenal function will be depressed by the lack of thyroxine, and adequate doses of hydrocortisone should be given. Patients are particularly sensitive to the effects of sedatives, hypnotics, analgesics and anaesthetics, which should be given in much reduced doses. The respiratory centre is said to be especially sensitive and depression sufficient to cause cyanosis has been reported following a 50 mg dose of pethidine.

The low BMR of course means a low CO_2 production, and if controlled ventilation is used, the minute volume used must be suitably reduced or a large artificial dead space included.

Hypotension and hypothermia are also common in this condition. Active warming is not indicated unless the temperature falls below 30°C, when there is a risk of an irreversible arrhythmia. Effective slow warming for myxoedema coma has been achieved by using humidified warmed air for artificial ventilation. The safest anaesthetic technique would be one based on N_2O/O_2 and relaxants.

PARATHYROID DISEASE [6, 7]

The parathyroid glands produce a single polypeptide hormone the release of which is controlled by feedback modulation directly on the glands by the level of calcium in the plasma. Parathyroid hormone acts on the small intestinal mucosa via vitamin D to increase the absorption of calcium, on the renal tubules to reduce the excretion of calcium and increase that of phosphorus, and on bone to stimulate osteoclasts and the release of calcium. The result of these actions is to maintain the level of plasma calcium within close limits (2·2–2·6 mmol/l). Changes in the level of plasma calcium must not be interpreted solely as the results of changes in parathyroid hormone because there are interrelationships with vitamin D, diet and renal function. The physiological role of calcitonin is still unclear but seems to be small.

HYPERPARATHYROIDISM [7]

There are four types of hyperparathyroidism. The only factor common to all of them is an increase in the blood of parathyroid hormone (or similar substances). The other features vary with the circumstances.

Primary hyperparathyroidism

This is the commonest type. It is caused by an oversecretion of parathyroid hormone because the system has escaped from physiological control. In over 80 per cent of patients the abnormality is in a parathyroid adenoma which is almost always benign. The other parathyroid glands are suppressed and consequently atrophy. In 10 per cent of patients the glands are all hyperplastic. This implies the presence of some stimulus to parathyroid tissue other than a reduced plasma calcium but the nature of this stimulus is unknown. Parathyroid hyperplasia and multiple adenomas may occur as part of the syndrome of familial multiple endocrine adenomatosis (Pleuriglandular syndrome). Adenoma cannot be distinguished clinically or biochemically from hyper-plasia (see below).

Presentation

The presentation of primary hyperparathyroidism is variable and the pattern has changed with developments in biochemistry. The condition now comes to light most commonly as a result of biochemical screening in patients with disorders such as thyroid disease or diabetes or in those with indefinite general symptoms. Presentation with renal calculus is common also. Some patients have major symptoms related to hypercalcaemia—these are likely to be nausea and anorexia, weakness, constipation, polyuria and thirst. Duodenal ulceration and pancreatitis may occur; hypertension with or without renal damage may be prominent. The classical presentation with skeletal changes causing bone pain, fractures or deformities is relatively uncommon.

Refined histological techniques can show bone changes in nearly all patients with hyperparathyroidism but often the changes are slight and many patients have neither skeletal symptoms nor radiological changes. The fully developed skeletal changes are called 'osteitis fibrosa' and the commonest radiological features are irregularity of the outer surface of the proximal phalanges from subperiosteal erosions and blurring of the bone texture of the vault of the skull. Tumours of giant cells and bone cysts may occur at any site. Disappearance of the laminar dura of the teeth is an unreliable sign.

Diagnosis

In the early or uncomplicated case the diagnosis is essentially made by exclusion and depends on the demonstration over several months of a persistently elevated level of plasma calcium in the absence of other causes. A raised level of urine calcium is common but not an essential feature. In borderline cases, the plasma calcium must be measured on blood drawn without venous stasis and with the patient fasting. Renal calculi or calcification increase the likelihood of the diagnosis, and typical radiological changes are diagnostic. Malignant disease, Paget's disease, calciferol administration, hyperthyroidism and sarcoidosis should be excluded.

A failure to suppress the level of plasma calcium by administering hydrocortisone by mouth, 40 mg 8-hourly for 10 days, will support a diagnosis of hyperparathyroidism rather than one of the alternatives given above. Measurement of plasma parathyroid hormone is now available. The lower limit of detection does not extend below the normal range. The measurement is not regarded as essential for diagnosis at present but may be helpful [4].

Management

Conservative

With earlier diagnosis it has become apparent that this disease may persist in a mild form for many years without complications and thus conservative management may have a place, particularly in the younger asymptomatic patient.

Surgical

The conventional treatment is surgical. Exploration of the neck destroys the natural planes of cleavage and second operations are particularly difficult. It is therefore most important that the diagnosis should be as certain as possible and that exploration is meticulous. If possible, all the parathyroid glands should be identified and an adenoma removed. For hyperplasia, most of the tissue should be removed leaving only a few fragments. Many techniques have been used to help in the localization of a parathyroid adenoma including arteriography, isotope scanning and methylene blue injection but none are satisfactory. Differential venous sampling from the neck for parathyroid hormone assay may prove to be more successful and will perhaps differentiate hyperplasia from adenoma.

Postoperatively, the level of plasma calcium should begin to fall within a few hours and is likely to reach subnormal levels after two to three days, particularly if the patient has osteitis fibrosa and the skeleton is avid for calcium. Thus tetany should be sought and treatment to raise the plasma calcium may be needed with intravenous calcium gluconate, with oral calciferol and calcium supplements (see below). A striking fall in plasma calcium is good evidence that sufficient parathyroid tissue has been removed. In most instances, after a few weeks the remaining parathyroid tissue regains control.

Secondary hyperparathyroidism

This condition is radically different from primary hyperparathyroidism. The secondary form arises as a normal physiological response to a persistently low level of plasma calcium from any cause, but most commonly vitamin D deficiency, intestinal malabsorption or chronic uraemia. Consequently, the plasma calcium level is *always* below normal although if the parathyroid response is vigorous the reduction of plasma calcium may be quite small. The main features will be those of the primary disorder coupled with some of the effects of excess parathyroid hormone. These will be most marked in the skeleton where radiological changes may appear and sometimes symptoms of pain or fractures. Biochemically, the plasma phosphate level falls as phosphate clearance is increased and there is an increased level in the plasma of bone alkaline phosphatase.

Tertiary hyperparathyroidism

In this condition, it is postulated that glands made hyperplastic in secondary hyperparathyroidism may give rise to an adenoma which becomes autonomous. The features then are those of primary hyperparathyroidism with a raised plasma calcium. Previous observation of a persistent low plasma calcium indicate the course of events. The management is as for primary hyperparathyroidism.

Pseudohyperparathyroidism

This term is applied to a condition resembling primary hyperparathyroidism with hypercalcaemia which occurs in association with a malignant tumour arising elsewhere than the parathyroid glands. It is therefore probably part of the spectrum of syndromes of ectopic hormone production in malignant disease.

Anaesthesia and hyperparathyroid disease

Because of early diagnosis, most patients with hyperparathyroidism have only mild hypercalcaemia (below 3·5 mmol/l) are in good general condition and no particular preoperative regime or anaesthetic management is indicated.

With severe hypercalcaemia however, the patient may be gravely ill. The accompanying nausea, vomiting and polyuria lead to dehydration and chloride depletion; renal damage with uraemia and hypertension may be additional features. The main stay of initial treatment is intravenous saline which not only corrects the water and electrolyte balance but also lowers the plasma calcium. Oral phosphate treatment should be started as soon as possible and is effective in further lowering the plasma calcium. Intravenous phosphate may be dangerous and other treatments which have been suggested, such as calcitonin, are effective only occasionally.

HYPOPARATHYROIDISM [6]

Total or partial removal of the parathyroid glands during surgery of the thyroid gland or larynx is by far the commonest cause of hypoparathyroidism. Spontaneous atrophy of the parathyroid glands (which may be familial) does occur but is a rare disease. A transient hypoparathyroidism due to suppression is manifest after removal of a parathyroid adenoma.

A state of relative hypoparathyroidism may be met in which the expected physiological response to a low level of plasma calcium is depressed or absent. Consequently, very low levels of plasma calcium are reached sometimes with tetany, and the usual bone changes of osteitis fibrosa do not appear. The reason for this failure of response is not known; it is most likely to be seen in chronic renal failure.

Clinical

The presenting symptoms of hypoparathyroidism are usually those of increased neuromuscular irritability, being heralded by paraesthesiae around the mouth or in the extremities followed by muscle cramps and stiffness and then tetany or epilepsy. Latent tetany may be sought by eliciting Chvostek's sign which consists of observing a contraction of the facial muscles at the corner of the mouth and in the cheek in response to a tap over the branches of the facial nerve as they emerge from the anterior border of the parotid gland on that side. A positive response should be interpreted with caution because some movement can be seen in many normal persons but a brisk contraction, particularly if it changes with time, is significant. Another test for latent tetany is Trousseau's sign. To elicit this, a sphygmomanometer cuff on the upper arm is inflated until the systolic blood pressure is exceeded and the pressure is then maintained. Muscle spasm in the forearm producing the 'main d'accoucheur' appearance of the hand, as in tetany, does not occur in normal persons in less than three minutes. If it occurs before that the test is positive. An epileptic fit due to hypocalcaemia is indistinguishable from the idiopathic type. Idiopathic hypoparathyroidism is commoner in females than in males and is usually identified in childhood. There may be developmental defects including mental retardation, poor teeth and ectodermal faults. Calcification of the basal ganglia may occur and other central nervous system abnormalities including papilloedema. Cataracts, intestinal dysfunction and psychosis are common. The postoperative form should of course be anticipated and forestalled.

Diagnosis

Diagnosis depends on the demonstration of a low level of plasma calcium in the absence of other causes such as vitamin D deficiency, renal failure or intestinal malabsorption. The level of plasma phosphate is raised above the upper limit of normal of 1·4 mmol/l, but this feature does not help the differentiation from renal failure in which the phosphate is raised also. Radiology of the skeleton is usually normal. Measurement of plasma parathyroid hormone is not yet sufficiently sensitive to detect low levels with certainty.

Treatment

The aim of treatment is to raise the level of plasma calcium to the lower part of the normal range (2·2–2·6 mmol/l) and maintain it there. This level is recommended as it is satisfactory in producing remission of symptoms while minimizing the risks of ectopic calcification and hypercalcaemia.

For urgent treatment a slow intravenous injection of 10 per cent calcium gluconate in a dose of 10 to 20 ml is suitable. In the mild transient postoperative case oral calcium supplements for a few weeks may suffice. In the more severe or permanent condition calciferol is the mainstay of treatment but it has to be used in a dose many times that of normal dietary needs. This uses the toxic property of calciferol of forcing excess intestinal absorption of calcium. The dose must be regulated carefully to individual needs as it is easy to produce hypercalcaemia but almost always 1·25 mg (50 000 units) to 2·5 mg/day is suitable. The standard British National Formulary tablets are 1·25 mg and 0·25 mg, so close adjustment of the dose is possible but requires care in prescribing and compliance. Calciferol is cumulative and very slow-acting. Rapid changes of dose are not useful and alterations once a month or so are better. Long-term follow-up with regular plasma calcium measurements is unavoidable as calciferol requirements may vary with apparently unrelated factors including emotional stress and ovarian function. It is preferable to use calciferol alone in the long term as calcium supplements are inconvenient because of their bulk and administration is likely to be unreliable; it is easier to adjust a single medication. Whether the metabolites of calciferol are superior for treatment remains to be seen. Parathyroid hormone preparations are impure, leading to allergic reactions, have a short duration of action and have to be injected so that they are useless for therapy.

Pseudohypoparathyroidism [6]

This very rare disorder is due to an inherited insensitivity of the renal tubules and the intestinal mucosa to the action of parathyroid hormone. Consequently, the patient presents the biochemical changes and their effects which characterize hypoparathyroidism but the level of parathyroid hormone in the plasma is raised.

REFERENCES

1 BRANSOM CJ, TALBOT CH, HENRY L, ELEMENOGLOU J. Solitary toxic adenoma of the thyroid gland. *Br J Surg* 1979; **66**: 590–5.

2 ECONOMOU SG. Foreword. Endocrine surgery. *Surg Clin North Am* 1979; **59**: 1.

3 EVERED D, HALL R. Foreword. Hypothyroidism and goitre. *Clin Endocrinol Metab* 1979; **8**: 1–2.

4 HABENER JF, SEGRE GV. Parathyroid hormone radioimmunoassay. *Ann Intern Med* 1979; **91**: 782–5.

5 IRVINE WJ, TOFT AD. The diagnosis and treatment of thyrotoxicosis. *Clin Endocrinol* 1976; **5**: 687–707.

6 LEWIN IG, PAPAPOULOS SE, TOMLINSON S, HENDY GN, O'RIORDAN JLH. Studies of hypoparathyroidism and pseudohypoparathyroidism. *Q J Med* 1978; **47**: 533–48.

7 MALLETTE LE, BILEZIKIAN JP, HEATH DA, AURBACH GD. Primary hyperparathyroidism: clinical and biochemical features. *Medicine* (Baltimore) 1974; **53**: 127–46

8 MILLER JM, HAMBURGER JI, KINI S. Diagnosis of thyroid nodules. Use of fine-needle aspiration and needle biopsy. *JAMA* 1979; **241**: 481–4.

9 VOPLE R. Foreword. Thyrotixicosis. *Clin Endocrinol Metab* 1978; **7**: 1–2.

10 ZONSZEIN J, SANTANGELO RP, MACKIN JF, LEE TC, COFFEY RJ, CANARY JJ. Propranolol therapy in thyrotoxicosis. A review of 84 patients undergoing surgery. *Am J Med* 1979; **66**: 411–16.

Chapter 17
Connective Tissue Diseases

B. McCONKEY

RHEUMATIC DISEASES

Connective tissue is not merely an inert supportive framework. Wherever found, from the extremes of the loose skin below the eye to dense tendon, it consists of three components—cells, fibres and ground substance. Different connective tissues are characterized by different proportions of these elements, by differences in their array or occasionally, as in bone, by the addition of mineral salts.

The cells. These are either (a) intrinsic—cells derived from embryonic mesenchyme with the capacity of differentiation to fibroblasts, chondroblasts or osteoblasts, or (b) extrinsic—granulocytes, plasma cells, lymphocytes. The role of the former is to synthesize connective tissue elements, of the latter to serve their usual functions of scavenging and antibody formation.

The fibres. There are three types, the most important being collagen, a fibrous protein consisting of helical chains of amino acids. The amount and array of collagen in connective tissue gives it its characteristics. The other fibres, elastin and reticulin, are present in small amounts and little is known of their function or their relation to collagen.

The ground substance. This is a watery gel of polymeric glycosaminoglycans (i.e. acid mucopolysaccharides) bound to globular protein molecules. The nature of the ground substance differs in different tissues. Its role is to provide a milieu for transport of ions, to contribute to some extent to the physical characteristics of a tissue and probably also to modulate collagen fibre maturation. All three components are involved in continuous turnover under control of physiological mechanisms including hormones such as growth hormone, corticosteroids and thyroxine.

Disorders of the connective tissue elements themselves comprise two contrasting groups, the very common degenerative diseases (osteoarthrosis and its consequences) and the rare, inherited connective tissue disorders. Most other connective tissue diseases have a vascular component as a major factor. Many of them are called 'collagen diseases' but this is a misleading term; collagen is seldom involved except incidentally.

Surveys of rheumatic complaints in various populations show that the most common is degenerative disease or its consequences. The real problem is, however, rheumatoid arthritis (RA); it accounts for about 10 per cent of all rheumatic complaints and its prevalence is probably about 3 per cent of the general population (although, adopting different diagnostic criteria, estimates have ranged from 0·5 per cent to 10 per cent). More than this, it is economically important in loss of working time and is a much more devastating disease than osteoarthrosis. Other disorders in this field, accounting for perhaps 10 per cent of all cases, are diverse and range from trivial to fatal.

INHERITED CONNECTIVE TISSUE DISORDERS

It would be tidy if one could group these by disorders of each of the main elements. Unfortunately this cannot be done as they are to some extent interdependent: collagen fibre array for instance probably being partly determined by the glycosaminoglycan matrix which is in turn dependent on the cell. However, certain syndromes have been delineated. The subject has been reviewed by McKusick [2] and only two of the commoner of these disorders will be described.

OSTEOGENESIS IMPERFECTA (FRAGILITAS OSSIUM)

This syndrome is characterized by brittle bones, blue sclerae, thin skin, deafness and a tam o'shanter deformity of the skull (i.e. prominent occiput). It is a fairly rare disorder and one of the few true *collagen* diseases. The bones are brittle because the collagen framework is defective and this defect has been observed in collagen in other parts of the body. The sclera is blue, for instance, simply because it is thin and pigment is easily seen through it. There is a tendency for the bones to become less brittle if patients survive the early years. Repeated fractures may lead to deformities of importance in anaesthesia, for instance a kyphoscoliosis from vertebral body collapse.

MARFAN'S SYNDROME

The features are an abnormal length of the extremities relative to the trunk (arachnodactyly, for instance) with a high, arched palate. There is often difficulty in deciding whether a tall patient has the Marfan defect or not. Probably the most reliable guide is comparison of crown to pubis, with pubis to heel measurements; if the lower segment exceeds the upper segment by more than three inches the diagnosis becomes more likely.

Patients with this defect, thought to be a fault in collagen array, are prone to dislocation of the lens of the eye, to spontaneous pneumothorax and, less often, to aneurysm of the aorta.

DEGENERATIVE DISEASE—'OSTEOARTHROSIS'

This group constitutes by far the largest cause for rheumatic complaints; nearly all of them, however, are either self-limiting or can be completely or largely controlled. Thus, though numerically important they do not prove as great a problem as the inflammatory arthropathies or other connective tissue diseases.

Connective tissue, like any other, changes with age. Such age changes are exacerbated by injury or wear and by other influences as yet ill-understood. Evidence is accumulating that in some instances hitherto regarded as 'degenerative', a chronic inflammatory process of unknown aetiology exerts a major effect. Though some people have thrown doubt on the importance of obesity it is probably still true to say that the knees of an obese elderly person are more likely to show degenerative change than those of someone who is young and thin. Similarly, age affects the connective tissue which retains the intervertebral discs, and probably the disc itself and a sudden strain may lead to rupture of the tissues with herniation of the disc. It is perhaps worth commenting that disc prolapse and age are not highly correlated so that more than one factor clearly operates. It is easy to see that a very wide range of disorders come into the group. However, certain common syndromes stand out.

PRIMARY OSTEOARTHROSIS

This common disorder was not really recognized as an entity till about 20 years ago. It most often affects middle-aged women, is polyarticular and characteristically affects the distal finger and first carpometacarpal joints; bony prominences (Heberden's nodes) at the distal finger joints are usual. It may however involve any joint. Patients usually complain of a variety of pains, seldom severe but worse in cold and damp weather. The disease is primarily a disorder of articular cartilage, probably an alteration in the collagen and glycosaminoglycans, though changes in nearby connective tissue structures such as joint capsules and bone are usual. The latter changes are thought to be due to the increased vascularity, itself a response to the changes in the joint. The aetiology and pathogenesis are not understood; age changes in the connective tissue elements are a major factor but an inherited predisposition is well documented and chronic inflammation has been shown to be present though its role is not clear (hence revival of the osteoarthrosis/itis argument). Environmental factors and diet have also been thought to play a part.

The diagnosis is a clinical one, which can often be confirmed by the X-ray changes —narrowing of joint spaces from thinning of articular cartilage, bone cysts and osteophytes. There are no helpful laboratory investigations.

Treatment often needs to be started with a warning; the remedy can be worse than the disease. Osteoarthrosis seldom cripples, it does not kill; some drugs do. Physiotherapy may help through the application of heat; warm tissues have a higher pain threshold than cold tissues. There may also be a need to strengthen muscle groups. Drug therapy is aimed at the relief of pain and this group of drugs is described in the section on rheumatoid arthritis.

Not infrequently, especially when a major weightbearing joint is involved, treatment has to be surgical, either by osteotomy to realign the joint, or more usually nowadays by joint replacement.

SECONDARY OSTEOARTHROSIS

If a joint surface is damaged by misalignment from a healed fracture, by infection or haemorrhage, or by an inflammatory arthropathy, then degenerative changes are hastened. The cartilage becomes thinner and the complex mechanism of joint lubrication becomes defective. As with primary osteoarthrosis, locally increased vascularity results in changes in nearby structures and osteophytes form by calcification in joint ligaments. Depending on the site of the joint there may or may not be symptoms. In the spine, gross changes on X-ray are often seen as incidental findings and it is better not to draw attention to them. In hips, knees or ankles, however, symptoms soon appear. Treatment is the same as for primary osteoarthrosis.

NONARTICULAR SYNDROMES

'Rheumatism'

Many patients complain of pains they describe as 'rheumatics' and for which there is no obvious explanation. The diagnoses of fibrositis or panniculitis which were formerly common are now thought to be no more meaningful than the term 'rheumatism'. The importance of this group, however, is that the pain may have some sinister origin and each case needs careful consideration. This must include a history paying particular attention to the duration and site of the pain and the factors affecting it. 'Rheumatism' as an entity of unknown cause, is a term used to describe a recurring pain aggravated by cold weather. It is self-limiting and treatment is rarely necessary. If the picture deviates from this then some other explanation must be sought, the most likely one being the commonest disorder—osteoarthrosis. However, many other conditions including inflammatory arthropathies, disorders of muscle, neurological disease, myelomatosis or a neoplasm might have to be considered. Screening procedures should include a chest X-ray and ESR; further investigation would depend on clinical clues.

Intervertebral disc lesions

Intervertebral discs consist of a gelatinous material composed of collagen and glycosaminoglycans; the material is retained above and below by the cartilage covering the end plates of the vertebral bodies and at the circumference by a tough fibrous ring (the annulus fibrosus) which is largely composed of collagen. Herniation of disc material into vertebral bodies, through the cartilage end plates is common; it leads to the X-ray appearance known as Schmorl's nodes and does not appear to be associated with symptoms. However, if the material protrudes anteriorly or laterally it may compress the spinal cord or a nerve root. This may occur at any age; when it occurs in younger patients it is usually because of an abnormally large strain. With increasing age, however, both the annulus and the disc material alter and the strain required to extrude disc material is less though disc problems are unusual after middle age.

Disc prolapse occurs more often in the lower lumbar region than other parts of the spine, leading to the syndromes of 'lumbago' or 'sciatica'. Backache is a common prelude; then, often abruptly, and without an obvious precipitating factor there is pain which can be recognized as being within the area of a myotome or dermatome. The commonest sites for a prolapsed disc are at the L4/5 and L5/S1 levels leading to the classic picture of sciatica, pain in the lower back, buttock, back of the thigh and often down to the lower leg. Physical signs may be merely those of nerve root irritation, pain on flexion of the spine and on stretching the sciatic nerve by 'straight leg raising'. Alternatively, with a large protrusion there may be signs of nerve root compression with the appropriate motor and sensory deficits and loss of reflexes; rarely there may be disturbances of bowel and bladder function. The diagnosis should be made on clinical grounds. X-rays usually show degenerative changes and may show a narrowed disc space. If the history is atypical and there is a suspicion of some alternative cause for the nerve root compression, myelography may help.

The treatment of a prolapsed disc, in the absence of a major cord or cauda equina compression, is to rest until the disc material has shrunk and fibrosed. Thus, bed rest for about ten days and then physiotherapy to restore muscle tone and strength followed by mobilization is a rational regime. Some authorities believe in earlier physiotherapy, some in traction, some in manipulation but the relative merits of these measures are not established.

In selected cases some have advocated extradural injections of various kinds by the caudal or lumbar routes, particularly in patients with lumbar or sacral root pain. Large volumes of saline (50 ml) have been advocated in an endeavour to break down 'adhesions'. Comparable quantities of dilute local analgesics have been employed to facilitate pain-free movement. There does not seem to be any difference in the results between these alternatives. Injection of methyl prednisolone has been found to be equally or more effective, and in such circumstances neither of the postulated mechanisms apply.

Although there have been suggestions that acute, recurrent, or chronic cases may respond differently, approximately 30 per cent of patients are completely relieved of residual pain, another 20 per cent are improved and about 50 per cent are not benefited whatever procedure is employed. It has recently been suggested that injection of chymopapain to disrupt the disc material may be beneficial.

It is difficult to be dogmatic about how long to persist with conservative treatment, but if after six weeks there are still signs of nerve root compression, surgery is probably indicated assuming that investigation confirms the diagnosis.

The second commonest part of the spine to be affected by degenerative disease is the cervical where, as with other areas of the spine, the proportion with abnormal X-rays exceeds the number with symptoms. A familiar syndrome is the middle-aged person with pain in the neck diagnosed as cervical spondylosis when the X-rays show osteophytes, narrowed disc spaces, and narrowing of the spinal canal or of the intervertebral foramina. The pain is characteristically on movement and is often troublesome at night. An important physical sign is diminished lateral flexion of the neck. When frank disc prolapse occurs there is the same pattern of symptoms and signs as in lumbar disc protrusion. The treatment either for spondylosis or disc prolapse is conservative, a collar may help, unless the severity of the lesion is such that surgery is necessary. Pain relief may be achieved with simple analgesics but they may have to be supplemented by so-called antirheumatic drugs (see below).

Other syndromes

As almost any tendon, bursa or ligament can be involved in traumatic or inflammatory lesions the number of possible conditions occurring in this group is rather large. Copeman [1] should be consulted for a comprehensive review. However, two conditions deserve comment here because they are common, often severely disabling, and treatable.

'*Frozen shoulder*' is familiar to most clinicians. Sometimes spontaneously, sometimes during the course of a connective tissue disease, sometimes after a period of bed rest for any disease (e.g. myocardial infarct) patients get pain in the shoulder with marked diminution in the range of movement; X-rays show no abnormality. There is inflammation of the joint capsule or nearby ligamentous structures but the reason why the shoulder, rather than any other joint, is so often involved is not known. Conservative treatment with physiotherapy and analgesics will usually result in spontaneous resolution after weeks or months. If a particularly tender area can be located, injection of a corticosteroid can speed recovery.

The '*carpal tunnel syndrome*' is often overlooked. It may occur as an isolated disorder or may complicate rheumatoid arthritis. Occasionally it is the first manifestation of a generalized connective tissue disease, and sometimes forms part of a disorder not usually thought of as rheumatic, such as, for example, myxoedema. It may even complicate pregnancy. The onset of this syndrome should be the signal to consider the patient as a whole even though the local symptoms dominate the picture.

The carpal tunnel is a channel formed by the carpal bones with the flexor retinaculum across it. Through this channel, with little space to spare, run a number of flexor tendons and the median nerve. The latter can easily be compressed. Presenting symptoms may be misleading; classically there is pain in the wrist and hand with paraesthesiae in the fingers (sparing the fifth). Actually pain is often of much wider distribution, sometimes affecting the whole arm; it is worse at night. The physical signs are those of a median nerve lesion at that point; sensory loss in the index, middle and ring fingers with weakness and wasting of the thenar muscles. If the diagnosis is in doubt, as is often the case, electromyography may help by showing delay in conduction. Treatment is a surgical division of the flexor retinaculum. Diuretics or corticosteroid injections occasionally help but these measures are almost always merely procrastination. It is worth reiterating that treatment should follow careful consideration of the cause.

INFLAMMATORY ARTHROPATHIES

RHEUMATOID ARTHRITIS

PRESENTATION

This disease affects perhaps 2 per cent of the population. Refinements of diagnostic criteria are of great importance to the epidemiologist; for him there may be a problem with, for instance, suspicious X-rays but not symptoms but this will not present as a clinical problem. Nevertheless, epidemiological work has made it possible to set out generalizations. Rheumatoid arthritis is, typically, a symmetrical arthropathy most often involving proximal interphalangeal joints, metacarpophalangeal joints, wrists and ankles. Knees are also often affected. Indeed any joint can be involved except the distal interphalangeal joints, and this distinguishes it from primary osteoarthrosis. Joints are painful, swollen and warm but seldom red. Morning stiffness is usual but occurs with any inflammatory arthropathy. These clinical features alone do not make the diagnosis certain though their presence for more than six weeks makes it highly likely. Nodules, most typically found just below the elbow on the ulnar surface, are pathognomic. Further evidence can be gained by X-raying the joints and examining serum for the presence of rheumatoid factor.

When the clinical picture and X-ray changes are typical and rheumatoid factor is present, there is no diagnostic problem. A proportion of patients, however, do not fulfil all these criteria; an example is a persistent monoarthritis when a biopsy of synovium may help. Even so there can be difficulties and it may be necessary to consider other causes of arthropathy such as sarcoidosis, the 'soluble complex arthritides', peripheral involvement in ankylosing spondylitis, Reiter's disease and systemic lupus erythematosus.

AETIOLOGY AND PATHOLOGY (WITH A NOTE ON SOLUBLE COMPLEX DISEASE)

It is not yet quite certain that rheumatoid arthritis is a single disease. Rheumatoid arthritis can start at any age but most often does so between 25 and 55 years, affecting women about three times as often as men. There is clearly a familial influence though it cannot be stated more strongly than that. Psychological stress and trauma have been considered as possible precipitating factors but remain unproven. Environment has not been shown to be an influence though it may modify the disease after onset. Endocrine and metabolic disorders have been exhaustively investigated—largely with negative results. The current view on the aetiology of rheumatoid arthritis involves the trio of infection, hypersensitivity and autoimmunity. An infective agent has long been sought and occasionally reported though such reports were never confirmed. By analogy with rheumatic fever it has been argued that an infective agent initiates the diseases in individuals who are susceptible, for instance via hypersensitivity. Further evidence to support this idea is that there is a correlation between rheumatoid arthritis and the tissue antigen HLA DrW4. If this were the case then a search for an initiating organism might well be unrewarding unless carried out very early or even in a hypothetical prodromal phase. Such a mechanism might account too for the familial influence and in general it would fit most of the facts. However, diseases such as rheumatic fever are not self-perpetuating; it is at this point that autoimmunity is invoked. One suggestion is that an initiating agent, perhaps one of several possible infective microorganisms, might precipitate a hypersensitivity reaction; in the course of this, antibody might be formed which reacted with complexes composed partly of the initiating agent and partly of antibodies to that antigen. Thus antibody would have been formed which reacted partly to 'self' tissue components. The stage for a perpetuating autoimmune disorder would then be set. There is no direct evidence for this hypothesis but it is in accord both with the association between rheumatoid arthritis and other diseases thought to be autoimmune (i.e. systemic lupus erythematosus, thyroiditis, Sjögren's syndrome), and with the phenomenon of rheumatoid factor.

Classical rheumatoid factor is a serum protein (M Wt approx. 900,000) of the IgM class, characterized by its property of reacting with altered IgG. The alteration in IgG is effected by heating or by application to the surface of a red cell or an inert particle such as latex. The tests usually carried out to demonstrate rheumatoid factor in serum depend on these properties. In the RA latex test rabbit IgG is applied to latex particles; if added serum contains rheumatoid factor this reacts with the altered IgG causing the latex particles to clump. A quantitative RA latex test can thus be done by serial dilutions of the serum. In the Rose-Waaler test rabbit IgG is applied to sheep's red cells but the principle is otherwise the same; reaction of rheumatoid factor with the 'sensitized' cells causes them to clump. The RA latex test is more sensitive and consequently less specific than the Rose-Waaler, but when suspect sera are diluted results for the two methods have a linear correlation. Thus either test may be used and many laboratories are now using the quantitative RA latex test rather than the classical Rose-Waaler because it is cheaper and quicker. The RA latex test is positive in a number of diseases other than rheumatoid arthritis (subacute bacterial endocarditis, some forms of liver disease).

It is now known that there is a 'family' of rheumatoid factors, which should be more accurately called antiglobulins, not all of them IgM. Methods for their assay are still at a development stage and the story is clearly far from complete; Holborow has provided a recent review [1].

Apart from being markers suggestive of an autoimmune process and apart from their use as a diagnostic, and to some extent prognostic, guide it is difficult to assign a pathological role to rheumatoid factors. Like any antibody they have been shown to be formed in plasma cells, often in synovial tissue, but the significance in pathogenesis is still debated.

Rheumatoid arthritis is a generalized disease which can affect any tissue, but two

18*

patterns of tissue response can be recognized. The main feature is, of course, the joint lesion; there is proliferation of synovial tissue accompanied by an increase locally in cells (lymphocytes and plasma cells) usually associated with immune phenomena. This proliferation, with an inflammatory response, accounts for the swelling, pain and warmth of an affected joint. Inflammation of any serious membrane usually leads to an exudate; hence joint effusions are common. At a later stage the proliferating synovium invades nearby tissue such as bones, tendons, and ligaments and this accounts for the local destructive changes of rheumatoid arthritis. The cause of this proliferation is unknown but is presumably a reaction to the inflammatory/immune process; the mechanism of destructive changes is, superficially at any rate, easier to explain since high concentrations of enzymes such as collagenases, which are normally intracellular can be shown by histochemical techniques at the leading edge of synovial proliferation. The enzymes are thought to be liberated from ruptured lysosomes.

The other, mainly extra-articular, lesions of rheumatoid arthritis are believed to be the consequence of vasculitis, itself probably resulting from deposition of immune complexes in the walls of small vessels with a subsequent inflammatory reaction. This process can occur anywhere and could account for such diverse extra-articular manifestations as neuropathy and pulmonary fibrosis. It may even be the factor initiating synovial proliferation; if so it would be central to the whole problem but this is, at this stage, mere speculation.

Soluble complex disease

Complexes between antigen and antibody, where there is excess antibody, are insoluble and eliminated without harm by the reticuloendothelial system. Where there is excess antigen, however, the complexes are usually soluble and may be deposited in blood vessels where they then evoke an inflammatory reaction. Such a mechanism is now thought to be at least a factor in diseases such as glomerulonephritis and rheumatoid arthritis. Moreover the mechanism probably explains the arthropathy following rubella or hepatitis and in serum sickness (e.g. penicillin sensitivity with arthropathy). In some such disorders, rubella, for example, the arthropathy may mimic, though transiently, rheumatoid arthritis; the antigen is a virus. The implications are obviously of great interest. The topic is discussed in greater detail later.

EXTRA-ARTICULAR MANIFESTATIONS

The reported prevalence of some extra-articular manifestations is closely correlated with the enthusiasm of the observer. It is valuable to keep a sense of proportion and remember that although this is a generalized disease, occasionally critically affecting the vasculature of a leg for example, it is most often a disease of joints.

Nodules

These are regarded as a hallmark of rheumatoid arthritis, occurring in about 25 per cent of clinically diagnosed cases. They are usually to be found at pressure points, specially just below the elbow on the ulnar surface. They are firm and usually mobile. Histologically, they consist of a central necrotic portion with a surrounding zone of lymphocytes, plasma cells and fibroblasts. They probably reflect the occurrence of vasculitis, and are only seen in patients who have positive rheumatoid factor tests.

Neurological disorders

These are so frequent as to affect nearly all cases of longstanding rheumatoid arthritis at some time. The commonest disorders have a mechanical cause and include the carpal tunnel syndrome, entrapment of the ulnar nerve at the elbow and involvement of the spine (most often cervical) leading to nerve root compression on myelopathy. A particularly important problem is that of subluxation at the atlanto-axial joint which may represent a special hazard during anaesthesia. Less often a neuropathy may be part of the rheumatoid arthritis, probably from vasculitis affecting the vasa nervorum; this type of neuropathy may be a mononeuritis, a diffuse sensory neuropathy or rarely a sensorimotor neuropathy. This last type is usually part of a particularly severe so-called malignant rheumatoid arthritis and widespread evidence of vasculitis is found; the prognosis is grave.

Pulmonary disorders

The commonest is probably pleural effusion, usually small and seen early in the disease. It is seldom even noticed at the time and only rarely requires treatment. Less often there may be pulmonary fibrosis which may be of any severity. Occasionally it is the presenting finding, the patient only subsequently complaining of joint symptoms. This type of lung involvement is particularly likely to occur in coal miners and it may be hard to differentiate it from pneumoconiosis. When the X-ray shows rounded opacities as well as fibrosis in a miner with rheumatoid arthritis it is given the name Caplan's syndrome. Solitary lung nodules sometimes lead to diagnostic difficulties and may be mistaken for a neoplasm.

Ocular

The commonest lesion is episcleritis; it is usually intermittent and mild and responds to simple local therapy. Less often a more serious scleritis may develop; it is more painful than episcleritis and if suspected an expert opinion is urgently necessary. Treatment is usually with corticosteroids which may, incidentally, sometimes be required even for the milder episcleritis.

A well-known ocular disorder, kerato-conjunctivitis sicca, occurs in up to 10 per cent of patients with rheumatoid arthritis as part of Sjögren's syndrome, the other complaints being aerostomia and salivary gland enlargement. Patients complain of dry, gritty eyes which easily become red. The cause is a loss of tears from involvement of lacrimal glands, and the same process involves salivary glands. Diagnosis is made by testing for tear production by a Schirmer strip; treatment is to lubricate the eye artificially with methyl cellulose, It has been observed that patients with this complication are more at risk from the adverse effects of various drugs.

Drugs account for another ocular problem; some antimalarials may, if administered over long periods at high dosage, lead to a severe retinopathy which does not recover when the drug is stopped. Corticosteroids occasionally lead to cataract.

Cutaneous vasculitis

Vasculitis may well be the fundamental tissue reaction in rheumatoid arthritis. Moreover, it is responsible for nearly all the extra-articular troubles, both those already mentioned and lesions in almost any other organ. When vasculitis affects the skin there are small (about 1 mm) areas of gangrene at the nail folds. The phenomenon is not very common, usually occurs in patients with nodules, a high RW titre and severe disease; it indicates a poor prognosis not merely for the rheumatoid arthritis but for life expectancy. Other cutaneous manifestations of vasculitis include leg ulcers and occasionally gangrene of extremities.

Haematological

The changes in the blood in rheumatoid arthritis result partly from the disease and partly from treatment. Anaemia is almost invariable; erythpoiesis is depressed, iron is probably not normally utilized and there is often blood loss from the gut due to the effects of drugs. There is also a high incidence of folate deficiency.

Felty's syndrome is a picture of hypersplenism complicating rheumatoid arthritis. Splenomegaly, neutropenia, anaemia, lymphadenopathy and sometimes thrombocytopenia occur. The cause is not known but it appears to be another of the disturbances of the immune system seen in rheumatoid arthritis. Splenectomy may sometimes be necessary.

MANAGEMENT OF RHEUMATOID ARTHRITIS

General measures

Rest is beneficial as in any inflammatory disorder. Putting patients with rheumatoid arthritis to bed is often helpful at an early stage but for obvious reasons can only be regarded as a temporary measure.

If there is anaemia an attempt should be made to correct it.

Drugs

All patients need, from the outset, adequate treatment with nonsteroid anti-inflammatory drugs (NSAID). All the NSAID's have three properties in common but to different degrees—analgesic, anti-inflammatory and maybe antipyretic. They are more effective than simple analgesics in the treatment of a rheumatic disorder; their greater efficiency is thought to be due to their anti-inflammatory effect. Various mechanisms, including stabilization of lysosomes and inhibition of prostaglandin synthesis, have been proposed to explain this effect. There are now many drugs in this group with fresh ones being added at the rate of two or three a year. It is never easy to know which is the best and, as with many groups of drugs, it is wise to become familiar with a few, sticking to those with a reputation not only for efficacy but also safety. Cost, of course, can also be a factor. Table 17.1 should help selection; most people would probably still choose soluble aspirin first, though the propionic acid derivatives are becoming popular. There is a commonly held impression that these drugs have an effect on the course of the disease, but one should not expect them to do more than alleviate symptoms and perhaps reduce swelling. Three points need emphasis. Firstly, phenylbutazone is an effective drug and is widely used because of this; there is however a risk of blood dyscrasia and alternatives ought to be considered. Secondly, nearly all the NSAID's displace anticoagulants from plasma binding sites and therefore must not be given to a patient receiving anticoagulants unless special

Table 17.1. Nonsteroid anti-inflammatory drugs.

Approved name	Trade name	*Cost of 7 days' treatment	No. of tabs/day	Tablet size	Comments	Other preparations available +other trade names
		p		mg		
Aspirin:						
Soluble	B.P.	42	16	300	Nausea+ indigestion common	Solprin Claradin Laboprin
Micro- encapsulated	Levius	59	8	500		
Glycinated	Paynocil	50	6	600	Large	
'Enteric-coated'	Caprin	158	16	324	number of	Breoprin, Nu-seals
Aloxiprin	Palaprin	130	10	600	tabs/day	
Bendrylate	Benoral	150	6	750		also suspension
Salgalate	Disalcid	90	8	500		—costly
Indomethacin	Imbrolin	155	4	50	? Risk of gastric ulcer	Suppositories +Indocid +Tannex
Tolmetin	Tolectin	943	9	200	New expensive	
Phenylbutazone	Butazolidin	28	3	100	Risk of marrow	Suppositories Butacote+injection
Oxphenbutazone	Tanderil	58	3	100	suppression	Parazolidin Suppositores Tandacote
Propionic acid derivatives:						
Ibuprofen	Brufen	97	3	400		Also syrup
Ketoprofen	Alrheumat	163	4	50		Suppositories+Orudis
Flurbiprofen	Froben	164	3	100		
Fenbufen	Lederfen	341	3	300	New drug	
Fenoprofen	Fenopron	382	5	600		Progesic
Naproxen	Naprosyn	248	2	500		Suppositories+ suspension+Synflex
Diclofenac	Voltarol	245	2	50		
Fenclofenac	Flenac	271	3	300	Rashes	
Sulindac	Clinoril	249	2	200		
Azopropazone	Rheumex	189	4	300		
Feprazone	Methrazone	203	3	200	Rashes	
Piroxicam	Feldene	210	2	10	New drug	

* Cheapest preparation—source MIMS 1980.

precautions are taken. Thirdly, studies have shown that there is marked individual variation in responsiveness to a particular drug; thus the alert clinician will have a wide repertoire.

If more is required of a drug, as is often the case, a different group of drugs ('second line', 'long-acting') have to be used. At a reasonable interval after starting treatment with NSAID's there are some questions needing answers

How well are symptoms controlled?
How active is the disease?
Is it likely to progress?

They are, of course, interdependent. Persisting inflammation in the joints, duration of morning stiffness, degree of functional disability, are all useful guides. A distinction has to be made between functional loss from inflammation and functional loss from tissue destruction; the former may be reversible whereas the latter is not amenable to drug therapy. The presence of nodules, and evidence of extra-articular manifestations in general, suggest a bad outlook.

Of the laboratory investigations, an ESR persistently raised above 40 mm/hr (by the Westergren method) suggests poorly controlled disease unless there is some other explanation such as an intercurrent infection. The ESR is occasionally misleadingly low. It is better to measure one of the 'acute phase proteins'; these are a class of serum proteins, mainly glycoproteins, whose levels in the blood are raised in inflammation. The best known is C-reactive protein; so long as measurements are accurate (usually by radial immunodiffusion) the test is more sensitive than the ESR. The rheumatoid factor test provides some information on prognosis, high titres being associated with a bad outlook.

The radiological changes in rheumatoid arthritis progress from periarticular osteoporosis at an early stage, to erosions (Fig. 17.1), cartilage thinning and later to

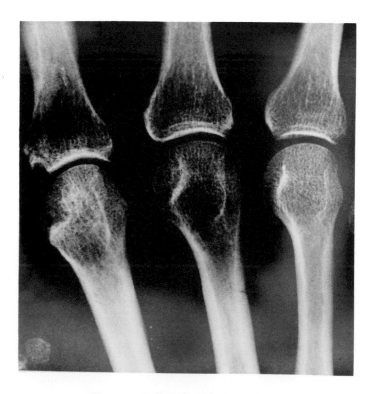

Fig. 17.1. Typical rheumatoid erosions.

severe deformities or bony ankylosis. If there is evidence of erosions at an early stage, the disease is likely to be severe.

Assuming control is inadequate and progression probable, it is necessary to proceed to what may be called second line drugs. Although some people have argued that no drug affects the course of rheumatoid arthritis, most experienced rheumatologists now believe that disease activity can be lowered; thus, though there is no cure, progression can be slowed, sometimes dramatically. There is argument about which drug to select at this point, but gold is probably still favourite. The drug, given as sodium aurothiomalate ('*Myocrisin*') has been shown to be superior to a placebo but its mode of action is unexplained. The usual dose is 50 mg weekly by intramuscular injection for 20 weeks then 50 mg fortnightly. Benefit from treatment is seldom detectable earlier than 12 weeks and is progressive up to about nine months in patients who respond. Long continued maintenance therapy is necessary and patients who stop the drug after less than a year usually relapse 3–4 months later. This is an important point for a second course of gold is less effective; if therefore gold is stopped because of some intercurrent event (e.g. herniorraphy) and not begun again soon, much may be lost. It is often difficult to judge how long to continue gold treatment; application of the same rules of assessment as described above helps greatly. Unfortunately gold is fairly toxic; about a third of all patients develop side-effects. Commonest are skin irritation, rashes and proteinuria. These are minor problems as a rule so long as gold is promptly stopped. The more serious side-effects are thrombocytopenia or even total marrow suppression. Opinions differ on how closely to monitor patients for adverse effects; a reasonable practical procedure is for the person giving the injection to make general enquiries about health and to test the urine each time. Some advocate weekly blood counts but monthly counts are usually sufficient; it is extremely rare to get warning of impeding thrombocytopenia and probably better to enquire about abnormal bruising than rely on platelet counts.

Some alternatives to gold are chloroquine, penicillamine, immunosuppressants or corticosteroids. Occasionally levamisole, dapsone and sulphasalazine will be used.

Chloroquine (or hydroxychloroquine) usually regarded as an antimalarial, was shown to be effective in systemic lupus erythematosus. Controlled trials later showed an effect in rheumatoid arthritis. The effect is, however, rather weak and the potential side-effect—retinopathy with permanent visual loss—is daunting. If used at all, it is wise to select a moderate dose (400 mg daily) for about six months and allow at least six months between courses of treatment. This drug is used much less than it used to be; the alert doctor will more often want to stop the patient having it than start it.

Penicillamine, an amino acid constituting part of the penicillin molecule was introduced rather tentatively as a treatment for rheumatoid arthritis ten years ago. The rationale at that time was that, apart from its well-known chelating effect in Wilson's disease, it has the property of dissociating macroglobulins; the assumption was made that if it dissociated rheumatoid factor, which it did, clinical benefit might ensue. Subsequent trials have confirmed it to be an effective drug but it is still too early to say what its place in a scheme of treatment should be. Recently it has rivalled gold as first choice among second line drugs. The starting dose should be no more than 125 mg daily, and increments small and widely spread. Side-effects are frequent, the most serious being nephrotic syndrome thrombocytopenia or leucopenia: a myasthenic syndrome has been described; fortunately they are usually reversible when the drug is stopped.

Whether penicillamine acts, as was originally supposed, by dissociation of rheumatoid factor, is not certain. It has a rather similar effect on collagen, is a chelating agent for copper and serum copper levels are said to be raised in rheumatoid arthritis, and may have antiviral properties.

Immunosuppressant therapy

The use of cyclophosphamide or azothioprine (i.e. cytotoxic drugs) is still a relatively new therapy for rheumatoid arthritis. Some trials suggest efficacy comparable with gold but it is too early to generalize. The risks are those attached to immunosuppressant therapy in general (marrow suppression, infections, malignancy) with the additional factor that the drugs may have been given for long periods; rheumatoid arthritis, unlike other diseases treated with these drugs, is not usually fatal. The rationale of immunosuppressant therapy is, of course, based on current theories of aetiology which invoke an autoimmune reaction.

Corticosteroids may have to be considered as an alternative. The discovery that cortisone was an effective remedy for rheumatoid arthritis nearly 30 years ago, injected new life into the field; the effects were dramatic and in potency far exceeded any other treatment. This is probably still the case at least in the short term. However, the side-effects are numerous and may be lethal.

If the decision is made to use oral steroids it is better to confine the choice to prednisolone for none of the numerous analogues have been shown to be superior and some have a greater incidence of side-effects. A suitable dose for long-term management would be not more than 7·5 mg prednisolone daily. It is unwise to alter the dose frequently; such action may increase the frequency of side-effects. Even with smaller doses the adrenals are suppressed; the dangers of sudden cessation of treatment are well known. As an alternative to oral therapy a depot intramuscular preparation can be used; methyl prednisolone ('Depomedrone') is helpful and a dose of 80 mg weekly, either as a single weekly injection or in two doses, is roughly equivalent to 10 mg prednisolone daily. The drug is useful when it is necessary to avoid oral therapy for, say, a week or two and frequent injections of hydrocortisone can be avoided. Some authorities prefer to use ACTH. This does have the advantage of a lower rate of side-effects but necessitates injections daily or on alternate days. A dose of 40 units ACTH gel on alternative days is roughly equivalent to 10 mg prednisone daily. On the whole long-term steroid treatment begun late in the disease is to be avoided if possible. The real place for these drugs is early in particularly severe disease, during especially severe exacerbations or to treat some extra-articular manifestations.

Physiotherapy

This plays a much smaller part in management than it used to. Warming the tissues either by lamps, short wave diathermy or wax baths for hands is comforting: pain is relieved probably by increasing the pain threshold. A more important role for physiotherapy is to strengthen muscle groups by selective exercises, for instance, to maintain power and tone in quadriceps muscles in a patient whose knee is painful. As the role of the physiotherapist diminishes that of the *occupational therapist* and *surgical appliance* makers increases. Much can be done to ease a patient's lot at home or at work by such things as night splints, special shoes and special gadgets in the kitchen.

Special situations

In some patients one joint, for example a knee, is so painful that it dominates the clinical picture. It is clearly illogical to give systemic therapy for a local problem. The first approach to consider is the injection of intra-articular corticosteroid. This is often a useful procedure but the benefit may be transient. If so the joint should be re-examined and X-rayed; removal of proliferating synovium (synovectomy) may be effective when there has been little bone damage.

A possible alternative, medical synovectomy by the injection of radioactive substances (e.g. yttrium, erbium), is undergoing trial and is said by some to be promising. It is not, however, only by synovectomies that the orthopaedic surgeon can help. Removal of nodules, repair of tendons, replacement of joints, are often strikingly successful; the surgical management of rheumatoid arthritis is a growing point in the subject.

ANAESTHESIA IN RHEUMATOID ARTHRITIS

The problems that confront the anaesthetist may arise both from the medical complaints and from their treatment; a personal preoperative evaluation is essential. Table 17.2 summarized the investigations that should be available.

Table 17.2. Preoperative assessment in rheumatoid arthritis.

All cases
Chest X-ray, neck X-ray
Blood picture
ECG
Urinalysis
Lung function tests—including blood gases
Drug history
Anaesthetic history

If indicated
Skeletal X-rays
Creatine clearance
Occult blood
Indirect laryngoscopy

The airway

Involvement of the temporomandibular joint may make visualization of the larynx difficult or impossible. This may be aggravated by limitation of movement in the cervical spine, atlanto-axial or low cervical luxation and hypoplastic mandible. Blind nasal intubation is often the method of choice. If there is doubt concerning the safety of the airway in the unconscious state, intubation under local anaesthesia with the patient awake may be necessary.

Airway problems may extend to the larynx itself. A significant incidence of crico-arytenoid arthritis is found in rheumatoid arthritis, recognized by redness and oedema of the tissues around the joint. There may be diminished or absent joint movement which results in narrowing of the laryngeal opening. This should be suspected if there is hoarseness, stridor, a feeling of fullness in the throat during speaking or dysphagia.

If a severe involvement is suspected and confirmed on indirect laryngoscopy, a preoperative tracheostomy may be indicated, particularly for major surgery.

Pulmonary function

Costochondral involvement may cause a restrictive defect, reduced vital capacity, and low total lung volume. This can be accentuated by a specific pulmonary fibrosis. Compliance is then reduced although few pulmonary function laboratories measure this as a routine. Ventilation/perfusion inequalities are common, leading to arterial hypoxaemia and reduced transfer capacity for carbon monoxide. Preoperative arterial blood gas measurements should be made in patients whose respiratory function may be adversely affected by the surgical procedure.

Other, rare, specific pulmonary complications include rheumatoid nodules and cysts with honeycombing of the lung and Caplan's syndrome (see page 543). Small pleural effusions are common but rarely give rise to symptoms.

Cardiovascular function

Pericardium, myocardium and endocardium can all be involved in the rheumatoid process. Arteritis may involve coronary vessels leading to ECG abnormalities, particularly of conduction. The functional assessment which anaesthetists commonly make may be misleading or impossible. Restriction of activity may be such that the patient will complain of neither breathlessness nor angina even though pulmonary function or coronary blood flow are severely affected. Bedridden patients may have rather inadequate circulatory reflexes.

Blood

Rheumatoid patients are frequently anaemic for one of several possible reasons. The disease process itself is associated with a hypochromic, normocytic anaemia usually refractory to iron by any route. It may be improved by transfusion of packed red cells and prior to major surgery, haemoglobin should be raised at least to 10 g/dl.

Drug therapy with aspirin, phenylbutazone and steroids, all in their various ways may cause gastrointestinal bleeding. Some are ulcerogenic whereas others can cause a bleeding tendency by systemic effects which include thrombocytopenia.

Plasma albumin may also be low, and this will be associated with hypovolaemia and altered distribution of plasma bound drugs.

Posture

Great care is necessary; the skin may be unusually fragile due to steroid therapy or associated with weight loss. Joint involvement with contractures may make it essential to adopt and support unusual postures. The most common need is for extensive support to the neck and head in the supine position. Manipulation of the neck, not only during intubation but thereafter, must be carefully controlled if subluxation is to be avoided.

Drug therapy

The usual precautions apply to patients who are receiving, or who have recently received, corticosteroids. Most anaesthetic agents are safe, but dosage must be moderated in the presence of muscle loss and hypoproteinaemia. Renal function can be impaired in some patients. Body weight may be so reduced that routine post-operative intravenous fluid regimes are inappropriate.

Postoperative problems are principally those involving lung function. Assisted ventilation may be required and should be anticipated in those with severe skeletal restrictive changes when diaphragmatic activity may be impaired by pain. Infection and atelectasis are the most common postoperative sequelae. The dosage of drugs which depress respiration should be carefully controlled. The principal problems are summarized in Table 17.3.

Table 17.3. Anaesthetic hazards in patients with rheumatoid arthritis.

Airway	*Cardiovascular*
Temporomandibular ankylosis	Pericardial and myocardial fibrosis
Restricted cervical spine movement	Coronary arteritis
Atlanto-axial subluxation	Dysrhythmias
Low cervical subluxation	Disseminating necrotizing arteritis
Crico-arytenoid arthritis	
Ventilation	*Haemopoietic, hepatic and renal*
Costovertebral joint fixation	Anaemia
Thoracic vertebral flexion deformity	Leucopenia
Interstitial fibrosis	Bleeding tendency (decreased platelets)
Rheumatoid nodules in lung	Renal amyloidosis
Drug therapy	*Posture*
Steroids	Skin fragility
Gold salts	Fixed deformities
	Postoperative chest complications

Causes of death

It is often said that patients with rheumatoid arthritis die of the same causes as other people but earlier. Regrettably this is not altogether true; a significant number die of causes related to treatment, and often with corticosteroids.

JUVENILE CHRONIC POLYARTHRITIS

Still's disease is a term which has now been largely abandoned. As with nearly all original descriptions, subsequent work suggests that more than one disease was then lumped together. Polyarthritis in a child has the same differential diagnosis as in adults so that infections, ankylosing spondylitis, psoriasis, and gut lesions known to be associated with arthropathy all need consideration, in addition to the chronic 'rheumatoid' types.

Juvenile chronic polyarthritis (JCP) is rare, affecting somewhat less than 0·1 per cent of children. The onset is often between the ages of 1–3 years, the prognosis being worse the earlier the onset, and as with the adult disease, it is commoner in females. The aetiology is no more clearly understood than in adults. Histological examination of synovial tissue shows changes resembling those of rheumatoid arthritis but the similarities end there for bone erosions seldom occur, nodules are uncommon and rheumatoid factor is not usually demonstrable; moreover sacro-iliitis is a common sequel.

Not infrequently the disease presents in acute form with high swinging fever, rash lymphadenopathy, splenomegaly and no joint involvement at first. More rarely, children may develop the adult form of RA but this diagnosis is only allowable when the presence of rheumatoid factor can be shown. The clinical picture differs from the 'sero negative' type for nodules occur, erosions and the extra-articular problems seen in adults.

The attitude to management of JCP is coloured by the knowledge that the outlook for most patients is good; thus drugs with potentially serious side-effects are used with more restraint than in adults. Management begins with adequate doses of an NSAID, aspirin being the drug of choice. Particular attention needs to be paid to avoiding permanent deformities so that when the disease eventually settles, as it usually does, a reasonable functional result will be the outcome. Exercises, splinting, surgery have if anything a larger place in juvenile disease.

The indications to give drugs other than NSAID's are persistence of symptoms and signs with raised ESR or acute phase proteins and radiological progression. Gold is perhaps the best second line choice. A particular problem presents with corticosteroid treatment—inhibition of growth. Some workers have explored ways of circumventing this by using alternate day dosage, anabolic steroids or growth hormone but without much success. It is better to attempt to stop steroids for a period before puberty; growth is then usually resumed and the puberty growth spurt may restore the situation. It is worth commenting that uveitis is not an uncommon feature and the choice may then rest between preserving vision or permitting growth.

Fortunately children seldom die with juvenile chronic polyarthritis. When they do the cause is likely to be either amyloidosis or infection, the latter sometimes related to steroid treatment.

ANKYLOSING SPONDYLITIS (WITH A NOTE ON GUT ASSOCIATED ARTHROPATHIES)

There has been revived interest lately in this disease and in certain arthropathies associated with bowel disease; the interest has arisen partly because of links between groups of diseases and partly because of associations with particular histocompatibility antigens, with implications that there may at last be clues about aetiology in what has been for long a rather stationary area.

Ankylosing spondylitis (AS) affects about 0·4 per cent of men and 0·05 per cent of women, with a maximum age incidence between 15 and 40 years. There is a strong familial influence. It usually begins with low back pain, gradually involving upper levels of the spine; iritis is seen in about 20 per cent of the patients and a peripheral arthropathy, which is often monarticular but occasionally polyarticular, in about 10 per cent. An important consequence of the disease is limitation of chest expansion by costo-vertebral involvement so that breathing becomes predominantly abdominal. The outlook is good; 80 per cent of patients are still at full-time work, so long as the type of work is suitable, many years after onset. This fact obviously influences treatment.

The pathological changes in the early stage resemble rheumatoid arthritis with localized accumulations of lymphocytes and plasma cells. Little tissue destruction occurs, however, and the inflammatory lesions are followed by progressive fibrosis.

The diagnosis depends mainly on a combination of the history with consistent X-ray appearances. The earliest radiographic changes are blurring of the sacro-iliac joint space; later, patchy osteoporosis and sclerotic changes round the joints proceed to obliteration of the joint. Subsequently the spine becomes involved with squaring of vertebral bodies and the classical bamboo appearance. It is, however, generally agreed that the changes in the sacro-iliac joints are not specific and are also seen in other sero-negative (i.e. negative RF test) arthropathies.

Similar changes of sacro-iliitis with or without peripheral joint trouble may occur in association with ulcerative colitis, Crohn's disease and Whipple's disease. Moreover, clinical and familial linkages are seen between the conditions already mentioned and psoriatic arthritis, Reiter's disease and Behçet's syndrome. Further evidence linking these disorders has come from studies of histocompatibility antigens (see page 573); several of the diseases are associated with an incidence of the HLA B27 antigen which is higher than in control groups. The association is highest with AS where 96 per cent of patients are HLA B27 positive. HLA B27 is present in about 4 per cent of the general population. Tissue typing may therefore help in a diagnostic problem. Beyond this we enter an area of speculation. It seems likely that inheritance of the antigen increases the risk of developing certain diseases, particularly AS; as some of the diseases (e.g. Reiter's) are thought to be infective and as certain infective diseases in mice are associated with particular histocompatibility antigens, new lines of thought about AS have been developing. Whilst the hypotheses are still evolving the general sense of this association, and of others (e.g. DrW4 and RA) is that the immune response to an external agent may be genetically determined.

The arthropathy associated with gut disease is of two types. With either ulcerative colitis or Crohn's disease a polyarthritis involving mainly large joints may be seen in about 20 per cent of patients. In ulcerative colitis the arthropathy tends to wax and wane with the gut lesion and improves after surgery. The same pattern may occur in Crohn's but is less obvious. In either disease, joint problems are much less important than the gut lesion. The other form of arthropathy which occurs with either ulcerative colitis or Crohn's is spondylitis. This resembles AS and does not have the same tendency to follow the course of the gut lesion as the peripheral type of arthropathy; sometimes indeed spondylitis precedes the bowel trouble. Links between AS and gut associated arthropathies are, therefore, through the spondylitis in particular.

It follows from the above that current thought on the aetiology of AS is that it may be infective. No agent has yet been found and, having regard to the good prognosis, treatment is generally a matter of using safe symptomatic measures. These are physiotherapy and NSAID's. Radiotherapy is now seldom used because of the long-term risk of leukaemia. Surgery to correct deformities may occasionally be needed.

Extra-articular manifestations are rare but two are worth mention. Peptic ulceration occurs more often than the expected frequency and can lead to difficulty with selecting a suitable NSAID. A particular type of pulmonary fibrosis has also been described; it tends to be apical in distribution and has been confused with tuberculosis.

Patients with AS may present for intercurrent surgery. Their principle disability is a restrictive pattern of changes in lung function, due to costochondral rigidity and severe flexion deformity of the thoracic spine, sometimes aggravated by pulmonary fibrosis. A technique involving controlled ventilation may be preferred, and assisted ventilation may well be necessary in the postoperative period.

There is also an appreciable incidence of valvular disease, commonly aortic incompetence due to thickening and shortening of the valve cusps and dilatation of the annulus fibrosis. It is of particular importance to avoid hypotension in such cases.

REITER'S DISEASE (WITH A NOTE ON PSORIATIC ARTHRITIS)

The clinical features are arthropathy, urethritis, conjunctivitis and skin rash, not necessarily all present at the same time. The disease is commoner in men and the maximum age incidence is between 20 and 40 years.

The aetiology is not fully understood. Early reports stressed how often it began after dysentery; more recently it has been assumed to be a consequence of sexually acquired genital infection. No particular organism has, however, been regularly implicated. In this connection it is worth remembering that here is another disease of the group which includes ankylosing spondylitis, characterized by frequent occurrence of sacroiliitis and by a high incidence of HLA B27. Thus infection may be only one factor and an inherited predisposition to react to that infection with an arthropathy may be another.

The first symptom is often urethritis. The arthropathy is usually polyarticular and may resemble rheumatoid arthritis. Sacro-iliitis occurs more often later in the disease though it can be the only joint manifestation; it is easily confused with AS. The conjunctivitis, which affects about 30 per cent of patients, is frequently mild but occasionally severe and associated with anterior uveitis. The rash (keratoderma blennorrhagica) in 10 per cent of cases, is on the soles and palms and evolves from macules to pustules to keratotic lesions. Circinate balanitis may be seen. There is no diagnostic test for Reiter's disease so that the clinical features may be the only guide though some help may be had from X-rays. Radiographically, the disease may show an erosive arthropathy resembling rheumatoid arthritis but more usually distal interphalangeal joints in the feet are involved and plantar spurs of rather fluffy appearance can be seen on the inferior surface of the os calcis. The sacro-iliitis may be seen on X-rays and does not differ from that seen in AS.

Reiter's disease is usually self-limiting. Though treatment with antibiotics has occasionally been said to be successful this is not the usual experience and most people would now treat the disease with NSAID's and await spontaneous improvement. Sometimes, however, the disease is found to be of such severity and persistence that corticosteroids or cytotoxic drugs may have to be used. This is particularly the case where iritis is severe.

Psoriatic arthritis is here included because of the links already referred to between this condition and the AS constellation; the links in this instance being more in terms of familial clustering and sacro-iliitis than in histocompatibility antigens. Psoriasis is, of course, very common; psoriatic arthropathy rather rare. The association between the nail changes of psoriasis (pitting) and arthropathy is closer than the skin/joint association. The arthropathy is bewilderingly diverse and may closely mimic rheumatoid arthritis so that occasionally diagnosis is a matter of opinion only. However, psoriatic arthropathy much more often affects distal interphalangeal joints and is usually asymmetrical. It is a destructive lesion, erosions soon appearing on X-rays, but fortunately is seldom rapidly so. Treatment is, generally speaking, as for rheumatoid arthritis.

RHEUMATIC FEVER

Not long ago this disease would have been regarded as the most important in this section. As is well known, its prevalence has greatly decreased, at least in the U.K., though in some other countries it still poses a considerable problem. Even in the U.K. rheumatic fever and heart disease still rank as an important cause of death between the ages of 5 and 20. Interestingly, evidence suggests that the apparent fall in prevalence is more a decline in the severity than in the frequency of the disease, and also that the decline began before the advent of penicillin, popularly supposed to account for the difference. Nevertheless, outbreaks of the disease in crowded conditions have been controlled occasionally by the use of prophylactic penicillin.

The evidence is quite clear cut that an infection with a β-haemolytic streptococcus always precedes rheumatic fever. The incidence of such infection is of course far greater than the incidence of rheumatic fever and we have to explain why some individuals develop the disease; there appears to be an individual susceptibility, partly inherited and partly the result of environmental factors. The mechanism is unknown but is thought to be some kind of sensitization to the organism, in effect a serum sickness. The explanation for cardiac involvement, the really serious aspect, is perhaps a cross-reaction between antibody to streptococcus and a component of the myocardium.

Histologically, the disease is characterized by lesions, in the vicinity of blood vessels, which are called Aschoff nodes when in the heart. The lesions are composed of proliferations of fibrous tissue and inflammatory cells. They differ from rheumatoid nodules in having a much smaller central necrotic area and a less clear cut margin. The fact that they are perivascular must again raise suspicion about the possible role of deposition of soluble complexes.

The clinical picture, usually seen in a child over the age of 4, but of either sex, is of a systemic illness with fever, headache and arthropathy of rather sudden onset but with a history of a sore throat preceding the illness by days or weeks. The arthropathy is, at an early stage, the dominant feature; it is very painful and 'flitting' but does not usually leave permanent joint damage in its wake. In a proportion of patients rashes are seen (erythema marginatum and erythema nodosum) and nodules may be felt. Cardiac involvement is signalled by cardiac murmurs, alterations in rhythm, pericarditis or even heart failure. The ECG may show prolongation of the PR interval. In cases of diagnostic doubt, measurement of the serum antistreptolysin O titre (ASOT) is helpful. There is no other diagnostic test.

On average the disease lasts six weeks but there is wide variation; it is uncertain to what extent treatment affects either the duration of the disease or the tendency to cardiac involvement. Standard treatment includes rest and salicylates. There is argument about how much salicylate to give and in what form but most people believe that soluble aspirin in a dose aimed at achieving blood levels of about 30 mg/100 ml is best. The role of corticosteroids is similarly uncertain; they undoubtedly have a major suppressing effect on clinical manifestations and the ESR, but when stopped rebound may occur. There is conflicting evidence of their effect on cardiac involvement. On balance the evidence is good enough to encourage one to use prednisone in the severe case. Treatment should be monitored by serial measurements of the ESR or acute phase proteins, as well as by clinical phenomena. Three other aspects of treatment need mention. Heart failure sometimes occurs and is treated in the usual ways. Sydenham's chorea, following involvement of corticostriate pathways, is best treated 'expectantly' if it occurs unless it is severe, when phenobarbitone may help. Penicillin should always be given, not for any effect on the acute attack but to lessen the chance of re-infection and to 'cover' the period of any operative procedure. Finally, of all diseases, rheumatic fever is perhaps the best example of the importance of preventive measures. These include social aspects as well as prompt treatment of throat infections.

COLLAGEN VASCULAR DISORDERS

As indicated previously, the name is merely a convenient label for a group of diseases; collagen is involved prominently in only one of them—scleroderma. The syndromes described below have certain distinguishing features; thus it may be possible to speak of 'typical systemic lupus erythematosus (SLE)', but it must be stressed that the degree of overlap between diseases in this group is considerable.

SYSTEMIC LUPUS ERYTHEMATOSUS

There are no reliable figures for prevalence but it affects women more often than men and its peak age incidence is 20–40 years. There is an impression that it is becoming more common. The clinical picture is enormously varied but the commonest features are fever, arthralgia, rashes, splenomegaly and proteinuria; in some recent series of cases neuropsychiatric findings were prominent. The rash is classically described as an erythema of the face of 'butterfly' distribution, but alopecia or livedo reticularis (marbled skin) are probably commoner. With such a varied clinical picture the diagnosis relies usually on laboratory investigation, the really relevant one being the demonstration in serum of antinuclear factor (ANF). ANF is an immunoglobulin with the property of combining with nuclear material, native double stranded DNA, that is to say it is an autoantibody. There are several ways it may be demonstrated but the usual method is an immunofluorescent technique.

The relevance of ANF in the pathogenesis of the disease is unknown. There is certainly more than one type of ANF and patients with SLE usually have a variety of other autoantibodies directed against other tissue constituents, for example, red blood cells, hence the haemolytic anaemia of SLE. The diversity of the clinical picture is readily explained on this basis. Many of the lesions, particularly those in the kidney, are likely to be the consequence of deposition of immune complexes.

The aetiology, in most cases, is not apparent but there is growing awareness that a number of drugs can lead to the SLE syndrome; examples are procaineamide and hydrallazine. Such cases have an ANF which reacts with single-stranded DNA.

Treatment depends on the cause, the activity of the disease, whether there are life threatening complications and perhaps on the type of SLE. So far as cause is concerned, clearly if a drug is implicated it must be stopped; drug-induced SLE has a good prognosis. The activity of the disease can be judged, as with rheumatoid arthritis, by a combination of clinical phenomena and the ESR. The phrase 'type of SLE' was used to draw attention to the clinical significance of positive ANF tests. A positive ANF test may be seen in a number of connective tissue diseases (e.g. rheumatoid arthritis, scleroderma) as well as in what is clinically SLE. To some extent they can be distinguished from each other by immunofluorescence when the pattern (speckled or homogeneous type; IgG or IgM) of ANF can be defined. Moreover it is now recognized that clinicians are seeing a larger number of mild variants of the disease and the concept of SLE with or without major organ involvement is gaining acceptance. The serious complications requiring vigorous treatment are renal involvement, CNS involvement and, less often, thrombocytopenia. The lines of treatment available are as follows.

Symptomatic treatment with NSAID's is only suitable for mild disease.

Chloroquine is effective but is used now mostly in the cutaneous discoid type.

Corticosteroids. These will be required in the majority of cases. Much the same general considerations apply as set out in the section on rheumatoid arthritis. However, in SLE bigger doses are often needed, perhaps prednisolone 60 mg daily at first which can later be reduced in accord with clinical and laboratory indices of prognosis.

Cytotoxic drugs. Where there has been failure to respond to corticosteroids and the more serious complications are evident it may be necessary to use these drugs though their efficacy is as yet uncertain.

POLYARTERITIS

This name is used here to cover three conditions which overlap and which may even be variants of the same disease.

Polyarteritis nodosa is characterized by lesions in medium sized arteries; the lesions in the arterial media consist of necrosis with an inflammatory response. Deposition of immune complexes seems the most likely explanation for the lesion and hepatitis β associated antigen has been demonstrated in the arterial wall in a high proportion of patients. As any vessel may be affected the clinical picture is correspondingly varied. However, the principal clinical features are usually systemic illness, weight loss, arthralgia and evidence of renal and pulmonary involvement. A muscle biopsy or renal biopsy may help but is often negative. The prognosis is usually very bad though treatment with corticosteroids and, in some cases cytotoxic drugs, can lead to dramatic improvement.

Polymyalgia rheumatica has been said to be at least as common as ankylosing spondylitis. Prevalence figures are not available, presumably because the diagnosis has no rigid criteria and there is no reliable specific test, but women are affected more often than men and the disease does not occur in patients aged less than about 60. The clinical picture, easy to confuse with depression or merely ageing, is general malaise, weight loss, muscle pains and stiffness. An ESR > 60 mm/hr in association with these clinical findings would be sufficient for a diagnosis. The pathological features and treatment are best discussed after describing the third condition of this group.

Giant cell arteritis will be more familiar under the name temporal or cranial arteritis. Classically, the disorder presents with systemic illness and headache; tenderness over a thickened temporal artery is the key sign. Histologically, the lesions differ from those of polyarteritis nodosa in that they are a panarteritis and giant cells are seen in the vicinity of areas of necrosis with inflammatory response. Although at one time the condition was thought to be confined to the temporal arteries it is now known that arterial involvement is much more widespread. Indeed the clinical picture then merges with that of polymyalgia rheumatica and there is considerable doubt whether distinctions should in fact be made between the two disorders. To confuse further, giant cell arteritis has itself been described as a variant of polyarteritis nodosa.

Treatment of either polymyalgia or giant cell arteritis should be prompt and with corticosteroids. Although it is said that in a proportion of patients recovery is spontaneous in about 18 months, the risk of sudden blindness in the giant cell type is not to be lightly dismissed. In an area where diagnosis has to be based on such vague criteria the risks of possibly giving corticosteroid treatment unnecessarily are small compared to the gains—great symptomatic relief and a reduced chance of losing sight.

DERMATOMYOSITIS/POLYMYOSITIS

These conditions, occurring alone or together in various proportions, present a variable picture. The skin lesion is a diffuse oedema and erythema; the muscle lesion widespread pain and weakness. Histology is not very helpful, showing necrotic and degenerative changes with an inflammatory response. It may be best to look on these disorders as a tissue reaction, probably immunologically mediated, to some underlying condition. Thus though dermatomyositis/polymyositis may have no identifiable cause in some patients, in others it occurs with a diffuse connective tissue disease (particularly scleroderma) and sometimes as a consequence of a neoplasm.

Management should, therefore, begin by looking for a cause. Treatment, other than for an identifiable cause, is with corticosteroids; occasionally, in resistant cases, cytotoxic drugs may be needed as well.

SCLERODERMA

Progressive thickening of the skin is the most obvious feature. Histology shows that the collagen content of the skin is increased and biochemical techniques confirm this. As with all of these diseases, however, there is clearly a vascular component (obliterative endarteritis and arteriolitis) and the changes are more widespread than at first clinically evident. Thus oesophageal, bowel and pulmonary lesions are well documented and lead to the symptoms that might be expected when fibrosis occurs in these areas, i.e. dysphagia, diarrhoea or progressive dyspnoea.

The aetiology is unknown; it is assumed to be a tissue reaction to some unidentified stimulus. One of the earliest clinical manifestations, Raynaud's phenomena, points to the importance of the vascular element and the frequent finding of ANF suggests a disorder of autoimmune type. The prognosis is very variable and treatment has so far not been found to affect the course of the disease. Corticosteroids help symptomatically only in the early stages. A more recent suggestion, based on its ability to dissociate macroglobulins by cleavage of disulphide bonds, is the use of penicillamine to 'break down' the collagen. No clear results have yet been shown.

MIXED CONNECTIVE TISSUE DISEASE

At first sight it might appear almost ludicrous, having stressed the overlap between these various conditions and then striven to identify separate patterns, to proceed to lump them together again under the above name. However, it has been claimed that there is a syndrome showing some of the clinical features of SLE, scleroderma and polymyositis and characterized by the finding of high titres of a specific antibody to an extractable nuclear antigen—probably an RNA protein. The response to corticosteroids in these patients is good and this fact, together with the 'specific' laboratory test, constitute reasonable grounds for regarding the disorder as an entity.

GOUT AND OTHER 'CRYSTAL ARTHROPATHIES'

From a theoretical point of view gout is of great interest because of the intricacies of the disturbances in protein metabolism, the interaction of excess urate production and decreased excretion, and the inflammatory response to crystals. From a strictly practical point of view the position is much simpler.

Gout usually presents as an acute arthritis of the first metatarsophalangeal joint; not infrequently the arthritis affects some other joint, less often it may be polyarticular. When the disorder has been present for a considerable time, accumulations of urate in the tissues may be evident as tophi either on the ears or in the vicinity of joints. The clinical phenomena are a response to deposition of crystals of sodium biurate. Ordinarily uric acid, in equilibrium with its sodium salt, is soluble. When concentrations in the extracellular fluids exceed about 0·36 mmol/l, crystals tend to form and then evoke an inflammatory response. Thus, considering the aetiology, we need to know why the levels of uric acid are raised and what causes crystals to form.

Serum uric acid can be elevated in the blood either from excess production (as in myeloproliferative disorders or psoriasis where there is a large turnover of nuclear material), diminished excretion (renal disorders, some drugs) or a combination of the two. In the common primary gout there is an inherited metabolic defect of protein metabolism leading to overproduction of uric acid and probably defective excretion as well. Secondary gout is the term given to the condition when it results from identifiable causes such as those mentioned above. Given an already raised serum uric acid other factors may aggravate the position; for instance, a meal with a high nucleoprotein content would further raise the level as would drugs interfering with urate excretion (pyrazinamide, thiazide diuretics, low dose aspirin). Factors precipitating deposition of crystals are numerous and hard to understand—trauma, infection, a myocardial infarct, for example.

The diagnosis is made by the clinical findings supported by a raised serum uric acid (normal values range from 0·12 to 0·36 mmol/l). Treatment can then be begun and it is important to emphasize that the first objective is to settle an acute inflammatory lesion, *not* to influence the serum uric acid. The inflammation, in the majority of patients, responds readily to indomethacin or colchicine; indomethacin 150 mg daily is probably best. Having treated the acute episode consideration would have to be given to pathogenesis. If it is secondary gout then the cause requires attention; if it is primary gout long-term treatment directed at lowering serum uric acid will be needed. The measures available are:

1   diet—exclusion of foods containing nucleoprotein is to some extent effective but now seldom if ever used;

2   uricosuric drugs—probenecid and sulfinpyrazone increase urinary excretion of uric acid;

3   allopurinol—this drug blocks the enzyme xanthine oxidase which degrades xanthine and hypoxanthine to uric acid. Thus instead of hyperuricaemia the patients have hyperxanthinaemia, but this state has not been shown to be associated with any untoward effects.

The measures outlined above are almost always successful. The prognosis is good and will probably be improved by better use of allopurinol though there is an association, as yet ill-understood between hyperuricaemia and ischaemic heart disease.

A number of other metabolic disorders are associated with joint pains resembling gout ('pseudogout'). They are generally the consequence of deposition of crystals of calcium pyrophosphate. These crystals, though needle-shaped like urate crystals, can be distinguished from them by polarized light microscopy. The disorder is rather more often polyarticular than is gout and can therefore lead to diagnostic difficulties; the crystals are derived from joint tissue, often being deposited in cartilage where they are then visible on X-ray (chondrocalcinosis). The commonest underlying disorder is osteoarthrosis but other less common conditions can present in this way, for example haemochromatosis. The diagnosis is made by demonstrating the crystals in joint fluid; treatment is with NSAID's and attention to the underlying disorder.

REFERENCES

1 HOLBOROW EJ. Rheumatoid factors and antinuclear antibodies. In: Scott JT, ed. *Copeman's textbook of the rheumatic diseases.* 5th ed. Edingburgh: Churchill Livingstone, 1978: 167–89.
2 McKusick V. *Heritable disorders of connective tissue.* 4th ed. London: Mosby, 1973.

FURTHER READING

SCOTT JT, ed. *Copeman's textbook of the rheumatic diseases.* 5th ed. Edinburgh: Churchill Livingstone, 1978.

Chapter 18
Immune Mechanisms Relating to Human Disease

R. J. POWELL AND B. McCONKEY

A knowledge of immune mechanisms is now essential to the practice of clinical medicine, not only to help us understand the response to infectious agents and transplanted organs, but also to comprehend diseases caused by disorders of immunity.

THE LYMPHOCYTES

At the centre of all immune responses are the lymphocytes because they can recognize, and specifically respond to, foreign antigens. It was demonstrated in the last decade that lymphocytes fall into two morphologically indistinguishable categories, B and T cells. There are more T cells (approximately 70 per cent) than B cells in the peripheral blood and therefore a lymphopenia usually indicates a reduced number of T lymphocytes.

B cells

These are derived from the bone marrow stem cells. Their characteristic feature is surface membrane immunoglobulin whose variable region (see immunoglobulin structure) provides the cell with its own individual antigen-specific receptor. Activation of these cells (when surface antibody reacts with the appropriate antigen) leads to maturation of the B cells into specific antibody secreting cells (*plasma cells*). Such antibodies form the effector mechanism of the *humoral immune response*, which is primarily involved in eliminating bacterial infections.

T cells (thymus derived)

The precursor cells of the T lymphocyte lineage are derived from haemopoietic stem cells in the blood forming organs. They migrate via the blood stream to the thymus where they proliferate and differentiate, eventually emerging as T cells capable of reacting in immune responses. Consequently neonatal thymectomy will lead to a marked reduction of T cells. T cells have no surface membrane immunoglobulin but develop antigen specific receptors. Mature T cells are a heterogeneous population, some developing into effector cells such as T cytotoxic cells and others into cells which produce factors (lymphokines) involved in the generation of the delayed hypersensitivity response. T cells mediate the *cellular immune response* which is particularly effective against parasite, virus, and fungal infections, malignant cells, and nonidentical transplanted tissue. T cells also regulate the antibody response of B cells (T helper and T suppressor cells).

A system of preprogrammed cells exists therefore to recognize a variety of antigens. In order that these cells have the maximum opportunity to meet their predetermined antigen they are mobile and recirculate in a nonrandom manner. The cell–cell co-operation which occurs is fundamental to the generation of the immune response. This is exemplified by the humoral part of the immune system in which macrophages usually present the antigen to B cells, and T cell facilitation controls the B cell response.

Location of lymphocytes

On leaving the marrow, B cells enter the recirculating pool of lymphocytes and are in a constant state of migration between the secondary lymphoid organs which are the gut, lymph nodes, spleen and bone marrow. The cells enter the lymphoid organs mainly via the blood stream and leave by the efferent lymphatics. They ultimately re-enter the blood stream by way of the thoracic duct. About 5 per cent of B cells are recirculating at any one time; the rest are clustered together to form discrete primary follicles in the secondary lymphoid organs which, when stimulated by antigen, may form germinal centres.

T cells also recirculate, but faster than B cells. They concentrate in the secondary lymphoid tissue in areas fairly distinct from the B cells, such as the lymph node medulla.

ANTIBODIES AND ANTIGENS

A multitude of foreign substances, both natural and synthetic, may provoke the production of specific antibodies. In some instances antibodies produced against one substance may react with a structurally similar but different second substance; this is termed a *cross-reaction*. In rheumatic fever, for example, antibodies produced against streptococci cross-react with human heart tissue. A single antibody molecule reacts only with a small well-defined structural area of an antigen, the *antigenic determinant*. Antigens usually have many such determinants which may all be different (as in the case of most proteins), or largely the same (particulate antigens, i.e. bacteria and viruses). Thus any given antigen molecule can be bound by many specific antibody molecules (as many as can be spatially fitted around it), to form a so-called *immune complex* (antigen-antibody complex).

The basic structure of immunoglobulin (antibody) was determined through studies of IgG (mol.wt 150,000). The IgG molecule (Fig. 18.1) is composed of two identical heavy chains (mol.wt 50,000) and two identical light chains (mol.wt 25,000) covalently linked by disulphide bonds. There are 5 classes of heavy chain (M, G, A, D, E) and 2 classes of light chains (Kappa (κ) and Lambda (λ)). Only one heavy chain class and one light chain class can be represented in one antibody molecule. This allows ten possible combinations of heavy and light chains, e.g. IgMκ, IgMλ, IgGκ, IgGλ, IgAκ, IgAλ, IgEκ, IgEλ, IgDκ and IgDλ.

The part of an immunoglobulin which binds to antigen is the terminal area of both arms of the Y shaped antibody molecule The terminal component of both the heavy and light chains forms the antigen binding site (*idiotype*). There are two arms on an IgG molecule and it follows therefore that there are two antigen binding sites per IgG molecule. IgM is a pentameric molecule and therefore has ten combining sites. The antigen combining sites of a given antibody molecule are always identical.

Great variability of antigen binding sites must exist between antibody molecules to allow recognition of all the possible antigens. The vast library of antigen combining sites can occur within any of the immunoglobulin heavy chain classes. Hence the antigen combining region of an antibody is often termed the *variable* region.

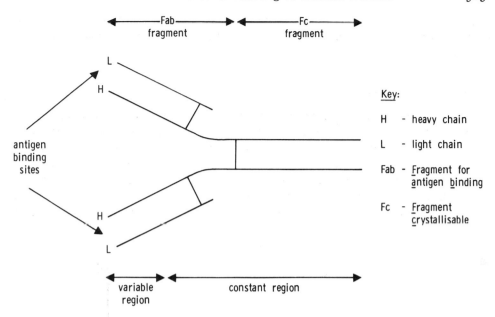

Fig. 18.1. Representation of an IgG molecule to demonstrate the relationship of the various parts.

The remainder of the antibody molecule is termed the '*constant*' region. It makes no contribution to antigen specificity but rather directs the biological activity of the antibody molecule.

The major properties of the heavy chain classes are:

IgG—complement fixation
　　—placental transfer
　　—combination with rheumatoid factor
IgM—complement fixation
IgA—seromucous secretion
IgE—mast cell and basophil binding, e.g. tissue sensitization
IgD—mainly B cell bound. The function of very small amounts in serum is unknown.

Generation of antibody diversity

It seems likely that an antibody response can be induced to any naturally occurring macromolecule and also to a vast number of synthetic molecules not present in the environment. An estimate of the minimum number of structurally unique antibody binding sites that an individual can generate must be in the region of five million. In classical genetic terms each different antigen binding site would be coded for by a structural gene and the antibody repertoire would be inherited directly in the germ-line (germ-line theory). However, if this were true a major portion or all of the available genome would be utilized. An alternative to this simple germ-line theory has been proposed: that we inherit only a small number of genes coding for different antigen binding specificities, and that the genes mutate as the stem cells divide and differentiate on their pathway to become antigen-specific lymphocytes (somatic mutation theory).

COMPLEMENT SYSTEM

The proteins of the complement system are a complex series of macromolecules which become activated sequentially, usually by proteolytic cleavage, in a manner analogous to the clotting cascade. There are two activating pathways, the 'alternate' and 'classical'. Their sole function is to produce a convertase which can cleave the central and major component of the complement cascade, namely C_3, into C_3b (activated C_3) (Fig 18.2). The generation of C_3b and its fixation at complement fixing sites (e.g. the

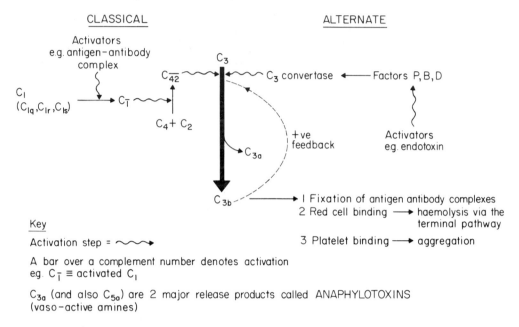

Fig. 18.2. Schematic representation of the early part of the human complement pathway.

Fc portion of IgG), is probably one of the most important roles of the entire cascade. Bacteria can be phagocytosed by neutrophil leucocytes but after they have been coated with antibody and C_3b (i.e. opsonized) then the efficiency of phagocytosis is increased more than one hundredfold. This explains why deficiencies of either immunoglobulin or C_3 can lead to increased susceptibility to infections.

Classical (conventional) pathway

The complement components C_1, C_4 and C_2 are activated in that sequence to produce a complex which functions as a C_3 convertase. C_1 activation occurs when IgG or IgM antibodies complex with antigen.

Alternate pathway

Endotoxin produced by gram negative bacilli is one of the activators of this pathway. It activates sequentially properdin (Factor P), Factor D and Factor B to produce the C_3 convertase of the alternate pathway. Activation of the complement cascade by this route is probably one of the major mechanisms involved in the generation of endotoxic shock.

Moreover, C_3b has the ability to cleave yet more C_3. The whole process is regulated by the inactivation and rapid decay of C_3b. The opsonic role of C_3b in phagocytosis has been mentioned, but it can also bind the platelets leading to their aggregation and to consequent vascular obstruction, and can bind to red cells leading to haemolysis. The red cell fixation of C_3b is facilitated by IgM and IgG anti-red cell antibodies and leads to the successive activation of the terminal complement components (C_5, C_6, C_7, C_8 and C_9) to form the red cell surface complex C_{56789} which is able to punch a hole in the red cell membrane leading to osmotic lysis.

Routine laboratories can measure serum C_3 and C_4 by radial immunodiffusion. Normal ranges are C_3 0·8–2·0 g/l; C_4 0·2–0·5 g/l. Low levels may indicate complement consumption in immune complex diseases. Thus, sequential C_3 and C_4 estimations in such immune complex diseases as SLE can provide a useful guide to the progress of disease activity.

Deficiencies

Clinically significant primary deficiencies of the complement components are rare. However in a proportion of patients with *angioneurotic oedema* there is a deficiency of the enzyme C_1 esterase inhibitor which inactivates activated C_1. This clinical syndrome, characterized by attacks of recurrent local oedema can affect the pharynx and larynx, occasionally leading to fatal airway obstruction.

Angioneurotic oedema

The attacks may be self-limiting and if there is no threat to maintenance of the airways, then it may be sufficient to observe the patient and perhaps administer antihistamines and adrenal corticosteroids. The only other measure which may need to be taken as an emergency procedure is intubation.

Fresh frozen plasma contains the deficient inhibitor and can be given to abort severe attacks. Danazol, a new androgen, may partially correct the C_1 esterase inhibitor deficiency and should be considered as prophylactic treatment in patients having recurring attacks of angioneurotic oedema.

HYPERSENSITIVITY REACTIONS

To understand this often confused term one must comprehend how sensitization occurs normally. A primary immune response occurs when an individual meets an antigen for the first time, for instance tetanus toxoid. After eight to ten days principally IgM antibodies against the toxoid appear in the blood and this indicates that the individual has now been sensitized. If a second exposure to tetanus toxoid occurs, the antibody response appears much faster (two to three days) and this time the major antibody class involved is IgG. This secondary response depends on recollection of the previous exposure by the immune system, i.e. immunological memory. However this further contact with antigen can sometimes lead to tissue damage, the so-called *hypersensitivity reaction*.

Hypersensitivity reactions have been usefully divided by Gell and Coombs into the following four basic types:

19

    I   Anaphylactic—so-called immediate hypersensitivity
    II   Antibody dependent cytoxicity
    III Complex mediated
    IV T cell mediated—delayed hypersensitivity

An antigen rarely elicits a hypersensitivity response of only one type.

I Anaphylactic hypersensitivity (type 1)

Predominantly IgE antibodies are responsible. They become bound via their Fc regions to mast cells and circulating basophils, and therefore are termed homocytotropic.

    When membrane bound IgE is cross-linked by a specific antigen, degranulation of mast cells occurs releasing a variety of vasoactive substances such as histamine, an eosinophil chemotactic factor, (ECF), platelet activating substance (PAF) and slow releasing substance A (SRSA) (Fig. 18.3 schematically represents type 1 or anaphylactic hypersensitivity).

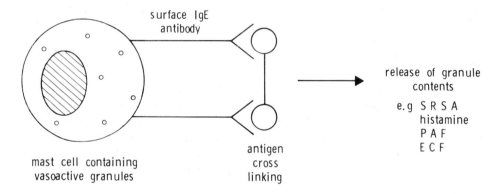

Fig. 18.3. Schematic representation of type I hypersensitivity.

    Anaphylactic responses are by definition immediate and for the most part are restricted to a few genetically prone individuals, who are termed 'atopic' and who produce an IgE response to antigens or allergens well-tolerated by the remainder of the population.

    It is useful to consider separately local and systemic forms of anaphylactic sensitivity depending on the portal of entry of the antigen.

Local (atopic allergy)

Localized anaphylactic reactions to extrinsic allergens such as grass pollens, animal danders, house dust mites, etc. occur in about 10 per cent of the population. The symptoms of rhinorrhoea, conjunctivitis and asthma are produced by contact of the allergen with cell bound IgE in the nasal mucosa, conjunctivae and bronchial tree respectively.

    Urticaria is also an anaphylactic phenomenon which can develop in sensitized individuals from the intestinal absorption of an antigen. Strawberries, nuts, eggs and shellfish are the common offenders.

Systemic (serum sickness)

Systemic anaphylaxis is induced when a guinea pig is injected with egg albumin. Nothing overt follows the primary injection, but if a second injection is given a few weeks later, then the animal rapidly dies from asphyxia. Intense bronchoconstriction will have occurred with dilatation of the capillaries as a result of the release of the contents of mast cell granules. Similar reactions can occur in humans after injections of penicillin, intravenous induction agents, procaine, contrast medium or even plasma substitute infusions. Previous antigenic challenge is *always* required to produce the sensitized state. Anaphylaxis in man is manifested by bronchospasm and laryngeal oedema resulting in extreme dyspnoea and cyanosis, and a marked fall in blood pressure. Diarrhoea, nausea and vomiting may be associated. It is a potentially fatal condition if not treated promptly with adrenaline and can also require antihistamines and adrenocorticosteroids.

Sensitization can be detected by intradermal skin testing, a positive test indicating the presence of specific IgE antibodies. The serum level of IgE may be elevated in patients with allergic asthma.

Treatment

Antihistamines remain a popular therapy. However some allergies, e.g. to house dust mite and grass pollens, can be modified by hyposensitization. The mechanism underlying hyposensitization is currently thought to be that small doses of allergen, injected subcutaneously in a suitable transport medium, lead to the production of IgG antibodies to the allergen. These circulating IgG antibodies could then react with antigen before it can bind with the IgE which is bound to mast cells; thus the patient's IgE hypersensitivity is modified.

II Antibody dependent cytotoxicity

This is a heterogeneous group of reactions whose common feature is the presence of circulating antibody to a tissue or cell-bound antigen. Binding of antibody to cell bound antigen leads to cell death by the enhancement of phagocytosis or activation of the whole complement cascade. Autoimmune haemolytic anaemia is a clear example of a type II reaction with antibodies to erythrocytes. These antibodies can be detected by the Coombs' test explained in Fig. 18.4.

In Goodpasture's syndrome (glomerulonephritis and haemoptysis) there are circulating antibodies to glomerular basement membrane. These antibodies bind to the basement membrane of both the kidney and lung and fix complement, thereby inducing an inflammatory response.

Hashimoto's thyroiditis is associated with complement-fixing IgG antibodies to thyroid secretory epithelium but they do not seem to be pathogenic on their own, possibly only being pathogenic when combined with a cell-mediated hypersensitivity. This example emphasizes the point that subdivision of the hypersensitivities into types is to a large extent artificial.

Transfusion reactions due to incorrect AB cross-matching are a further example of

19*

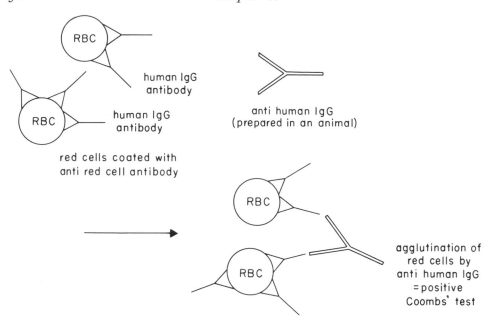

NB Agglutination can only occur if red cells are
already coated with human anti red cell IgG

Fig. 18.4. Coombs test—schematic representation.

antibody mediated cytotoxicity. AB cells transfused into an individual of group O
will react with circulating anti-A and anti-B antibodies. These anti-red cell antibodies
are of the IgM type and will agglutinate the cells and fix complement, leading to
intravascular sludging and inflammation respectively. Anti-rhesus antibodies, in
distinction to the IgM anti-ABO antibodies, are of the IgG class and can traverse the
placental barrier. This has obvious importance in haemolytic disease of the newborn
and demonstrates how different effector mechanisms between the classes of heavy
chain immunoglobulins can be relevant.

Circulating antibodies may be detected by immunological techniques such as red
cell and latex particle agglutination, complement fixation tests and indirect immunofluorescence.

III Immune complex mediated hypersensitivity

Antigen-antibody complexes (immune complexes) activate complement and consequently excite an inflammatory response. Irreversible vascular damage, the hallmark
of this hypersensitivity process, may then follow.

Two broad types of immune complex disease can be distinguished, depending on
the absolute amounts of antigen and antibody present and their relative proportions.
We discuss below, under separate headings, examples from each end of the spectrum
of possibilities; some important diseases such as rheumatoid arthritis and systemic
lupus erythematosus show features of both, or even intermediate, types. The actual
size of the immune complex so formed is recognized to be the most important factor.
The reaction of a divalent antibody, e.g. IgG, with a multivalent antigen may result in

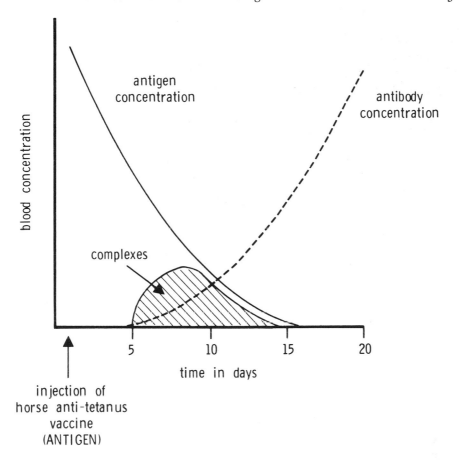

Fig. 18.5. Circulating complex formation after antigen injection in type III hypersensitivity.

the formation of large aggregates leading to the precipitation of insoluble proteins. At other ratios soluble complexes form (Fig 18.5).

Antibody excess

A vast excess of circulating antibody leads to rapid complex formation and precipitation; an erythematous response with oedema at the site of the reaction occurs after 3 to 8 hours. Pigeon fancier's lung and Farmer's lung are good examples of this reaction occurring locally in the lungs after inhalation of pigeon droppings, and *Micropolyspora Faeni* and *Thermoactinomyces Vulgaris*, respectively. This type of local response is called the *Arthus reaction*.

Antigen excess (serum sickness)

The classic example of serum sickness in man can be provoked by horse antidiphtheria or antitetanus injection. About eight days later the patient's temperature rises, usually associated with lymphadenopathy and arthralgia. Investigations reveal albuminuria, marked depression of serum complement levels and the presence of immune complexes. The clinical picture results from the formation of small complexes and their consequent deposition in the vascular bed.

Small circulating immune complexes form in antigen (Ag) excess, e.g. Ab_1, Ag_2 (IgG antibodies (Ab) divalent). Large complexes form as the relative amounts of antibody increase—$Ab_2 Ag_3$, $Ab_3 Ag_4$, etc. (Fig 18.6). Larger complexes are rapidly removed from the circulation and rendered harmless by the reticuloendothelial system (now increasingly referred to as the macrophage monocyte system) but the smaller complexes persist in the circulation, excite the complement cascade and

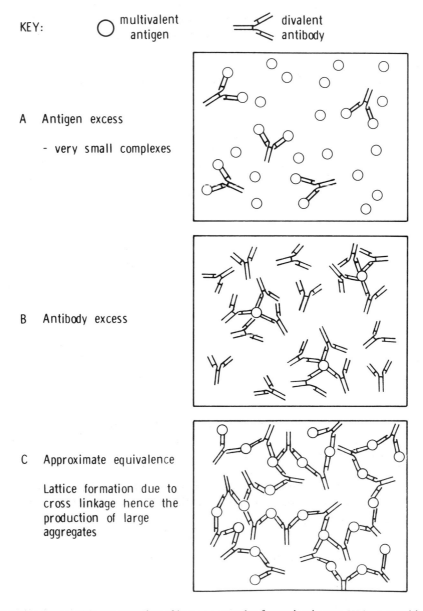

KEY: ◯ multivalent antigen   divalent antibody

A Antigen excess
   – very small complexes

B Antibody excess

C Approximate equivalence
   Lattice formation due to cross linkage hence the production of large aggregates

Fig. 18.6. Diagrammatic representation of immune complex formation in type III hypersensitivity when the relative proportions of antigen and antibody are varied.

produce the clinical picture of serum sickness. The complexes are eventually deposited in different parts of the vascular bed, for example kidney glomeruli.

Other disease states may simulate a comparable picture, e.g. systemic lupus erythematosus (DNA anti-DNA complexes), polyarteritis nodosa (hepatitis B antigen-antibody complexes). In subacute bacterial endocarditis nonthrombotic extracardiac manifestations are related to streptococcal antigen-antibody complexes.

IV Cell mediated (delayed) hypersensitivity

Free antibody plays no part in these T lymphocyte mediated reactions. Characteristically intracellular infectious agents such as viruses (measles, smallpox, herpes) and some bacterial infections (tuberculosis, brucellosis and syphilis) elicit the cell mediated immune response.

The time-hallowed example of this type of hypersensitivity is the tuberculin response in sensitized individuals who, about 18 to 48 hours after inoculation show an 'indurated' area at the site of inoculation; biopsy shows a predominantly mono-nuclear 'infiltration', i.e. cell-mediated immunity. These mononuclear cells are mainly T lymphocytes. These T cells carry antigen specific receptors on their surface, and after appropriate antigen recognition release lymphokines which nonspecifically activate macrophages to promote phagocytosis and killing. The specificity of the whole reaction is the property of the T cell, the macrophages being only nonspecifically armed.

Characteristics of some T cell lymphokines

Lymphokine	Properties
Macrophage chemotactic factor (CF)	Attracts macrophages *in vitro*
Macrophage migration inhibition factor (MIF)	Inhibits macrophage movement *in vitro*
Macrophage aggregation factor (MAF)	Agglutinates macrophages *in vitro*
Lymphocyte blastogenic factor (BF)	Induces lymphocyte DNA synthesis *in vitro*
Interferon	Prevents viral replication in target cells
Transfer factor	Transfers delayed hypersensitivity to specific antigens from one person to another.

Type IV reactions can also occur on skin contact with a variety of chemicals, notably antibiotics such as penicillin, and heavy metals such as nickel in the fastenings of ladies' underwear. These substances become antigenic by binding to proteins in the skin and lead to the clinical picture of contact dermatitis.

Homograft rejection is thought to be mediated predominantly by a cell-mediated hypersensitivity, but circulating antibodies to the graft components can be detected and may have an as yet undefined role.

Other 'hypersensitivity responses'

Stimulating antibody

Certain IgG antibodies have a stimulating action on an end organ, e.g. TSH receptor antibodies in the thyroid. These stimulate their target cells rather than damage them.

Excess of these antibodies leads to thyrotoxicosis, and placental transfer can lead to neonatal hyperthyroidism.

Cell-mediated antibody dependent cytoxicity

Killer cells (K cells) are a subgroup of lymphoid cells or monocytes which can destroy target cells coated with antibody *in vitro*. This is a complement independent mechanism and K cells do not require the thymus for their development. No definitive role for such a mechanism has yet been documented but K cell mediated cytotoxic reactions may be important in tumour rejection and defence against parasitic infections, e.g. schistosomiasis.

AUTOIMMUNITY

An individual does not normally show an immune response against components of his own tissues; this is the state of *immunological tolerance*. When this state of tolerance breaks down it is referred to as an *autoimmune reaction*. The antibodies responsible are called autoantibodies and may be directed against tissue antigens or free molecules such as immunoglobulins or coagulation factors.

The autoantibody mediated diseases can be divided into organ specific (e.g. antiglomerular basement membrane, or antiadrenal) and nonorgan specific where the antigenic determinants are present in numerous organs, e.g. antinuclear antibodies in SLE.

It is often difficult to decide whether autoantibodies are the cause of the clinical manifestations, an associated phenomenon or are only a consequence of the disease. For example, antierythrocyte antibodies are responsible for the anaemia observed in autoimmune haemolytic anaemia, but antiheart antibodies are probably only secondary to tissue damage after myocardial infarction.

Factors that favour the development of autoimmunity are

Increasing age
Females > males
Genetic factors—near relatives of patients with autoimmune diseases often exhibit the same disease
Immunological background—complement deficiency states (C_2 deficiency is often associated with SLE)
Association of autoimmune diseases—they tend to be associated (pernicious anaemia is 50 times more frequent in subjects with Hashimoto's thyroiditis).

Possible mechanisms of autoimmunity

All the theories explain some of the clinical and experimental data but none completely explains all the currently known facts.

Altered antigens

An antigen to which tolerance exists might be chemically changed and bypass the state of tolerance. Antibodies to the rhesus antigens are not normally present but methyldopa can bind to the red cell membranes, alter the D antigen, and provoke anti-D antibody formation.

Loss of tolerance to autoantigens

If B cells are exposed to antigens at a very early state of development when their antigen receptors are IgM alone, they can easily be rendered immunologically non-reactive, i.e. tolerant. Failure of this switch-off mechanism could then lead to harmful autoimmune disease. In recent years it has become clear that a subset of T cells play an important role in suppressing activation of both T and B cells by antigen. Hence a lack of T suppressor cells may lead to autoimmunity. This latter mechanism is suspected in SLE and has been demonstrated in the SLE-like syndrome of New Zealand black mice.

Sequestered antigen

Certain auto-antigens are not usually available to sensitize the immune system—some proteins of the lens of the eye for instance. Release of such antigens into the circulation following trauma may result in activation of otherwise quiescent clones of autoreactive cells and thus produce sympathetic ophthalmia.

Cross-reactions with autoantigens

Certain haemolytic streptococci have antigenic determinants shared between myocardium and glomerular basement membrane. An immune response generated against streptococcal antigens may therefore also react with these self antigens (*cross-reactivity*) and poststreptococcal nephritis or rheumatic fever result.

HLA SYSTEM

The importance of transplantation in modern surgery has given great impetus to the study of the major histocompatibility complex in man which is known as HLA (human leucocyte antigen). The HLA antigens are found on most tissues but differ quantitatively in their distribution. The part of the genome which codes for the antigens is on chromosome 6. Peripheral blood can be used for tissue typing (HLA typing) because the HLA antigens are present on leucocytes, their source of discovery, and platelets but not on red cells.

There are four main series of antigens in the HLA system—HLA: A, B, C and D, the first three being defined serologically and the latter requiring lymphocyte culture techniques. There are many antigens in each series, approximately 20 in each of the HLA-A and HLA-B categories alone, and therefore a vast number of combinations of antigens are possible. The chance of any two individuals being identical for a given HLA haplotype is very small.

Disease associations related to HLA type have been found (Table 18.1); the strongest association is between ankylosing spondylitis and HLA B27.

Recently some antigens close to HLA-D, 'D related' or DR, have been identified. The newer, less well-defined antigens still have the prefix W (workshop) so that the full title of this new group of antigens would be HLA DRW, followed by the number of the antigen in that series, e.g. HLA DRW4. It is now recognized that HLA DRW4 is associated with rheumatoid arthritis and HLA DRW3 haplotype associated with an increased susceptibility to adverse reactions to gold in the treatment of rheumatoid arthritis.

Table 18.1. Disease and HLA typing.

Disease	HLA type	% frequency in patients	% frequency in controls
Ankylosing spondylitis	B27	90	8
Reiter's disease	B27	80	9
Rheumatoid arthritis	DRW4	56	15
Coeliac disease	DRW3	96	27
	B8	67	20
Active chronic hepatitis	DRW3	41	15
	B8	52	17
Haemachromatosis	A3	72	21
Multiple sclerosis	DRW2	41	22
Myasthenia gravis	DRW3	32	17
	B8	39	17

IMMUNODEFICIENCY DISEASES

These are probably rare because an intact immune system is vital for survival: we have not therefore attempted a comprehensive review. Possible mechanisms responsible for the cellular defects in the various primary immunodeficiency diseases is schematically represented in Fig. 18.7.

The term 'combined immunodeficiency states' relates to defects in both T and B cell development, and these defects probably occur during the early common development pathways of T and B cells.

The following brief notes exemplify some of the defects seen in the immunodeficiencies.

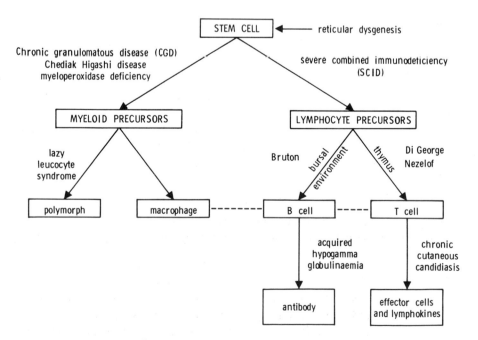

Fig. 18.7. Cellular basis of immunodeficiency states.

Severe combined immunodeficiency (SCID)

The affected infants appear normal at birth but in the first few months of life develop recurrent diarrhoea and weight loss. Recurrent candida and pyogenic infections are common and if the children are vaccinated, progressive necrotic vaccinia occurs. There is thymic hypoplasia, IgG levels drop from birth (as the maternal antibody is metabolized), IgA and IgM levels remain low, and blood lymphocytes do not respond to antigen. There is often an associated neutropenia. A severe and very rare form of combined immunodeficiency occurs called reticular dysgenesis in which both granulocyte and lymphocyte production is defective.

Immunodeficiencies predominantly associated with T cell failure

Di–George syndrome

This syndrome is characterized by the absence of parathyroid and thymic tissue associated with abnormalities of the heart and great vessels. This absence is related to a maldevelopment of the 3rd and 4th pharyngeal pouches which occurs before 8 weeks gestation and is possibly related to intrauterine damage by a drug or virus. The affected infant has tetany, no thymic shadow on X-ray, cardiovascular problems, cleft palate and micrognathia and is especially prone to infections such as candida. The immunoglobulin levels are usually normal. Transplantation of thymic tissue in this syndrome is a recent major advance.

Nezelof syndrome

This is similar to the Di George syndrome but the parathyroid tissue is present and vascular abnormalities are absent.

Immunodeficiencies associated with B cell failure

Congenital cross-linked hypogammaglobulinaemia (Bruton)

The affected infant is well until three to four months of age because maternal IgG offers some protection. However upper and lower respiratory infections and chronic diarrhoea from *giardia lamblia* and bacteroides infections soon become a major problem. An interesting polyarthritis can develop. Low immunoglobulin levels are found and treatment with pooled gamma globulin injections weekly improve both the infective and, sometimes, the arthritic problems.

Common variable, unclassifiable immunodeficiency

This is an acquired hypogammaglobulinaemia in which T cell function may also deteriorate. Infections are again the main problem especially giardia lamblia in the gut.

Selective IgA deficiency

This occurs in 1 in 700 of the population in Europe and USA, is the commonest immunodeficiency and is often found by chance. However this selective IgA deficiency is found more in atopic individuals and those with autoimmune diseases, for example, RA, SLE, thyroiditis and pernicious anaemia.

Transient hypogammaglobulinaemia of infancy

Prematurity often results in low fetal IgG levels at birth because the maternal IgG is transferred across the placenta in the third trimester. Fetal immunoglobulin is not produced for the first months of life and this can lead to a transient immunodeficient state.

IMMUNOGLOBULIN IN DISEASE

Measurement of immunoglobulin levels can help in the investigation of a variety of conditions.

1 Intrauterine infection may result in antibody production and hence IgM in the fetal circulation may provide evidence for such infection.

2 Atopic individuals often have elevated levels of IgE antibodies. Specific IgE response to a variety of allergens can be monitored.

3 Definition of the class of antibody produced in response to an infection can be of importance, for example in putative rubella infection during pregnancy. The presence of IgM antirubella antibodies would indicate current infection (primary antibody response) whereas IgG antirubella antibodies would point to a past infection.

4 Increased polyclonal immunoglobulin levels are found in chronic infections, chronic liver disease and certain other chronic inflammatory conditions, e.g. collagen diseases.

5 An increased level of one immunoglobulin type (monoclonal) is seen in patients with plasma cell abnormalities. In these there is an expansion of a single clone of plasma cells all producing the same immunoglobulin—referred to as a *paraprotein* which appears on protein electrophoresis as a dense band usually in the gamma region. The most common reason for such a paraprotein is myelomatosis, a plasma cell malignancy If the associated light chain is produced in excess of the given heavy chain it can appear in the urine, the so-called *Bence-Jones* protein. Benign paraproteins do exist especially in people over 70 years of age. In myelomatosis there is suppression of the production of other immunoglobulins leading to secondary immunodeficiency but in benign paraproteinaemia there is no such suppression. Other causes of secondary immunodeficiency include nephrotic syndrome, malnutrition, cytotoxic drugs, many lymphoproliferative disorders, etc.

METHODS OF FACILITATING THE IMMUNE RESPONSE

Plasma-exchange

The patient's blood is separated into plasma and cellular elements, the latter then being returned to the patient in a plasma solution such as plasma protein fraction. The term 'plasmapheresis' is often used interchangeably with plasma-exchange but in fact refers to exchange of plasma for crystalloid solution. Four sequential one-litre exchange cycles are usually performed using a large vein or arteriovenous fistula.

Plasma-exchange removes damaging immune complexes and also any free antigen and antibody, thus altering the ratio of antigen to antibody which is so important in determining the size and hence pathogenicity of these complexes. Current knowledge suggests that blockade of the reticuloendothelial system by excess complexes may be important in the build-up of these pathogenic complexes in the circulation, and plasma-exchange would help restore the phagocytic capacity of the reticuloendothelial system. Plasma-exchange thus allows suitable diseases to be controlled fairly rapidly in the short-term while long-term control with other agents is established.

Plasma-exchange can play a useful role in a wide range of diseases, for example in myasthenia gravis to remove the autoantibody to a modulating receptor near the acetylcholine receptor, in Goodpasture's syndrome to remove the antiglomerular basement membrane antibody, in systemic lupus erythematosus to remove anti-DNA antibody complexes and in Rhesus haemolytic disease to remove anti-D antibodies.

Immunosuppressive agents

High doses of steroids seem to alter the short-lived B lymphocyte population and will help produce a remission in B cell neoplasia, for example chronic lymphocytic leukaemia. They are also powerful anti-inflammatory agents and will minimize the tissue damage caused by immune complexes.

Antilymphocytic globulin (ALG)

By injecting human thoracic duct lymphocytes into horses, a horse antihuman lymphocyte serum can be obtained. The IgG fraction of this horse serum can be injected into transplant recipients and will lead to a rapid depletion of T cells, predominantly, and hence graft rejection can be reduced.

X-irradiation

The rate at which a particular dose of X-irradiation is given and the time intervals between doses, rather than the total dose given, determine its effectiveness. Proliferating cells are particularly sensitive to X-irradiation but are not necessarily killed outright, and resting cells are in fact stimulated to divide. Therefore tissues where there is active proliferation will be most radiosensitive. Consequently bone marrow, digestive tract, skin, and reproductive tissues are those that suffer; hence some of the radiation side-effects like bone marrow depression, diarrhoea, alopecia and sterility.

Cytotoxic agents

These are probably immunosuppressive by their effect on the dividing lymphocyte population of the effector side of the immune response.

Alkylating agents. These are the derivatives of mustine, for example cyclophosphamide, chlorambucil and malphalan. They act by interfering with DNA replication.

'Antimetabolites'. Analogues of a wide range of vital nuclear materials compose this group, for example:

Analogue	Nuclear substrate
Methotrexate	folic acid
6-mercaptopurine	Purines
Azathioprine	
5-fluorouracil	Pyrimidines
Cytarabine	

These drugs act by substitution during DNA synthesis and thereby reduce cell division.

IMMUNIZATION

The vaccination with cowpox to protect against smallpox by Jenner in 1796 was the beginning of modern immunization. Immunization can be effected either passively by transfer of immune products or actively by exposing the individual to the antigen (usually altered).

Passive immunization

By transferring immunoglobulins from an immune to a nonimmune subject a degree of protection can be achieved. These acquired immunoglobulin antibodies disappear gradually by either combination with antigen or catabolism, hence passive immunity is *temporary*.

Passive immunization through transfer of immune cells and transfer factor (see delayed hypersensitivity) has recently been tried but this method is still at the developmental stage.

The immunoglobulin used can be heterologous (animal→human) or isologous (human→human).

Heterologous

Horse antitetanus and antidiphtheria antisera were used extensively in the past. Unfortunately with all heterologous antisera there is a danger of serum sickness after the first injection and anaphylaxis after the second.

Isologous

Human hyperimmune sera are available for prophylaxis against tetanus and rubella (for seronegative mothers). Pooled human gammaglobulin can be utilized for passive immunization against hepatitis A and poliomyelitis, and is extensively used in hypogammaglobulinaemic individuals.

Active immunization

The generation of a protective long lasting immunity is the aim of active immunization programmes. Generally two types of vaccine are used.

Live preparations

The uncultured organism has been used in the past, e.g. variolation with smallpox virus or exposure of young girls to rubella. However, the development of avirulent strains (live attenuation) which was pioneered by Pasteur, has reduced the risk of severe infections while maintaining the advantage over killed vaccines of a dividing inoculum; this ensures a large eventual antigenic dose and hence a good immune response. Even this is not always safe; immunodeficient individuals can get life-threatening infections if given live-attenuated vaccines, e.g. BCG.

Killed preparations

Inactivated/killed vaccines produce a poorer immune response compared to live vaccines owing to a smaller antigenic load. Frequent booster doses are consequently often required. However, the purification of killed/inactivated antigens reduces the untoward reactions which continue to be a problem with live vaccines.

Examples of killed/inactivated vaccines are:
1 heat killed whole organisms, e.g. Salmonella Typhi;
2 inactivated toxin, e.g. diphtheria and tetanus toxoid.

Active immunization can be used to evoke responses both in the humoral and in the cellular arms of the immune response. Most of the examples given generate an antibody response, but BCG (Bacillus Calmette + Guerin) elicits a cellular response. BCG is given to Mantoux-negative normal children in their early teens. This sensitizes these children to tubercle bacilli so that if they encounter *M. tuberculosis* again, a secondary type immune response will occur. Such a secondary response leads to a marked local reaction at the site of inoculation (usually pulmonary), but greatly reduces the likelihood of spread to the lymph nodes and even miliary tuberculosis. Because a TB-sensitized patient would produce a violent skin reaction to BCG, all patients to receive BCG must be previously skin tested with tuberculin (crude heat-concentrated filtrate of a liquid culture of TB) or PPD (proteins from the tubercle bacilli culture fluid). Both PPD and tuberculin will elicit the delayed hypersensitivity response to tubercle bacilli but will not sensitize the individual to TB.

FURTHER READING

1 HAYWARD AR. *Immunodeficiency*. Current topics in immunology. Series No 6. London: Edward Arnold, 1977.
2 HOOD LE, WEISSMAN IL, WOOD WB. *Immunology*. Menlo Park Calif: Benjamin/Cummings, 1978.
3 ROITT IM. *Essental immunology*. 3rd ed. Oxford: Blackwell Scientific Publications, 1977.

Chapter 19
Psychological Aspects of Anaesthesia

CHRISTINE EVANS AND D. E. N. EVANS

Throughout the rest of this book an understanding of disease relevant to the anaes-thetist has involved examining each body system individually. In isolation, these various systems are merely parts of a whole: a full rounded assessment of the individual involves linking these systems together in such a way that their interdependence and interrelationship are appreciated. But even with this complete physical profile, the picture is still incomplete. The missing link centres around the fact that each individual is unique: each person has his own private internal world that colours reality for him. External events are not assessed in a purely objective manner; they also have a personal symbolic meaning.

The practising anaesthetist needs to be aware that each individual person will have his own notion of what hospitalization, anaesthesia and surgery mean to him and that, as a result, he will react in his own special manner. The spectrum of emotional reac-tions ranges from moderate fear and anxiety at one end, through to acute confusional states and psychosis at the other.

The manner in which an individual responds to the whole experience is not solely governed by his own characteristics, however; the surroundings, both the hospital environment and the people he meets in it, are additional potent influences that require consideration.

THE NORMAL INDIVIDUAL

To understand the various responses of individuals to hospitalization, anaesthesia and surgery, two underlying theoretical concepts need to be clarified: the concept of psychological stress and the concept of coping. A diagramatic representation of the relationship of these concepts is given in Fig. 19.1.

PSYCHOLOGICAL STRESS

The word 'stress' has a number of different meanings but in this chapter the concept of stress is synonymous with that of threat.

Engel[4] has defined psychological stress as all the processes which impose a challenge or demand upon the organism, whether originating in the external environment or within the individual. He described three principle categories of stress.

1 Loss, or threat of loss, of 'psychic objects' such as personal relationships, prestige, body functions or image, social roles, job, valued possessions or indeed anything or person which is experienced as 'part of themselves'.

2 Injury or threat of injury involving notions of pain and mutilation whether actual or threatened.

3 Frustration of biological drive satisfaction, especially basic nutrient and libidinal needs and avenues for discharging aggression.

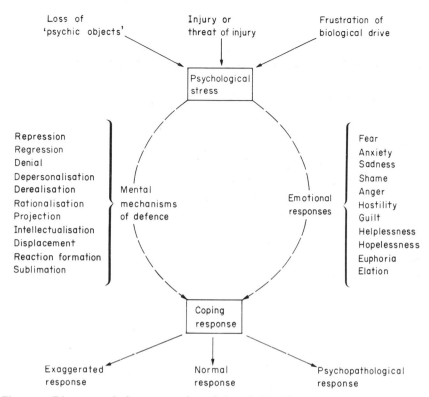

Fig. 19.1. Diagrammatical representation of the relationship between stress and coping.

Entering a hospital to become a patient includes all these categories of stress. It involves leaving behind family, job, friends and possessions. It necessitates a change in status, an alteration in the way of life and personal expression. The dehumanizing experience includes accepting a number, a diagnostic label, and surrendering responsibility for survival and existence to medical personnel. In addition, illness and treatment may include pain, discomfort, nausea or other unpleasant symptoms.

For a number of people the prospect of a general anaesthetic is particularly stressful. The patient may be frightened of needles or that he might feel pain. He may be worried by the fact that someone else will be responsible for his breathing or other vital functions. 'Will I hear, feel or see anything during the operation?', or 'Will I say or do anything of which I will be ashamed?' are common questions put to the anaesthetist, and just as commonly left unasked even though consciously considered. A general anaesthetic and the thought of suffocation are sometimes linked together. For some people the concept of their own death, symbolically expressed by the anaesthetized state, is very disturbing, so that the anaesthetist will frequently meet patients who express a fear that they will not wake up.

Stress is a very personal matter, and its strength cannot be estimated from its external features alone. Any individual may recognize certain aspects as being more highly charged than others, and certain parts will have more meaning. This personal significance is determined by the individual's internal world which contains his complete life history, a complete catalogue of past experiences and development with all that individual's strengths and weaknesses. Past experience colours present reality—the present triggers and revitalizes similar earlier experiences which, if they were satisfactory, serve as a strong support from which to approach the present. If, however, the past experience was unsuccessful or incomplete, then the residual emotional charge surfaces and is re-experienced in the present. A mature adult may be surprised at the distress he feels on admission to hospital, until he realizes that he is re-experiencing an earlier more painful separation carrying with it the emotional distress of a child. Similarly, when anticipating a modern general anaesthetic, a patient may be re-living an earlier anaesthetic experience under less sophisticated conditions.

Intelligence and social and cultural background are other factors which affect how the stressfulness of any event is perceived. With advancing age there is less resilience, energy and recuperative ability, so that stresses may have a greater impact. For children there are a number of very difficult mental tasks which are discussed later.

The type of illnesses, its onset, rate of progression and expected outcome colour the picture still further. Certain organs carry a greater emotional charge than others: the heart is known to be central to physical functioning and is felt to be central to one's very being, so that operations on the heart may appear to be attacks on a person's very soul. Amputations or other disfiguring operations can, in their alteration of body image, also alter self-esteem. Women tend to be more affected by the prospect of disfigurement and men more by disablement with associated dependency.

COPING

Psychological stress disrupts a person's equilibrium and so challenges that person to find ways of coping in order to overcome the threat. People tend to have more or less enduring modes of stress response—they have a 'coping style'. A person free of major mental conflict will have a more resilient, more flexible repertoire. Conversely, individuals with considerable internal conflict are restricted by their neurotic difficulties and are unable to adapt further. An individual who is free of conflict can learn from a totally new challenge and enhance his repertoire for responding to stress so that the end result is emotional growth.

An individual's characteristic coping style is determined by biological make-up, early social experience and relationships, developmental progress, especially the level of maturation achieved, and by previous experience of psychological stress and successful ways of dealing with it.

Although the perception of stress and the manner of coping is uniquely individual, it is possible to identify some common responses which are related to personality:

1 the *dependent* personality generally responds to stress with increased demands;
2 the *orderly* compulsive person cannot tolerate human failings or changes in routine;
3 the *dramatizing histrionic* person reacts with excessive emotional responses;
4 the *long-suffering masochist* awaits yet another painful experience;
5 the *guarded paranoid* individual misinterprets and mistrusts the world;
6 the *narcissistic* person dreads any alteration in body image;
7 the *schizoid* personality remains aloof.

Coping involves both mental mechanisms of defence and emotional responses.

Mental mechanisms of defence

The mental (cognitive) mechanisms, if used appropriately and in moderation, serve to absorb, reduce, deflect and eliminate the threat or the effects of that threat. They are therefore adaptive, and restore the mental equilibrium. However, when they are used to excess or inappropriately, they are maladaptive and fail to protect the individual who may then be overwhelmed and present with a psychopathological response. There are several mental mechanisms which can be identified.

Repression is the basic mechanism whereby material that cannot be tolerated consciously is pushed into the unconscious; it finds expression in indirect ways.

Regression involves retreating to earlier more infantile ways of behaving and relating to others. A moderate degree of regression is required of all patients: they have to surrender part of their adult independence to accept help and treatment. Excessive regression, however, leads to increased dependency and demanding behaviour that cannot be satisfied by the hospital staff so that the patient feels ignored and uncared for, whilst the staff feel the patient is uncooperative.

By denial a fact, its implications, or the feelings it arouses are ignored or denied. Denial is frequently used for short periods at times of crisis such as the death of a loved one. A moderate degree of denial of an illness or its significance may be conducive to healthy adjustment if it allows a sick patient to continue a full life. Complete denial, however, suggests serious psychopathology.

Depersonalization is a mechanism whereby the distinction between self and nonself is blurred. The experience has a dreamlike quality so that it seems not to be really happening. *Derealization* involves distortion of the environment so that it seems changed or strange.

Rationalization involves making plausible, more socially acceptable, explanations to hide the real story. Facts, feelings or symptoms are ascribed to causes that are less threatening so that chest pathology is rationalized as a cold or gastrointestinal disease as food upset.

Projection is a process of ascribing to others that which belongs to the self. Unpleasant or unacceptable feelings are often externalized and ascribed to others. A patient unable to accept or express his own discontent with his treatment may describe staff as being discontented.

With intellectualization ideas and painful feelings are separated in an attempt to understand at an intellectual level, facts that at a feeling level are very frightening. A patient may read avidly about his illness yet show no upset.

Thoughts or feelings directed at one person can be shifted by *displacement* onto another or expressed as the opposite by *reaction formation* whilst by *sublimation* impulses can be translated and expressed in a socially acceptable form.

It is unusual for a single mechanism to be relied upon and Lipowski[10] distinguishes two general modes of dealing with the facts and feelings of illness and injury. *Minimization*, where the person uses selective inattention, denial and rationalization, and *vigilant focussing*, where the person insists on detailed information and meticulously observes all treatment regimes.

Emotional responses

The appearance of unpleasant emotions is the first indicator of the disruption of the dynamic state of mental equilibrium. These emotional responses are experienced subjectively as 'feelings' but they may be accompanied by physiological or biochemical changes. The *cognitive* coping mechanisms discussed above, if effective, will influence the intensity of the emotional responses favourably but some degree of anxiety or other emotion usually appears.

Fear is the normal emotional response to threat. *Anxiety* is a state of apprehension or uneasiness, related to fear. Janis[7] has linked the degree of preoperative fear with the degree of postoperative adjustment. He notes that people who experienced a moderate degree of preoperative anticipatory fear were least likely to develop emotional disturbance during or after the stress exposure. Preoperatively they were able to establish good relationships, ask for information, and so comfortably do some 'worry work' or mental rehearsal and build up adaptive ways of coping. Persons who experienced a low degree of preoperative fear were likely to show poor postoperative adjustment and displayed anger and resentment towards staff. They had not re-hearsed the experience but rather used denial as a protective coat preoperatively and when this defence was removed by reality they were more upset during the actual threat period. The task for the staff is how to initiate some worry work in such patients and at the same time provide reassurance. Patients with high preoperative fear tend to be neurotically anxious people with a high degree of anxiety regularly present. They try to build up reassuring relationships and inner defences but even with repeated reassurance they fail and postoperatively may still be very anxious.

Sadness or grief is commonly aroused when the threat is construed as one of loss whether it be real, threatened or fantasized. Actual loss of limb or breast requires considerable internal realignment but this is only achieved after the grief has been fully felt and worked through to its natural conclusion of acceptance.

Shame is the emotion felt when a person judges that he has failed to live up to the performance required by his own self-imposed standards. It may be precipitated by the feeling of being exposed to the eyes of others. Shame is often felt when there has been an alteration in body image as a result of deformity or disfigurement, but a person may also be ashamed of nakedness, smallness, feelings or weakness.

Anger and hostility are the natural and normal emotions experienced by any organism under threat. They are part of the 'fight or flight' pattern of response associated with self-protection.

Guilt feelings in the face of danger are more difficult to understand. It is the emotion felt when the standards of the harsh, critical, 'superego' are transgressed. It brings with it the need for punishment. A person may feel that his illness is punishment for his innate badness. Janis[7] puts forward two possible explanations. First, that a person may feel guilty when he perceives that he has emotions which he feels are un-acceptable. Second, that when a threat is consciously appraised as intimidation then it is unconsciously linked with earlier intimidating experiences. These earlier ex-periences centre around threats of parental punishment for bad behaviour. The in-dividual will then strive to be the perfect patient to mitigate the fear of punishment.

Feelings of helplessness and hopelessness is ominous since these emotions herald a general 'giving-up' which may lead to death, in spite of treatment. Feelings of despair and futility override all other emotions with pervasiveness and the patient resists attempts to overcome them. Conversely, courage and the will to live can master and conquer what is sometimes assessed as an insuperable difficulty.

Euphoria or elation are occasionally seen postoperatively. The experience of these emotions may be related to emotional relief after the danger period has passed, or they may represent a defensive reaction to ward off guilt or other unpleasant emotions.

Abnormal emotional responses

If the stress is brief, or if the mental processes are quickly able to find a solution, then the unpleasant emotions are mild. When, however, the stress is prolonged, the emotional response may be more intense. Similarly, when the appropriate mental processes are not available, or are unsuccessful, then there is an escalation and distortion of response. The emotions may persist for an inappropriate length of time or intensity, or may be replaced by others. The picture is then further complicated by the biochemical and physiological changes generated by intense or sustained emotions. These physiological changes may then precipitate further pathological changes in a susceptible person. For instance, anxiety or rage in an individual with an already damaged heart can result in a coronary thrombosis, so increasing the amount of stress further. Occasionally, the attempts to overcome the stress and dissipate the emotions become so disordered that the response becomes pathological and a neurotic or psychotic picture appears.

In patients with pre-existing psychiatric disorder, physical illness and treatment usually worsen the condition. Neurotic anxiety can increase, and pre-existing affective psychosis and obsessional disorders worsen. Relapses in recurrent affective psychosis and schizophrenia can occur. However, although physical illness and treatment can precipitate the first episode or a relapse of schizophrenia, they can sometimes lead to improvement or remission. Similarly, neurotic anxiety can also remit when the patient has a physical illness. Acute confusional states that appear after hospital admission should lead one to suspect alcoholism, drug addiction or an organic mental illness. In any patient who has pre-existing psychiatric disorder or in whom a psychopathological response emerges, it is advisable to seek the advice of a psychiatrist, especially when interruption of established drug therapy is necessary. The anaesthetist should, however, have a working knowledge of common psychiatric symptoms and syndromes and some practical guidelines. The speedy treatment of symptoms not only brings relief to the patient but enables the staff to continue with physical care: a disturbed psychotic patient, for example, will not be likely to tolerate infusions or drains. The natural, exaggerated and pathological responses seem to lie on a continuum but the boundary between them is harder to define than to recognize.

Anxiety

Healthy anxiety is experienced by most people as a response to a threatening situation and is an adaptive response. The individual experiences a feeling akin to fear accompanied by autonomic disturbances such as tachycardia and sweating. *Morbid* anxiety, however, pervades the whole life of the individual and serves no useful purpose. The term 'anxiety neurosis' or 'anxiety state' is used for conditions in which anxiety is the predominant symptom either as constant tension, bodily responses, or as attacks of panic. Phobias are a form of anxiety when the response is localized to particular environments or objects. Anxiety may be a prominant feature in many different psychiatric disorders such as depressive illness or in the early stages of schizophrenia. Treatment includes psychotherapy, behaviour therapy and the anxiolytic drugs such as chlordiazepoxide and diazepam.

Affective disorders

Affective disorders refers to those abnormal states in which there is predominantly and primarily an altered mood. It may be lowered, as in depression, or elevated, as in hypomania and mania. *Depression* means, merely, lowered or sad mood. It can be a normal emotional reaction particularly to loss, a symptom of some physical or psychiatric illness, or an 'illness' in itself, but the borderline between these categories is blurred. Depressive illness, the commonest affective disorder, is a syndrome in which depression of mood is accompanied by feelings of worthlessness, guilt, hopelessness and helplessness. There is usually also a loss of interest in work or other social activities, poor concentration, hypochondriasis, sleep disturbance, anxiety, crying and suicidal tendencies. Physical changes include anorexia, weight loss and constipation. Treatment may involve psychotherapy, antidepressant drug therapy (tricyclic antidepressants and less commonly monoamineoxidase inhibitors), or electroconvulsive therapy (ECT).

Mania and hypomania are much less common affective disorders but present a more dramatic picture. The clinical features include elevated mood, irritability, hostility or belligerence, increased self-esteem, poor judgement, overactivity, flight of ideas and decreased sleep. Phenothiazines, butyrophenones, lithium carbonate and ECT are effective in treatment.

What is most relevant to the anaesthetist is that he should recognize quantitative and qualitative changes in mood and refer the patient appropriately. In addition, a note must be taken of concomitant drug therapy and any implications for anaesthesia.

Schizophrenia

This psychosis is characterized by disorders of perception, thinking, emotion and behaviour. Physical illnesses and operations can precipitate a first episode or relapse of schizophrenia although sometimes they can lead to remission or improvement. Hallucinations may occur in any sense modality but auditory ones and most common. The voices may be intermittent or continuous, abusive, hostile or reassuring. They may talk to the patient, or about him in the third person. Patients may hear voices commenting on their actions or speaking their own thoughts aloud. In schizophrenic thought disorder the power of conceptional thinking is altered. Thought blocking and alienation of thought, either insertion, withdrawal or broadcasting are also characteristic. Delusions, disorder of thought content, may be primary, arising *de novo*, or secondary when they are explicable in the light of the patient's altered mood or hallucinations. Their content depends to a considerable degree on cultural factors. Passivity feelings, where the patient feels that this thoughts, feelings, speech and actions are not his own, but under the control of external influences, are diagnostic of schizophrenia. Although elation or depression may occur, flattering or incongruity of affect are more characteristic. The inability of these patients to form or maintain human contact is often described as 'a glass wall' shutting the patient off from the world. A decrease in total activity usually occurs although states of ecstasy, wild excitement, impulsive behaviour or stupor can occur. Clinically, schizophrenia may be divided into hebephrenic, catatonic, simple or paranoid, according to the predominant mode of presentation.

The phenothiazines and butyrophenones exert a specific therapeutic effect in schizophrenia when given in doses which may seem unusually large to anaesthetists.

For example, chlorpromazine is administered in divided daily doses ranging from 150 to 600 mg, trifluoperazine from 5 to 15 mg daily and haloperidol from 1 to 12 mg daily. Maintenance is now more reliable with the use of intramuscular injections of fluphenazine decanoate (Modecate) 12·5–25 mg every 2–4 weeks. Extrapyramidal reactions to these drugs respond to anti-parkinsonian drugs. ECT also has a place in the treatment of certain types of schizophrenia.

Acute paranoid psychoses

These disorders can occur during any physical illness, after childbirth and in the postoperative period. Clouding of consciousness helps with the diagnosis but this is not invariably present. These acute psychoses usually remit with appropriate treatment and should be referred for expert advice without delay.

Organic disorders

These mental illnesses are the result of anatomical or physiological changes in the brain. These changes are either reversible or irreversible. *Acute* and *subacute delirium* (*the confusional state*) are temporary, reversible conditions in which clouding of consciousness is the salient feature. In subacute delirium, attention and grasp are diminished with disorientation for time and place. The mood is usually anxious or fearful and physical symptoms include tremor and restlessness. A fluctuating course is characteristic with symptoms more severe at night. If, in addition, there is severe restlessness, hallucinations and illusions, the condition is known as delirium. The hallucinations are most commonly visual and often take the form of small animals moving across the visual field. Illusions take the form of either misidentification of objects in the environment or misinterpretation of bodily sensations. Acute or subacute delirium are more readily precipitated at the extremes of life. Common causative factors include cardiovascular disease, acute infection, intoxications especially those due to alcohol or barbiturates, metabolic disorders such as hepatic or renal insufficiency, water and electrolyte imbalance, vitamin deficiency and cerebral disease or injury. Treatment is symptomatic and that of the underlying cause. The patients should be nursed in a brightly lit room by calm reassuring staff. Attention should be paid to diet and fluid balance, and vitamin supplements (Parenterovite) are particularly indicated in alcoholic patients. Chlorpromazine is the drug of choice.

In *dementia* there is usually a progressive intellectual deterioration as a result of brain damage. Recent memory is impaired, general information faulty, concentration and grasp reduced with disorientation for place and time. Disorders of speech and language may be present. A loss of inhibition occurs in the personality and behaviour. Interest, practical performance and appearance decline. Emotional lability is common but anxiety or depression may be the predominant picture, particularly in the early stages when the patient may have insight into his lack of ability. Dementia is of two main types, senile and arteriosclerotic. Other less common causes include, cerebral tumours or other space occupying lesions, chronic alcoholism, trauma, myxoedema, Vitamin B_{12} deficiency and normal-pressure hydrocephalus.

ALCOHOLISM AND DRUG ABUSE

Addiction is characterized by psychological dependence, change in tolerance and a specific withdrawal syndrome. In general, drugs are abused either to obtain oblivion or excitement. Common aetiological factors are psychiatric illness, personality disorder and social factors; more rarely, injudicious use of drugs in medical treatment can be the initiating cause although in the acute treatment of illness in surgery, anaesthesia and intensive care, well-documented examples of this are notably absent. For the purpose of this chapter, only those drugs of addiction and their possible complications relevant to the anaesthetist are discussed. These drugs are alcohol, narcotics, barbiturates, amphetamines, lysergic acid diethylamine (LSD) and certain solvent and glues that are sniffed. It should be remembered that many addicts abuse more than one drug.

In a known addict it is advisable to maintain the drug therapy in the immediate pre- and postoperative periods; this is not the time to attempt to wean the patient off his addiction and it may only serve to precipitate an acute withdrawal reaction. But the drug abuser does not always admit to his addiction, and the first sign may be the appearance of the withdrawal or abstinence syndrome. The symptoms of withdrawal in the barbiturate addict usually commence with convulsions followed by an acute confusional state characterized by anxiety, tremulousness, disorientation and visual hallucinations. Unless recognized and treated this specific barbiturate abstinence can be fatal. Treatment consists of diazepam to control the convulsions and, on a trial-and-error bases, doses of pentobarbitone or a benzodiazepine sufficient to maintain a mild degree of intoxication, which are then reduced gradually over several days.

Delirium tremens is the specific withdrawal syndrome of alcohol addiction and is characterized by an emotional state of fear or terror which is accompanied by vivid and frightening hallucinations. The level of consciousness is impaired and there is disorientation for time, place and person. Delirium tremens usually occurs within 3–4 days of the withdrawal of alcohol and is a serious illness which may result in death. Treatment includes very careful attention to fluid balance, the giving of vitamins (particularly thiamine), and adequate sedation with chlordiazepoxide or chlormethiazole.

The abstinence syndrome in narcotic addicts presents a varied and prolonged picture of restlessness, irritability, lacrymation, rhinorrhoea, perspiration and paroxysms of yawning. The symptoms rise to a peak within 2–3 days when painful cramps develop together with vomiting, diarrhoea, loss of appetite and extreme weakness. Although uncomfortable, this specific withdrawal syndrome of narcotic addiction is rarely fatal. Phenothiazines and diazepam play an important part in the management of such cases.

Specific organ damage may result from drug addiction. Alcohol addiction gives rise to liver damage which can progress to cirrhosis with altered protein synthesis, inadequate glycogen storage and subsequent susceptibility to hypoglycaemia and hypoxaemia. In addition, alcoholics are prone to bleeding, especially from the gastrointestinal tract, and there may be hypomagnesaemia. A cardiomyopathy with resultant cardiovascular instability may be present. Solvent or glue-sniffers may have hepatic or renal damage and bone marrow suppression. In narcotic addiction contamination of needles and syringes produces a high incidence of serum hepatitis which frequently results in hepatic damage.

Anaesthetizing addicts can present the anaesthetist with several problems. Patients addicted to alcohol are said to be resistant to anaesthesia, need large doses of barbiturates to induce sleep, and require higher concentrations than usual of anaesthetic agents. Cross-tolerance occurs with ether, halothane, cyclopropane, methoxyflurane and nitrous oxide. If severe liver damage is present, there may be increased sensitivity to suxamethonium due to lowered plasma cholinesterase, although this requires a fall in enzyme activity below about 10 per cent of normal. Resistance to tubocurarine has been described, and attributed to altered protein patterns. There may be an underlying cardiomyopathy. The need for increased amounts of anaesthetic agents due to tolerance and cross-tolerance also occurs in barbiturate and narcotic addicts, and this may result in overdosage. Hypotension has occurred in narcotic addicts under anaesthesia, and has responded to intravenous morphine when other causes have been excluded[14]. Narcotic antagonists are contraindicated in opiate addicts and this also includes the use of pentazocine and other drugs which have antagnonistic properties. Amphetamine addiction produces a similar increased requirement for anaesthetic agents and in addition may be associated with cardiac dysrhythmias. L.S.D. possesses a mild degree of anticholinesterase activity so that prolongation of suxamethonium block can occur in the chronic abuser. Finally, difficulty may be encountered establishing intravenous infusions because of widespread sclerosis of veins in addicts who use this route of administration.

Psychiatric drugs and the anaesthetist

The use of certain drugs in psychiatric practice may present problems when patients are anaesthetized.

Monoamine oxidase inhibitors (MAOIs) possess many potentially toxic effects. To the anaesthetist the most significant are the interactions with pethidine and sympathomimetic amines, particularly those that release noradrenaline from nerve terminals or which are themselves normally metabolized by monoamine oxidase[13]. Any drug with α-adrenergic blocking properties such as droperidol will also exhibit synergism with MAO inhibitors. Other narcotic analgesics besides pethidine may produce interactions, but morphine is the least likely to cause untoward effects[5]. The interaction with pethidine may cause hypotension, respiratory depression and coma, or a severe hypertensive crisis with hyperpyrexia, convulsions and coma[13]. Interaction with sympathomimetic amines produces hypertension together with restlessness, agitation, hallucinations, convulsions, severe headaches, coma and hyperpyrexia. Because of these unpredictable toxic side-effects, surgical operations should be postponed 10–14 days until the effects of these drugs have been eliminated and fresh enzyme generated. If, however, the operation cannot be postponed, obviously pethidine and sympathomimetic amines must be avoided. A sensitivity test to pethidine may be conducted before embarking on anaesthesia or even pain relief[3]. Initially 10 mg of pethidine is given, and the patient is carefully observed with particular attention to pulse and blood pressure. If these remain stable and the patient is not comatosed or cyanosed, then the dose is repeated at 15 minute intervals to a total dose of 50 mg. Should local anaesthesia or regional block be required, local analgesic solutions containing felypressin as a vasoconstrictor should be employed. Felypressin is not a catecholamine and does not potentiate MAOIs.

The tricyclic antidepressant drugs which include imipramine and amitriptyline may cause nonspecific electrocardiographic changes following long-term therapy. Similar ECG changes, notably dysrhythmias and conduction defects, may be encountered following prolonged courses of phenothiazines. Patients receiving phenothiazines are also more susceptible to the hypotensive action of general anaesthetics, particularly the rapidly acting barbiturates, and are also unduly sensitive to blood loss. Finally, of interest is the reported potentiation of suxamethonium in a patient receiving lithium therapy[6].

Some of the drugs used in anaesthesia may have psychiatric symptoms as side-effects. Ketamine is the most obvious example of such a drug. In the immediate postoperative period following ketamine anaesthesia disorientation, restlessness and agitation, irrational speech and uncontrolled crying or moaning are seen. Physically disturbing the patient at this stage can accentuate these side-effects. Vivid dreams and hallucinations can occur up to 24 hours after administration of the drug. Their morbid content and vivid colours can be very distressing to the patient. It has been asserted that these sequelae are not so disturbing to children: they probably are, but as they seem to fit into their rich world of fantasy, magic and monsters, they are less complained about. The acute psychological side-effects of ketamine can be prevented by giving droperidol or diazepam intravenously towards the end of the surgical procedure. Lorazepam premedication is also particularly effective in reducing these unpleasant side-effects of ketamine[9].

When droperidol is used alone the patient appears outwardly calm and tranquil but is frequently inwardly very disturbed. The unpleasant side-effects include hallucinations, loss of body image, apprehension and restlessness. In addition dystonic reactions have been reported 24 hours after administration. The combination with analgesics reduces these side-effects of droperidol. Its use alone cannot be recommended. Pentazocine is also capable of producing psychomimetic symptoms particularly when used in doses at the top end of the therapeutic scale (40–60 mg). These side-effects vary from mild thought disturbances and bizarre dreams to feelings of impending death and agitation.

THE ENVIRONMENT

This chapter has so far focussed on the very personal experience of stress and the individual's response to it. One must, however, give some attention to the reality of the outside world. The hospital environment, with its strange sights, sounds and smells, bombards the sensory system of the individual. Even so-called routine procedures such as examinations, ward rounds and investigations can be new and frightening experiences. Ward size can be important; some people are more settled in a large ward whereas others prefer a more private setting.

The ability to cope with new and strange environments decreases with advancing age so that an elderly person, although self-sufficient at home, may quickly become confused, disorientated and agitated on admission to hospital. Phenothiazines produce symptomatic improvement but the introduction of familiar objects and people and a speedy return home is called for.

Changes in the amount of stimulation from the environment affect everyone. Too much input leads to sensory overload, and too little to sensory deprivation when hallucinations quickly develop. The sensory isolation of deafness or blindness combined with mild senile brain changes can result in the development of a paranoid psychosis.

The strangeness of the hospital environment increases in the specialized areas and of these, the recovery room, operating theatre, and anaesthetic room are relevant. Patients are not usually asleep when they leave the comparative sanctuary of the ward and familiar nurses are not always available as escorts. The anaesthetist can therefore be an important buffer, lessening the impact of the anaesthetic room on the patient.

His preoperative visit, by making personal contact with the patient as an individual, is vital in this respect.

The patient receiving regional or local anaesthesia is usually sedated but may still be aware of his surroundings in the operating room. He may also hear and misinterpret remarks inadvertently made by the operating team.

The real nightmare, however, is the experience of awareness during general anaesthesia. Neuromuscular blocking agents permit surgery to proceed when the concentrations of anaesthetics reaching the brain are insufficient to produce unconsciousness or even analgesia. Obstetric patients are particularly at risk because of the light level of anaesthesia which is employed to prevent adverse effects to the fetus. Patients requiring cardiopulmonary bypass procedures are also at risk since anaesthetic agents depress myocardial activity in proportion to dose and are, therefore, used sparingly, and also because the oxygenator may acutely alter plasma concentrations of anaesthetic agents especially if volatile agents are used.

Whilst some reports have described a condition of wakefulness without pain or undue anxiety, this is probably dependent on the vagaries of other medication and cannot be relied upon. On the contrary, reports by other patients who have experienced awareness under general anaesthesia are horrific; mere words are inadequate to describe the mounting panic, fear and searing pain that comprise this living death[1]. Blacher[2] has used the term 'acute traumatic neurosis' to describe the symptoms that can arise as a result of being aware whilst paralysed. The neurosis is characterized by anxiety, irritability, preoccupation with death and repeated nightmares from which the patient awakes with a sense of unreality and an uncertainty as to whether he is alive or dead. Blacher's patients were often unclear as to whether they had really been awake but their symptoms improved when their suspicions were confirmed.

There is no doubt that patients benefit from modern techniques of light anaesthesia combined with muscle relaxants but there is, as yet, no reliable means of monitoring awareness in a paralysed patient. Several authors have described techniques involving isolating a limb from the effects of muscle relaxants in order to elicit conscious responses. The ethics of conducting anaesthesia at such a light level seem dubious, since the consequences of adequate levels of narcosis have not been shown to be harmful in the situations in which the techniques are employed. In the view of the authors, awareness is a totally unacceptable complication of general anaesthesia.

The recovery room is full of distressing scenes but fortunately few patients recall the experience. Winkelstein *et al.*[15] demonstrated that patients are, however, not oblivious to events in the recovery room. Patients were able to relate clearly shortly after surgery and were able to recall the interview 24 hours later. Amnesia may therefore be pharmacologically and psychogenically induced. Reassurance and reorientation are clearly needed by patients postoperatively in this setting.

As the name Intensive Care Unit suggests, the nursing and medical care within these units is intensive. All the specialized medical and technological skills are focused and concentrated in these areas. Patient care is individual yet paradoxically can be the most impersonal, and dehumanizing. Patients may feel helpless and personally annihilated in a jungle of electronics.

Serious illness, immobility, passivity, dependence on people and machines for survival, sensory monotony, social and sensory deprivation and interrupted sleep are all contributory factors in the development of the many psychiatric symptoms that can arise. Anxiety and depression are almost the norm, but psychotic symptoms and delirium can also occur. The physiological, metabolic and pharmacological changes found in these seriously ill patients are obvious causes of delirium, but of particular interest is the high frequency with which delirium occurs following cardiac surgery. Here the delirium arises after a lucid period of a few days and improves when the patient is returned to a more normal ward setting. Kornfield[8] therefore concluded that although the severity of the illness and length of time on cardiopulmonary bypass are contributory factors, the impact of the environment is also significant.

The anxiolytics and phenothiazines will provide symptomatic improvement, but making the environment more real can prevent the emergence of symptoms. Using rooms with windows, introducing clocks and calendars and following the usual natural day-night rhythm with as few interruptions as possible for nursing procedures, facilitates orientation and reduces the incidence of hallucinations. Monitoring equipment with rhythmic bleeping can be stationed away from the patient and any monotonous background noise reduced to a minimum. Radios and television sets can relieve sensory monotony but the only really meaningful sensory stimuli are the touch of another human being and conversation. Talk is particularly important, even when the patient cannot respond. The patient may be paralysed and sedated but still be aware of his surroundings. Explanations of machinery and procedures help the patient to make sense of his alien environment and so reduce his anxiety. Anticipating and verbalizing what one imagines a person might be feeling, provides the comfort and reassurance that someone understands, and that someone is there.

The psychological trauma of the intensive care unit can also result in emotional difficulties after discharge. Indeed depression and anxiety could be considered normal after such an experience. It is also important to remember that such units can be highly stressful for the staff concerned: just as the patient cannot leave his machine, so the nurse cannot leave her patient.

THE PROFESSIONAL STAFF

All hospital staff need to be able to combine efficiency and objectivity with the emotional warmth that provides a more relaxed, comfortable and generally supportive atmosphere.

Nurses and doctors have to develop psychological defences to enable them to work in a hospital environment. How else could they tolerate the pain and suffering of others? Unfortunately, the defence mechanisms used by the hospital staff serve not only to protect that staff member, but may also prevent him or her from appreciating the emotional impact of the hospital experience on a patient.

Whilst it is not appropriate to identify completely with the patient, it is not helpful to remain remote, aloof, and unaware of a patient's emotional distress. The appropriate emotional distance from a patient is somewhere between these extremes. The ideal situation occurs when the doctor can integrate within himself, his medical objective self, and his more human, caring and spontaneously warm self. If the doctor behaves as a whole, he is more likely to treat, and relate to a patient as a whole person with a physical, and a feeling self.

From discussions earlier in this chapter, it will be clear that the stress of becoming a patient within a hospital and requiring an anaesthetic, put simply, releases the child within the adult. From his regressed dependent position, the patient projects onto the medical staff a parental image. Janis[7] has likened this to a transference reaction, where the emotional attitude adopted is determined by earlier relationships with parents. The patient, therefore, develops a childlike trust in what Janis calls the 'danger control figures'. Statements made by such figures assume greater emotional significance than would be ordinarily expected. If the doctor remains distant or absent, then the patient is left with his fantasies of either an all powerful 'good' parent or an all powerful 'bad' destructive parent. It is important that the patient sees the operating team as 'good' since the ability to tolerate stress depends to a large degree on that person's ability to maintain high confidence in protective figures. The ideal parental figure is not one that commands, 'Don't worry' or dismissively says, 'I know best', but rather is the doctor who conducts himself with obvious competence and conveys his trustworthiness and understanding in his approach.

It might be argued that this has little relevance to the anaesthetist since in comparison, his contact with any one patient is brief. But paradoxically it is of paramount importance, since it is the anaesthetist who renders the patient completely dependent with a general anaesthetic. Furthermore, because the time available is limited, he needs greater interpersonal skills to achieve the desired relationship quickly.

One might expect that to develop a trusting relationship, the doctor and patient need to meet on several occasions. Fortunately, the anaesthetist does not need to establish a long-term relationship since the patient is in a highly charged emotional state and waiting to be emotionally carried through a short but traumatic experience by a 'good' competent parent.

The anaesthetist's interview with a patient begins with introductions. The patient needs to feel he is known, and needs to know who is going to anaesthetize him. There is far less danger from someone who has given his name, and touched you, than from some faceless, nameless figure. Subsequently, the interview can be divided into three parts—the receiving of information in the form of history-taking, the ventilation and sharing of fears and feelings, and the giving of information in the form of explanations.

History-taking usually involves direct questions and answers, but this alone is not conducive to ventilation of feelings or fears. Some patients have no difficult expressing their feelings—they just flow out. Others, however, need help: they need to be given permission. The anaesthetist can facilitate this ventilation by making empathic statements (not questions) based on chance remarks made by the patient, or on non-verbal cues he may have observed whilst taking the history. It is at these times that the anaesthetist needs to know all the various ways anxiety can be disguised. If a patient honours us by sharing his innermost fears then it follows that our response should be respectful, empathic and warm, and without judgment.

The patient not only needs to feel understood, he also needs to be informed. A patient will find emotional support if he knows what to expect, i.e. if he has a realistic view of the crisis. A realistic view reduces fantasy, corrects erroneous beliefs, and initiates the mental rehearsal that is so necessary for building up immunity. Awareness of events and their sequence acts as a desensitizing agent, gives the patient a feeling that he is party to decision-making, and leaves him with some sense of control over events. Making accurate predictions for the patient enhances his sense of security and maintains and confirms the trustworthiness of the doctor.

This sort of interview emotionally supports a patient, reduces anxiety and facilitates and strengthens appropriate ego defence mechanisms. Difficulties can arise with either the patient who denies fears, or the overanxious patient. Direct confrontation with the patient who denies any upset can precipitate further disturbance. Patience, support and suggestion may help such a person face some unpleasant future experiences. The overanxious patient will require repeated explanations and reassurance, but firmness

20*

in an authoritative, yet caring, manner may also be required, since limits have to be set.

In intensive care units explanation of what is, or might be, happening is even more vital especially when the patient cannot respond. Providing a running commentary makes real contact with a patient. It can be likened to the way a mother intuitively talks to a helpless child, commenting, explaining and anticipating possible feelings without expecting a response.

Doctors should never lose sight of the fact that the manner in which they approach patients acts as a model for other staff and, if well handled, can also generate a feeling of security throughout the ward. It is not only the patient but also his family and nursing attendants who need support. The key to such support centres around open, trusting communication between staff members and between staff and patients.

CHILDREN

A child's internal world, and his view of the external world, is so different from that of an adult that some brief separate discussion is warranted. A child's reaction will be determined not only by his own personality and past history, but also by his level of intellectual and emotional development, and by the quality of his relationship with his parents.

At birth an infant's personality is unintegrated; he is vulnerable and totally dependent upon his mother. With what Winnicott[16] describes as a 'good enough mother' a special relationship exists whereby the mother is completely in tune with the needs of her infant. A mother knows her infant. This 'primary maternal preoccupation' enables the mother to do what is right for her infant. This relationship is dynamic, changing appropriately to match the different needs of the developing child, so facilitating emotional growth.

It is difficult to assess the impact of surgical procedures on small infants but they do undoubtedly suffer as a result of separation from their mothers during hospitalization. Not only may they lack stimulation and become subdued and quiet, but separation may disrupt or prevent the establishment of a bond between the mother and infant so that the future parent-child relationship may be strained or distorted. Mothers and babies need close physical contact, so that even if separated infants do respond to strange nurses and do not protest when separated, it is important that mothers handle and care for their infants as much as possible.

Between three and six months a baby recognizes his mother, and by seven months of age he not only shows clear signs of distress when separated from her, but resists approaches from strangers. Separation anxiety can be a problem throughout childhood, but is experienced most intensely by children under the age of four years. It is a grief reaction; the child mourns the loss of his mother. Initially the child protests vehemently, crying loudly and searching for sight or sound of his mother. This stage of protest[12] is gradually followed by two further phases of despair and denial when the child deceptively appears to have 'settled in'. In the phase of despair the child is less active, withdrawn and apathetic, but if the separation is prolonged he may show more interest in his surroundings and appear happy. During this phase of denial he may appear to hardly know his mother, and once this drastic stage has been reached, it can take some considerable time for the child to thaw out on returning home.

The toddler has no experience or understanding of the world and no conception of time. If his mother leaves him she is gone for ever. He is left undefended and bombarded by new and frightening experiences. During the stage of autonomy the toddler is learning that not only does he have power over his own neuromusculature but also over his environment. The necessary submission to anaesthesia, surgery or other procedures is diametrically opposed to the developmental needs of this age group. At the point when he is beginning to experience himself and his own power, he is rendered powerless and no matter how loudly he shouts his cherished 'No', he cannot win.

Children between the third and sixth year of life are struggling with basic developmental crises and in addition their thinking and reasoning are different from that of an adult. They see themselves as the centre of the world, everything has feelings, there is no logic and crime deserves punishment. Separation is therefore construed as their fault, and just punishment for their badness. Illnesses and painful procedures can be misinterpreted and seen to fit in with their rich fantasy world so that anxiety and guilt can easily be generated.

Older children have mastered these early developmental crises, have stronger ego defences and are capable of rational thinking. They are therefore less vulnerable and can be more satisfactorily prepared for unpleasant procedures.

Understanding the possible traumata to children has resulted in humanizing paediatric services. Children over four years of age benefit from open visiting; they need warm, considerate staff and facilities that permit expression and working through of experiences through play. Below this age children react particularly badly, displaying various symptoms not only during their hospital stay but also afterwards. They are unresponsive to anything other than their mother's presence[11]. Only she can help the child make sense of an alien environment and prevent the child from being overwhelmed by anxieties he cannot cope with.

The natural corollary must therefore be that the mother of a young child should be encouraged to stay in the hospital with her child, or at least to visit frequently and be present at times of maximum stress. Without his mother the child may appear to be 'better behaved', the ward quieter and the task for nursing and medical staff easier. But to create an experience which safeguards a child's psychological health the mother's presence is important as is allowing the child to protest and be upset.

The situation is complicated by the fact that parents bring with them their own misconceptions and anxieties which may be based on fact or fantasy. These fears are then transferred to the child even though he may be told 'that there's nothing to be frightened of'. During his preoperative visit the anaesthetist can elicit and resolve the mother's anxieties by clear explanation of the sequence of events, procedures and experiences in an understanding and emotionally supportive manner. Trust and confidence are then established between the parent and anaesthetist and these positive feelings are then transferred to the child. A bridge then exists from the anaesthetist via the parent to the child. If this satisfactory end point can be reached the mother can accompany her child into the anaesthetic room for the induction of general anaesthesia and also be present immediately the child wakes up, and both will benefit from the experience.

Unfortunately, there are some mothers who are so anxious that in the time available their fears cannot be resolved, they cannot really trust the staff. Such parents are unable to support their children with feelings of confidence and reassurance but continue to inject their children with confusion, fear and general upset. Under these circumstances the presence of the mother in the anaesthetic room can be detrimental. An anaesthetist who has seen a mother clutching her child in frozen panic will not want such a situation to develop again. The anaesthetist has therefore to exercise considerable skill preoperatively. He will need to assess how much stress a mother can tolerate and decide at what point the mother must be separated from her child. His attention can then be focused on helping the mother leave her child rather than stay with him.

With older children the anaesthetist's interview may include a parent, but it is principally directed towards the child. Using language and/or play appropriate to the child's intellectual and emotional development the anaesthetist can help a child understand and be prepared for his anaesthetic. During this meeting the anaesthetist is not only communicating with the child and building up a relationship, he is also assessing the child with a view to deciding which anaesthetic technique would be most suitable. Ideally both the degree of sedation used as a premedication and the mode of induction of anaesthesia will be matched to the individual child. There is no hard and fast rule, but it is the opinion of the authors that wherever possible a child's fears should be 'worked through' and resolved. Time and understanding are safer both physically and psychologically than heavy premedication.

The preparation of a child needs on the one hand to be simple, yet on the other, thorough, so leaving little to his fantastic imagination. For instance, the word 'sleep' is simple enough, yet to a child it can have an added meaning. Adults often use 'sleep' as a euphemism for death when attempting to explain the death of a relative, friend or pet animal. The word therefore needs to be qualified—the child reassured that he will wake up.

If the child is to be awake or drowsy in the anaesthetic room then he will need to know something about the route from the ward to the operating theatre, e.g. he will be wheeled along on the trolley, or taken in a lift. Detailed descriptions can be too confusing, obvious signposts are probably sufficient. He will also need to be told about the clothing he and the staff wear. Arranging to collect a very anxious child can be enormously helpful and once such promises are made it is important to keep them. Some anaesthetists prepare a child by taking him along the expected route and showing him the anaesthetic room and operating theatre. In general that amount of preparation seems extreme, except perhaps where a child is to spend time in an intensive care unit postoperatively. In that event, frequent visits may be necessary until the room and staff become familiar.

When a child is to receive inhalation induction of anaesthesia, he can be introduced to the mask at the preoperative visit, encouraged to practise breathing through it and be told of the dizziness he will experience as he goes to sleep. Some children can be so well prepared that when the time comes they can hold the mask themselves during the induction. Active participation by the child is the most effective way of relieving him of feelings of being a passive recipient of an overpowering force. A child to receive an intravenous induction cannot actively participate but he can be prepared in an honest manner so that a point of trusting acceptance can be reached. In addition every anaesthetist will have his own personal way of relating to children—the games, toys, stories, songs, etc. are infinite.

Most children have some form of special object which is vitally important to them. It may be a piece of blanket, silk scarf, sheet, teddy-bear or other doll, etc. Winnicott[16] has emphasized the importance of these 'transitional objects' in the normal development of a child and described them as intermediate between the self and the outside world. They are used particularly when the child goes to sleep, is sad, lonely or anxious and enables the child to withstand upset of whatever cause. Children should therefore be allowed to bring such comforts with them to the anaesthetic room.

Postoperatively the use of play materials that allows a re-enactment of the experience or expression of feeling aroused by the experience, facilitates mastery of that experience. Postoperative ventilation of fears through words or play is the key to resolving anxieties.

REFERENCES

1 ANONYMOUS. Editorial. *Br J Anaesth* 1979; **51**: 711–12.

2 BLACHER RS. On awakening paralysed during surgery. *JAMA* 1975; **234**: 67–8.

3 CHURCHILL-DAVIDSON HC. Anaesthesia and monoamine oxidase inhibitors. *Br Med J* 1965; **1**: 520.

4 ENGEL GL. *Psychological development in health and disease*. Philadelphia: WB Saunders, 1962.

5 EVANS-PROSSER CDG. The use of pethidine and morphia in the presence of MAOI's. *Brit J Anaesth* 1968; **40**: 279–82.

6 HILL GE, WONG KC, HODGES MR. Potentiation of succinylcholine neuromuscular blockade by lithium carbonate. *Anesthesiology* 1976; **44**: 439–42.

7 JANIS IL. *Psychological stress. Psychoanalytic and behavioural studies of surgical patients*. London: Chapman and Hall, 1958.

8 KORNFIELD DS, ZIMBERG S, MALM JR. Psychiatric complications of open-heart surgery. *N Engl J Med* 1965; **273**: 287–92.

9 LILBURN JK, DUNDEE JW, NAIR SG, FEE JPH, JOHNSTON HML. Ketamine sequelae. Evaluation of the ability of various premedicants to attenuate its psychic actions. *Anaesthesia* 1978; **33**: 307–11.

10 LIPOWSKI ZJ. Physical illness, the individual and the coping process. *Psychiat Med* 1970; **1**: 91–102.

11 PRUGH DG, STAUR EM, SANDS HH, KIRSCHBAUM RM, LENIHAM EA. A study of the emotional reactions of children and families to hospitalisation and illness. *Am J Orthopsychiat* 1953; **23**: 78–104.

12 ROBERTSON J. *Young children in hospital*. London: Tavistock Publications, 1958.

13 SJOQVIST F. Psychotropic Drugs (2). Interaction between MAOI's and other substances. *Proc Roy Soc Med* 1965; **58**: 967–78.

14 The Experts Opine. What are your most important considerations in the management of the drug addict who requires general anaesthesia for a surgical procedure? *Survey of Anesthesiology* 1973; **17**: 376–9.

15 WINKELSTEIN C, BLACHER R, and MEYER B. Psychiatric observations on surgical patients in recovery room. *NY St J Med* 1965; **65**: 865–70.

16 WINNICOTT DW. *The family and individual development*. London: Tavistock Publications, 1965.

Index

Initials of diseases, drugs, procedures, etc. are not *normally* used as main headings in this index though they are *sometimes* used in the subheadings.

21*